Essentials of Canine and Feline Electrocardiography:

Interpretation and Treatment

Essentials of Canine and Feline Electrocardiography:

Interpretation and Treatment

SECOND EDITION

LARRY PATRICK TILLEY, D.V.M.

Diplomate, American College of Veterinary Internal Medicine
(Internal Medicine)
Staff (Consultant)
Department of Medicine—Cardiology
The Animal Medical Center
President, Cardiopet, Inc.
New York, New York

Lea & Febiger   1985   Philadelphia

Lea & Febiger
600 South Washington Square
Philadelphia, Pa. 19106-4198
U.S.A.
(215) 922-1330

Notice

Medicine is a science that is constantly changing. Changes in treatment and drug therapy are required with new research and clinical experience. The author and the publisher of this textbook have made every effort to ensure that the drug dosage schedules are accurate. The drug dosages are based on the standards accepted at the time of publication. The product information sheet included in the package of each drug should be checked before the drug is administered to be certain that changes have not been made in the recommended dose or in the contraindications for administration. This advice is especially appropriate for new or infrequently used drugs.

Library of Congress Cataloging in Publication Data

Tilley, Lawrence P.
   Essentials of canine and feline electrocardiography:
   Interpretation and treatment

   Bibliography: p.
   Includes index.
   1. Veterinary electrocardiography. 2. Dogs—Diseases.
3. Cats—Diseases. I. Title.
SF811.T54 1984   636.7′0896161207547   83-24837
ISBN 0-8121-0920-1

PRINTED IN THE UNITED STATES OF AMERICA

Print Number: 3 2 1

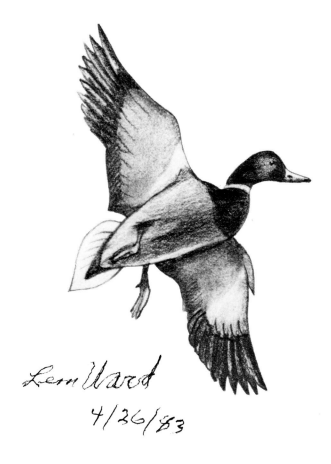

Lem Ward
4/26/83

*"To wake at dawn with a winged heart
and give thanks for another day of loving"*

(Kahlil Gibran - The Prophet)

*Dedicated to Jeri, my mother, brother, grandparents,
and in loving memory of my father*

Foreword

In recent years, practicing veterinarians have demonstrated considerable interest in clinical electrocardiography. This, in turn, has stimulated cardiologists who are concerned with the teaching of electrocardiographic interpretation to students and practitioners of companion animal medicine. During the past decade, a number of publications and textbooks have dealt with fundamental aspects of clinical electrocardiography in animals. These data have served as a basis for clinical interpretation, yet, have been incomplete in certain areas. For example, although the experimental literature abounds with discussions of canine and feline cardiac arrhythmias, little of this information is presented in most standard textbooks of veterinary medicine. Specifically, there is a paucity of information concerning feline electrocardiography and advanced cardiac rhythm diagnosis in the dog. Happily, many of the gaps in our current electrocardiographic literature have been filled with the publication of this textbook, *Essentials of Canine and Feline Electrocardiography*, by Larry Patrick Tilley, D.V.M.

This work is authored by an experienced clinician who has practiced at an exciting, progressive institution with a large cardiology case load. Dr. Tilley has correlated the clinical and pathologic features of many of his cases via collaboration with Dr. Si-Kwang Liu. The advantageous merging of clinical science and pathology is evidenced by their numerous papers in various areas of clinical cardiology, particularly feline myocardial diseases. This environment has provided the author with a wealth of clinicopathologic experience and substantially enhances the value of his electrocardiographic interpretations. The breadth of his experience is attested by a study of the electrocardiograms found in this volume.

This textbook provides a comprehensive review of the most important aspects of clinical canine and feline electrocardiography. Significant to this format are practical explanations pertaining to recording and interpreting electrocardiograms in dogs and cats. A consistent, pragmatic approach to interpretation is emphasized throughout the text and provides a continuity that is appreciated by students and clinicians alike. Dr. Tilley has provided a satisfying mixture of electrophysiologic principles, diagnostic implications, and practical applications. His discussions of basic electrocardiographic principles are complemented by the subsequent chapter on "The Electrophysiologic Basis of Cardiac Arrhythmias" by Drs. Boyden and Wit.

The reader will be pleased with the quality and variety of electrocardiograms in this textbook. The chapters devoted to analysis of canine and feline P-QRS-T deflections and common arrhythmias are filled with lucid well-explained illustrations. The introduction into the text is well organized and appears immediately adjacent to the topic being considered. In most cases, the author has provided numerous clinical examples to illustrate and reinforce the principles under discussion. The veterinary clinician will find important diagnostic and therapeutic information throughout this volume since Dr. Tilley includes salient pathologic correlations and therapeutic principles as they relate to each electrocardiographic disorder. In some cases, the author presents syndromes that are, as yet, unreported in the veterinary literature.

Almost every imaginable cardiac rhythm disturbance is included in the chapters on common and uncommon cardiac arrhythmias. Of particular interest is the array of rhythm disturbances illustrated in the chapters on feline electrocardiography. Experienced internists will be challenged by many of the electrocardiograms found in Chapter 12. Due to the complexity of some of these ECGs, the thoughtful reader will undoubtedly offer alternative rhythm diagnoses for some cases. Such divergent opinions are unavoidable—as the author, himself, concedes—when the rhythm diagnosis is obtained via the surface electrocardiogram. In this setting, the value of intracavitary electrocardiography is explored in theory and demonstrated with selected examples. The use of laddergrams ("Lewis diagrams") in the analysis of complex rhythm disturbances is particularly welcome. The self-assessment section offers helpful autodidactic materials and reinforces many of the principles presented in this textbook.

Advances in veterinary electrocardiography are an important facet in the rapid development of companion animal medicine. Much work remains to be completed—particularly in the areas of electrocardiographic-pathologic correlations, complex rhythm diagnosis, intracavitary electrocardiography, and antiarrhythmic therapy. This textbook provides an excellent foundation for the advancement of clinical veterinary electrocardiography. Dr. Tilley is to be commended for his timely work. I am happy, indeed, to add a short foreword to such an important contribution.

It has been five years since the first edition of this textbook was published. *Essentials of Canine and Feline Electrocardiography* was, at that time, the most complete and comprehensive textbook of small animal electrocardiography available. With this second edition, Dr. Tilley has expanded the scope of veterinary electrocardiography and has provided the student and practitioner with a complete and useful reference work.

While maintaining the readable and well-illustrated format of the previous volume, Dr. Tilley has expanded the text with a chapter describing the pathophysiologic basis and hemodynamic consequences of arrhythmias (with Dr. Si-Kwang Liu) and a chapter detailing special methods for analyzing and treating cardiac arrhythmias, including cardiac pacing. Drs. Boyden and Wit have updated their chapter on cellular electrophysiology and pathophysiology, while Dr. Muir and I have included a chapter describing cardiac antiarrhythmic therapy in the dog and cat. The complex arrhythmia chapter contin-ues to be interesting reading for the advanced student and internist. In short, my previous comments about the quality of the original textbook are quite applicable to this second edition, and I am confident that the reader will appreciate and use this textbook for both study and practice.

John D. Bonagura, D.V.M., M.Sc.

Diplomate, A.C.V.I.M.
(Cardiology, Internal Medicine)
Department of Veterinary Clinical Sciences
College of Veterinary Medicine
The Ohio State University
Columbus

Preface

Ever since Waller first reported the electrical activity of the canine heart with Einthoven's string galvanometer (1909), we have come to know more and more about the function and activity of this vital organ. Electrocardiography has become established as an atraumatic, relatively inexpensive, and extremely useful technique for gaining information about the heart and is now generally accepted as a necessary part of the cardiac examination of a dog or cat. Electrocardiography can serve two purposes: (1) the understanding of the biologic processes of the heart and (2) the diagnosis of problems in cardiac structure and function. Once the tool only of the cardiologist, the electrocardiogram is now commonly used by the internist, surgeon, and general practitioner alike. More veterinary hospitals each year are purchasing electrocardiographs, thereby increasing the number of tracings taken by veterinarians and necessitating a book with a simplified approach toward accurately interpreting these electrocardiograms.

This book explains the basic elements of electrocardiography in the simplest terms, utilizing a large number of illustrations. Most of the electrocardiograms are presented as almost full-sized tracings. The reader will be able to gain experience in interpreting electrocardiograms by being presented with them in much the same way as they are presented to the veterinarian in a clinical setting. To draw attention to important points for quicker recognition and easier understanding, identifying marks and arrows are used. One important feature is that all electrocardiograms have been painstakingly touched up, resulting in increased clarity. Many published canine electrocardiograms do not show the R wave clearly, primarily because of the large amplitude of the recording or the poor quality of the machine. The sections on canine and feline electrocardiographic interpretation are arranged so that each double page describes only one subject or part of one subject. Each double page has full-sized tracings on the right page and the corresponding descriptive text on the left. **Throughout the book, except where noted, electrocardiograms are lead II and were recorded at a paper speed of 50 mm/sec and a standard amplitude of 1 cm = 1 mv.** Because the difficulty in interpreting many electrocardiograms can often be attributed to the confusing and varied terminology and nomenclature, I have attempted to use widely accepted standards.

The primary objective of the first edition of *Essentials of Canine and Feline Electrocardiography* was to provide a practical and complete approach to the interpretation of canine and feline electrocardiograms for the purpose of establishing a diagnostic and therapeutic regimen.

My fondest dream was realized when the textbook was chosen as a comprehensive reference source for canine and feline electrocardiography by veterinary students, practicing veterinarians, and board-certified cardiologists. The textbook has also been translated into Italian and Japanese.

Over the last few years, numerous articles in the veterinary and human medical literature have described new findings in the field of electrocardiography. There is major interest in the development of new therapeutic approaches to the treatment of arrhythmias, such as the use of pacemakers and the administration of new antiarrhythmic drugs. In addition, investigative studies of intracardiac electrocardiography are under way, to enable us to better understand these complex abnormalities. Dr. Charles Fisch of the Krannert Institute of Cardiology, in his Lewis A. Conner Memorial Lecture, "The clinical electrocardiogram: a classic" (53rd Scientific Session, American Heart Association, 1980), summarized it well: "He who maintains that new knowledge of electrocardiography is no longer possible or contributive, ignores history."

Since the first edition of this textbook was published in 1979, there has been tremendous growth in the field of canine and feline electrocardiography. The aims of the second edition basically remain the same as those of the first edition, that is, to provide a concise but complete text of information needed by clinicians interested in the diagnostic and therapeutic aspects of veterinary electrocardiography. My intention is for the book to be useful to a wide audience, but comprehensive enough to serve as a reference for the advanced student and the electrocardiographic interpreter. The entire textbook has been revised, updated, and expanded. At least 150 new illustrations and electrocardiographic strips have been added to provide more complete coverage of their respective subjects. Some of the more recent advancements in electrocardiography that have been included in the textbook are: transtelephonic electrocardiography, computerized electrocardiography, electrocardiographic equipment, pacemakers, His bundle electrocardiography, causes of cardiac arrhythmias (including neurologic disorders), and antiarrhythmic therapy.

Two new sections have been added to the second edition: Section Four—Pathophysiologic Basis and Effects of Cardiac Arrhythmias and Section Five—Management of Cardiac Arrhythmias. As part of their knowledge of cardiology, today's veterinarians are expected to be able to identify the various electrocardiographic patterns. These patterns are discussed in detail in the interpretation sections of the textbook. It is also important for the veterinarian to understand the inherent consequences of these patterns because such knowledge provides a more comprehensive understanding of what may be happening to the animal as well as a rationale for the therapeutic regimen. The electrocardiogram serves as a focus for discussing various cardiac drugs and cardiac diseases. The hemodynamic effects and clinical features of various arrhythmias have been added to the chapters on interpretation and to the section on self-assessment tracings when appropriate.

My experience in evaluating large numbers of cats and dogs with electrocardiographic abnormalities at the Animal Medical Center and at Cardiopet, Inc., a transtelephonic electrocardiographic firm, has made it possible for me to correlate accurately the anatomic and electrophysiologic bases of the various electrocardiographic abnormalities with their clinical and hemodynamic manifestations, together with a rational approach to therapy.

More than 170 years ago, Dr. Robert Watt of Glasgow wrote: "To obtain correct views of medicine, it is necessary to have recourse to original authors, to such as write from actual observation, who have seen and treated the disease they describe" (From F.A. Willus and T.E. Keys: *Cardiac Classics*, St. Louis, C.V. Mosby, 1941). In accordance with Dr. Watt's view, I have been fortunate to have both John D. Bonagura, D.V.M., M.Sc., Dip. A.C.V.I.M. (Cardiology, Internal Medicine), and William W. Muir, D.V.M., Ph.D., as authors of the chapter on antiarrhythmic therapy for the dog and cat. Both men are pioneers in the field of veterinary cardiac therapeutics and have numerous publications to their credit. Also pioneers in their field, Penelope A. Boyden, Ph.D. and Andrew L. Wit, Ph.D. have written the chapter on the cellular electrophysiologic basis of cardiac arrhythmias. Si-Kwang Liu, D.V.M., Ph.D., my friend and colleague in cardiology, has written a section on the pathologic analysis of cardiac arrhythmias

and conduction disturbances. Knowledge of cardiac pathology is important for the clinician who wishes to understand the electrocardiogram. This knowledge can only be gained by studying the heart at necropsy and by correlating pathologic findings with electrocardiographic interpretations.

A special section (Six) on complex arrhythmias has been included, but should be left for later study until the beginner gains confidence with simpler recordings. A self-assessment section (Seven) aims at providing the reader with additional opportunities to evaluate his own understanding by interpreting electrocardiograms and by solving problems of arrhythmias as they occur clinically. Each tracing is accompanied by a short case history and a question on interpretation. The tracing is then again shown on the reverse side of the page with appropriate labeling and interpretation. The interpretation of the electrocardiogram is the most important and often the most difficult aspect of electrocardiography. It is not uncommon to find that even after prolonged and careful study, many practitioners and even cardiologists differ considerably in their interpretations of the same electrocardiogram. I welcome constructive criticisms and comments in this regard.

An appendix added to the textbook includes normal electrocardiographic values for the dog and cat, tables for deriving the mean electrical axis, and two client-education charts for use in private practice. The references, which have been updated and placed at the end of each chapter, include some of the books and journal articles that I have found particularly helpful and significant. The interested reader is encouraged to consult these works as much as possible.

New York   Larry Patrick Tilley

Acknowledgments

I would like to express my appreciation to all who made this edition possible: John D. Bonagura, D.V.M., Diplomate A.C.V.I.M. (Cardiology, Internal Medicine), for his patient and thorough review of portions of the manuscript and for his many suggestions and helpful criticism; Robert Glassman, M.D., of the Krannert Institute of Cardiology, Indianapolis; Lawrence Frame, M.D., of the Department of Cardiology, University of Pennsylvania, Philadelphia; Steve Scheidt, M.D., Department of Cardiology, New York Hospital-Cornell University, New York for their constructive criticism of portions of Chapter 11 (Uncommon Complex Arrhythmias). Michael Schollmeyer, D.V.M. of Medtronics, Inc., Minneapolis, was helpful in the discussion of artificial pacemakers.

Several physicians and veterinarians have graciously provided illustrations for the original text and for this edition: M. Rosenbaum, M.D.; A.L. Wit, Ph.D.; R.E. Phillips, M.D.; H.J. Attar, M.D.; H.H. Friedman, M.D.; C.W. Lombard, D.V.M.; F.B. Hembrough, D.V.M.; D.B. Coulter, D.V.M.; R. Lazzara, M.D.; G.H. Bardy, M.D.; W.P. Nelson, M.D.; E. Besterman, M.D.; J. Fenoglio, M.D.; C. Kvart, D.V.M.; F. Navarro-Lopez, M.D.; W.H. Werhrmacher, M.D.; H.J.L. Marriot, M.D.; D.C. Harrison, M.D.; G. Jacobs, D.V.M.; A. Tidholm, D.V.M.; N. Belic, M.D.; M. Ishijima, D.V.M.; T. Bauer, D.V.M.; and P. Fox, D.V.M.

All new illustrations and retraced electrocardiograms in this edition are the work of Mrs. Denise Donnell. Ms. Leslie Orgel and Mrs. Pamela Faber typed the revised manuscript. I am grateful to them for their excellent work. I would like to especially thank Ms. Christine MacMurray, Ms. Cynthia Fazzini, and Mrs. Nancy Baumoel for their thorough editorial supervision of the entire manuscript. Recognition should also be given to my colleagues in cardiology and to all the personnel at Cardiopet, Inc. for their support during the preparation of this book.

In addition to thanking veterinarians who have referred cases to me, I would like to express my gratitude to each of the veterinary students, interns, and residents whom I have had the privilege of teaching. Their curiosity and intellectual stimulation have enabled me to grow and have prompted me to undertake the task of writing this book.

I am deeply grateful to Lemuel Ward for the pencil drawing on the dedication page. Lemuel Ward, 86 years old and from Crisfield, Maryland, is beyond praise among his peers for his wildlife drawings and carvings.

Finally, Christian C. Febiger Spahr, Jr., Veterinary Editor, Mrs. Dorothy Di Rienzi, Mrs. Janet Nuciforo, Mr. Thomas J. Colaiezzi, and their colleagues in the Production and Copy Editing Departments of Lea & Febiger are meticulous workers and kind people who have made the final stages of preparing this book both inspiring and fun.

L.P.T.

Contributors

John D. Bonagura, D.V.M., M.Sc.
Diplomate, A.C.V.I.M. (Cardiology, Internal Medicine)
The Ohio State University
College of Veterinary Medicine
1935 Coffey Road
Columbus, Ohio

William W. Muir, D.V.M., Ph.D.
Diplomate, A.C.V.A.
Chairman, Department of Veterinary Clinical Sciences
The Ohio State University
College of Veterinary Medicine
1935 Coffey Road
Columbus, Ohio

Si-Kwang Liu, D.V.M., Ph.D.
The Animal Medical Center
510 East 62nd Street
New York, New York

Penelope A. Boyden, Ph.D.
College of Physicians & Surgeons
Columbia University
Department of Pharmacology
630 West 168th Street
New York, New York

Andrew L. Wit, Ph.D.
College of Physicians & Surgeons
Columbia University
Department of Pharmacology
630 West 168th Street
New York, New York

Contents

Appendices

1 Generation of the electrocardiogram: basic principles

I was almost tempted to think with Fracastorius that the motion of the heart was only to be comprehended by God.[1]

WILLIAM HARVEY
De motu cordis, 1628

. . . demonstrates by the structure of the heart that blood is continually passed through the lungs into the aorta, as by two clacks of water bellows to raise water. The passage of blood from arteries to veins is shown by means of a ligature. So it is proved that a continual movement of the blood in a circle is caused by the beat of the heart.*

WILLIAM HARVEY
Prelectiones Anatomiae Universalis, 1616

A history of electrocardiography

That the heart beats to circulate the blood was an important discovery made by Harvey in 1616. Physiologists later found that the

---

*The first notation of the discovery of the circulation of blood in animals, from Harvey's 1616 *Lecture notes.*

heartbeat was also an electrical process: each time the heart muscle contracted, electrical currents flowed through it. Science was called on to facilitate the investigation of the heartbeat as an electrical event. An understanding of the general concepts of electrochemistry is important as a basis for this chapter.

The early investigators explained the electrical processes of the heart on the basis that the body fluids are good conductors of electricity. Augustus D. Waller[2] (Fig. 1–1) in 1887, using the capillary electrometer, reported the first recording of electrical changes accompanying the heart's beat in man; he later reported similar findings in the cat (Fig. 1–2A). A light beam interrupted by the mercury column of the Lippman electrometer enabled photographic records to be made on plates mounted on slowly moving toy train wagons (Fig. 1–2B). Waller was the first to demonstrate that the electrical impulses of the heart could be recorded from the surface of the body. This historic event, witnessed by Willem Einthoven, took place in 1887. In 1895, Einthoven introduced the terms P, Q, R, S, and T for the electrocardiographic deflections.[3] Waller was the first to use the term electrocardiogram.[4] Einthoven (1903) developed the string galvanometer, which gave more accurate tracings of the heart's electrical activity.

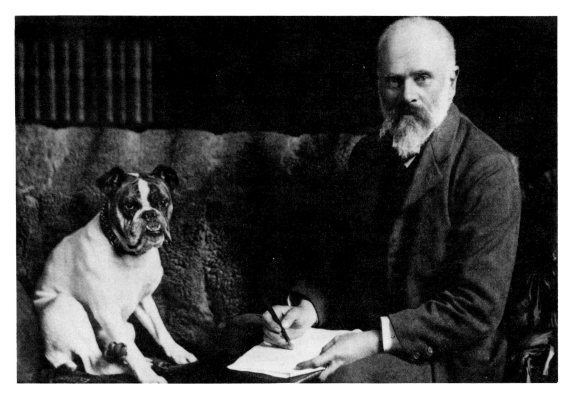

Fig. 1–1. Augustus Desire Waller with his pet Bulldog, Jimmie. Waller obtained the first electrocardiograms in man, the cat, and the dog. Jimmie was used in many of Waller's studies with the capillary electrometer. (See Fig. 1–3.) (From Burch, G.E., and DePasquale, N.P.: *A History of Electrocardiography.* Chicago, Year Book Medical Publishers, Inc., 1964, courtesy Yale University Medical Library, New Haven, Conn.)

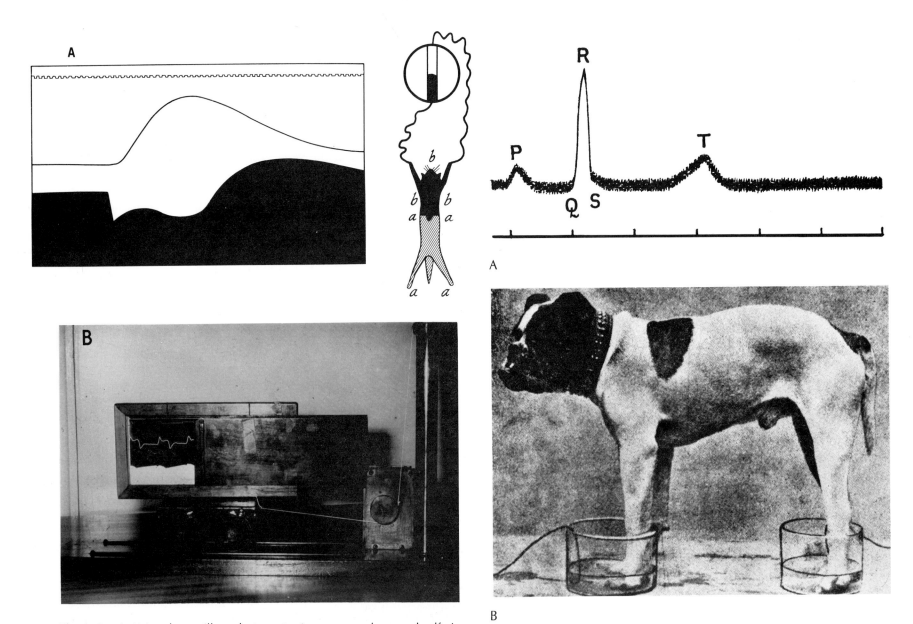

Fig. 1–2. **A,** Using the capillary electrometer (a mercury column and sulfuric acid column) on the right, Waller was first to record the electrical changes accompanying the heart's beat in the cat. The tracing on the left (middle line) was recorded with electrodes placed directly on the exposed heart of a kitten. Methods were later developed to calibrate and correct these records; to formulate the electrocardiogram as it is presently recognized. Top bracketed line is the time scale. (From Waller, A.D.: A demonstration on man of electromotive changes accompanying the heart's beat. J. Physiol., *8:*229, 1887; reprinted in Burch, G.E., and DePasquale, N.P.: *A History of Electrocardiography.* Chicago, Year Book Medical Publishers, Inc., 1964.) **B,** Toy train wagon carrying photographic plate used by Waller to record the "electrogram" shown above in **A.** (From Besterman, E., and Creese, R.: Waller—pioneer of electrocardiography. Br. Heart J., *42:*61, 1979, with permission.)

Fig. 1–3. **A,** One of Waller's original electrocardiograms of the dog, using Einthoven's galvanometer. Einthoven experimented with the capillary electrometer and improved the instrument by making alterations in circuitry and resistance levels. **B,** The method of recording the electrocardiogram in a dog with the capillary electrometer is shown on the right. The Bulldog is Jimmie, shown with Waller in Figure 1–1. (**A** from Waller, A.D.: Lancet, *1:*1448, 1909; **B** from Waller, A.D.: *Physiology, the Servant of Medicine.* London, University of London Press, 1910; reprinted with permission of Hodder & Stoughton, Ltd., Sevenoaks, Kent, England.)

Nürr, in 1922, was the first to approach electrocardiography in the dog from a clinical point of view.[5]

One of Waller's original records of the first electrocardiogram of his dog Jimmy and his recording technique are shown in Figure 1–3. Jimmy, who had a "Churchillian" quality, had the distinction of having had a question put to Waller about him in the House of Commons:

Question: "At a conversazione of the Royal Society at Burlington House on May 12th last, a bulldog was cruelly treated when a leather strap with sharp nails was wound around his neck and his feet were immersed in glass jars containing salts in solution, and the jars in turn were connected with wires to galvanometers. Such a cruel procedure should surely be dealt with under the "Cruelty to Animals Act" of 1876?"

Answer: "The dog in question wore a leather collar ornamented with brass studs, and he was placed to stand in water to which sodium chloride had been added, or in other words, common salt. If my honorable friend had ever paddled in the sea, he will appreciate fully the sensation obtained thereby from this simple pleasurable experience!"[6,7]

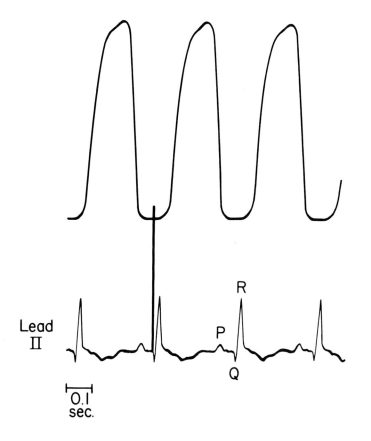

Fig. 1–4. Simultaneous recording of the electrocardiogram and left ventricular pressure tracing in a dog. Note how the onset (vertical line) of the QRS complex precedes the rise in left ventricular pressure.

Introduction

The P-QRS-T deflections described by Einthoven are associated with the wave of excitation that spreads throughout the heart and releases the contractile forces of the heart. *P* corresponds to atrial depolarization or contraction, and *QRS* corresponds to ventricular depolarization or contraction. The *T* wave represents ventricular repolarization or relaxation. The onset of the P-QRS precedes the onset of contraction. Figure 1–4 shows a simultaneous recording of the electrocardiogram and the left ventricular pressure tracing in a dog. The events leading to the generation of these electrical and hemodynamic changes will be considered at three levels: (1) the cell—its electrical activity, (2) cardiac muscle—electrical and contractile properties, and (3) cardiac muscle fiber—generation of the "electrogram."

In addition to the cardiac muscle cells (which have electrical and contractile properties), the heart also possesses certain "specialized" cells whose primary function is the genesis and conduction of electrical impulses. The latter cells form the conduction system of the heart. The gross anatomy of these specialized tissues or cells will be discussed for both the dog and the cat, and the generation of the electrocardiogram will be explained in terms of its relationship to the conduction system. The various lead systems for accurately recording the heart's electrical field also will be discussed. This chapter, then, provides a basis for the electrocardiographic diagnosis of arrhythmias and cardiac disease.

ELECTRICAL ACTIVITY IN THE CELL

If the cell is penetrated by a capillary microelectrode, a negative potential of 90 mv (resting membrane potential) is recorded[8] (Fig. 1–5). The inside of the cell is negative with respect to the surface of the cell because of a gradient of potassium ions (K^+) across the cell membrane. The intracellular concentration of K^+ is approximately 30 times higher than the extracellular concentration. A reverse concentration gradient exists for sodium ions (Na^+) and for calcium ions (Ca^{++}).[9] The resting cell membrane is also relatively permeable to K^+, but less so to Na^+ and Ca^{++}. Two active transport mechanisms, the sodium pump and the potassium pump, are responsible for maintaining the resting membrane potential. Na^+ is pumped to the outside of the cell; K^+ is pumped to the inside of the cell. The sodium-potassium pump is a protein complex that utilizes ATP to transport these ions against their energy gradients. The sodium-potassium pump is also important because it appears to be a site of binding and action of digitalis.[9–11]

When a single cardiac muscle cell of appropriate strength is stimulated, the resting membrane potential is reduced to a critical level, called the threshold potential (Fig. 1–5). The permeability of the cell membrane to Na^+ and K^+ is suddenly altered. Because of these ions' electrical and concentration gradients, Na^+ enter the cells rapidly, and K^+ move to the outside of the cell. The result of this abrupt change in cell permeability is an action potential (Fig. 1–5), an electrical event that initiates muscle contraction.

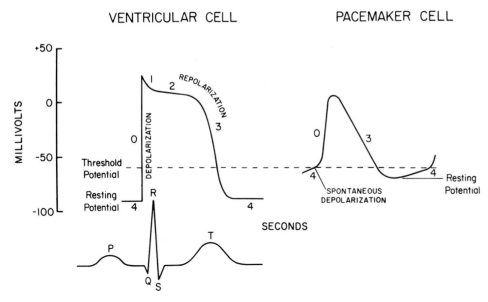

VENTRICULAR CELL   PACEMAKER CELL

Fig. 1–5. Diagram of the action potential of a nonpacemaking cell (on the left) with the relationship of the electrocardiogram (on the bottom). The action potential of a pacemaking cell is illustrated on the right.

The electrocardiogram basically represents the summation of many such action potentials recorded from the entire heart. The various slopes of the action potential have been designated 0, 1, 2, 3, and 4 (Fig. 1–5). Phase *0* is the initial rapid upstroke or depolarization; phases *1* through *3* are the stages of repolarization (depolarization results in the QRS complex of the electrocardiogram, repolarization in the ST-T wave); phase *4* is the period between action potentials during electrical diastole.[12]

The action potential results from an influx and an efflux of ionic charges across the cell membrane. Phase 0 is dependent on the rapid inward Na^+ current. Phase 1, early rapid repolarization, is associated with a decrease in Na^+ entry and a passive shift of chloride (Cl^-) into the cell. Phase 2, slow repolarization, is due to a slow inward Ca^{++} current as well as a slow Na^+ entry. Phase 3, rapid repolarization, is associated with an efflux of K^+ and a return to the resting membrane potential.[11]

All myocardial and specialized conducting cells are excitable. If a stimulus of appropriate strength and duration is applied to a cell, an action potential will result. The cells in the specialized conducting system, called pacemaker cells, are also capable of initiating their own impulses in the absence of an extrinsic stimulus. Pacemaker cells can depolarize spontaneously during phase 4 until threshold potential is reached and an action potential occurs (Fig. 1–5). There is a slow leak of Na^+ into the cell throughout phase 4. This capacity for impulse formation is a unique property called automaticity. The dominant pacemaker cells are located in the sinus node. Automaticity is also a property of atrial specialized conducting fibers, various fibers on the

atrial surface of the mitral[13] and tricuspid[14] valves, fibers in the lower or nodal-His region of the atrioventricular (AV) node, and fibers in the His-Purkinje system.[15] Any one of these automatic cells may demonstrate automatic activity and act as a pacemaker of the heart (a site at which the impulse originates).

The more rapid pacemaker activity of the sinoatrial (SA) node normally activates the atria first and then the ventricles. The intrinsic pacemaker activity of the lower regions is normally obscured by the SA node activity. The overall normal rate of impulse formation in the SA node is 70 to 160 beats/min in the dog. The SA rate in the cat and in puppies is normally much faster, with the average being 160 to 240 beats/min.[16,17] If the SA node were to become inactive, a lower pacemaker would become active. The cells in the lower region of the AV node are the most rapid of the lower pacemakers, with an approximate rate of 40 to 60 beats/min. If an electrical impulse fails to be transmitted through the AV node and bundle of His and into the ventricles, the pacemaker cells in the Purkinje fibers begin to discharge impulses. Their intrinsic discharge rate is approximately 20 to 40 beats/min. The normal order of electrical activation from an impulse arising in the sinoatrial node is shown in Table 1–1. The corresponding conduction velocities and intrinsic pacemaker rates also are outlined.[18,19]

PROPERTIES OF CARDIAC MUSCLE

There are three types of cardiac muscle: atrial, ventricular, and noncontractile (the last being fibers of the specialized conduction system). There are five fundamental physiologic properties of cardiac muscles: automaticity, excitability, refractoriness, conductivity, and contractility.[9,20] As will be discussed in Chapters 9 and 12, explanations of arrhythmogenesis are dependent on these physiologic properties.

Table 1–1. Normal order of cardiac electrical activation in the adult canine heart

Normal order of activation	Intrinsic pacemaker rate (beats/min)	Average conduction velocity (mm/sec)
Sinoatrial (SA) node	70–160	—
↓ Atrial myocardium	None	800–1000
↓ Atrioventricular (AV) node (high or low midnodal region)	None	50–100
↓ AV node-His bundle region	40–60	800–1000
↓ Bundle branches	20–40	2000–4000
↓ Purkinje network	20–40	
↓ Ventricular myocardium	None	400–1000

Automaticity (rhythmicity)

As discussed in the previous section, the cells in the specialized conduction system are capable of initiating their own impulses. Figure 1–5 illustrates that these cells can depolarize spontaneously during phase 4 until a threshold potential is reached and an action potential results. Any of these cells in the proper set of conditions can demonstrate automatic activity and act as a pacemaker of the heart (Table 1–1).

Excitability

Cardiac muscle is excited when the stimulus reduces the resting potential to a certain critical level, the threshold potential (Fig. 1–5). The degree of the resting potential within the cell therefore determines its excitability. The cardiac response to a stimulus obeys the "all-or-none" law.[21] Once the threshold is reached through a proper stimulus, a complete action potential is produced. If the stimulus intensity is increased, there is no change in the action potential. The action potential will not occur if the stimulus is below the threshold potential.

Refractoriness

Refractoriness is a property of all types of cardiac muscle. Heart muscle will not respond to external stimuli during its period of contraction. The contraction must be completed and the cell recovered before another can occur. If the heart did not possess this important property, it would fail as a pump because it would be constantly undergoing continued contractions.

Conductivity

Conductivity is the property of heart muscle whereby the activation of an individual muscle cell produces activity in the neighboring muscle cell. The heart is essentially a true anatomic syncytium. Every cardiac muscle fiber is separated at each end from its neighbor by intercalated discs that cross the short axes of the cells and are thought to represent low-resistance pathways between the myocardial cells (Fig. 1–6). A humoral transmitter also may be involved in the electrical transmission from cell to cell.[19]

Conduction velocity varies in the different portions of the specialized conduction system and the myocardium (Table 1–1). The velocity

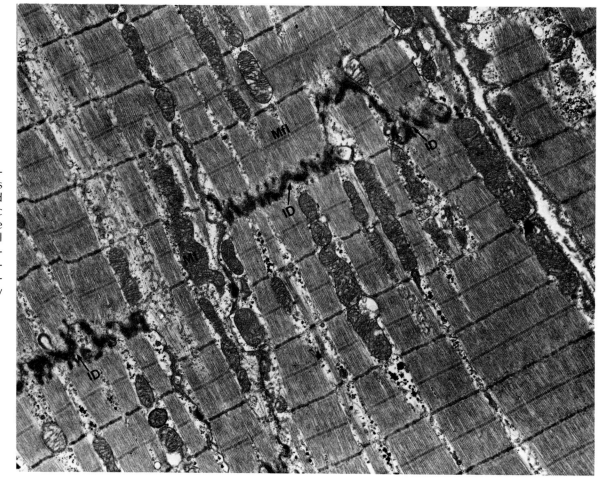

Fig. 1–6. Electron microphotograph of normal canine cardiac muscle cells, showing the myofibrils *(Mfl)* and the intercalated discs *(ID)*. The intercalated discs provide a strong union between the cardiac muscle fibers—true cell-to-cell junctions—and have the ability to pass charged particles freely from cell to cell. They thus allow for the rapid spread of electrical activity between adjacent cells. *Mt,* Mitochondria. (Courtesy of J. Fenoglio, M.D., Columbia University College of Physicians and Surgeons, New York, N.Y.)

is greatest in the Purkinje fibers and least in the mid-portion of the AV node. This activation sequence for the different portions of the specialized conductive tissue is so arranged that the maximum mechanical efficiency is provided from each corresponding contraction.[22]

Contractility

Contractility occurs in response to electrical current (Fig. 1–4). The physiology of cardiac contractility is dependent on many factors. These factors will not be discussed, for they comprise a large subject area and have little relevance to the analysis of the electrocardiogram.

THE ELECTROGRAM

We now are ready to record electrical activity from the surface of a single cardiac muscle fiber or cell and study the generation of the "electrogram." The electrocardiogram, which will be discussed later, is a graph of the variations in voltage produced by a mass of associated cardiac muscle cells or bundle of muscle fibers.

To understand the genesis of the electrocardiogram, we must consider the potential differences that occur when a single muscle fiber (Fig. 1–7) is stimulated.[23] The electrogram recorded from the cell surface consists of two parts: (1) a wave of depolarization after the cell membrane surface is stimulated and (2) repolarization (recovery) of the cell to its original resting state. The electrogram and electrocardiogram are recorded from outside the cells, not from within as previously discussed when an action potential is recorded.

The surface of a resting cardiac muscle fiber, then, is positively charged, whereas the inside of the cell has a negative resting potential. Figure 1–7A illustrates a resting cardiac muscle fiber; all portions of the cell surface are positively charged. There is no difference in recorded potential, so the electrogram remains at the baseline. When

the muscle fiber is stimulated (Fig. 1–7B), a wave of depolarization passes over the cell from left to right. The surface of the depolarized area (shaded area) is negatively charged, so the positive electrode (on the right) is facing a region of greater potential than is the negative electrode (on the left). The electrogram will record an upward deflection if the depolarization wave flows toward the positive electrode. The muscle fiber is now fully depolarized, and the external surface is negative in relation to the interior (Fig. 1–7C). Because there is no potential difference between various portions of the cell surface, the recording returns to the baseline. Both electrodes now face the same degree of negativity. Repolarization, or recovery of the cell, begins at the same point on the muscle fiber where depolarization began (Fig. 1–7D). A potential difference opposite in polarity to that seen during depolarization is recorded. Since the left surface charge on the cell is positive to the right surface charge, a downward deflection occurs. The recording will return to the baseline as repolarization is completed.

RECORDING THE ELECTRICAL ACTIVITY OF THE HEART—THE ELECTROCARDIOGRAM

The true electrical activity within the heart can be depicted as a quantity produced by a mass of associated cardiac muscle cells or bundles of muscle fibers. The total electrical activity can be determined

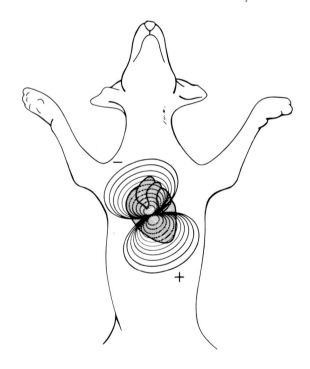

Fig. 1–8. The total electrical activity of the heart can be determined at an external point and resolved into a single electrical force or charge, as a dipole. One half of the dipole or electrical field is positive, and the opposite half is negative. When electrodes are attached to the skin on the legs, the electrical activity of the heart can be recorded by an electrocardiograph.

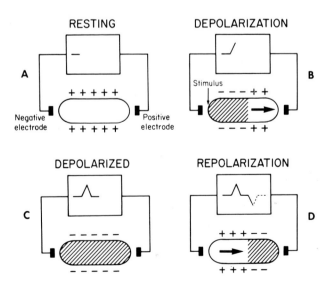

Fig. 1–7. The "electrogram" recording the electrical activity that occurs when a single muscle fiber is stimulated.

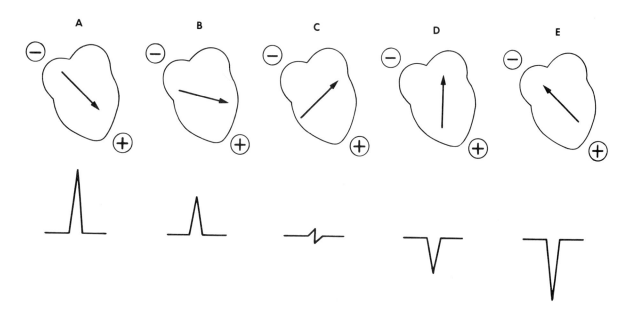

Fig. 1–9. Effect of the depolarization wave on the deflections of the electrocardiogram, determined by wave direction. Each lead has a positive and a negative pole. By tradition, the electrocardiogram is generated in such a way that it shows a positive wave when the depolarization wave is flowing *toward* the positive electrode (**A** and **B**). A negative deflection is recorded when the depolarization wave moves *away* from the positive electrode (**D** and **E**). The deflection is *isoelectric* when depolarization is perpendicular to an imaginary line connecting the two electrodes (**C**).

at an external point and resolved into one electrical force or charge—a theory termed the "dipolar hypothesis"[9] (Fig. 1–8). The dipolar hypothesis assumes that each instantaneous vector is the result of an electrical potential that acts as a dipole. True electrical activity within the heart rises from multiple dipoles, each vital cell acting as a dipole. If the body tissue and fluids are homogeneous conductors of electrical potential, a single dipole summating all the dipoles can be measured at the body surface.

The model of the heart as a dipole in the center of a conducting medium is not incorrect; it is only oversimplified. For example, all the body tissues are not equally good conductors. As will be discussed later, the lungs of wide-chested dogs act as regions of high electrical resistance and the electrocardiographic complexes are often smaller than normal in deflection.

The cardiac vector

Electrical forces are vector quantities whose magnitude is represented by the length of the arrow and whose direction and polarity are represented by the arrowhead (Fig. 1–9). The term cardiac vector signifies all electrical forces of the heart cycle. A resultant *mean vector* is recorded for each portion of the heart cycle. The majority of potentials are cancelled out by opposite forces. Thus the mean vector for atrial (P) and ventricular (QRS) depolarization and ventricular repolarization (T) are recorded. Repolarization of the atria (T_a wave) is usually not seen because it is buried in the QRS complex.

Figure 1–9 illustrates the effect of the depolarization wave on the deflections of the electrocardiogram. When the depolarization wave moves *toward* the positive electrode, a *positive* deflection is recorded; when the depolarization wave moves *away* from the positive electrode, a *negative* deflection is recorded. The deflections will obviously be very small or absent when the depolarization is *perpendicular* to the imaginary line connecting the electrodes. This rule is the basis for under-

standing the various lead systems that will be discussed at the end of the chapter. By using the various lead systems and the different angles at which they record the heart's electrical activity, one can determine the angle of the mean electrical impulse traveling through the ventricle—called the mean electrical axis of the electrocardiogram (Chapter 3).

From the preceding discussion, the basic principles of cardiac vectors for electrocardiographic interpretation are the following:

1. Forces moving towards a positive electrode cause an upward deflection on the electrocardiogram.
2. Forces moving away from a positive electrode cause a downward deflection on the electrocardiogram.
3. Forces moving at right angles to a recording lead (a negative electrode and positive electrode) or to the positive electrode over a short distance cause very small or absent deflections on the electrocardiogram.
4. The magnitude of the electrocardiographic deflection is proportional to the thickness of the muscle activated and to the proximity of the electrode to it.

ANATOMY OF THE CONDUCTION SYSTEM

The heart is composed of muscle fibers with a well-coordinated conduction system. The conduction system consists of the sinoatrial

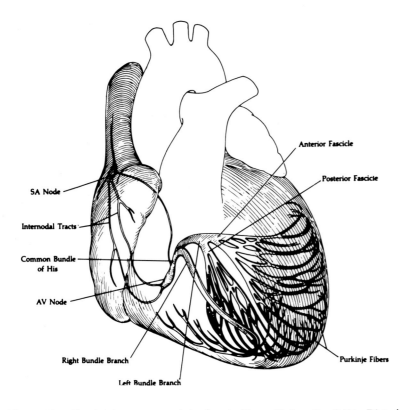

Fig. 1–10. Conduction system of the heart. (From DeSanctis, R.W.: Disturbances of cardiac rhythm and conduction. In *SCIENTIFIC AMERICAN MEDICINE.* Edited by E. Rubenstein. New York, Scientific American, 1982, with permission.)

(SA) node, the internodal atrial tracts, the atrioventricular (AV) node, the bundle of His, the right and left bundle branches, and the Purkinje system (Fig. 1–10). The anatomy of the cardiac conduction system in the dog and that in the cat have been reviewed.*

Before the conduction system can be discussed, the anatomic terms used to describe direction should be established. The terms for direction are the same as those used in human anatomy. Because of man's upright position, however, confusion may result when these terms describe canine and feline positions. A structure at or toward the head end of the body of a dog or cat is *cranial* or *anterior* (e.g., cranial vena cava); one at or toward the tail end is *caudal* or *posterior*. Comparable positions in man are superior (e.g., superior vena cava) and inferior. A structure at or toward the spine of a dog or cat is *dorsal;* one toward the belly, *ventral*. The terms dorsal and ventral are rarely used in human anatomy, the comparable directions being posterior and anterior.

The anatomic terms used in this text to describe the cardiac conduction system will be based on those used in man, as has been done in veterinary electrocardiography.[32–34] For example, the two divisions

of the left bundle branch are described as anterior and posterior. Comparable positions in the dog and cat would be ventral and dorsal.[35,36]

The *SA node* is the primary pacemaker of the heart and is located in the upper part of the right atrium, close to the entry of the cranial vena cava. Conduction through the atria occurs via three internodal tracts: anterior, middle, and posterior. A direct fiber-to-fiber connection exists in all three pathways between the SA and AV nodes.

The remaining specialized conduction tissues of the heart form essentially a single structure connecting the atria to all parts of the ventricles. The *AV node* lies on the right side of the lower part of the interatrial septum and is continued as the *bundle of His*. The bundle of His penetrates the fibrous AV ring, providing the only normal electrical link between the atria and the ventricles. The bundle of His courses along the edge of the membranous septum toward the aortic valve and bifurcates at the valve into the left and right bundle branches. The *right bundle branch* passes down the right ventricular side of the muscular septum to the anterior papillary muscle. A network of conducting fibers radiating from the right bundle branch then extends over the right ventricular wall. The *left bundle branch* passes down the left ventricular side of the septum just below the cusps of the aortic valve. At its junction with the upper third of the septum, it divides into two widely interconnected pathways: the *anterior fascicle* and the *posterior fascicle*, which pass to the bases of the corresponding papillary muscles. An interconnection of these two fascicles, the *septal fascicle*, distributes over the midseptal area. All three fascicles divide into a complex network of fibers, called Purkinje fibers, which are distributed to the ventricular myocardium.[37]

With an understanding of these anatomic facts, one can better appreciate the frequency of many electrocardiographic abnormalities in both the dog and the cat. For example, a small lesion of the right midseptal surface in the path of the right bundle most likely would cause a right bundle branch block. The same lesion at the same level on the left side probably would not cause a left bundle branch block because there are more opportunities for bypassing the lesion owing to the extensive network of the left bundle. This could possibly help to explain the greater clinical frequency of right bundle branch block in the dog.

Direct visualization of the conduction system

The peripheral conduction system of the left ventricle can actually be visualized. It has a high content of glycogen and therefore is stained easily with Lugol's iodine applied to the endocardial surface by means of a cotton swab. The left bundle branch and its fascicles in the left ventricle of the dog can be sharply defined by this technique (Fig. 1–11). The same technique will also show the right bundle and its conducting fibers (Fig. 1–12). The glycogen rapidly undergoes postmortem autolysis, rendering the conduction system nonstainable after approximately 2 hours. These rapid changes in the conduction system may explain the bizarre conduction abnormalities seen in the electrocardiograms of dying animals.[31]

---

*References 24, 25, 26, 27, 28, 29, 30, 31

The electrocardiograph can now be used to measure the electrical potential of the heart at the body surface. The electrocardiograph as a galvanometer has a delicate writing instrument that will indicate a single positive or negative charge. As discussed, the genesis of the electrocardiogram involves a number of factors: (1) initiation of impulse formation in the primary pacemaker (SA node), (2) transmission of the impulse through the specialized conduction system of the heart, (3) activation or depolarization of the atrial and ventricular myocardium, and (4) recovery or repolarization of the preceding three areas. The six diagrams in Figure 1–13 depict the electrocardiogram on the basis of these factors.[8,22,38,39]

A positive electrode (located over the left ventricle in all six diagrams) is used for recording the genesis of the entire electrocardiogram. Depolarization waves spread from the SA node through the right atrium toward the left atrium and the AV node (Fig. 1–13A). The result is a positive wave (P wave), the depolarization or activation force directed toward the positive electrode. The rest of the P wave is recorded when the left atrium is depolarized (Fig. 1–13B). The left atrial activation forces are directed slightly away from the positive lead. Since the two atrial processes overlap, the result is an upright P wave. The P wave thus records depolarization of the right atrium and then of the left atrium. This anatomic fact will be important later when right atrial and left atrial enlargements are diagnosed on the electrocardiogram. Transmission of the impulse into the ventricles is prevented by a nonresponsive fibrous ring that supports the valves and great vessels. The only normal pathway into the ventricles is through the bundle of His.

Three phases or waves of electrical activity produce the Q, R, and S deflections on the electrocardiogram. The depolarization force is directed first toward the right bundle branch and also away from the positive electrode (Fig. 1–13C). Most of the early impulses are transmitted by the left bundle branch, with forces directed from the left to the right side of the septum, resulting in a negative deflection and a Q wave.

The Q wave represents the first phase of ventricular depolarization.

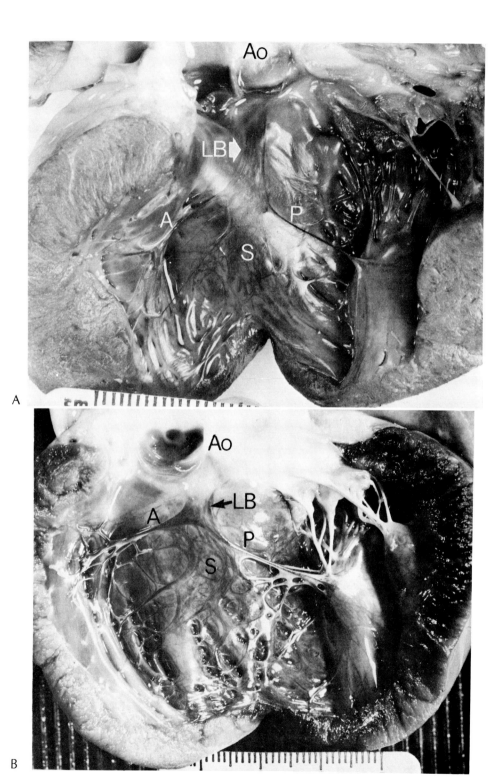

A

B

Fig. 1–11. Left ventricular conduction system in two canine hearts. These photographs were made of the left ventricular septal surface after iodine staining of the endocardium. The left bundle branch (LB) emerges as a bandlike structure below the aortic valve (Ao) in both cases. The left bundle branch bifurcates into the anterior (A) and posterior (P) fascicles, which are attached to the apical portions of the papillary muscles. A network of midseptal Purkinje fibers (S) is distributed throughout the septal surface bordered by the two major fascicles. In **B,** the septal fibers are extensive and the contribution of the posterior fascicle is predominant. Many of the strands on the unstained heart are, in effect, portions of the peripheral and terminal branches of the conduction system.

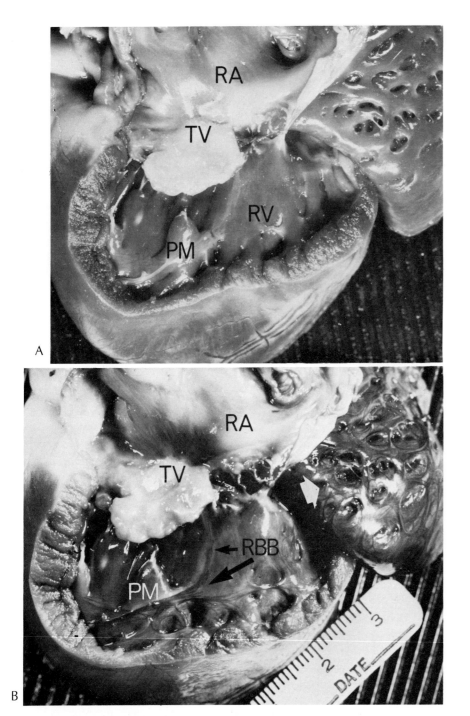

Fig. 1–12. Heart of a dog, **A,** opened to expose the right ventricular cavity and, **B,** stained with iodine solution to bring out the conduction system. The right bundle branch *(RBB)* appears beneath the leaflet of the tricuspid valve *(TV)*. It continues down the septum and at the halfway point deviates to the anterior papillary muscle. It then divides into two or three primary branches, which terminate in the free wall. The network of conduction fibers radiating from the primary branches of the right bundle is extensive (white arrow). *RA,* Right atrium; *PM,* papillary muscle.

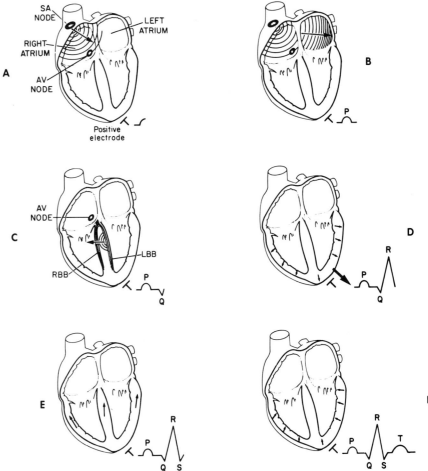

Fig. 1–13. Electrocardiogram and the cardiac conduction system as an electrical impulse travels from the sinoatrial (SA) node to the ventricular Purkinje network.

The P-Q or P-R interval is the measurement from the beginning of the P wave to the beginning of the Q or R wave of the QRS complex. This delay between the P and the Q or R wave represents atrial depolarization and the slow conduction of atrial impulses through the AV junction. The delay allows the ventricles time to fill with blood before they contract. During this time, the electrocardiographic tracing returns to the baseline and the isoelectric P-R (P-Q) segment is inscribed.

A positive deflection, called the R wave, represents the second phase of ventricular depolarization (Fig. 1–13D). The conduction system branches subendocardially, with the apex and free walls of both ventricles simultaneously depolarized from the endocardium toward the epicardium. Because the mass of the left ventricle exceeds that of the right, leftward electrical forces predominate over those directed to the right. The spread of the impulse toward the positive electrode through the left ventricular muscle mass causes the upward deflection.

The third phase of ventricular depolarization produces the S wave (Fig. 1–13E). The basal regions of the free walls and septum are the last part of the ventricles to be activated. Since the depolarization wave moves away from the positive electrode, a negative S wave is recorded.

After depolarization of the ventricles, the complex usually returns to the baseline, producing an isoelectric S-T segment. Repolarization of the ventricles results in a T wave (Fig. 1–13F). The orientation of the T wave in the dog is quite variable, and the normal limits are not well established. Repolarization is shown to begin at the epicardial surface of the ventricle and to spread toward the endocardium.[40]

INNERVATION OF THE HEART

The autonomic nervous system, the sympathetic and parasympathetic branches (Fig. 1–14), are responsible for the innervation of the heart.[41] The autonomic nervous system regulates the rate of intrinsic impulse formation or heart rate, affects the conduction of impulses, and influences the contractility of both the atria and the ventricles.[42–45]

The nerve impulse in both sympathetic and parasympathetic systems is transmitted by a chemically mediated neurotransmitter. The preganglionic neuron of the sympathetic and parasympathetic divisions as well as the postganglionic neuron of the parasympathetic division have acetylcholine as their neurotransmitter and thus are

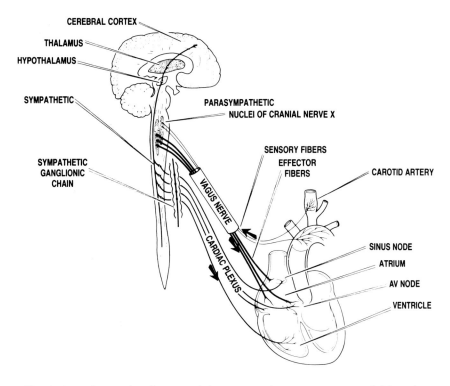

Fig. 1–14. Composite diagram of the autonomic nervous system divisions innervating the heart. (From Phillips, R.E., and Feeney, M.K.: *The Cardiac Rhythms.* Philadelphia, W.B. Saunders, 1980, with permission.)

called cholinergic fibers. The postganglionic neuron of the sympathetic system utilizes norepinephrine as its neurotransmitter and is called an adrenergic fiber.[46]

The sympathetic preganglion nerves originate in the first four to five thoracic segments of the spinal cord and extend to the sympathetic chains.[46] The cardiac sympathetic nerves arise from the corresponding upper thoracic sympathetic ganglion and innervate the following areas of the heart: SA node, atria, AV nodal region, bundle of His, and the ventricles. Sympathetic stimulation causes an increase in the sinus rate (a positive chronotropic effect) as well as an increase in the force of myocardial contraction (positive inotropic effect).[47]

It is well established that the right and left sympathetic nerves to the ventricles differ in their cardiac effects in the dog and the cat,[48–51] the left sympathetic nerves being dominant. Fibers from the right sympathetic nerves supply mainly the anterior ventricular wall, whereas those from the left sympathetic nerve supply the posterior ventricular wall.[49] Stimulation of the left sympathetic nerves produces AV junctional and/or ventricular arrhythmias, prolongation of the Q-T interval, and alternation of the T wave.[48,52] Naturally elicited emotional behavior or strenuous exercise after ablation of the right sympathetic nerves also causes these effects.[51] Epinephrine released into the bloodstream from the adrenal glands has similar actions on the myocardium.

The cardiac parasympathetic nerves originate in the medulla oblongata, forming the vagus nerves, whose fibers terminate primarily in the SA node, the atria, and the AV node.[50] The right and left vagi have different distributions to the SA and AV nodes: the right vagus nerve affects the SA node predominantly, whereas the left vagus nerve exerts its greatest influence on the AV conduction tissue.[9] The major effects are supraventricular, causing a slowing of the heart rate and a decrease in rate of conduction through the AV node.[9] A pronounced variation in heart rate, or sinus arrhythmia, is often observed in dogs with respiratory disorders. The vagi are responsible for mediating this respiratory arrhythmia. Vagal tone has less influence on the cat's heart rate, and pronounced sinus arrhythmia is uncommon.

LEAD SYSTEMS

The electrocardiograph can now be used to look at the electrical activity of the heart from different angles to get a complete picture. Each different angle or pair of electrodes is called a lead. The different leads can be compared to radiographs taken from different angles (e.g., lateral and dorsoventral thoracic radiographs taken for evaluation of cardiac chambers). Selecting which lead to use to get the best view of the heart is difficult, since the heart is hidden within the thoracic cavity. The following lead systems* are necessary to view the heart from different directions:

---

*Terminology based on committee proposal for standards on canine and feline electrocardiography.[34,53]

Bipolar standard leads
  Lead I—right arm (−) compared with left arm (+)
  Lead II—right arm (−) compared with left leg (+)
  Lead III—left arm (−) compared with left leg (+)

Augmented unipolar limb leads
  Lead aVR—right arm (+) compared with left arm and left
    leg (−)
  Lead aVL—left arm (+) compared with right arm and left
    leg (−)
  Lead aVF—left leg (+) compared with right and left arms
    (−)

Special leads
  Unipolar precordial chest leads
    Lead CV_5RL (rV_2)—fifth right intercostal space near edge
      of sternum
    Lead CV_6LL (V_2)—sixth left intercostal space near edge of
      sternum
    Lead CV_6LU (V_4)—sixth left intercostal space at costo-
      chondral junction
    Lead V_{10}—over dorsal spinous process of seventh thoracic
      vertebra
  Modified orthogonal lead systems
    Lead X—lead I; right (−) to left (+)
    Lead Y—lead aVF; cranial (−) to caudal (+)
    Lead Z—lead V_{10}; ventral (−) to dorsal (+)

Invasive leads
  Esophageal leads
  Intracardiac leads

Five separate wire electrodes are connected to the electrocardiograph by the patient cable. The lead selector switch on the electrocardiograph selects the different combinations of these electrodes.
The three bipolar standard leads and the three augmented unipolar
limb leads represent the minimum leads to be recorded in the dog
and cat. Other lead systems are used for specific conditions and provide increased electrocardiographic accuracy.

Standard bipolar leads

The standard leads (I, II, and III) have been used since the beginning of electrocardiography. Much of what is known about electrocardiography in the dog and cat is based on studies of these three
leads.

To obtain the three standard leads, electrodes are applied to the
left arm *(LA)*, right arm *(RA)*, and left leg *(LL)* (Fig. 1–15). The right
hindleg *(RL)* connects the animal to the ground. Only two extremities
are used for each lead. The electrocardiograph records the difference
in electrical activity between the two electrodes used. In lead I, *RA* is
the negative terminal and *LA* is the positive terminal. In lead II, the
right arm is the negative terminal and the left leg is the positive
terminal. In lead III, the left arm is the negative pole and the left leg
is the positive pole (Fig. 1–15). As illustrated in Figure 1–16 and

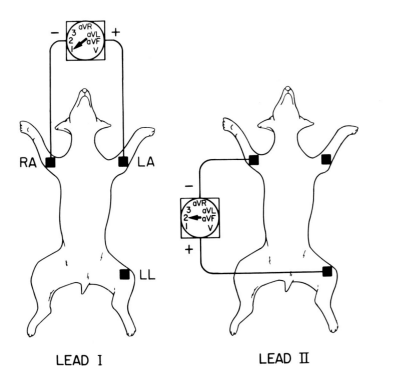

LEAD I   LEAD II   LEAD III

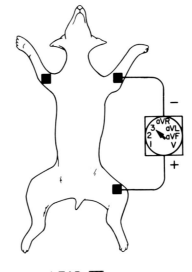

Fig. 1–15. Three bipolar standard leads. By means of
a switch incorporated in the instrument, the galvanometer can be connected across any pair of several electrodes. Each pair of electrodes is called a *lead*. The leads
illustrated here are identified as *I*, *II*, and *III*.

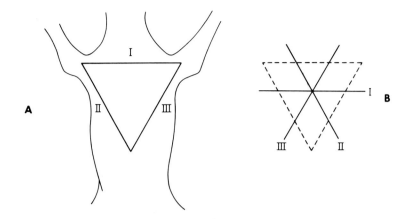

Fig. 1–16. A, The equilateral triangle of Einthoven, formed by leads *I, II,* and *III.* **B,** The triaxial lead reference system is produced by transposing the three sides of the triangle (leads *I, II,* and *III*) to a common central point of zero potential. This triaxial lead system will later be used to formulate the hexaxial lead system.

originally proposed by Einthoven, the area between the leads forms roughly an equilateral triangle. The midpoint of each lead is marked at the center of the triangle. The leads are superimposed at their midpoints to form the triaxial lead system (Fig. 1–16). The three standard leads are bipolar (i.e., they show the activity of the heart from two different locations).

The standard leads are especially useful for (1) studying abnormalities in the P-QRS-T deflections, (2) diagnosing cardiac arrhythmias, and (3) determining the mean electrical axis.

Augmented unipolar limb leads

The augmented unipolar limb leads use the same electrodes as are used in recording the three standard leads, but now the lead selector switch *(aVR, aVL, aVF)* connects them together in different combinations. The heart can thus be studied from three new angles. The augmented unipolar limb lead compares the electrical activity at the reference limb to the sum of the electrical activities at the other two limbs. For example, in Figure 1–17, lead *aVR* shows both LA (left arm) and LL (left leg) electrodes connected to one wire of the electrocardiograph by the lead selector switch. This makes the machine "think" it is looking at a point halfway between both electrodes. The remaining electrode is connected to the other electrocardiographic wire, and the electrocardiogram recorded is the voltage between the heart and the right arm, i.e., the aVR lead. The left arm *(aVL)* and left leg *(aVF)* recordings are obtained in the same way (Fig. 1–17). In lead *aVR,* the RA is the positive pole and the negative pole is the LA and LL. In lead *aVL,* the LA is the positive pole and the negative pole is the RA and LL. In lead *aVF,* the LL is the positive pole and the negative pole is the RA and LA.

The augmented unipolar limb leads are especially useful for (1) determining the mean electrical axis or the position of the heart and (2) confirming information obtained from other leads.

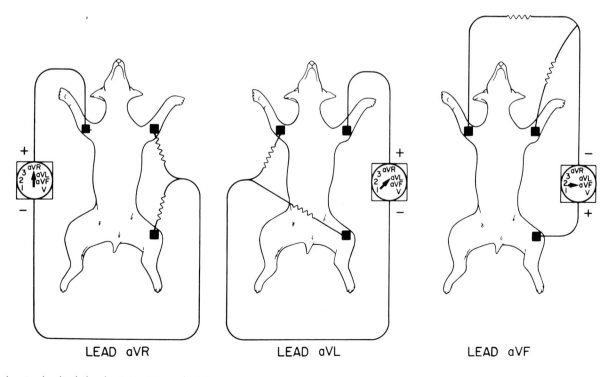

LEAD aVR   LEAD aVL   LEAD aVF

Fig. 1–17. Augmented unipolar limb leads *aVR, aVL,* and *aVF.*

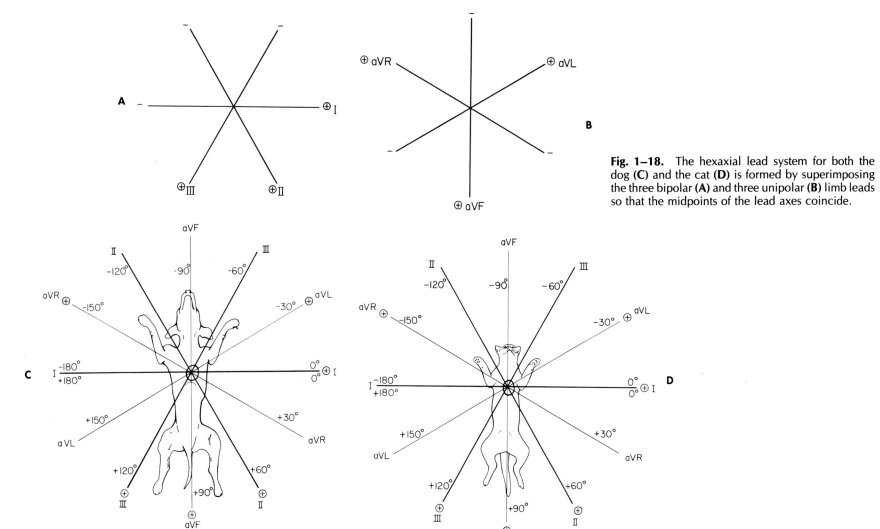

Fig. 1–18. The hexaxial lead system for both the dog (**C**) and the cat (**D**) is formed by superimposing the three bipolar (**A**) and three unipolar (**B**) limb leads so that the midpoints of the lead axes coincide.

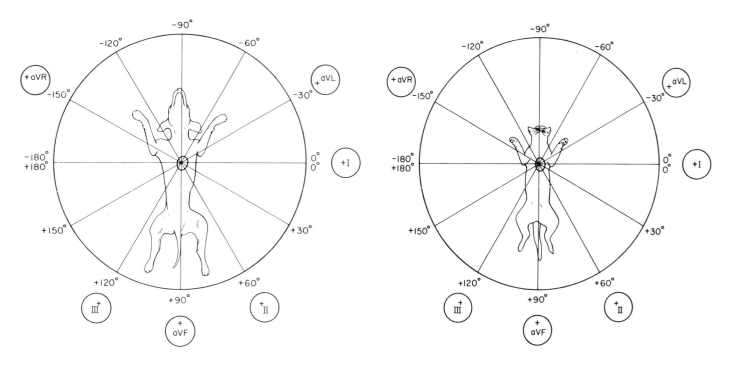

Fig. 1–19. The hexaxial lead system for both the dog and the cat in Fig. 1–18 can be enclosed in a circle. The circular field will be used in this textbook for determining the direction and magnitude of the electrical axis of the heart. The positive pole of each lead is indicated by a circle.

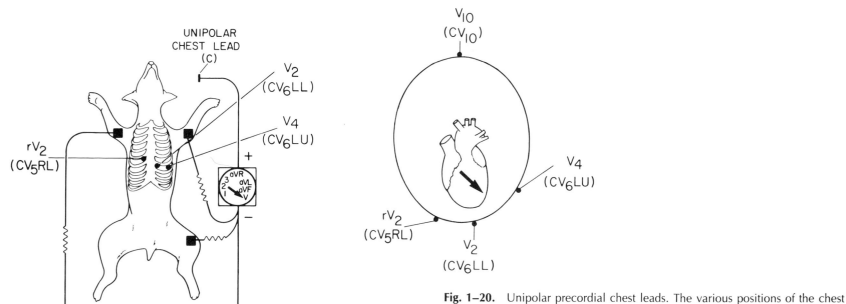

Fig. 1–20. Unipolar precordial chest leads. The various positions of the chest electrodes on the thoracic cavity are viewed from the ventral aspect (left diagram) and in cross section (right diagram). V_{10} is located over the seventh dorsal spinous process, CV_5RL on the right edge of the sternum at the fifth intercostal space, CV_6LL and CV_6LU both over the sixth intercostal space, CV_6LL near the sternum, and CV_6LU at the costochondral junction.

The unipolar augmented limb leads can be represented as a triaxial system to be superimposed on a triaxial system of the standard limb leads (Fig. 1–18), resulting in a frontal plane hexaxial lead system. Each lead has a positive and a negative pole, and each pole an angle value. The adjacent angles of the hexaxial system are all 30° (Fig. 1–18). The circular field of the hexaxial system applied to the dog and cat as viewed from the ventral aspect is useful in determining the direction and magnitude of the electrical axis of the heart (Fig. 1–19) (Chapter 3).

SPECIAL LEADS

Unipolar precordial chest leads

The unipolar precordial chest leads are exploring electrodes that can record electrical activity from the dorsal and ventral surfaces of the heart. When the lead selector switch is set to the various "V" positions, the electrocardiograph connects the RA, LA, and LL electrodes to form a zero reference equivalent to the potential at the center of the heart. The machine will now measure the voltage from the heart to the selected location of the chest electrode (Fig. 1–20). The chest electrode (C) is the positive pole of each unipolar precordial lead. The unipolar precordial leads are not well established in canine and feline electrocardiography; the V_{10} lead is used most frequently among the precordial leads.

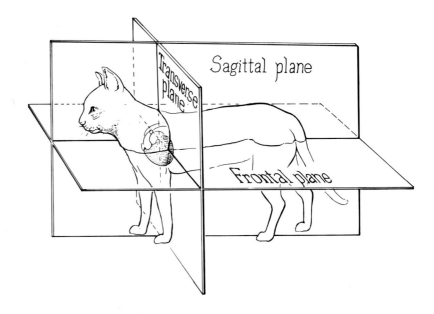

Fig. 1–22. The three orthogonal planes of a cat. The frontal plane is actually horizontal as the cat stands. (From Coulter, D.B., and Calvert, C.A.: Orientation and configuration of vectorcardiographic QRS loops from normal cats. Am. J. Vet. Res., *42*:282, 1981, with permission.)

The precordial leads are particularly valuable for (1) detecting right and left ventricular enlargement, (2) diagnosing myocardial infarction and bundle branch block, (3) diagnosing cardiac arrhythmias (P waves are often more obvious in the precordial leads), and (4) confirming the data obtained from the six hexaxial leads.

Modified orthogonal lead systems

These special leads are directed perpendicular to each other and view the heart in three planes (leads X, Y, and Z) (Figs. 1–21 and 1–22). The X lead axis measures a frontal plane directed from right to left and is roughly represented by lead I. The Y lead axis indicates a midsagittal plane directed craniocaudally and is roughly represented by lead aVF. The Z lead axis indicates a transverse plane directed ventral to dorsal and is roughly equivalent to lead V_{10}. The orthogonal leads can be used to generate a vectorcardiogram[33,54] These orthogonal leads, derived from an anatomic relationship, may produce a somewhat distorted representation of the true X, Y, and Z axes. Corrected orthogonal lead systems (McFee, Schmidt, and Frank lead systems) require the utilization of several electrodes at precise placements.[33,34]

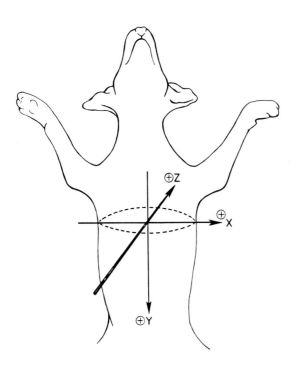

Fig. 1–21. Orthogonal lead system. The heart can be viewed in three planes: frontal (X), midsagittal (Y), and transverse (Z). This system can be used to generate a vectorcardiogram, a more accurate measurement of the cardiac vector than can be obtained by using the standard limb leads and precordial chest leads.

REFERENCES

1. Harvey, W. (1628): Exercitatio anatomica de motu cordis et sanguinis in animalibus (English translation by C.D. Leake, 1958). In *Anatomical Movement of the Heart and Blood in Animals.* 4th Edition. Springfield, Ill., Charles C Thomas, 1958.
2. Waller, A.D.: A demonstration on man of electromotive changes accompanying the heart's beat. J. Physiol., *8*:229, 1887.

3. Burch, G.E., and DePasquale, N.P.: *A History of Electrocardiography.* Chicago, Year Book Medical Publishers, 1964.

4. Waller, A.D.: The electrocardiogram of man and dog as shown by Einthoven's string galvanometer. Lancet, *1*:1448, 1909.

5. Lannek, N.: A clinical and experimental study of the electrocardiogram in dogs (thesis). Stockholm, 1949.

6. Marshall, R.: Early days in Westmoreland Street. Br. Heart J., *26*:140, 1964.

7. Besterman, E., and Creese, R.: Waller—Pioneer of electrocardiography. Br. Heart J., *42*:61, 1979.

8. Hamlin, R.L., and Smith, C.R.: Electrophysiology of the heart. In *Duke's Physiology of Domestic Animals.* 9th Edition. Ithaca, N.Y., Cornell University Press, 1977.

9. Berne, R.M., and Levy, M.N.: *Cardiovascular Physiology.* 3rd Edition. St. Louis, C.V. Mosby, 1977.

10. Ettinger, S.J.: Cardiac arrhythmias. In *Textbook of Veterinary Internal Medicine.* Edited by S.J. Ettinger. 2nd Edition. Philadelphia, W.B. Saunders, 1983.

11. Hoffmann, B.F., and Cranefield, P.F.: *Electrophysiology of the Heart.* New York, McGraw-Hill, 1960.

12. Parker, J.L., and Adams, H.R.: Drugs and the heart muscle. J. Am. Vet. Med. Assoc., *171*:78, 1977.

13. Wit, A.L., et al.: Electrophysiological properties of cardiac muscle in the anterior mitral valve leaflet and the adjacent atrium in the dog, possible implications for the genesis of atrial dysrhythmias. Circ. Res., *32*:731, 1973.

14. Bassett, A.L., et al.: Ectopic impulses originating in the tricuspid valve and contiguous atrium. Fed. Proc., *33*:445, 1974.

15. Rosen, M.R., and Hordof, A.J.: Mechanisms of arrhythmias. In *Cardiac Arrhythmias in the Neonate, Infant and Child.* Edited by N.K. Roberts and H. Gelband. New York, Appleton-Century Crofts, 1977.

16. Gompf, R.E., and Tilley, L.P.: Comparison of lateral and sternal recumbent position for electrocardiography of the cat. Am. J. Vet. Res., *40*:1483, 1979.

17. Hill, J.D.: The significance of foreleg position in the interpretation of electrocardiograms and vectorcardiograms from research animals. Am. Heart J., *75*:518, 1968.

18. Goldman, M.J.: *Principles of Clinical Electrocardiography.* 11th Edition. Los Altos, Calif., Lange Medical Publications, 1982.

19. Katz, A.M.: *Physiology of the Heart.* New York, Raven Press, 1977.

20. Fozzard, H.A.: Cardiac muscle: excitability and passive electrical properties. Prog. Cardiovasc. Dis., *19*:343, 1977.

21. Ganong, W.F.: *Review of Medical Physiology.* 6th Edition. Los Altos, Calif., Lange Medical Publications, 1973.

22. MacLean, W.A., Waldo, A.J., and James, T.N.: Formation and conduction of the cardiac electrical impulse. In *The Conduction System of the Heart.* Edited by H.J.J. Wellens, K.I. Lie, and M.J. Janse. Philadelphia, Lea & Febiger, 1976.

23. Tilley, L.P.: *Basic Canine Electrocardiography.* Milton, Wis., The Burdick Corp., 1978.

24. Baird, J.A., and Robb, J.S.: Study, reconstruction and gross dissection of the atrioventricular conducting system of the dog heart. Anat. Rec., *108*:747, 1950.

25. Davies, F., and Francis, T.B.: The conducting system of the vertebrate heart. Biol. Rev., *20*:12, 1945.

26. James, T.N.: Anatomy of the conduction system of the heart. In *The Heart.* Edited by J.W. Hurst. New York, McGraw-Hill, 1974.

27. Kulbertus, H.E., and DeMoulin, J.C.: Pathological basis of concept of left hemiblock. In *The Conduction System of the Heart.* Edited by H.J.J. Wellens, K.I. Lie, and M.J. Janse. Philadelphia, Lea & Febiger, 1976.

28. Liu, S.-K., Tilley, L.P., and Tashjian, R.J.: Lesions of the conduction system in the cat with cardiomyopathy. Recent Adv. Stud. Cardiac Struct. Metab., *10*:681, 1975.

29. Myerberg, R.J., Nilsson, K., and Gelband, H.: Physiology of canine intraventricular conduction and endocardial excitation. Circ. Res., *30*:217, 1972.

30. Truex, R.C., and Smythe, M.Q.: Comparative morphology of the cardiac conduction tissue in animals. Ann. N.Y. Acad. Sci., *127*:19, 1965.

31. Uhley, H.N., and Rivkin, L.: Peripheral distribution of the canine A-V conduction system—observations on gross morphology. Am. J. Cardiol., *5*:688, 1960.

32. Bolton, G.R.: *Handbook of Canine Electrocardiography.* Philadelphia, W.B. Saunders, 1975.

33. Ettinger, S.J., and Suter, P.F.: *Canine Cardiology.* Philadelphia, W.B. Saunders, 1970.

34. Hahn, A.W. (chairman), Hamlin, R.L., and Patterson, D.F.: Standards for canine electrocardiography. The Academy of Veterinary Cardiology Committee Report, 1977.

35. International Committee on Veterinary Anatomical Nomenclature: Nomina anatomica veterinaria, Vienna, 1968, Adolf Holzhausens Nachfolger. (Distributed in the United States by the Department of Anatomy, New York State Veterinary College, Ithaca).

36. Walker, W.F.: *A Study of the Cat with Reference to Man.* 2nd Edition. Philadelphia, W.B. Saunders, 1972.

37. Anderson, R.H., and Becker, A.E.: Gross anatomy and microscopy of the conducting system. In *Cardiac Arrhythmias—Their Mechanisms, Diagnosis, and Management.* Edited by W.J. Mandel. Philadelphia, J.B. Lippincott, 1980.

38. Hamlin, R.L., and Smith, C.R.: Anatomical and physiologic basis for interpretation of the electrocardiogram. Am. J. Vet. Res., *21*:701, 1960.

39. Hamlin, R.L., and Smith, C.R.: Categorization of common domestic animals based upon their ventricular activation process. Ann. N.Y. Acad. Sci., *127*:195, 1965.

40. Spach, M.S., and Barr, R.C.: Ventricular intramural and epicardial potential distributions during ventricular activation and repolarization in the intact dog. Circ. Res., *37*:243, 1975.

41. Silverman, M.E., and Schlant, R.C.: Anatomy of the cardiovascular system. In *The Heart.* Edited by J.W. Hurst. 3rd Edition. New York, McGraw-Hill, 1974.

42. Agostini, E., et al.: Functional and histological studies of the vagus nerve and its branches to the heart, lungs, and abdominal viscera in the cat. J. Physiol., *135*:182, 1957.

43. Armour, J.A., and Randall, W.C.: Functional anatomy of canine cardiac nerves. Acta Anat. *91*:510, 1975.

44. Kaye, M.P., Geesbreght, J.M., and Randall, W.C.: Distribution of autonomic fibers to the canine heart. Am. J. Physiol., *218*:1025, 1970.

45. Muir, W.W.: Effects of atropine on cardiac rate and rhythm in dogs. J. Am. Vet. Med. Assoc., *172*:917, 1978.

46. Anderson, M., and del Castillo, J.: Cardiac innervation and synaptic transmission in the heart. In *Electrical Phenomena in the Heart.* Edited by W.C. DeMello. New York, Academic Press, 1972.

47. Phillips, R.E., and Feeney, M.K.: *The Cardiac Rhythms.* Philadelphia, W.B. Saunders, 1980.

48. D'Agrosa, L.S.: Cardiac arrhythmias of sympathetic origin in the dog. Am. J. Physiol., *233*:H535, 1977.

49. Lown, B., Verrier, R.L., and Rabinowitz, S.H.: Neural and psychologic mechanisms and the problem of sudden cardiac death. Am. J. Cardiol., *39*:890, 1977.

50. Mizeres, N.J.: The anatomy of the autonomic nervous system in the dog. Am. J. Anat., *96*:290, 1966.

51. Schwartz, P.J., Verrier, R.L., and Lown, B.: Effect of stellectomy and vagotomy on ventricular refractoriness in dogs. Circ. Res., *40*:536, 1977.

52. Schwartz, P.J., Periti, M., and Malliani, A.: The long Q-T syndrome. Am. Heart J., *89*:378, 1975.

53. Tilley, L.P. (Chairman), Gompf, R.E., Bolton, G., and Harpster, N.: Criteria for the normal feline electrocardiogram. The Academy of Veterinary Cardiology Committee Report, 1977.

54. Coulter, D.B., and Calvert, C.A.: Orientation and configuration of vectorcardiographic QRS loops from normal cats. Am. J. Vet. Res., *42*:282, 1981.

Section One

General Principles of
Electrocardiography

2 Principles of electrocardiographic recording

*The time is at hand, if it has not already come, when an examination of the heart is incomplete if this new method is neglected.**

SIR THOMAS LEWIS, 1912

As early as 1912, the electrocardiogram was considered an important method of studying the heart. Today the electrocardiogram is well established as an essential tool in the clinical evaluation of the veterinary patient with cardiac disease. It is easy to obtain an electrocardiographic tracing from a dog or a cat, and interpretation of the recording is facilitated by following the systematic method recommended in this book.[2,3]

PLACE OF THE ELECTROCARDIOGRAM IN CLINICAL PRACTICE

In clinical practice, the electrocardiogram must be evaluated in conjunction with a complete data base. The data base for the cardiovascular system consists of (1) history, (2) physical examination, and (3) laboratory profile (Fig. 2–1). The laboratory examination includes the electrocardiogram, thoracic radiography, and an analysis of blood, urine, and extravascular fluids. Other special laboratory techniques that may be indicated to evaluate a particular cardiovascular abnormality are phonocardiography, fluoroscopy, cardiac catheterization, angiocardiography, echocardiography, and central venous pressure. Electrocardiography is the most widely used laboratory test in cardiology.

Many times, the electrocardiographic findings alone are used in diagnosing cardiac disease. The general principles of electrocardiography should be discussed only from the standpoint of their relation to the clinical diagnosis of heart disease. *In general, the person best qualified to read the electrocardiogram is the clinician in charge of the patient.*

VALUE OF ELECTROCARDIOGRAPHY

Electrocardiography is a useful tool in two major areas:[4–6] (1) diagnosing most cardiac arrhythmias, since the electrocardiogram can determine the source of the rhythm and the frequency with which the impulse arises, and (2) providing information on the status of the myocardium, since the P-QRS-T deflections of the electrocardiographic tracing are often altered by either pathologic or physiologic factors.

The electrocardiogram, then, can be used as an aid in a cardiac evaluation to establish an etiology, an anatomic and physiologic diagnosis, and a prognosis. Some of the important indications for taking an electrocardiogram are as follows:

1. Tachycardia, bradycardia, or arrhythmia heard on auscultation (a more exact diagnosis can be made)
2. Acute onset of dyspnea
3. Shock
4. Fainting or seizures
5. Cardiac monitoring during and after surgery (for depth of anesthesia as well as cardiac complications)
6. All cardiac murmurs
7. Cardiomegaly found on thoracic radiographs
8. Cyanosis
9. Preoperatively in older animals
10. Evaluating the effect of cardiac drugs—especially digitalis, quinidine, and propranolol
11. Electrolyte disturbances, especially potassium abnormalities (e.g., diseases related to renal physiology, endocrine disturbances [Addison's disease, diabetic ketoacidosis]), and effects of drug reactions (digitalis, diuretics, steroids)
12. Periocardiocentesis, for monitoring purposes as well as for locating the needle

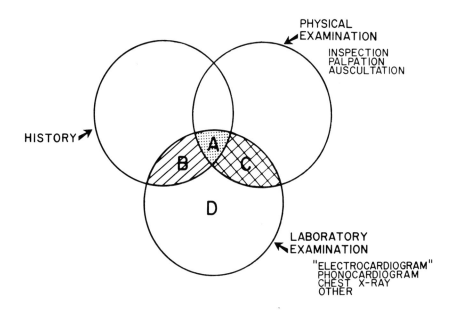

Fig. 2–1. Venn diagram illustrating the method(s) by which a cardiovascular abnormality can be identified. **A,** Abnormality identified by history, physical examination, and laboratory examination. **B,** Abnormality identified by history and laboratory examination. **C,** Abnormality identified by physical examination and laboratory examination. **D,** Abnormality identified by laboratory examination only. (Modified from Hurst, J.W.: *The Heart.* 3rd Edition. New York, McGraw-Hill, 1974.)

---

*Lewis, T.: *Clinical Disorders of the Heart Beat.* London, Shaw, 1912. Sir Thomas was one of the first to apply electrocardiography to the study of cardiac arrhythmias.[1]

13. Systemic diseases that affect the heart (e.g., pyometra, pancreatitis, uremia, neoplasia), with toxic myocarditis and arrhythmias as a result
14. Basis for records and for consultation
15. Serial electrocardiograms as an aid in the prognosis and diagnosis of cardiac disease

LIMITATIONS OF ELECTROCARDIOGRAPHY

The clinician should be aware of the limitations of electrocardiography and should resist the tendency to read too much into an electrocardiogram. The following limitations of the electrocardiogram are to be considered:[4]

1. The electrocardiogram should always be interpreted as part of the clinical picture and not without the benefit of clinical knowledge, experience, and judgment.

2. The electrocardiogram tells nothing about the mechanical status of the heart, since an animal with congestive heart failure may have a normal electrocardiogram, and a perfectly normal animal may show nonspecific electrocardiographic abnormalities. The electrocardiogram must always be evaluated in conjunction with the clinical findings. Serial tracings over a period of time are of greater value in evaluating the functional status of the heart.

3. The electrocardiogram cannot always evaluate the prognosis. In general, however, the more severe the electrocardiographic abnormality, the less favorable the prognosis. Certain individual animals with markedly abnormal electrocardiograms may live out their full life expectancies.

4. The electrocardiogram does not record the pathology of valves, coronary arteries, endocardium, or pericardium; only of the myocardium.

5. The division between normal and abnormal electrocardiograms must be considered as a broad zone rather than a sharp line. It is important that the clinician avoid trying to read too much into an electrocardiogram if borderline changes are present.

6. The veterinary literature lacks adequate studies on necropsy follow-ups to obtain exacting standards for electrocardiographic and anatomic correlations.

7. The wide variations in body conformation and breeds of dogs may alter the accepted standard measurements. Body conformation is probably the only major factor that alters measurements in the cat.

8. Electrocardiograms must be recorded properly. The recordings must be complete and accurate with a stable baseline.

THE ELECTROCARDIOGRAPH

Every veterinary practice should have at least an oscilloscope (Fig. 2–2) and a single-channel electrocardiograph (Figs. 2–3 and 2–4). The electrocardiograph should meet the 1975 standards set forth by the Committee on Electrocardiography of the American Heart Association.[7] The choice of a machine depends primarily on the repair service in your locality. The electrocardiograph is essentially a sensitive voltage-metering device for determining the electrical potential of the

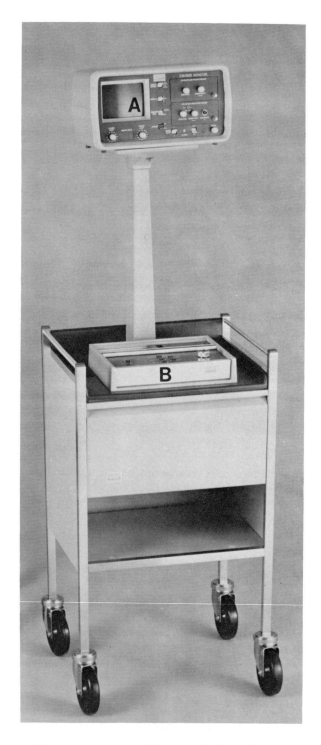

Fig. 2–2. Mobile stand with an oscilloscope (A) (Burdick two-channel CS-525 monitor for monitoring electrocardiogram and blood pressure) and a single-channel electrocardiograph (B). (Courtesy of Burdick Corp., Milton, Wis., and J. Weintraub, Inc., Bronx, N.Y.)

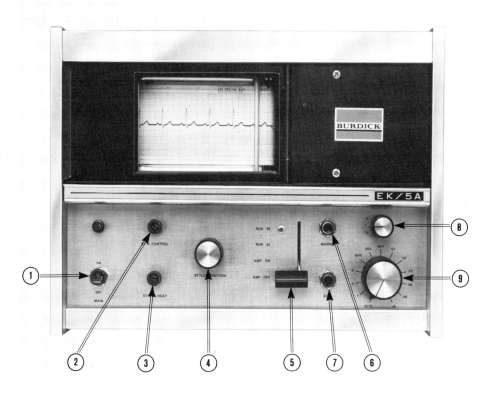

Fig. 2–3. Control panel for the electrocardiograph. When the on-off switch (1) is turned on, the electrocardiograph is ready for operation. (Some units require a warm-up time.) The paper speed lever (5) has four positions: amp off; amp on; run 25, paper speed of 25 mm/sec; run 50, paper speed 50 mm/sec. The lead selector switch (9) can be dialed to each lead: I, II, III, aVR, aVL, aVF, and V. The stylus position control (4) adjusts the stylus to be centered on the paper. Stylus heat control (3) can be adjusted to darken the tracing. The ST'D control (2) is used to calibrate stylus deflection when the ST'D button (7) is depressed. The sensitivity switch (8) can either double the height of the complexes or cut them in half. The marker button (6) can be pushed to mark the lead or to note events. (Courtesy of the Burdick Corp., Milton, Wis.)

heart. The voltage meter or amplifier is combined with a strip recorder, which gives a permanent record. The record is usually produced by the movements of a heated stylus on wax-coated electrocardiographic paper.

The patient monitor, or oscilloscope, produces a constant electrocardiographic pattern on a fluorescent screen. Permanent records can be obtained by connecting the oscilloscope to a direct-writing apparatus. Nowadays, these monitors are practically routine in intensive care units and in surgery.

The electrocardiograph control panels of the various manufactured units are basically the same (Fig. 2–3). The instruction manual for each electrocardiograph should be consulted for any differences. Whichever electrocardiograph you choose, it should be able to run electrocardiograms at a paper speed of 50 mm/sec (Fig. 2–3, 5). The heart rates of both cats and dogs are so rapid that, at slower speeds of 25 mm/sec, many measurements would be inaccurate. The faster speed will "stretch out" the electrocardiogram because the paper is moving twice the normal speed (Fig. 2–5).

The sensitivity switch (Fig. 2–3, 8) controls how much amplification or gain the amplifier has. The normal setting for this switch is position 1. By international agreement, it has been established that 1 mv input should cause the stylus to move 1 cm or 10 small boxes on the paper graph (Fig. 2–6). Position 2 will make the electrocardiogram twice the normal size, and position 1/2 will make the electrocardiogram half the normal size (Fig. 2–6).

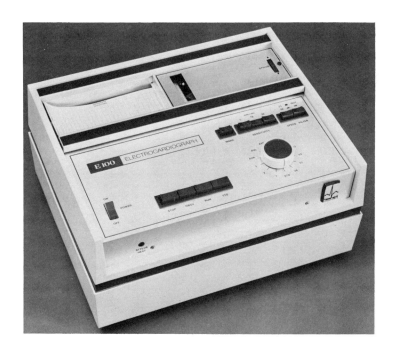

Fig. 2–4. New single-channel electrocardiograph (Burdick E100) with push-button operating controls arranged for optimum operator convenience. (Courtesy of Burdick Corp., Milton, Wis.)

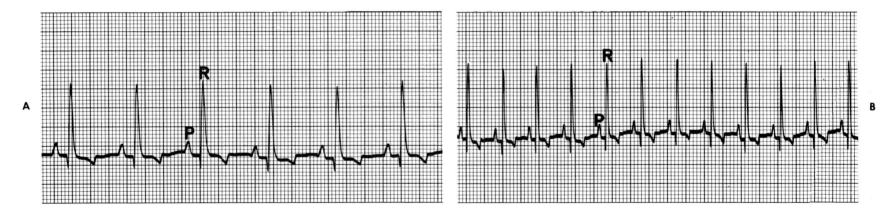

Fig. 2–5. Comparison of two paper speeds of the same electrocardiogram. **A,** 50 mm/sec; **B,** 25 mm/sec. Note how the faster paper speed allows for an easier interpretation of the electrocardiogram. The standard paper speed in veterinary medicine is 50 mm/sec.

Fig. 2–6. Effect of the various positions of the sensitivity switch on the electrocardiogram (positions *1/2, 1,* and *2*). The normal standard position of the switch is position 1; the middle tracing indicates that a 1 mv input will produce a deflection of 1 cm (or 10 small boxes). The corresponding electrocardiograms are changed accordingly.

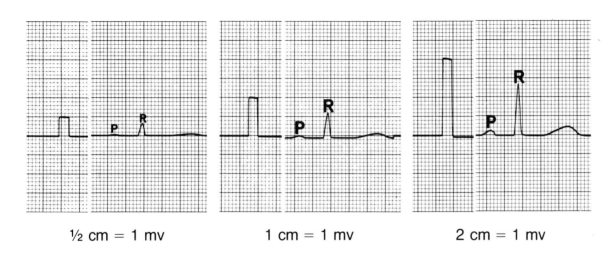

½ cm = 1 mv   1 cm = 1 mv   2 cm = 1 mv

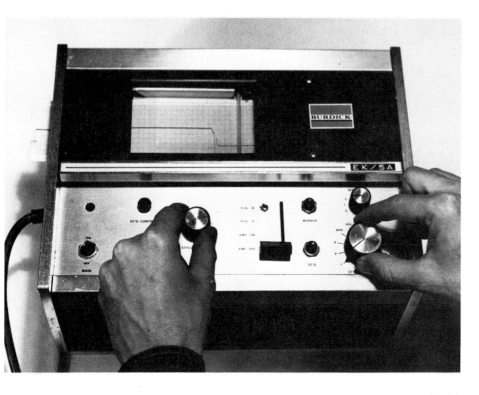

Fig. 2–7. When running the electrocardiographic tracing, the operator should maintain his left hand always on the stylus position control to keep the complexes in the center of the paper. The right hand dials the lead selector, depresses the marker button to mark each lead, changes the paper speed, and starts and turns off the electrocardiograph.

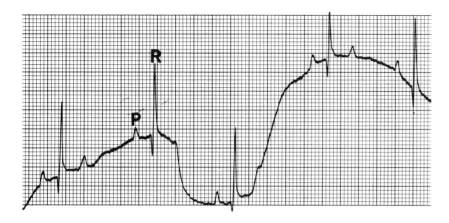

Fig. 2–8. The left hand should always be on the stylus position control to keep the complexes in the center of the paper. Without this constant adjustment the complexes will wander off the paper.

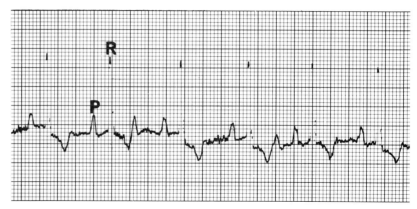

Fig. 2–9. Low stylus heat or a dirty stylus will make the QRS complexes difficult to see. The stylus heat control should be turned clockwise.

The position control (Fig. 2–3, *4*) is used to keep the electrocardiograph recording in the center of the paper (Fig. 2–7). When running the electrocardiographic tracing, the operator should always put his left hand on the stylus position control to keep the complexes in the center of the paper (Figs. 2–7 and 2–8). The right hand is used to dial the lead selector (Fig. 2–3, *9*) and to depress the marker button to mark each lead (Fig. 2–7). Some of the new electrocardiographs record a lead code on the paper automatically. The lead code most commonly used is as follows: lead I (–), lead II (– –), lead III (– – –), aVR (—), aVL (— —), and aVF (— — —). The stylus heat control (Fig. 2–3, *3*) adjusts the stylus temperature. If the heat is too low, the stylus does not melt the plastic coating quickly enough (Fig. 2–9).

CHOICE OF ELECTRODES

The standard electrocardiographic cable is made up of five separate wire electrodes (Figs. 2–10 and 2–11, *A* and *B*) labeled right arm *(RA)*, left arm *(LA)*, right leg *(RL)*, left leg *(LL)*, and the V lead or exploring precordial chest lead *(C)*. Alligator clips or flat contact electrodes with bands are used to attach the leads to the dog or cat.[8,9] To relieve the discomfort of pinching, the jaws of the clips can be flattened, filed, or bent out slightly with pliers (Fig. 2–11*D*). The clips should all be made of the same material, preferably copper. If not, artifacts affecting the baseline or amplitude or no recorded tracing will result. Small electrode plates may be attached to the jaws of the clip; these provide even less discomfort, especially to cats (Fig. 2–11*C*). The pin electrode of the electrocardiographic cable can also be fitted with an enlarging adapter to give a low-contact resistance (Fig. 2–11*A*).

PREPARATION FOR THE ELECTROCARDIOGRAPHIC RECORDING

Position and restraint

The animal ideally should be positioned on a nonconductive surface to eliminate electrical interference and to ensure its comfort. A For-

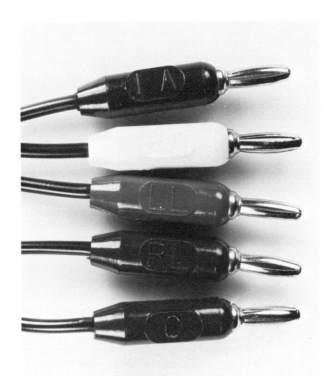

Fig. 2–10. Standard electrocardiographic cable with five separate wire electrodes: *LA,* left arm; *RA,* right arm; *LL,* left leg; *RL,* right leg; and *C,* V lead. Alligator clip electrodes are used for attachment to the skin. (See Fig. 2–11.)

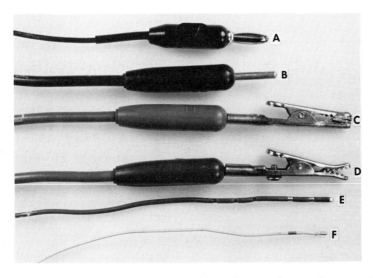

Fig. 2–11. Various types of wire electrodes, alligator clips, and intracardiac electrode catheters. **A,** Cable tip electrode fitted with an enlarging adapter so that alligator clips can be easily positioned for low-contact resistance; **B,** cable tip without an alligator clip attached; **C,** alligator clip with electrode plates attached to the jaws of the clip to relieve the discomfort of pinching; **D,** alligator clip with jaws bent slightly to relieve pinching; **E,** hexapolar intracardiac electrode catheter; **F,** bipolar intracardiac electrode catheter. (**C** courtesy of Spevack Surgical Supply, Brooklyn, N.Y.)

mica table or a metal table covered with a blanket or rubber mat will serve the purpose. The dog or cat is held by an attendant in the standard position, right lateral recumbency (Fig. 2–12). The right arm of the attendant rests over the animal's neck, while the left arm rests over its hindquarters. Both hands should hold the legs so they do not touch. Since improper positioning can change the mean electrical axis of the QRS, the forelimbs must be perpendicular to the long axis of the body.[6,10]

The majority of dogs and cats need no chemical restraint. The owner's presence at the end of the table will usually calm the older animal after a few minutes. This is in sharp contrast to puppies or kittens, which often are difficult to restrain. The electrocardiogram should be obtained quickly while the younger animal is held as tightly as possible. The use of drugs for restraint purposes is not advised. If

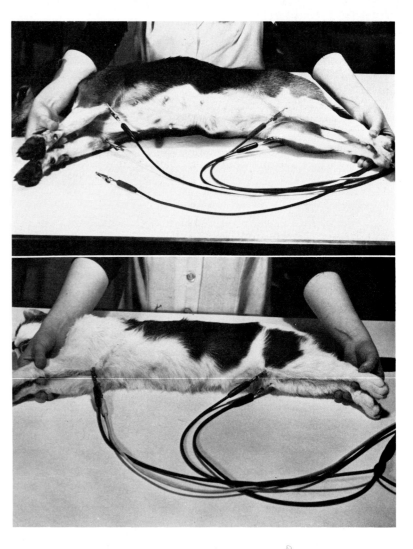

Fig. 2–12. Right lateral recumbency, the standard position for canine and feline electrocardiography.

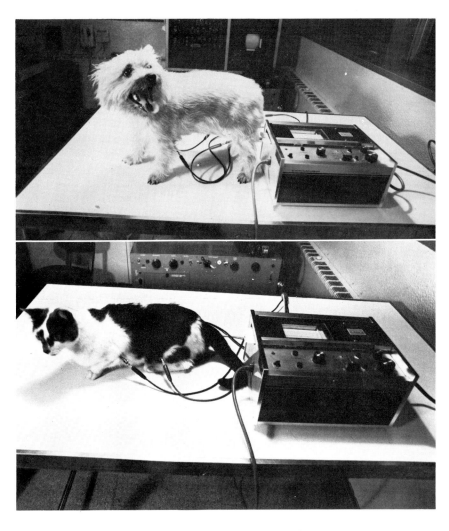

animals with severe respiratory distress, when restraint would be hazardous.

Placement of the electrodes

The electrode clips are attached directly to the animal's skin (Fig. 2–14). The RA and LA clips are attached proximal to the olecranon on the caudal aspect of the appropriate foreleg. The RL and LL clips are attached over the patellar ligament on the anterior aspect of the appropriate hindleg. The skin and electrode should be moistened with a commercial conductive gel or paste, alcohol, or pHisoHex (Fig. 2–14).

Alcohol works well clinically as a conductive medium, although it has been reported to decrease recording accuracy by not consistently

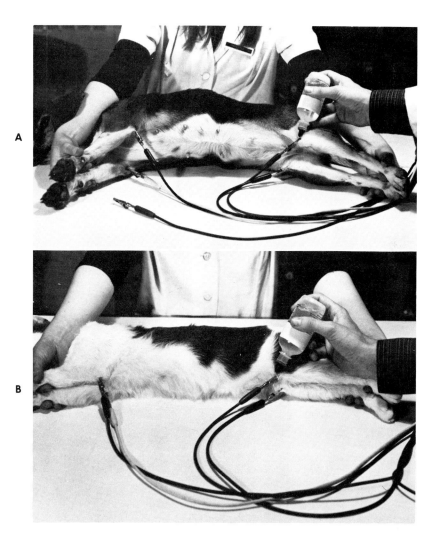

Fig. 2–13. Positioning of the animal is not critical for daily monitoring of the electrocardiogram (analysis of the cardiac rhythm and/or electrocardiographic intervals), when restraint is difficult, or when restraint would be hazardous to an animal in respiratory distress. The strip may be recorded with the animal restrained in a standing, sitting, or recumbent position on the floor, table, or even in the cage.

tranquilizers are needed, the electrocardiogram must be interpreted with regard to the possible cardiac actions of the drug. For example, ketamine hydrochloride and diazepam both are considered to have significant antiarrhythmic activity.[11-14] Tranquilizers for purposes of restraint should be used only when P-QRS deflections and electrical axis calculations are required, since they will not significantly affect these measurements. Tranquilizers, however, can affect the rhythm of the heart and should not be used for the analysis of arrhythmias. The normal position of the dog or cat (e.g., standing or sternal recumbency) can be used for the analysis of the cardiac rhythm and/or electrocardiographic intervals (Fig. 2–13) and is especially useful in

Fig. 2–14. The hair and skin surrounding the electrode should be moistened with a commercial conductive gel or alcohol. With a plastic bottle, alcohol is being applied to the electrodes of this dog and cat.

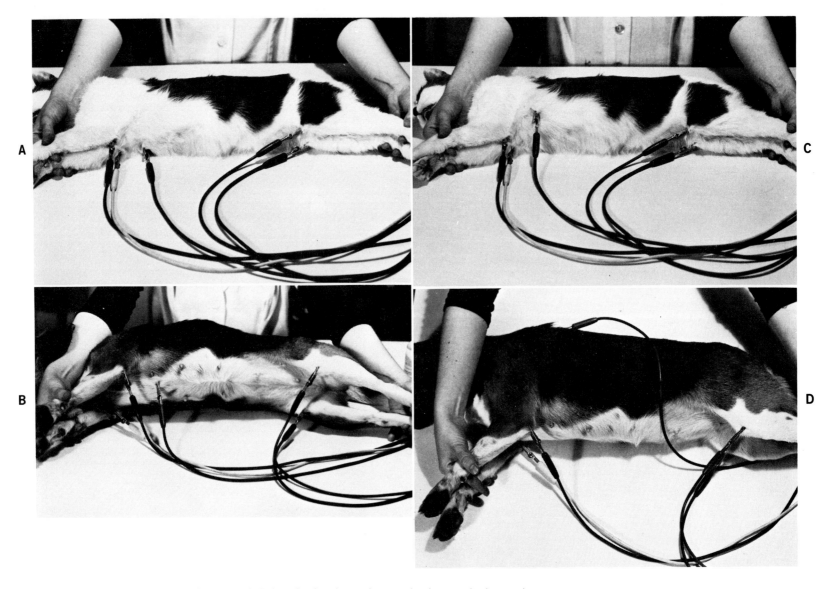

Fig. 2–15. Various positions for the unipolar precordial chest leads. The C clip or V lead is attached to each designated position: **A,** CV_5RL (also termed rV_2), located at the right fifth intercostal space at the edge of the sternum; **B,** CV_6LL (also termed V_2), located at the left sixth intercostal space at the edge of the sternum; **C,** CV_6LU (also termed V_4), located at the left sixth intercostal space at the costochondral junction; **D,** V_{10}, located over the dorsal spinous process of the seventh thoracic vertebra.

lowering electrical resistance.[8] It does not have to be cleaned off the hair as do many electrode pastes. Creams that are less messy to use (e.g., Liquicor, Burdick Corp., Milton, Wis.) have been developed. Creams or pastes should be used in surgery because alcohol evaporates quickly.

The clip for the V lead (C) is attached to those locations for the unipolar precordial chest leads: $CV_5RL(rV_2)$, $CV_6LL(V_2)$, $CV_6LU(V_4)$, and V_{10} (Fig. 2–15).

PROCEDURE FOR RECORDING THE ELECTROCARDIOGRAM

As soon as the animal is in proper position and the electrodes have been attached, the electrocardiogram can be recorded. The following procedure for taking the electrocardiogram can be used:

1. Turn on the power switch. The new machines are transistorized, so they are ready to record immediately after the power switch is turned on. For machines requiring a warm-up period, the

power switch should be turned on before restraining the animal.

2. Position the stylus to the center of the chart with the left hand. The left hand should remain on the stylus position control throughout the recording to keep the complexes centered on the paper (Fig. 2–7). Check that sensitivity switch is at position 1.
3. Turn on the record switch to a paper speed of 25.
4. Push the standardization button to check sensitivity.
5. Move the record switch to a paper speed of 50.
6. Record the leads of the electrocardiogram:
   a. Set the lead selector to 1 with the right hand and record three to four good complexes of that lead.
   b. Without turning the record switch off, move the lead selector to 2 and record three to four good complexes.
   c. Repeat this procedure for leads III, aVR, aVL, and aVF.
   d. Set the lead selector next to 2 and record at least 15 to 20 inches of lead II rhythm strip.
   e. If the precordial chest leads are being run, stop the recording.
   f. Prepare the electrode position for $CV_5RL(rV_2)$. Move the lead selector to V. Turn on the recorder.
   g. Repeat this procedure for the other V positions. The machine must be turned off each time to reposition the electrode.
   h. Move the lead selector to O or STD and push the standardization button again.
   i. Turn off the record switch.
   j. Turn the machine to off.
7. Remove the electrode clips from the animal.
8. Write the animal's case number, owner's name, and date on the tracing.
9. File the electrocardiogram.

The electrocardiographic tracing should be observed closely while it is being recorded.

Centering. The recording should always be near the center of the paper. The position control is adjusted with the left hand throughout the recording. The electrocardiogram will wander when the animal breathes heavily or when there is movement.

Amplitude. When the QRS complexes go off the paper, the sensitivity switch must be set at position 1/2 to reduce the amplitude. If the P-QRS complexes are too small, the sensitivity switch can be set at position 2 to increase the amplitude. In most cases, especially in cats, the increase in amplitude will also magnify any artifacts (e.g., muscle tremor or respiratory movements). A standardization mark should always be made to indicate the change in sensitivity.

Length of tracing. If an arrhythmia is recognized during the recording, a longer lead rhythm strip should be taken. If an arrhythmia is being looked for, longer leads are also necessary.

Polarity. The R waves should normally be positive in lead I. The lead wires should be checked first to determine whether they are connected to the correct electrodes. If the electrodes are properly connected and R waves are negative in this lead, an abnormality truly exists.

TRANSTELEPHONIC ELECTROCARDIOGRAPHY

The system of transtelephonic electrocardiography involves the use of a small ($4 \times 2\frac{1}{2}$ inches), portable, battery-powered, transistorized electrocardiographic preamplifier that converts electrocardiographic signals into tones that can be transmitted over the telephone line (Fig. 2–16). The animal is first positioned in right lateral recumbency. Two electrodes from the transmitter are first attached to the caudal aspect of the forelegs near the elbow, and both skin and electrodes are moistened with alcohol. The electrocardiographic data center is then contacted by telephone, where a technician records relevant clinical information. The veterinarian supervising the transmission places the telephone mouthpiece on the transmitter and switches the unit to the "on" position for approximately 5 to 10 seconds to transmit lead I. The procedure is repeated twice with the electrodes positioned to transmit the other two leads—lead II (right front leg and left rear leg) and lead III (left front leg and left rear leg) (Fig. 2–16). A 60-second lead II rhythm strip is transmitted.[15,16]

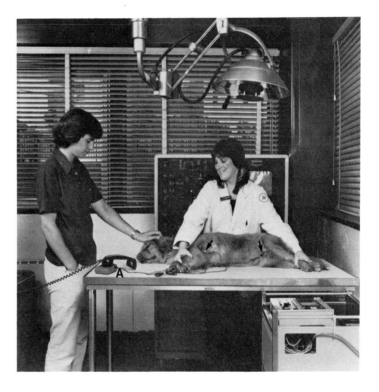

Fig. 2–16. Electrocardiographic transmitter (preamplifier) **(A)** capable of converting electrocardiographic signals into tones that can be transmitted over the telephone line. Lead III is being recorded; electrodes (arrows) have been positioned on the left forearm and left rear leg of the dog. (From Chiert, A., and Tilley, L.P.: Techniques for recording an electrocardiogram. Canine Pract., 9:26, 1982, with permission.)

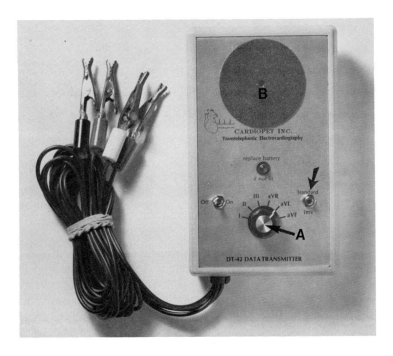

Fig. 2–17. Six-lead transmitter (preamplifier) with four wires and a standardization button (arrow). The lead selector (**A**) allows the transmission of the six basic limb leads. During the transmission, the telephone mouthpiece is placed on the transmitter (**B**). (Courtesy of Wolff Industries, San Marino, Calif.)

A six-lead transmitter with four wires and a standardization button can also be used (Fig. 2–17). A 1-mv reference is provided, which will be injected at the point of the electrode input to the preamplifier. By moving the lead selector, the six basic limb leads, I, II, III, aVR, aVL, and aVF, can be transmitted without moving the electrodes. If the veterinarian already has an electrocardiograph, a small adapter permits simultaneous telephone transmission of the electrocardiogram as it is recorded at the doctor's office as well as at the electrocardiographic data center.

A demodulating device (Fig. 2–18), located at an electrocardiographic data center, converts the sound with a frequency range of 1200 to 2100 Hz into electrocardiographic signals. Each electrocardiogram is reviewed for arrhythmias or conduction disturbances. A written interpretation and a mounted portion of the actual electrocardiographic strip is mailed to the veterinarian. In an emergency, the interpretation can be given at the time of the transmission. Transtelephonic electrocardiography has been established as an accurate technique for the diagnosis of cardiac arrhythmias and conduction disturbance.[15,17–19] Waller or Einthoven probably did not expect that, in such a short time period, their electrocardiograph would be used to help evaluate the cardiac condition of an animal from any state in the United States or from any country. Einthoven, however, did use the term "Le Télécardiogramme."[20]

MONITORING THE ELECTROCARDIOGRAM

Monitoring the electrocardiogram is essential for identifying the critical arrhythmias during surgery, as well as for the daily evaluation of a canine or feline electrocardiogram. Continuous electrocardiogram monitoring must be established as soon as possible on all animals who are suspected of having an irregular pulse, severe heart

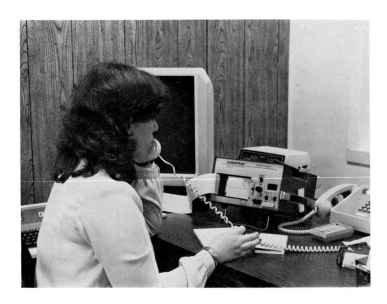

Fig. 2–18. Demodulating device and electrocardiographic recorder located at the electrocardiographic data center that converts electrocardiographic signals into sound and records the electrocardiogram. (From Chiert, A., and Tilley, L.P.: Techniques for recording an electrocardiogram. Canine Pract., 9:26, 1982, with permission.)

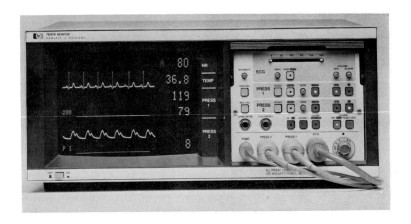

Fig. 2–19. Hewlett-Packard 78342A multichannel monitor for monitoring the electrocardiogram, blood pressure, and temperature. This monitor features an audible heart rate meter with a wide range at both 25- and 50-mm sweep speeds. A nonglare CRT screen eliminates light reflection problems, and the heart rate meter has both upper and lower limit alarm controls. (Courtesy of Hewlett-Packard Co., Waltham, Mass.)

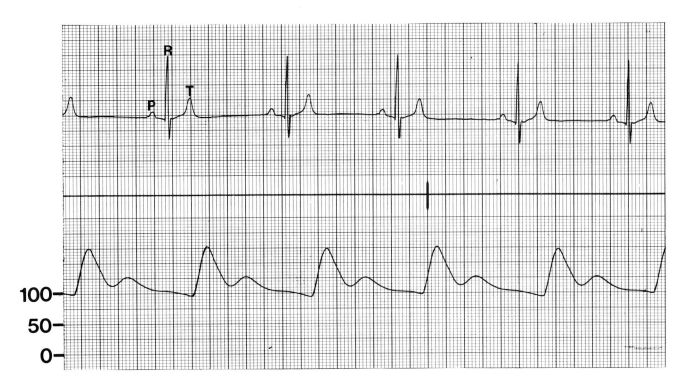

Fig. 2–20. By combining a multichannel electrocardiograph and a monitor, a permanent record can be obtained during the monitoring period. The top tracing is the lead II electrocardiogram, and the bottom tracing is the femoral arterial blood pressure; systolic pressure is 175 mm Hg and the diastolic pressure is 100 mm Hg.

failure, hypotension, or cardiac arrest. The oscilloscope (Fig. 2–19) used in surgery displays the electrocardiogram in a continuous pattern on a fluorescent screen. Many oscilloscopes also provide an additional channel for monitoring blood pressure (Fig. 2–19). By combining a multichannel electrocardiograph and a monitor, a permanent record can be obtained (Fig. 2–20).

For continuous electrocardiographic monitoring and arrhythmia detection, a single lead is recorded. Three electrodes are usually employed to obtain an electrocardiographic lead for monitoring. One electrode is designated as positive, the second electrode is negative, and the third is called ground. The positive and negative electrodes are positioned on the body so that well-defined P-QRS-T deflections are obtained; lead II is usually obtained by positioning the negative electrode on the right foreleg and the positive electrode on the left hindleg. The placement of the ground electrode is not critical except that it should be placed as far away from the other two electrodes as possible. The position of the dog or cat is not critical for monitoring electrocardiograms.

An auditory alarm is incorporated into many cardiac monitoring oscilloscopes and is activated by heart rate above or below a set limit (Fig. 2–19). The instrument senses any vertical oscillation beyond a certain amplitude, with sensitivity adjusted so that one deflection of each cardiac cycle is of a magnitude that will provide one signal to the pulse sensor. A single, tall, upright QRS deflection (the R wave) is the most suitable component of the cardiac cycle to fall within the sensitivity range of the device. If the sensitivity is set too low, some of the cardiac cycles will not be counted, and a slower rate will be counted.

FILING THE ELECTROCARDIOGRAM

For protection, reference, and consultation, the electrocardiogram should be filed properly. It should be so filed and stored that the serial tracings and different leads can be compared. Either of the following methods can be used:

1. The electrocardiogram can be stored in a file folder (15 × 3⅝ inches, Fig. 2–21), which can then be filed in an appropriate filing cabinet (Fig. 2–22). (Any stationery company will make these file folders for a nominal fee.)
2. The electrocardiogram can be cut into sections and mounted (Fig. 2–23). These 8½ × 11 inch sheet mounts can easily be filed in medical record folders. Several different types of mounts are available through most electrocardiograph companies.

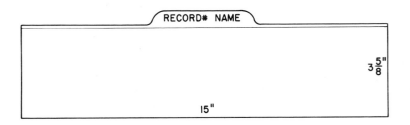

Fig. 2–21. File folder to store electrocardiograms in a file cabinet. (See Fig. 2–22.)

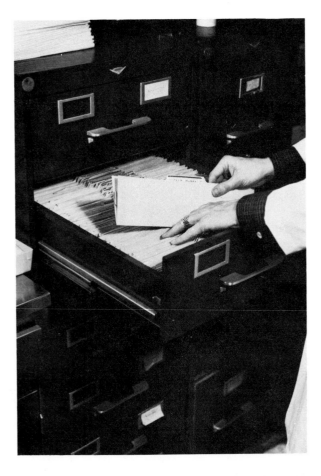

Fig. 2–22. File cabinet for the file folders. The electrocardiographic strips are filed as to the animal's case number and owner's name.

COMMON ARTIFACTS AND THEIR CORRECTIONS

Since the electrocardiogram is a mechanical recording, a number of technical or mechanical problems can occur while it is being obtained. These technical or mechanical problems superimposed on the normal cardiac complexes cause distortions of the electrocardiogram, known as artifacts, which often interfere with interpretation of the electrocardiogram by causing abnormalities that are not due to cardiac disorders.

Electrical interference

Electrical interference appears as a regular sequence of 60 sharp up-and-down waves/sec, also called 60-cycle artifact (Figs. 2–24 and 2–25). The electrocardiogram cannot be interpreted with 60-cycle artifact, so the cause of the artifact must be found and eliminated. To correct:

1. Make sure the power cord is properly grounded into a three-hole wall outlet. The proper outlet will automatically ground the electrocardiogram. The right leg (RL) electrode (the ground electrode) carries alternating current from the animal. The power cord of older-model electrocardiographic units should be converted to the modern three-prong plug. If this cannot be done, an auxiliary ground lead wire from the ground jack of the machine to a water pipe or an object with a common ground can be attached.
2. Reapply the electrode clips, making sure that all are securely attached to the animal. The electrode should be placed on a "fleshy" part of the leg, staying away from large folds of skin often seen with cats. The leads should not be saturated with alcohol but merely dampened.
3. Make sure the clips are clean and securely attached to the cables. Sandpaper can be used to remove any material that builds up on the clip.
4. Pull the plug on all other electrical equipment in the room. Fluorescent lights should be turned off.
5. Make sure the animal's legs are held apart so the clips do not touch each other.
6. Be certain that the attendant is not touching any of the clips.
7. If a metal table is being used, ground it by connecting the auxiliary ground wire between the table and the ground jack of the electrocardiograph. Use a rubber mat so the animal does not touch any metal portion of the table.
8. Make sure no electric cords (including the power cable) are touching the table.
9. Move the table away from walls that may contain electrical wiring. It may be necessary to move the table to another room. Electrical equipment in use in another room can also cause interference. If the electrical interference cannot be eliminated, contact the respective electrocardiograph company for service.
10. Be certain that the hospital "ground" has been adequately set up in the first place.

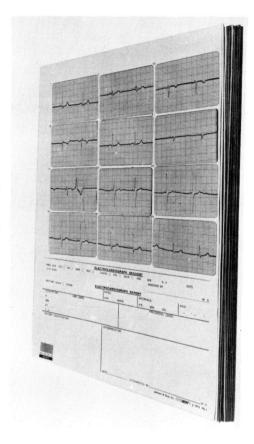

Fig. 2–23. Electrocardiographic systems pattern mounts with pressure-sensitive surfaces. These standard mounts provide space for interpretation, history, and medical records identification. The convenient 8½ × 11 inch size fits standard photocopiers, clinical chart holders, and files. (Courtesy of Burdick Corp., Milton, Wis.)

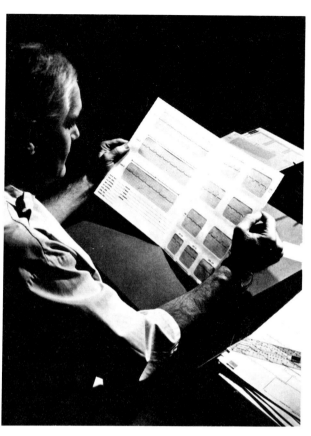

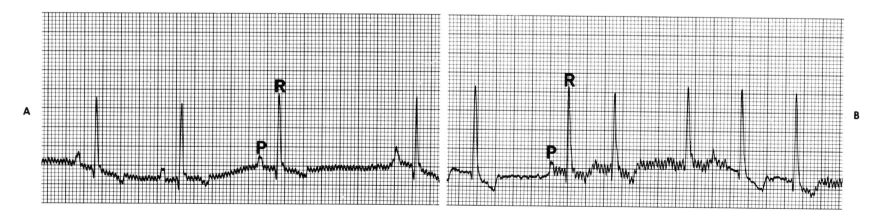

Fig. 2–24. **A,** 60-Cycle interference on this canine lead II electrocardiogram caused by an inadequately grounded electrocardiograph. **B,** 60-Cycle interference produced when the clip electrodes connected to this dog were intermittently touched by the handler.

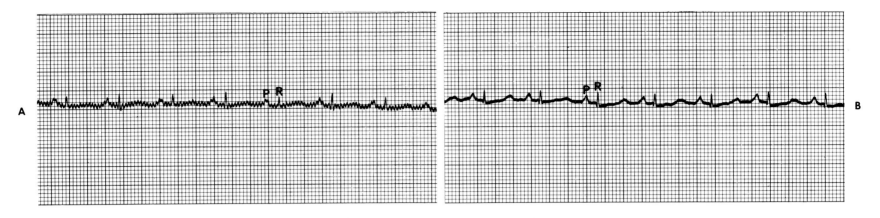

Fig. 2–25. **A,** Electrocardiogram (feline) recorded with inadequate electrode solution and/or electrode clip contact. **B,** Tracing from the same cat after electrode clips were reapplied to the skin (not just the hair) and after application of greater quantities of alcohol.

Muscle tremor

Muscular and/or body movements by the animal can produce artifacts (Fig. 2–26), rapid and irregular vibrations of the baseline. The greater the movement, the greater will be the amplitude of the artifact. This same artifact is also seen when a cat is purring during recording of the electrocardiogram. To correct:

1. Make sure the animal is in a comfortable position. The table must be large enough to adequately support the limbs.
2. If the animal shows signs of nervousness or tension, try to gain its confidence. Sometimes having the owner in the room will relax the animal.
3. Mild tranquilization is safe in most cases, but its effects must be considered when interpreting the electrocardiogram. Tranquilizers can affect the rate and other rhythms of the heart.

4. Patience, gentle manipulation of the larynx, and blowing into a cat's face are helpful if purring is a problem.
5. Readjust or reapply the electrodes. The clips can sometimes be uncomfortable on thin-skinned dogs.
6. Placement of your hand over the chest wall with moderate pressure during the recording will often minimize muscular tremor.
7. Reducing the amplitude by setting the sensitivity switch at position 1/2 will sometimes reduce the artifact enough to make the remainder of the electrocardiogram legible.

Wandering baseline

Changes in resistance between the electrode and the patient's skin can cause an up-and-down wandering of the baseline. Respiratory movements are the most common cause, resulting in a cylindrical

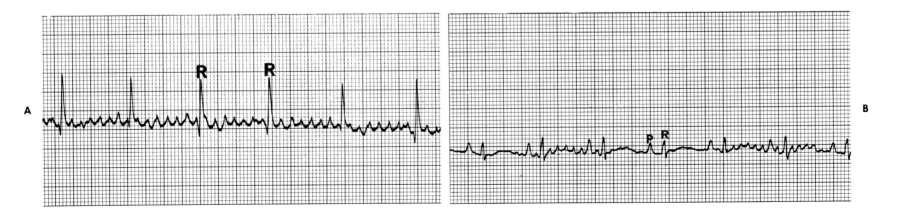

Fig. 2–26. Artifact from a muscle tremor. **A,** Electrocardiogram recorded from a nervous dog that is trembling. The rapid and irregular vibrations of the baseline resemble atrial ectopic waves. The true sinus P waves cannot be identified. **B,** Electrocardiogram recorded from a cat that is intermittently purring.

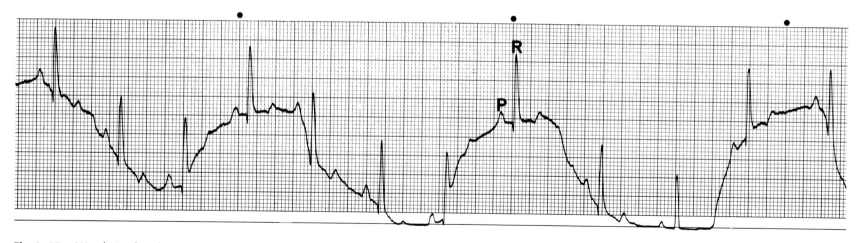

Fig. 2–27. Wandering baseline. Respiratory movements in this dog cause the electrodes to be moved with each breath. The rise and fall of the baseline coincide with the phases of respiration.

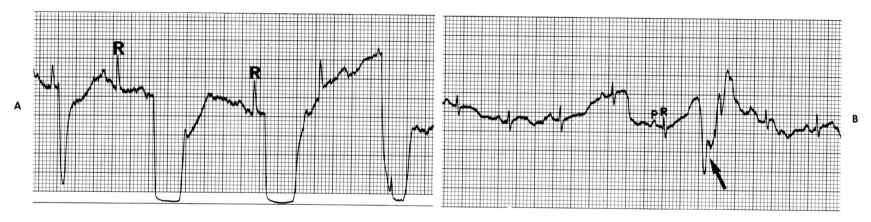

Fig. 2–28. **A,** The sudden shifts of the baseline in this electrocardiogram are produced when the cat moves or coughs. **B,** The baseline drifts up and down on this electrocardiographic tracing because of the cat's respiratory movements. The large artifact (arrow) due to the cat's jerking one leg could easily mimic a ventricular premature complex.

rising and falling of the baseline that coincides with the phases of respiration (Fig. 2–27). Coughing or panting also causes an interruption in the baseline (Fig. 2–28). Respiratory movements are most often evident in the precordial leads. To correct:

1. Make the animal as comfortable as possible. If the animal is in heart failure, the electrocardiogram should not be done in right lateral recumbency because this position will further stress the animal. In such situations, the electrocardiogram should be done in the position the animal assumes. Then the analysis of heart rate and rhythm is of priority, and these values will not be affected by the animal's position.
2. The animal's mouth can be held closed for 3 to 4 seconds, which is all the time needed to obtain a good recording of each lead.

Poorly defined baseline

If the baseline is not well defined, the P-QRS-T deflections will be difficult to measure. This especially pertains to complexes that are large in amplitude, such as R waves (Fig. 2–29). To correct:

1. Increase the stylus heat.
2. If the stylus is dirty, burn off the accumulated plastic. This can be done by turning on the machine for a short period with the paper roll removed from the machine.
3. The stylus arm should be checked by the manufacturer of your electrocardiograph. A stylus that gives a heavier baseline is used by some electrocardiograph manufacturers; a thick baseline should be avoided (Fig. 2–30).

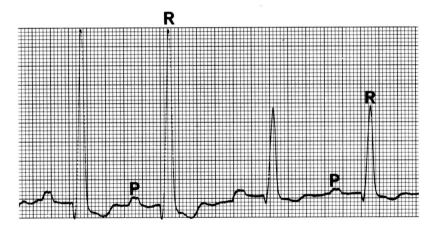

Fig. 2-29. Poorly defined P-QRS-T deflections often are present if complexes are large. Reducing the amplitude (switch position at 1/2) in the latter half of the strip makes the complexes easier to see. The standardization button should be pressed to note this change.

4. If complexes are not well defined because of their large amplitude, reduce the amplitude by setting the sensitivity switch at position 1/2 (Fig. 2-29).

Inadequate frequency response

The quality and accuracy of the deflections of the P-QRS-T are affected by the frequency response. Frequency response is the ability of the unit to reproduce accurately all of the frequency applied to it, resulting in a true reproduction of the electrocardiogram. The electrocardiographic signal is a very small electrical potential that contains high-frequency (QRS complexes and notch-like wave forms) and low-frequency (P wave, ST segment, and T wave) signals. An amplifier is needed to make the complexes larger. An electrocardiograph that has poor high-frequency response records an amplitude of the output

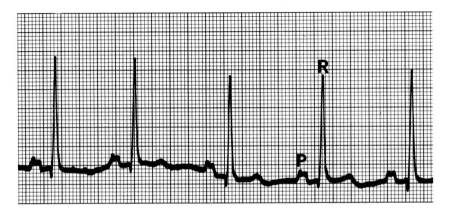

Fig. 2-30. The thick baseline on this canine electrocardiogram makes it difficult to accurately measure the P-QRS-T deflections. The stylus heat should be decreased.

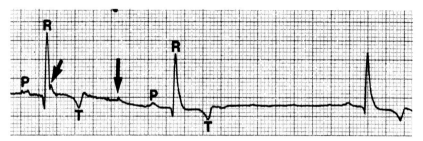

Fig. 2-31. Electrocardiogram of consecutive cardiac cycles recorded at different frequency responses (500 Hz and 70 Hz). The large arrow indicates where a filter is introduced to reduce the frequency response. Note the slurred or notched end of the QRS complex (small arrow) in the high-frequency recording. The P wave is also distorted. Note that the height of the QRS complex is reduced and that the notch in the QRS is now not present. This represents reduction in amplitude as higher-frequency components are lost in the filtered record. (Courtesy of Dr. C. Kvart, College of Veterinary Medicine, Uppsala, Sweden).

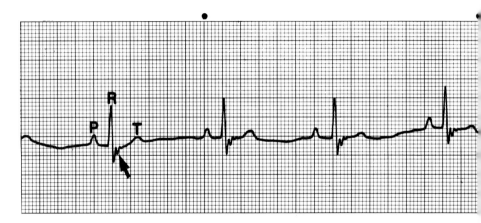

Fig. 2-32. A transmitted transtelephonic electrocardiogram from a normal dog. Note the distorted and depressed ST segment (arrow) secondary to the poor low-frequency response of the transmitter. Arrhythmias and conduction disturbances can be accurately evaluated. ST segment depression and QRS width measurements may be difficult to define, as the J point (termination of ventricular depolarization) can sometimes be difficult to define in the depressed ST segment.

signal less the input. The height of the QRS complex is reduced, and any "notch-like wave forms" present will be minimized (Fig. 2-31). If the electrocardiograph has a poor low-frequency response, the ST segment will not be faithfully reproduced (Fig. 2-32), and there is also the possibility that distortion will occur in the P and T waves.[15,21,22]

The specification of the American Heart Association is a band width of 0.05 to 100 Hz, to ensure accuracy for measurements used clinically such as wave amplitude. All electrocardiographs should be checked for proper frequency response standards.[7] The low-frequency response of 0.17 Hz in new transtelephonic transmitter units presently being used by an electrocardiographic data center are satisfactory, especially for the analysis of cardiac arrhythmias. The ST segment is minimally distorted.

REFERENCES

1. Lewis, T.: *Clinical Disorders of the Heart Beat*. London, Shaw, 1912.
2. Bolton, G.R.: *Handbook of Canine Electrocardiography*. Philadelphia, W.B. Saunders, 1975.
3. Tilley, L.P., and Gompf, R.E.: Feline electrocardiography. Vet. Clin. North Am., 7:257, 1977.
4. Riseman, J.E.: *A Guide to Electrocardiographic Interpretation*. 5th Ed. New York, Macmillan, 1968.
5. Rubin, G.J.: Applications of electrocardiography in canine medicine. J. Am. Vet. Med. Assoc., 153:17, 1968.
6. Tilley, L.P.: *Basic Canine Electrocardiography*. Milton, Wis., The Burdick Corp., 1978.
7. Pipberger, H.V., et al.: Recommendations for standardization of leads and of specifications for instruments in electrocardiography and vectorcardiography. Report of the Committee on Electrocardiography, American Heart Association. Circulation, 52:11, 1975.
8. Almasi, J.J., Schmitt, O.H., and Jankus, E.F.: Electrical characteristics of commonly used canine ECG electrodes. Proceedings of the Twenty-third Annual Conference on Engineering in Medicine and Biology, Washington, D.C., 1970.
9. Hahn, A.W., Hamlin, R.L., and Patterson, D.F.: Standards for canine electrocardiography. Academy of Veterinary Cardiology Committee Report, 1977.
10. Hill, J.D.: The significance of foreleg position in the interpretation of electrocardiograms and vectorcardiograms from research animals. Am. Heart J., 75:518, 1968.
11. Muenster, J.J., Rosenburg, M.S., Carleton, R.H., and Graettinger, J.S.: Comparison between diazepam and sodium thiopental during DC countershock. JAMA, 10:168, 1967.
12. Muir, W.W., Werner, L.L., and Hamlin, R.L.: Antiarrhythmic effects of diazepam during coronary artery occlusion in dogs. Am. J. Vet. Res., 36:1203, 1975.
13. Smith, R.D., and Pettway, C.E.: Absence of sensitization to epinephrine-induced cardiac arrhythmia and fibrillation in dogs and cats anesthetized with CI744. Am. J. Vet. Res., 36:695, 1975.
14. Stanley, V., Hunt, J., Willis, K.W., and Stephen, C.R.: Cardiovascular and respiratory function with CI-581. Anesthes. Analg., 47:760, 1968.
15. Tilley, L.P.: Transtelephonic analysis of cardiac arrhythmias in the dog; diagnostic accuracy. Vet. Clin. North Am., 13:395, 1983.
16. Chiert, A., Tilley, L.P., and Cohen, R.B.: Techniques for recording an electrocardiogram. Canine Pract., 9:19, 1982.
17. Capone, R.J., Grodman, R.S., and Most, A.S.: Transtelephonic surveillance of cardiac arrhythmias. J. Cardiovasc. Med., 6:57, 1981.
18. Carp, C.: Transtelephonic diagnosis of transient arrhythmias, a new practical method. Med. Interne, 17:393, 1979.
19. Hasin, J., David, D., and Rogel, S.: Diagnostic and therapeutic assessment by telephone electrocardiographic monitoring of ambulatory patients. Br. Med. J., 2:612, 1976.
20. Burch, G.E., and DePasquale, N.P.: *A History of Electrocardiography*. Chicago, Year Book Medical Publishers, 1964.
21. Berson, A.S., and Pipberger, H.V.: The low frequency response of electrocardiographs, a frequent source of recording errors. Am. Heart J., 71:779, 1966.
22. Berson, A.S., et al.: Distortions in infant electrocardiograms caused by inadequate high-frequency response. Am. Heart J., 93:730, 1977.

3 The approach to the electrocardiogram

What you or I think is not important.
*What is important is the truth.**

WILLEM EINTHOVEN (1860–1927)

To obtain the "electrocardiographic truth," Einthoven was essentially stressing the fact that the interpretation of an electrocardiogram must always be preceded by a systematic approach to the electrocardiogram, or marked variations in its interpretation will occur. Even with a systematic approach, variations in interpretation can occur—not only among the readers of the electrocardiogram but also with the same clinician on successive readings.[2] The interpretation of the electrocardiogram is the most important and most difficult aspect of electrocardiography.

The clinician should appreciate the potential inaccuracy of the electrocardiogram. To take full advantage of the electrocardiogram as a valuable aid in clinical diagnosis, he should consider three conditions:[3,4]

1. In general, the person best qualified to read the electrocardiogram is the clinician in charge of the patient. If someone else reads the electrocardiogram, he should then become a consultant in a manner similar to that of a radiologist. Before the first interpretation is made, this consultant should discuss the clinical picture with the clinician.

2. It must be understood that the electrocardiogram records just the sum of activity generated by action potentials of the heart. Any conclusions from the electrocardiogram regarding anatomic abnormalities or changes in the physiologic state are not always accurate. The clinician should appreciate the fact that the interpretation does not represent a firm diagnosis, but merely suggests a condition that with the highest probability is indicated by the electrocardiogram.

3. The clinician should recognize the broad variations in the normal and the overlap between the various entities producing abnormalities in the electrocardiogram.

There are three levels of electrocardiographic "readers": the veterinarian recording and interpreting tracings of his own animals; the veterinarian who interprets electrocardiograms for veterinary hospitals, research institutions, or other veterinarians, thus acting as a consultant; and the veterinarian whose chief interest is in electrocardiography and who acts as a teacher, investigator, and expert in electrocardiography.[5] Certification by the American College of Veterinary Internal Medicine and by the Specialty Board of Cardiology requires extensive knowledge in the field of electrocardiography. The criteria for competence of electrocardiographers in the human field have been well defined. A list of essential recommended skills and knowledge has been prepared by the American College of Cardiology.[6]

ROUTINE APPROACH TO THE ELECTROCARDIOGRAM

The complete electrocardiogram should include at least three to four complexes of each bipolar standard lead (I, II, III), three augmented unipolar limb leads (aVR, aVL, aVF) and at least 15 to 20 inches of a lead II rhythm strip. The unipolar precordial chest leads (CV_5RL, also termed rV_2; CV_6LL or V_2; CV_6LU or V_4; and V_{10}) can also be recorded for added electrocardiographic accuracy in specific conditions. The minimum electrocardiographic recording is a lead II rhythm strip (Fig. 3–1) and the six basic limb leads (Fig. 3–2). This recording in both the dog and the cat is the primary basis for discussion in this textbook. The precordial leads are discussed only in certain specific conditions.

After the complete electrocardiogram has been recorded, it must be analyzed to determine whether it is normal or abnormal by measuring the various complex heights and interval lengths and comparing them with the normal values (canine, Chapter 4; and feline, Chapter 5).

Every electrocardiogram should have at least four features examined systematically: heart rate, heart rhythm, P-QRS-T complexes and intervals, and mean electrical axis. Following are the steps in analysis (Fig. 3–1):

1. Calculate the heart rate.
2. Evaluate the heart rhythm.
3. Measure the complexes and intervals.
   a. P wave
   b. P-R interval
   c. QRS complex
   d. S-T segment
   e. T wave
   f. Q-T interval
   g. Basic limb leads (I, II, III, aVR, aVL, and aVF) (Fig. 3–2)
4. Determine the mean electrical axis.

ELECTROCARDIOGRAPHIC PAPER

The electrocardiographic paper (Fig. 3–3) is lined into boxes that can be used to make quick and accurate measurements. There are two sets of boxes on the electrocardiographic paper: one large and one small. For convenience and accuracy in measuring, every fifth vertical and horizontal line is darker than the others. The horizontal lines are 1 mm apart and represent 0.1 mv when the electrocardiogram is standardized at 10 mm = 1 mv. Ten small boxes vertically are equal to 1 mv. The vertical lines are time lines with each interval

---

*Einthoven himself settled an argument involving electrocardiography with this statement.[1] When he was awarded the Nobel Prize in 1924, the citation read that the prize was for "the discovery of the mechanism of the electrocardiograph."

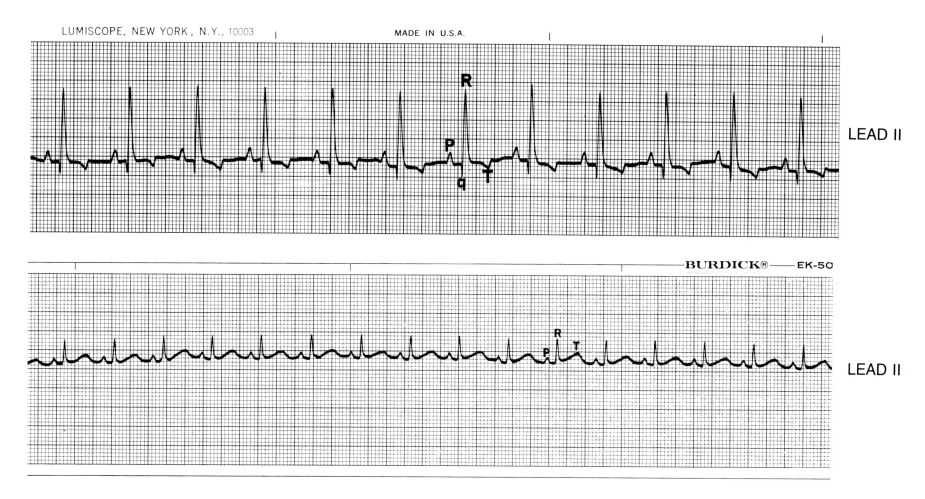

LEAD II

LEAD II

Fig. 3–1. A lead II rhythm strip taken at the end of a complete electrocardiographic recording is used in both dogs and cats for the first three steps in an analysis. The steps include (1) heart rate, (2) heart rhythm, and (3) complexes and intervals. The analysis of these two lead II electrocardiographic strips is normal. The clinician can readily see that the feline electrocardiogram (bottom tracing) has a faster heart rate and smaller complexes when compared with the canine electrocardiogram (top tracing). Paper speed, 50 mm/sec; standardization, 1 cm = 1 mv.

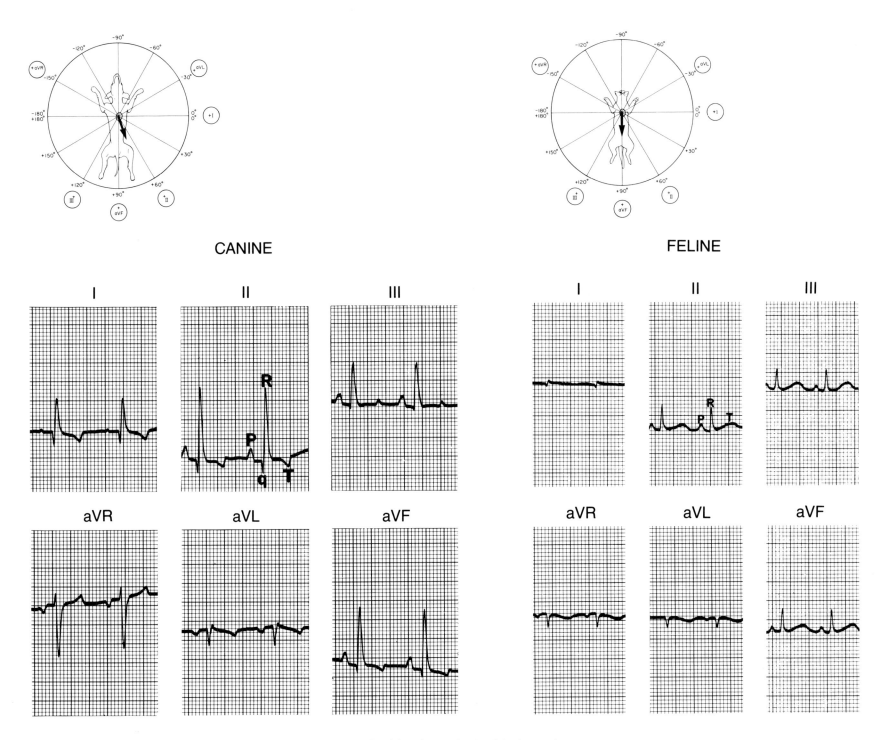

CANINE

FELINE

Fig. 3–2. For the systematic analysis of the direction and magnitude of the electrical axis of the heart, the six basic limb leads *(I, II, III, aVR, aVL,* and *aVF)* are arranged in a circular field according to the direction of each lead and the location of the positive electrodes. The mean electrical axis for this dog is +70°, and for this cat, +90°.

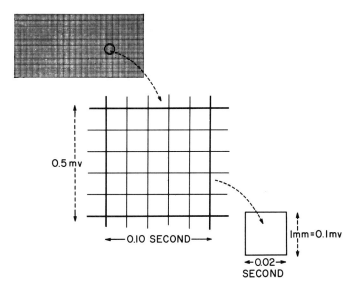

Fig. 3–3. Electrocardiographic paper and grid lines. At the standard paper speed of 50 mm/sec in veterinary medicine, the interval between two heavily drawn vertical lines is 0.10 second and between two fine vertical lines, 0.02 second. At the normal standardization setting (position 1), 5 mm (5 small boxes) is equal to 0.5 mv, so each box is 0.1 mv going up or down.

0.02 second when recorded at the standard paper speed of 50 mm/sec. Five small boxes, then, are equal to 0.10 second. Electrocardiographic complex values of magnitude are expressed in millivolts (mv) whereas values of duration are expressed in seconds. Electrocardiographic paper also has time markings in the margin for every 75 mm (15 large boxes) (1.5 sec) (Fig. 3–1).

ELECTROCARDIOGRAPHIC REPORT FORM

The electrocardiographic report form is used to record the measurements and conclusions found as the electrocardiogram is analyzed (Fig. 3–4). One section provides space for specific numerical measurements, e.g., rate, rhythm, P wave, P-R, QRS, Q-T, and S-T.

ELECTROCARDIOGRAPHIC INTERPRETATION

The second section is blank for interpretation, which is based on the various measurements and observations as well as on the results of the other clinical laboratory techniques (phonocardiography, radiography, and analysis of the blood, urine, and extravascular fluids). The interpretation should include statements on the rhythm and diagnosis and comparison with previous tracings. The final interpretation can include the following possibilities[7]:

1. The tracing is normal.
2. Borderline record; there are minor changes, the significance of which will depend on the clinical findings and serial electrocardiograms.

THE ANIMAL MEDICAL CENTER
510 East 62nd Street
New York, New York 10021
CARDIOVASCULAR LABORATORY DATA SHEET

CLIENT

CASE NO.

SPECIES

BREED _____ AGE _____ SEX _____

HISTORY:

ECG INTERPRETATION:

CHEST X-RAY:

OTHER LABORATORY DATA:

ELECTROCARDIOGRAM:
Rate
Rhythm
P
P · R
QRS
Q · T
ST · T
Other

PLAN

PROBLEM LIST · DIAGNOSIS	TREATMENT · SUMMARY

Date: _____ Doctor: _____ Consultation Fee $ _____

LAWRENCE P. TILLEY, D.V.M.
DIPLOMATE A.C.V.I.M.

Fig. 3–4. Cardiovascular laboratory data report form. The top right-hand section is designed for recording the electrocardiographic findings.

3. Abnormal tracing typical of (name of condition).
4. Abnormal tracing consistent with (name of conditions).
5. Abnormal tracing not characteristic of any specific entity.

As has been stated, it is important to correlate the features of the electrocardiographic tracing with the whole clinical picture. This correlation, however, should be made only after a complete study of the electrocardiographic record. It must be remembered that a normal electrocardiogram does not imply a normal heart and that an abnormal electrocardiogram does not always imply organic heart disease.

CALCULATION OF HEART RATE (Figs. 3–5 and 3–6)

The heart rate is the number of beats per minute. In some cardiac arrhythmias, the atria and ventricles do not beat at the same rate, necessitating that atrial and ventricular rates each be calculated. The method used to calculate the heart rate depends on whether the rhythm is regular or irregular. When the rhythm is regular, the heart rate can be calculated by either of the following three methods (paper speed = 50 mm/sec) (Figs. 3–5 and 3–6):

1. Since one small box is 0.02 second in width, the number of small boxes equaling 1 minute is 60 divided by 0.02 (or 3000). Therefore the number of small boxes in one R-R interval divided into 3000 gives the heart rate per minute (Fig. 3–5).

2. A large box is equal to 0.02×5, or 0.10 second in width, so the number of large boxes equaling 1 minute is 60 divided by 0.1 (or 600). Therefore the number of large boxes in one R-R interval divided into 600 gives the heart rate per minute (Fig. 3–6).

3. A heart rate calculator ruler provides a means for a rapid accurate determination of the heart rate (Fig. 3–7). There are many different kinds of calculators using several different methods for cal-

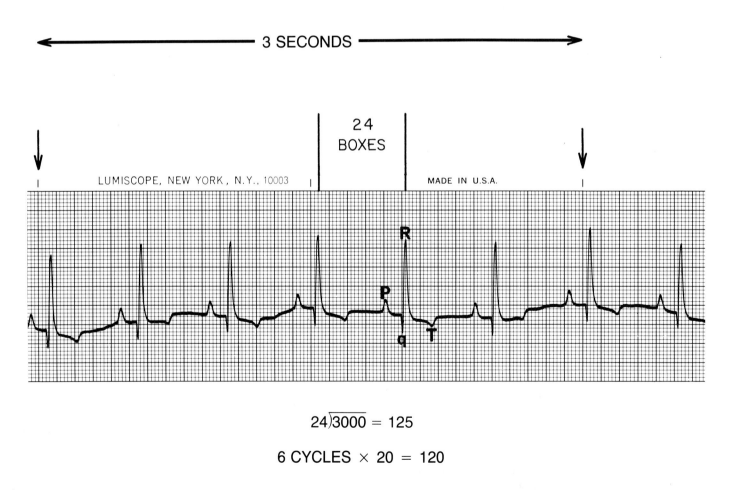

$$24\overline{)3000} = 125$$

$$6 \text{ CYCLES} \times 20 = 120$$

Fig. 3–5. Calculation of the heart rate from a normal canine electrocardiogram. When the ventricular rate is regular, the number of small 0.02 second boxes divided into 3000 equals the heart rate ($3000 \div 24 = 125$). When the rhythm is irregular, the approximate number of cycles (R-R intervals) between two sets of marks (arrows) multiplied by 20 equals the heart rate ($6 \times 20 = 120$). Paper speed, 50 mm/sec.

culating the heart rate. They should be used according to printed directions.

When the rhythm is irregular, the ventricular heart rate can be calculated by counting the number of cycles (R-R intervals) between two sets of marks (3 sec) in the margin and multiplying by 20 (Figs. 3–5 and 3–6). In very slow rates, greater accuracy will be achieved by counting the cycles in four of the 1.5-second intervals (6 seconds) and multiplying by 10. The fraction of the last cycle should be estimated in tenths. At a paper speed of 50 mm/sec, these marks are spaced 1.5 seconds apart. When the heart rate is calculated this way, the result is always slightly less than the actual heart rate.

EVALUATION OF HEART RHYTHM

In evaluating the heart rhythm, the clinician must analyze the electrocardiogram systematically (see Chapter 6 for details).[2,3,8]

General inspection. This will show whether the rhythm is a normal sinus rhythm or is characteristic of a type of cardiac arrhythmia. The term *arrhythmia* denotes all deviations from normal in the origin (automaticity) and sequence (conductivity) of heart action. It should be determined whether the arrhythmia is occasional, frequent, or continuous; regular or irregular; and repetitive or occurring with various combinations.

Identification of P waves. This should also include determining whether the atrial activity is uniform or irregular.

Recognition of QRS complexes. The complexes should be characterized as to their configuration, uniformity, and regularity. A QRS complex that is normal in width and configuration most often indicates a supraventricular mechanism. If the QRS complex is widened, however, all available criteria must be used to decide whether this is ectopic ventricular activity or abnormal intraventricular conduction.

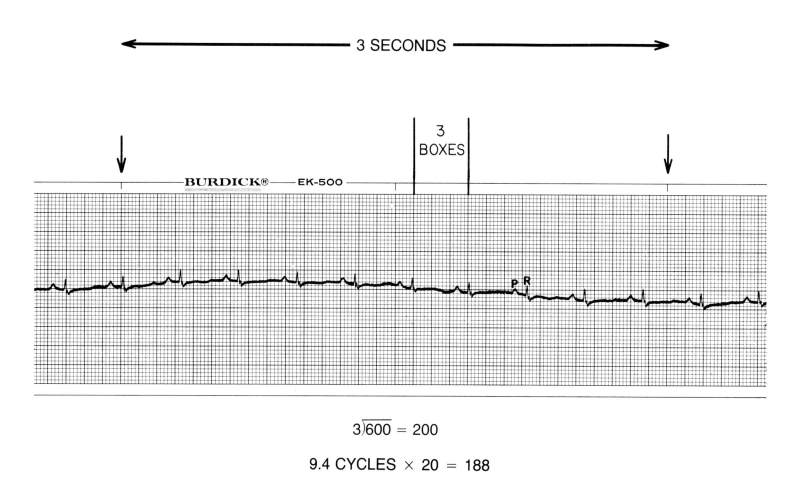

$$3\overline{)600} = 200$$

$$9.4 \text{ CYCLES} \times 20 = 188$$

Fig. 3–6. Calculation of the heart rate from a normal feline electrocardiogram. When the ventricular rate is regular, the number of large 0.10 second boxes divided into 600 can also equal the heart rate (600 ÷ 3 = 200). Paper speed, 50 mm/sec.

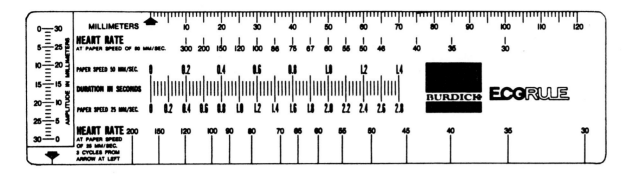

Fig. 3–7. Heart rate calculator ruler. (Courtesy of Burdick Corp., Milton, Wis.)

Fig. 3–8. Use of an electrocardiographic caliper for plotting P-P and/or R-R intervals to determine whether rhythm is regular or for locating P-QRS complexes. The QRS complexes occur at a regular rhythm in this canine electrocardiogram.

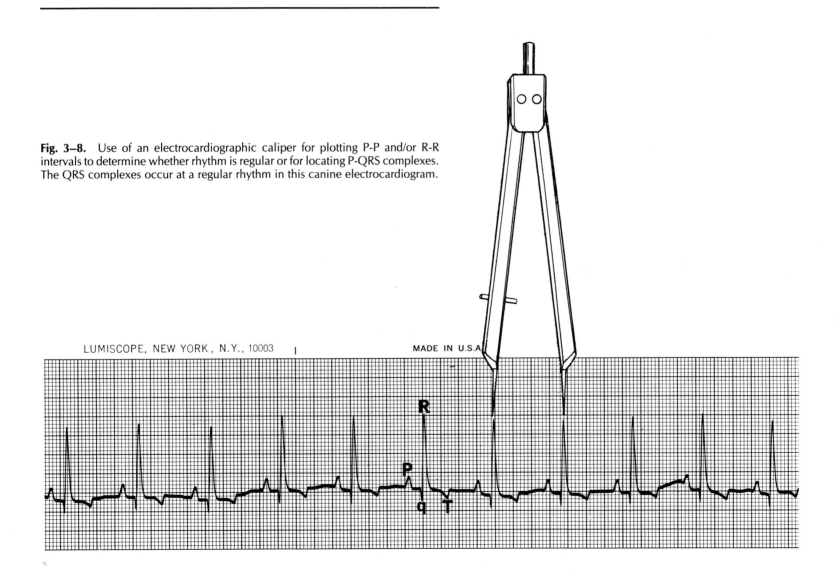

Analysis of the relationship between P waves and QRS complexes. If the initial inspection of the electrocardiogram suggests the presence of an arrhythmia, a long rhythm strip should be taken. The lead (usually lead II) should be carefully selected to illustrate discrete P waves. The crucial part of the electrocardiographic examination is identification and analysis of the P wave. Doubling the sensitivity of the electrocardiograph will sometimes be helpful in magnifying the P waves. The analysis of arrhythmias can also be facilitated by the availability of an electrocardiogram prior to the onset of arrhythmias. The configurations of P waves and QRS complexes can then be compared.

The clinician can also use electrocardiographic calipers for plotting intervals (Fig. 3–8). The needle points of each of the two legs are positioned over the apex of two successive P waves (or QRS complexes). If calipers are not available, a simple method is to place a card immediately beneath the apex of the P waves (or QRS complexes) that are recognized (Fig. 3–9); then make a mark on the card in conjunction with each apex of two or three P waves (or QRS com-

plexes); the card (or caliper) can be shifted to the right or left so the first mark falls on the next P wave (or QRS complex); if the rhythm is regular, all the marks on the card or two needle points will fall under the appropriate complexes. This method can often be used to find P waves in arrhythmias in which the P waves are hidden in the QRS complexes.

DIRECTIONS FOR MEASURING COMPLEXES AND INTERVALS
(Figs. 3–10 and 3–11)

Measurement of complexes and intervals is done on the lead II rhythm strip. The amplitude of deflections, as already stated, is recorded in boxes or millivolts. Measurements of upward deflections are made from the upper edge of the baseline to the peak of the wave; downward deflections, from the lower edge of the baseline to the lowest point of the wave. The duration of waves, complexes, intervals, and segments can be measured in practically every instance from the beginning to the end of that specific deflection.

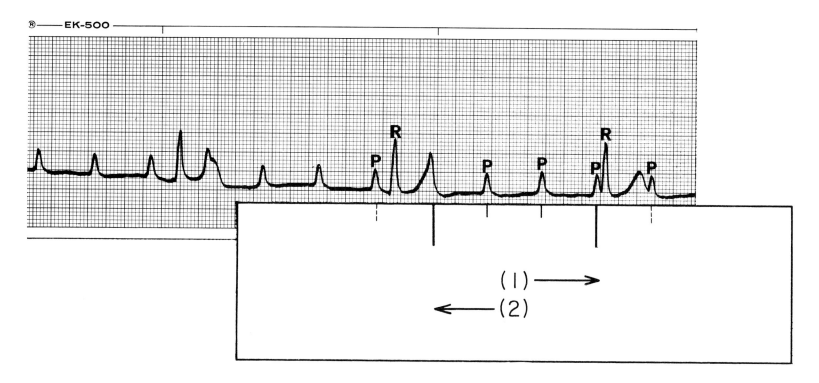

Fig. 3–9. Card method for examining arrhythmias. A card has been marked at two places (small dark lines) beneath the apex of two waves. By moving the card to the right (1), the examiner can see that a P wave (heavy dark line) falls within an R wave. By moving the card to the left (2), he determines that a P wave (heavy dark line) falls within a T wave (explaining its increased amplitude). This electrocardiogram is an example of complete heart block.

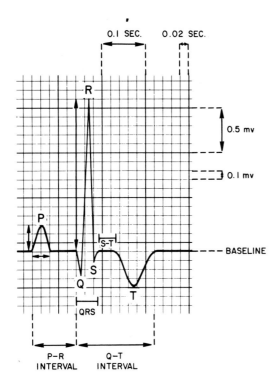

Fig. 3–10. Close-up of a normal canine lead II P-QRS-T complex with labels and intervals. Measurements for amplitude (millivolts) are indicated by positive and negative movement; time intervals (hundredths of a second) are indicated from left to right. Paper speed, 50 mm/sec; 1 cm = 1 mv.

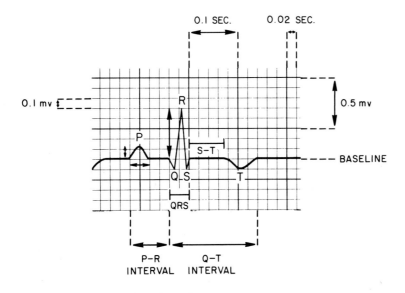

Fig. 3–11. Close-up of a normal feline lead II P-QRS-T complex with labels and intervals. Measurements for amplitude (millivolts) are indicated by positive and negative movement; time intervals (hundredths of a second) are indicated from left to right. Paper speed, 50 mm/sec; 1 cm = 1 mv.

Figures 3–10 and 3–11 are close-up views of the P-QRS-T complexes as to measurements for amplitude and time intervals in the dog and cat. Measurements include the amplitude and width of the P wave, the length of the P-R interval, the amplitude and width of the QRS complex, the S-T segment and T wave, and the length of the Q-T interval.

The calipers (Fig. 3–8) can also be used to measure the various time intervals and amplitudes of P-QRS-T complexes. To use the calipers, place one needle point at the beginning of the measurement to be made and open the other leg until the needle point is at the end of the time interval; without changing the distance between the two legs, move the calipers so one of the needle points rests on a heavy dark line on some other part of the paper. The number of boxes between the two needle points can now be counted easily. The number of boxes multiplied by 0.02 second, or 0.1 mv, equals the measurement, depending on whether amplitude (millivolts) or a time interval (seconds) is measured. These measurements apply to the standard paper speed of 50 mm/sec and a standardization of 1 cm = 1 mv (10 small boxes = 1 mv).

P wave (Figs. 3–10 and 3–11)

The P wave represents depolarization of the atria, and its duration indicates the time required for an impulse to pass from the sinoatrial (SA) node to the atrioventricular (AV) node. The P wave may be positive, notched, biphasic, or negative depending on the particular lead being recorded (Fig. 3–12). The normal P wave in lead II is usually a small rounded wave. Positive P waves are measured from the upper edge of the baseline to the top of the P. Negative P waves are measured from the lower edge of the baseline to the bottom of the P. Biphasic P waves are measured by adding the amplitudes above and below the baseline. The width of the P wave is measured in hundredths of a second at its inside, from the start to the end of the deflection from the baseline.

P-R interval (Figs. 3–10 and 3–11)

The P-R interval represents the time required for an impulse to travel from the SA node to the ventricle. It is measured from the beginning of the P wave to the beginning of the Q wave (R wave, if no Q wave is present). The P-Q interval is equivalent to the P-R interval. The P-R interval should be approximately the same from

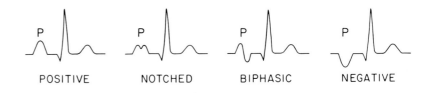

Fig. 3–12. Type of P wave depending on the particular lead being recorded or the abnormality present.

complex to complex; if the P-R varies from beat to beat, an arrhythmia or conduction disturbance could be responsible. The P-R interval does vary with heart rate: the higher the rate, the shorter the conduction time through the atria and the AV node to the bundle of His.[9]

QRS complex (Figs. 3–10 and 3–11)

The QRS complex represents depolarization of the ventricles. Its various components are defined as follows (Fig. 3–13).

Q wave. The first negative deflection which precedes an R wave.

R wave. The first positive deflection.

S wave. The first negative deflection which follows an R wave.

R′ wave. The second positive deflection.

S′ wave. The second negative deflection following an R wave.

QS wave. A single negative deflection representing the QRS complex.

QRS complexes with W forms and R′ and S′ waves are common in the cat. Capital and lower case letters are used to indicate the approximate size of the various deflections. A capital letter represents a deflection of large amplitude; a lower case letter, a deflection of low amplitude. Notching and slurring are two changes in the QRS complex that do not cross the baseline.

The width of the QRS complex is measured from the beginning of the first deflection to the end of the final deflection of the complex. The height of the R wave is measured from the top edge of the baseline to the peak of the R wave. The depth of the Q or S wave is measured from the bottom edge of the baseline to the lowest part of the Q or S, respectively.

S-T segment (Figs. 3–10 and 3–11)

The S-T segment represents the time interval from the end of the QRS interval to the onset of the T wave, the early phase of ventricular repolarization. It may be above (elevated), at, or below (depressed) the level of the baseline.

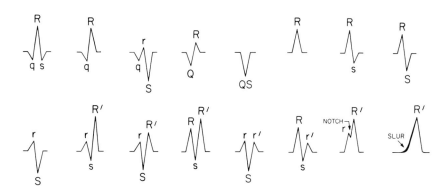

Fig. 3–13. Components and nomenclature of the various QRS complexes.

T wave (Figs. 3–10 and 3–11)

The T wave is the first major deflection following the QRS complex and represents repolarization of the ventricles. It may be positive, notched, negative, or biphasic.

Q-T interval (Figs. 3–10 and 3–11)

The Q-T interval is measured from the onset of the Q wave to the end of the T wave. It is the summation of ventricular depolarization and repolarization and represents ventricular systole. The Q-T interval should be measured from a lead in which the T wave is seen clearly.

The Q-T interval varies inversely with the heart rate: the faster the heart rate, the shorter the Q-T interval. Formulas and tables define the relationship of the Q-T interval to heart rate and age and sex in humans.[10] The calculation of the corrected Q-T interval for the various heart rates has been discussed in the dog.[11] The Q-T interval alone in veterinary medicine is not often helpful in diagnosis. The comparison of the Q-T intervals with those on previous electrocardiographic strips at approximately the same heart rates may be more helpful. A useful rule is that the Q-T interval should be less than half the preceding R-R interval[12] for normal sinus heart rates. If the heart rate slows below the approximate normal range (below 70 in the adult dog and below 160 in puppies and the cat), the maximal normal Q-T duration decreases accordingly, below half the preceding R-R interval. As the rate increases above the approximate normal range (above 160 in the adult dog and above 220 in puppies and the cat), the normal Q-T duration gradually exceeds half the preceding R-R interval.

The deviation of the Q-T interval is chiefly determined by an interplay of autonomic influences. Recent findings suggest that the heart rate and Q-T interval are governed separately by different sympathetic neurons that may or may not be activated together.[13] Corrections of the Q-T interval for heart rate appear to be applicable under circumstances such as exercise. During neurally mediated cardiovascular adjustments that do not involve exercise, the Q-T interval is maintained within narrow limits.[13]

MEAN ELECTRICAL AXIS

The electrical activity of the heart produces simultaneously many potentials of many directions in a three-dimensional field. The electrical axis refers to the average direction of this activation process during the cardiac cycle. Using the six limb leads (I, II, III, aVR, aVL, and aVF) and the different angles at which they record the heart's electrical activity, one can estimate the mean electrical axis (Fig. 3–2) in the frontal plane.

In the normal canine heart, the axis will be found to lie between +40° and +100°[14–15a] (Fig. 3–14). In the normal feline heart, the axis will be found to range widely between 0° and +160° (rounded off, −1.83° to +160°)[16] (Fig. 3–15). The latter axis range was determined by adding and subtracting 1.96 standard deviations from the mean in 48 normal cats. Values calculated from standard deviations are

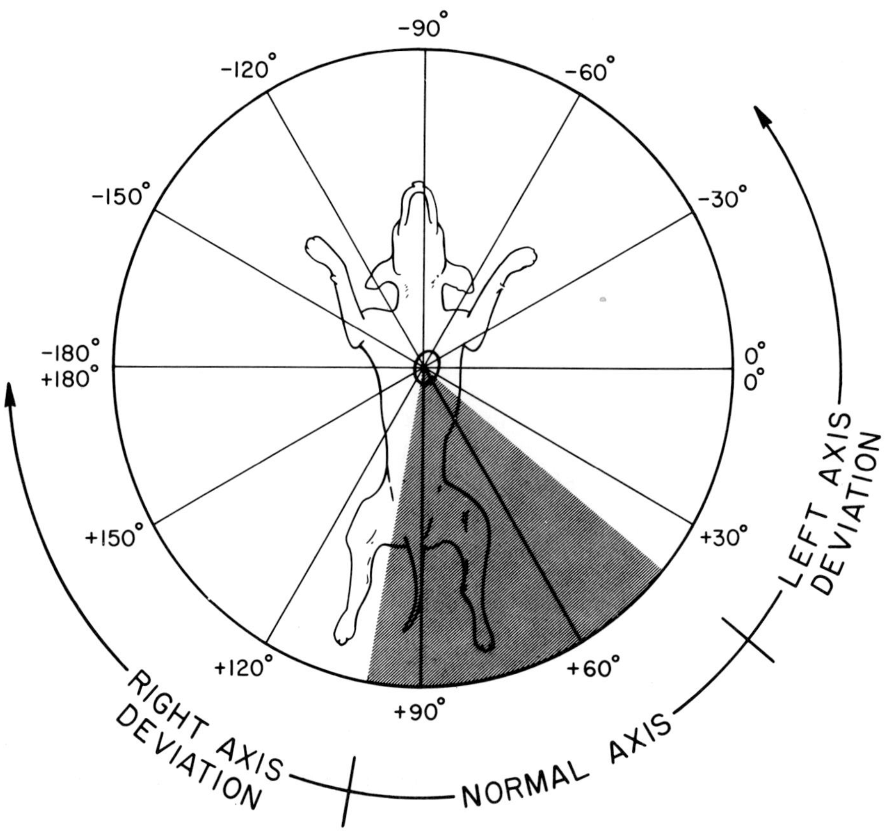

Fig. 3–14. In the dog, the normal mean electrical axis in the frontal plane is from +40° to +100°. If the axis becomes less than +40°, this is called left axis deviation; if greater than +100°, right axis deviation.

accurate especially if data are "normally" distributed. The data from this study of 48 cats were "normally" distributed.[16] Such a wide range in the electrical axis is consistent with the findings of other studies in the literature.[14,17–20]

The primary clinical significance of the mean electrical axis in dogs and cats is to establish criteria for right ventricular enlargement and for various intraventricular conduction defects.[19,21] If the axis becomes less than +40° in the dog, this is called left axis deviation. If the axis shifts to greater than the normal range, such as greater than +100° in the dog, this is called right axis deviation. When the axis deviation is so severe, such as −90°, it could represent either severe left axis deviation or very severe right axis deviation. The type of axis deviation can sometimes be determined by evaluating the clinical picture (e.g., the thoracic radiograph may indicate the chamber that is enlarged). Left or right axis deviation may indicate a conduction abnormality or enlargement of the respective ventricle. For example, in cats with hypertrophic cardiomyopathy, a left axis deviation of −60° indicates either a block of the left anterior fascicle of the conduction system and/or left ventricular hypertrophy.

The thoracic shape of various dog breeds affects the mean electrical axis.[22] Narrow-chested dogs, e.g., Collies, Poodles, and German Shepherds, have a more vertical and constant axis. Broad-chested dogs, e.g., Cocker Spaniels and Boxers, have a more horizontal and variable heart axis. The broad-chested Dachshund is an exception; its axis is usually vertical.

The reason for the variation of the cat's mean electrical axis as compared with the dog's is unknown. The most likely explanation is that the ventricular activation process from cat to cat is just different.[23] The absence of a strong mediastinum in the cat may make the heart easily susceptible to positional changes.[18] This positional change can be aggravated by changes in total weight of the heart (hypertrophy or dilatation), pneumothorax, abdominal distention, and even heart rate. Further studies may later show the electrical axis to be more accurate in sternal recumbency. The electrical axis of cats in sternal recumbency (−8° to +148°) tends to be slightly leftward compared with that in lateral recumbency, but the difference is not significant. The axis calculation is still quite useful in the cat, however, especially when serial electrocardiograms are compared.

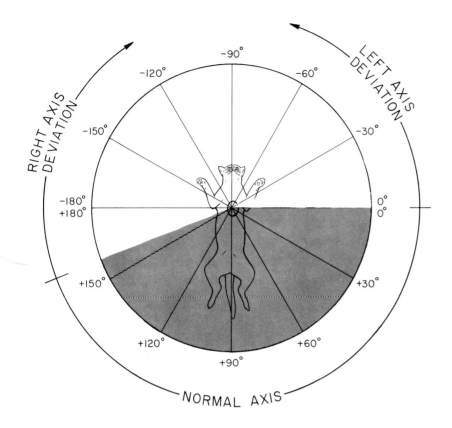

Fig. 3–15. In the cat, the normal mean electrical axis in the frontal plane is from 0° to +160°. If the axis becomes less than 0°, this is called left axis deviation; if greater than +160°, right axis deviation.

METHODS FOR DETERMINING THE ELECTRICAL AXIS

The most accurate method for determining the mean electrical axis of the QRS complex is to measure the net area rather than the amplitude of the various waves of the QRS complex. The determination of the net areas of the QRS complex is quite difficult, however. The size of the deflections is then used to calculate the mean electrical axis. When comparing deflections in the bipolar leads with those in the augmented unipolar limb leads, remember to multiply the voltages in the augmented unipolar leads (aVR, aVL, aVF) by 1.15 for the dog and 1.26 for the cat.[14]

There are three basic methods for estimating the mean electrical axis in the frontal plane:

1. Find an isoelectric lead, the algebraic sum of the QRS deflections being zero.
2. Choose the lead with the largest net QRS deflection.
3. Measure the algebraic sum of the QRS deflections in lead I and lead III and plot the values on the triaxial system. Since this method can be too cumbersome for routine use, the values can be plotted using the tables in Appendix B.[10]

Finding the isoelectric lead (Figs. 3–16 and 3–17)

All six standard leads should be inspected to see whether one can be found where the algebraic sum of the QRS deflections is zero. This is called the isoelectric lead. If this lead is found, the mean electrical forces must be directed perpendicular to the axis of the lead (Figs. 3–16 and 3–17). The lead perpendicular to the isoelectric lead can then be taken as the electrical axis. For example, if the isoelectric lead is found in lead I, the electrical axis is parallel with aVF. The net value (plus or minus) of the major deflection in aVF determines the deviation of the electrical axis, which would be the +90° or −90° (Fig. 3–16). This is the simplest and most practical method of obtaining the electrical axis. If two leads are isoelectric, the smaller isoelectric lead is preferable. When no isoelectric lead is present, one of the other two methods should be used.

All the leads will often be isoelectric in the cat and occasionally in the dog (Figs. 3–18 and 3–19). When this happens, the electrical axis cannot be calculated in the frontal plane.

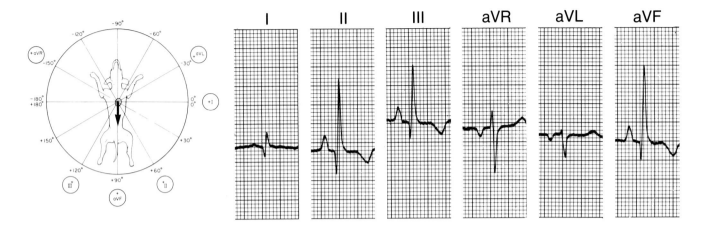

Fig. 3–16. The mean electrical axis in this canine electrocardiogram is +90°. Lead *I* is isoelectric. The lead perpendicular to lead I is *aVF* (see axis chart). Since lead aVF is positive, the axis calculates to be +90° (a normal axis).

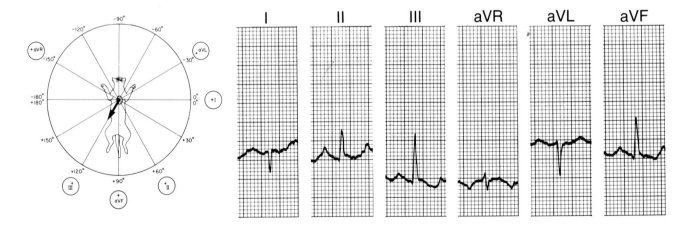

Fig. 3–17. The isoelectric lead in this feline electrocardiogram is *aVR*. On the axis chart, lead aVR is perpendicular to lead *III*. Since lead III is positive on this tracing, the axis is directed toward the positive pole of lead III (or +120°). An axis of +120° is normal in the cat.

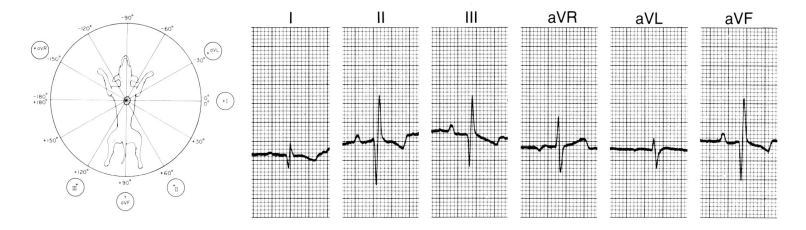

Fig. 3–18. Since all leads in this canine electrocardiogram are essentially isoelectric, the electrical axis cannot be calculated. Precordial chest leads can often be used to provide some information on the true cardiac vector.

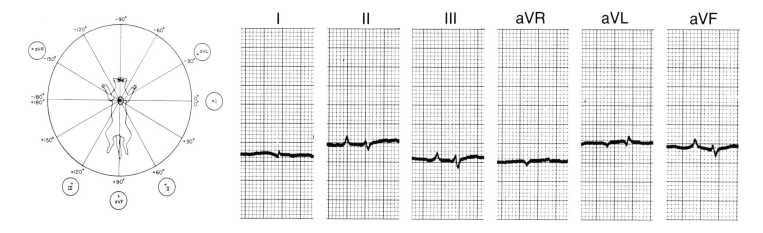

Fig. 3–19. The electrical axis in this feline electrocardiogram cannot be calculated because all leads are isoelectric.

Estimating the axis by major deflection (Figs. 3–20 and 3-21)

The mean electrical axis can be estimated to the nearest 30° by a simple general inspection of leads I, II, and III. The procedure involves choosing the lead with the largest net QRS deflection. This QRS deflection will be relatively parallel with the axis of this lead (Fig. 3–20). If the QRS deflection is upward, the axis is projected along the positive half of the lead axis. If the QRS deflection is downward, the axis is directed along the negative half of the lead axis. The same method can be applied when the QRS deflections in two of the leads are equal; the axis will be between the two lead axes (Fig. 3–21).

The QRS deflection method of estimating the mean electrical axis is only a general indicator and is not always precise. Greater accuracy in determining the electrical axis is possible by using the next method outlined.

Plotting the lead I and lead III values (Fig. 3–22)

A precise method for determining the mean electrical axis involves measuring the net amplitudes in lead I and the net amplitudes in lead III. When the triaxial system (Fig. 3–22) is used, the point representing the net value obtained is marked off from the zero point on lead I; this procedure is repeated for the sum of the deflections in

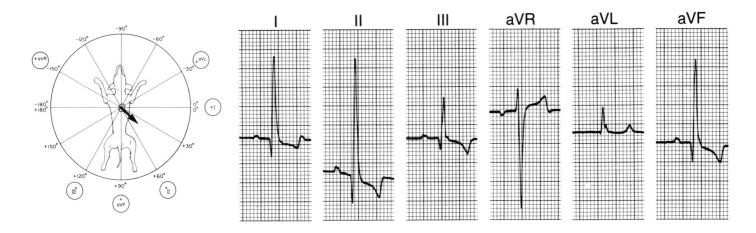

Fig. 3–20. In this canine electrocardiogram, no lead is isoelectric. Lead *II* has the largest QRS deflection. The electrical axis should be relatively parallel with the axis of lead II. Since lead II is positive, the axis is directed toward +60°. Lead *aVL* is perpendicular to lead II. Since aVL is more positive than negative, the axis is less than +60° or toward the positive pole of lead aVL. The axis is closer to +40°.

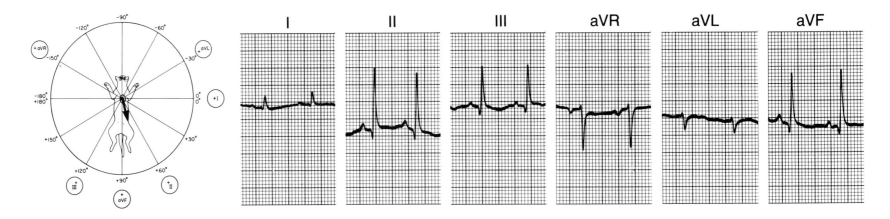

Fig. 3–21. In this feline electrocardiogram, leads *II* and *aVF* QRS complexes are of almost equal amplitude. The electrical axis will be between the two lead axes (or +75°).

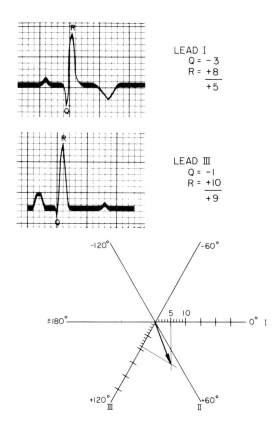

LEAD I
Q = −3
R = +8
――――
+5

LEAD III
Q = −1
R = +10
――――
+9

Fig. 3–22. Plotting the lead *I* and lead *III* values for calculating the mean electrical axis. The positive and negative deflections for each lead are added (I = +5; III = +9). Perpendicular lines are then followed from the positive or negative point determined for each lead on the triaxial system. A line drawn from the center of the triaxial system to the point of the intersected perpendicular lines gives the direction and relative magnitude of the mean QRS vector (approximately +70°).

lead III. Perpendiculars are then followed from these two points to their intersection. A line drawn from the center to this intersection represents the QRS axis. Since this method can be cumbersome for routine use, the values can be plotted using the tables in Appendix B.[10]

REFERENCES

1. Burch, G.E., and DePasquale, N.P.: *A History of Electrocardiography.* Chicago, Year Book Medical Publishers, 1964.
2. Silber, E.N., and Katz, L.N.: *Heart Disease.* New York, Macmillan, 1975.
3. Selzer, A.: *Principles of Clinical Cardiology: An Analytical Approach.* 2nd Edition. Philadelphia, W.B. Saunders, 1983.
4. Johnson, J.C., Horan, L.G., Flowers, N.C.: Diagnostic accuracy of the electrocardiogram. Cardiovasc. Clin., *8*:25, 1977.
5. Resnekov, L. (chairman), et al.: Task Force IV: Use of electrocardiograms in practice. Am. J. Cardiol., *41*:170, 1978.
6. Listing of Essential Knowledge and Skills for Electrocardiographic Readers and Teachers. Bethesda, Maryland, American College of Cardiology, 1976.
7. Goldman, M.J.: *Principles of Clinical Electrocardiography.* 11th Edition. Los Altos, Calif., Lange Medical Publications, 1982.
8. Tilley, L.P.: *Basic Canine Electrocardiography.* Milton, Wis., The Burdick Corp., 1978.
9. Hamlin, R.L.: Relationship between PP and PQ intervals in the electrocardiogram of dogs. Am. J. Vet. Res., *33*:2441, 1972.
10. Friedman, H.H.: *Diagnostic Electrocardiography and Vectorcardiography.* 2nd Edition. New York, McGraw-Hill, 1977.
11. Musselman, E.E., and Hartsfield, S.M.: Complete atrioventricular heart block due to hypokalemia following ovariohysterectomy. Vet. Med. Small Anim. Clin., *71*:155, 1976.
12. Marriott, H.J.L.: *Practical Electrocardiography.* 6th Edition. Baltimore, Williams & Wilkins, 1977.
13. Davidowski, T.A., and Wolf, S.: The QT interval during reflex cardiovascular adaptation. Circulation, *69*:22, 1984.
14. Dubin, S., Beard, R., Staib, J., and Hunt, P.: Variation of canine and feline frontal plane QRS axes with lead choice and augmentation ratio. Am. J. Vet. Res., *38*:1957, 1977.
15. Hill, J.D.: The electrocardiogram in dogs with standardized body and limb positions. J. Electrocardiol., *1*:175, 1968.
15a. Musselman, E.E.: Computer analysis of the spatial angular parameters of the canine QRSsÊ loop from necropsy—verified normal dogs. J. Electrocardiol., *16*:253, 1983.
16. Gompf, R.E., and Tilley, L.P.: Comparison of lateral and sternal recumbent position for electrocardiography of the cat. Am. J. Vet. Res., *40*:1483, 1979.
17. Robertson, B.T., Figg, F.A., and Ewell, W.M.: Normal values for the electrocardiogram in the cat. Feline Pract., *2*:20, 1976.
18. Rogers, W.A., and Bishop, S.P.: Electrocardiographic parameters of the normal domestic cat. A comparison of standard limb leads and an orthogonal system. J. Electrocardiol., *4*:315, 1971.
19. Tilley, L.P., and Gompf, R.E.: Feline electrocardiography. Vet. Clin. North Am., *7*:257, 1977.
20. Coulter, D.B., and Calvert, C.A.: Orientation and configuration of vectorcardiographic QRS loops from normal cats. Am. J. Vet. Res., *42*:282, 1981.
21. Hahn, A.W. (chairman), Hamlin, R.L., and Patterson, D.F.: Standards for canine electrocardiography. The Academy of Veterinary Cardiology Committee Report, 1977.
22. Chastain, C.B., Riedesel, D.H., and Pearson, P.T.: McFee and Parungao orthogonal lead vectorcardiography in normal dogs. Am. J. Vet. Res., *35*:275, 1974.
23. Hamlin, R.L., and Smith, C.R.: Categorization of common domestic animals based upon their ventricular activation process. Ann. N.Y. Acad. Sci., *127*:195, 1965.

Section Two

Interpretation of P-QRS-T Deflections

4 Analysis of canine P-QRS-T deflections

NORMAL CANINE ELECTROCARDIOGRAM

The first and most important step in electrocardiographic interpretation is differentiating between normal and abnormal. The second step is differentiating between the various abnormal electrocardiographic patterns and their correlation with known cardiac entities. Reports on the normal canine electrocardiogram[1-6] have provided a basis for comparing electrocardiograms of dogs with cardiac lesions. Most of the publications on canine electrocardiography are related to cardiac disease processes. Therefore, more is known about the electrocardiograms of diseased dogs than about those of normal dogs.

Abnormalities in cardiac enlargement that are detected on the electrocardiogram require further definition with thoracic radiography or angiocardiography. Echocardiography in veterinary medicine recently has been proved useful in the noninvasive assessment of structure and function of such intracardiac structures as the ventricular chambers, left atrium, right and left atrioventricular valves, and aortic valves.[6a]

The establishment of valid normal electrocardiographic limits for the dog is more complex than most clinicians realize. The determination of valid normal electrocardiographic limits in man has been discussed in great detail by Simonson.[7] The main prerequisites for determining normal limits are (1) adequate sample size, (2) composition of the sample representative of the average healthy population, (3) use of a standard technique in recording values, and (4) adequate statistical evaluation. In most studies of canine electrocardiograms, at least one of these principles has been disregarded. A summary of the electrocardiographic normal limits[1-5] appears on p. 58.

Before the electrocardiogram can be interpreted, the terms abnormal, borderline, and criteria must be defined.[8] For each electrocardiographic measurement there is a normal zone, an abnormal zone, and a borderline zone. These zones can be selected only on the basis of electrocardiographic criteria.

Abnormal is used to describe an electrocardiographic feature that is outside the normal limit and has significantly greater prevalence in diseased than in otherwise similar but healthy animals. *Borderline* is used as a modifier for normal and abnormal. *Criteria* for describing the various electrocardiographic patterns can be used only when there are established sharp boundaries between "normal" and "abnormal." A list of criteria for the electrocardiogram not only should be absolutely complete and well established but also should include indications of the sensitivity and specificity of the patterns. To list the absolute criteria for the various electrocardiograms is beyond the scope of this textbook.

An important application of statistics is expressed by Bayes' theorem, which states that the probability that certain electrocardiographic criteria are indicative of a specific disease entity depends not only on the sensitivity and specificity of such criteria but also on the prior probability of that animal having such a disease as assessed by other nonelectrocardiographic criteria.[9] For example, assume that certain electrocardiographic criteria for right heart enlargement have a sensitivity of 95% and a specificity of 95% (false positives = 5%). This criteria appears to be excellent. The criteria is now applied to a survey of 1000 animals in whom the estimated prior probability of right heart enlargement (by nonelectrocardiographic, epidemiologic criteria) is 10%. Therefore, 95% (sensitivity) of the 100 abnormal cases = 95; 5% (false positives) of the 900 normal cases = 45. The total abnormal electrocardiograms = 140. The positive predictive accuracy, however, = 45/140, or 68%.[9,10] The same criteria can be used to evaluate a group of 100 animals with pulmonic stenosis. The prior probability of right ventricular enlargement by nonelectrocardiographic criteria is at least 95%. Therefore, 95% (sensitivity) of 95 animals (90.25) plus 5% (false positive) of 5 animals (0.25 animals) gives a total recognition rate of 90.5. In this example, the positive predictive accuracy = 90.25/90.5, or over 99%. It is thus rather obvious that prior probability is a major factor in predictive accuracy, even though sensitivity and specificity remain constant.[9,10]

This book's primary purpose is to present the clinician with features that are essential to electrocardiographic diagnosis. Based on the numerous publications on electrocardiography (see "References") and my experience with a large case load, the electrocardiographic features, associated causes, and therapy are outlined for each entity. They are discussed only when there is an important basis for diagnostic experience.

Rate
  70 to 160 beats/min for adult dogs
  Up to 180 beats/min for toy breeds
  Up to 220 beats/min for puppies

Rhythm
  Normal sinus rhythm
  Sinus arrhythmia
  Wandering SA pacemaker

Measurements (lead II, 50 mm/sec, 1 cm = 1 mv)
  P wave
    Width: maximum, 0.04 second (2 boxes wide)
    Height: maximum, 0.4 mv (4 boxes tall)
  P-R interval
    Width: 0.06 to 0.13 second (3 to 6½ boxes)
  QRS complex
    Width: maximum, 0.05 second (2½ boxes) in small breeds
          maximum, 0.06 second (3 boxes) in large breeds
    Height of R wave*: maximum, 3.0 mv (30 boxes) in large breeds
          maximum, 2.5 mv (25 boxes) in small breeds
  S-T segment
    No depression: not more than 0.2 mv (2 boxes)
    No elevation: not more than 0.15 mv (1½ boxes)
  T wave
    Can be positive, negative, or biphasic
    Not greater than one fourth amplitude of R wave
  Q-T interval
    Width: 0.15 to 0.25 second (7½ to 12½ boxes) at normal heart rate; varies with heart rate (faster rates have shorter Q-T intervals and vice versa)

Electrical axis (frontal plane)
  +40° to +100°

Precordial chest leads (values of special importance)
  CV_5RL (rV_2): T wave positive
  CV_6LL (V_2): S wave not greater than 0.8 mv (8 boxes), R wave not greater than 2.5 mv (25 boxes)*
  CV_6LU (V_4): S waves not greater than 0.7 mv (7 boxes), R wave not greater than 3.0 mv (30 boxes)*
  V_{10}: negative QRS complex, T wave negative except in Chihuahua

*Not valid for thin deep-chested dogs under 2 years of age.

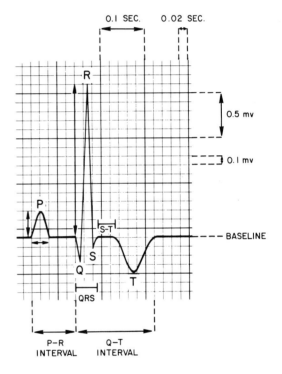

Fig. 4–1. Close-up of a normal canine lead II P-QRS-T complex with labels and intervals, *P*, 0.04 second by 0.3 mv; *P-R*, 0.1 second; *QRS*, 0.05 second by 1.7 mv; *S-T* segment and *T* wave, normal; *Q-T*, 0.18 second.

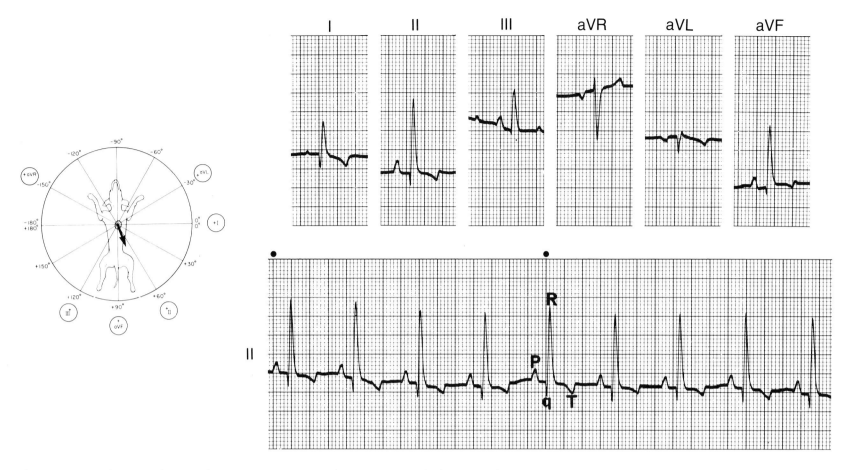

Fig. 4–2. Normal canine electrocardiogram. Heart rate, 165 beats/min. Heart rhythm, normal sinus. Complexes and intervals: *P*, 0.04 second by 0.3 mv; *P-R*, 0.08 second; *QRS*, 0.05 second by 1.9 mv; *S-T* segment and *T* wave, normal; *Q-T*, 0.16 second. Mean electrical axis, +70°.

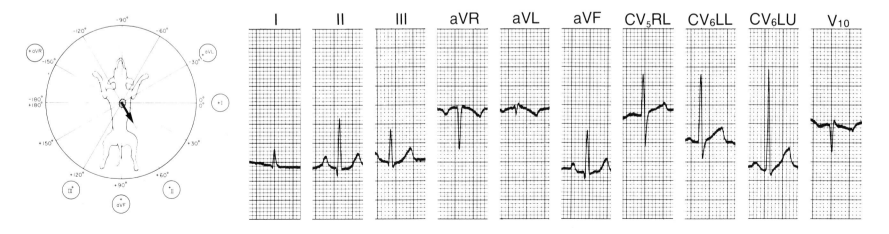

Fig. 4–3. Normal canine electrocardiogram illustrating the bipolar standard leads *(I, II, III)*, the augmented unipolar limb leads *(aVR, aVL, aVF)*, and the unipolar precordial chest leads *(CV₅RL, CV₆LL, CV₆LU, and V₁₀)*. Mean electrical axis, +60°.

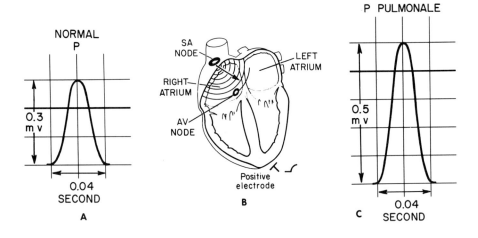

Fig. 4–4. The initial portion of the P wave is produced primarily by the right atrium (B). In right atrial enlargement (C) the mean P vector is of increased magnitude and is rotated more to the right.

Right atrial enlargement

The P wave represents atrial depolarization. In right atrial enlargement, it is of increased amplitude in leads II, III, and aVF. The term *enlargement* is used because tall P waves are seen in conditions causing right atrial hypertrophy and/or dilatation.

Electrocardiographic features

1. The P wave is greater than 0.4 mv (4 boxes).[2]
2. The P wave is of 0.04 second (2 boxes) or less duration.
3. The P wave is usually tall, slender, and peaked, especially in chronic pulmonary disease (often called *P pulmonale*).
4. A slight depression of the baseline following the P wave is sometimes seen in atrial enlargement. This represents atrial repolarization and is called the T_a wave. The T_a wave can also be seen in very rapid heart rates.[11]

Associated conditions

The term P pulmonale is not always specific for right atrial enlargement or pulmonary disease; for example, a rapid heart rate alone can cause an increase in amplitude of the P wave and simulate P pulmonale.

1. Chronic respiratory disease, e.g., bronchitis, pneumonia, and especially collapsed trachea
2. Various congenital heart defects, e.g., interatrial septal defect and tricuspid dysplasia[12,13]

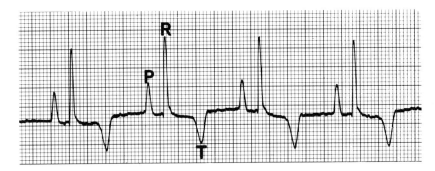

Fig. 4–5. Right atrial enlargement in a dog with collapsed trachea. The P waves are 0.7 mv (7 boxes) in amplitude.

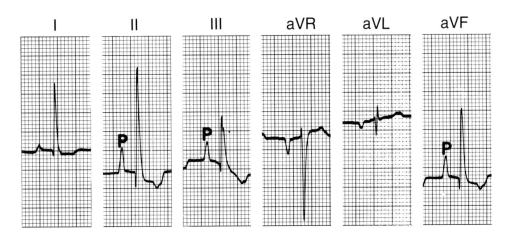

Fig. 4–6. Right atrial enlargement in a dog with severe chronic bronchitis. The P waves are tall in leads *II, III,* and *aVF.*

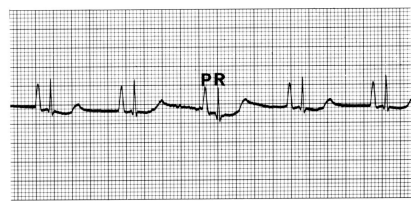

Fig. 4–7. Right atrial enlargement in a dog with collapsed trachea. Note the T_a wave (depression of the baseline following the P wave).

Left atrial enlargement

The latter portion of the P wave is produced primarily by the left atrium (Fig. 4–8). In left atrial enlargement, the P wave is of increased duration, best seen in lead II. The P wave pattern, which is most often associated with mitral valvular disease, is called *P mitrale*. The P wave is often notched from superimposition of the asynchronous right and left atrial conduction. In man, P wave morphology has been correlated with left atrial appendage cell size, atrial fibrosis and echocardiographic measurement of left atrial size. Mitral valve disease leads to a hemodynamic insult to the left atrium that injures and destroys some cells. The increased pressure and/or volume load leads to cellular hypertrophy and atrial dilatation which results in death of some atrial cells with replacement fibrosis. The percent of fibrosis is roughly correlated with the length of the P wave.[13a]

Electrocardiographic features

1. The duration of the P wave is greater than 0.04 second (2 boxes).[2]
2. Notching of the P wave itself is not abnormal unless the wave is also wide.

Associated conditions

1. Wide and notched P wave, also attributable to disturbances in the conduction pathway from the SA to the AV node.[14] The term P mitrale can be misleading since mitral valvular disease is not always present. In most cases, however, mitral valvular disease is the usual cause of P mitrale.
2. Acquired mitral valvular insufficiency
3. Various congenital heart defects, e.g., mitral valvular insufficiency, aortic stenosis, ventricular septal defect, and patent ductus arteriosus[12]

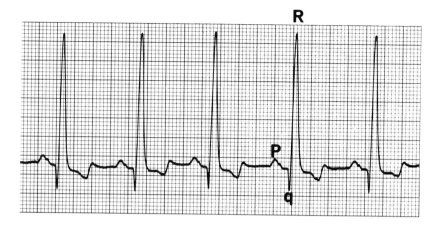

Fig. 4–9. Left atrial enlargement in a dog with chronic mitral valvular insufficiency. The P waves are wide (0.06 sec, or 3 boxes) and notched.

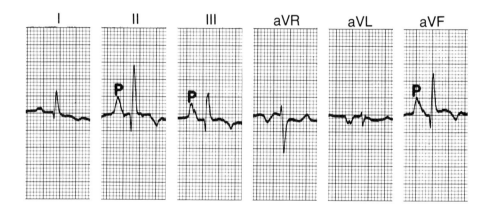

Fig. 4–10. Left atrial enlargement in a dog with chronic mitral valvular insufficiency. The P waves are wide and notched in leads *II, III,* and *aVF.*

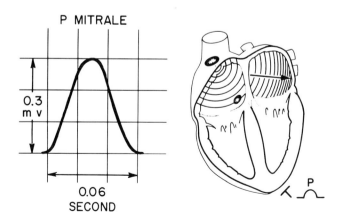

Fig. 4–8. Left atrial enlargement. The mean P vector is shifted somewhat posteriorly and is of increased duration because the left atrium is activated later.

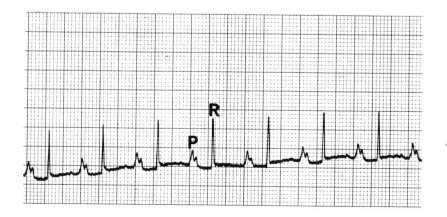

Fig. 4–11. Left atrial enlargement. Notching of the P waves can easily be seen. The P waves are also wide.

Biatrial enlargement

In biatrial enlargement, the P wave is of increased amplitude and duration. These changes could also occur in right atrial enlargement with an intra-atrial or interatrial conduction defect in the left atrium. The diagnosis of atrial enlargement from the electrocardiogram is not always accurate. There is considerable normal variation in the voltage, duration, morphology, and direction of the P wave. For example, giant breeds (e.g., St. Bernards) can sometimes have normal P waves that are 0.045 second (2½ boxes) in duration. The P wave is also very sensitive to autonomic influences. An increase in the heart rate alone may cause increased voltage of the P wave. Because conditions other than hypertrophy or enlargement cause P wave changes, the term *abnormality* may be more correct to indicate changes in P wave morphology.[14]

Electrocardiographic features

1. The P wave is greater than 0.4 mv (4 boxes) and wider than 0.04 second (2 boxes).[1]
2. Notching or slurring of the P wave is often present.

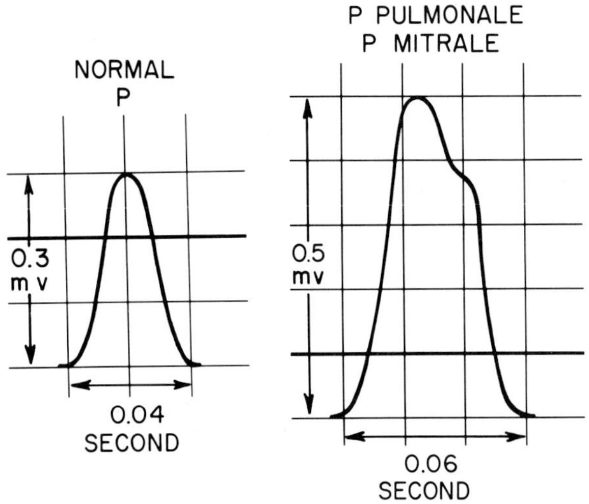

Associated conditions

1. Chronic mitral and tricuspid valvular insufficiency, or chronic mitral valvular insufficiency with accompanying pulmonary congestion, causing secondary pulmonary hypertension and right atrial enlargement
2. Various congenital heart defects, especially those in combinations

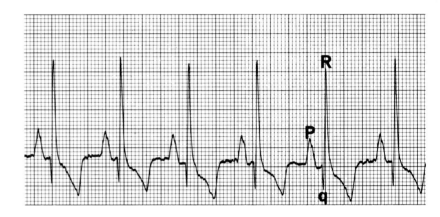

Fig. 4–13. Biatrial enlargement in a dog with chronic mitral and tricuspid valvular insufficiency. The P waves are both abnormally wide (0.06 sec, or 3 boxes) and abnormally tall (0.7 mv, 7 boxes).

Fig. 4–12. Biatrial enlargement. There is both increased amplitude and increased duration of the P wave.

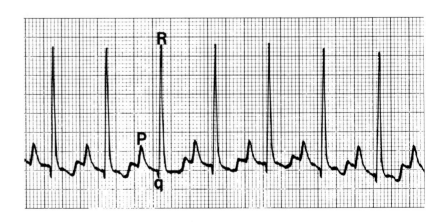

Fig. 4–14. Biatrial enlargement. Note the tall and wide P waves. The depression of the baseline (T$_a$ wave) following the P wave can be associated with the fast heart rate, or it can represent atrial repolarization.

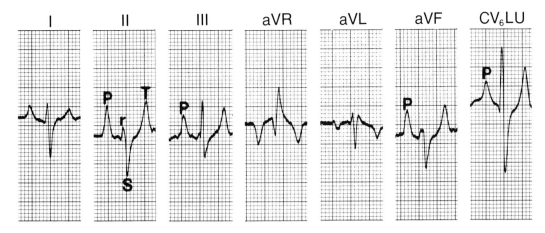

Fig. 4–15. Biatrial enlargement in a dog with more than one congenital heart defect. Note the tall and wide P waves in leads *II, III, aVF,* and *CV₆LU*.

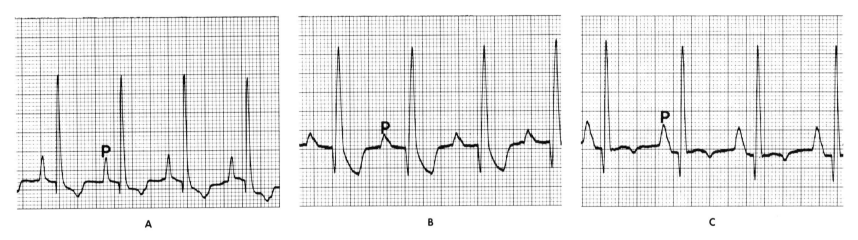

Fig. 4–16. **A,** Right atrial enlargement, tall P waves. **B,** Left atrial enlargement, wide and notched P waves. **C,** Biatrial enlargement, combined criteria for **A** and **B,** wide and tall P waves. A Tₐ wave is present (depression of the baseline following the P wave), indicating right atrial enlargement.

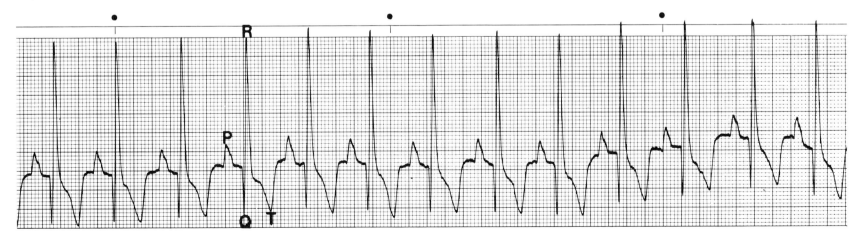

Fig. 4–17. Biatrial enlargement in a large-breed dog with primary myocardial disease (dilated cardiomyopathy).

Right ventricular enlargement

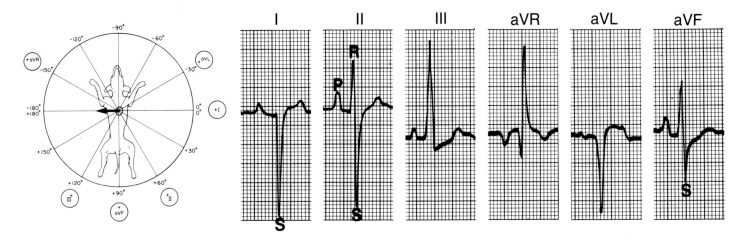

Fig. 4–18. Severe right ventricular enlargement in a dog with tetralogy of Fallot. There is abnormal right axis deviation ($-180°$). The S waves are large in leads *I, II,* and *aVF.*

Usually it is not possible to distinguish between ventricular hypertrophy and dilatation on the electrocardiogram, so the term *enlargement* is preferred. The heart is composed mainly of left ventricle. Because of the order of depolarization and the dominance of the left ventricle, the right ventricle must be markedly enlarged to cause changes on the electrocardiogram. Right ventricular enlargement therefore is often not detectable by electrocardiography.

Electrocardiographic features*

1. When any three of the following features are present, right ventricular enlargement can be diagnosed with a low incidence of false-positive results.[17]
   a. S wave in lead CV_6LL greater than 0.8 mv (8 boxes)
   b. Mean electrical axis of the QRS complex in the frontal plane 103° and clockwise
   c. S wave in lead CV_6LU greater than 0.7 mv (7 boxes)
   d. S wave in lead I greater than 0.05 mv (½ box)
   e. R/S ratio in CV_6LU less than 0.87
   f. S wave in lead II greater than 0.35 mv (3½ boxes)
   g. S waves in leads I, II, III, and aVF
   h. Positive T wave in lead V_{10} (except in Chihuahua)
   i. W-shaped QRS complex in V_{10}

2. Other patterns are characteristic of right ventricular enlargement:
   a. Right atrial enlargement (tall P waves)
   b. Right bundle branch block often difficult to differentiate from right ventricular enlargement
   c. Right ventricular enlargement, suggested by the presence of deep Q waves in leads I, II, III, and aVF greater than 0.5 mv (5 boxes), especially in leads II and aVF (This pattern may be normal in certain thin-chested breeds[13] [Fig. 4–21].)
   d. Acute cor pulmonale[9] (Fig. 4–22), a right ventricular enlargement pattern with secondary repolarization changes S-T segment and T wave (P pulmonale and sinus tachycardia are sometimes seen.)

Associated conditions

1. Certain congenital cardiac defects, e.g., pulmonic stenosis, tetralogy of Fallot, reverse-shunting patent ductus arteriosus, and tricuspid dysplasia[12,13,20]
2. Heartworm disease, most often severe or in congestive heart failure[20a]
3. Mitral and tricuspid valvular insufficiency
4. Acute cor pulmonale secondary to pulmonary embolism, e.g., after chemotherapy for adult heartworms, right atrial hemangiosarcoma, or renal amyloidosis[21,22]
5. Occasionally, chronic diffuse pulmonary disease

*References 2, 13, 15–19.

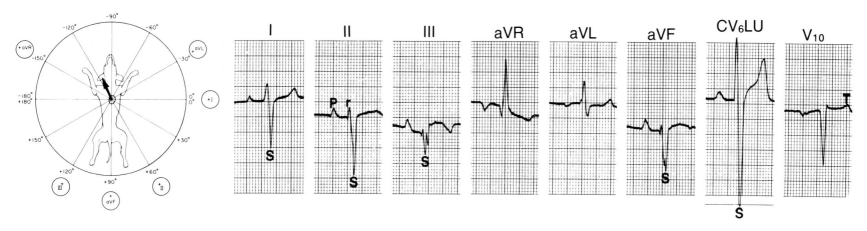

Fig. 4–19. Severe right ventricular enlargement in a dog with pulmonic stenosis. There is a right axis deviation of approximately −110°. Note the large S waves in leads *I, II, III, aVF,* and *CV₆LU*. The T wave is positive in *V₁₀*.

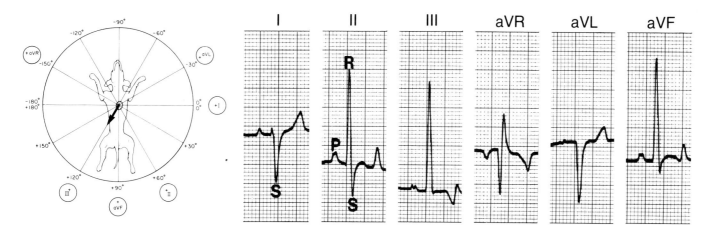

Fig. 4–20. Right ventricular enlargement in a dog with pulmonic stenosis. There is abnormal right axis deviation (+120°). The deflection of the S waves in leads *I* and *II* is large.

Right ventricular enlargement—cont'd

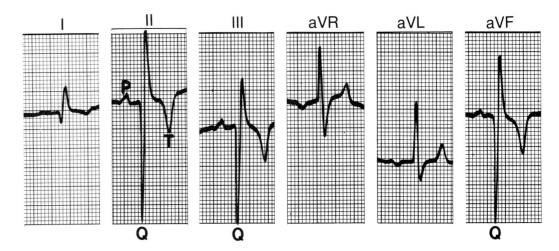

Fig. 4–21. Probable right ventricular enlargement in a Doberman Pinscher with primary myocardial disease (dilated form). There are deep Q waves, in leads *II*, *III*, and *aVF*. This pattern is sometimes associated with the dilated form of cardiomyopathy.

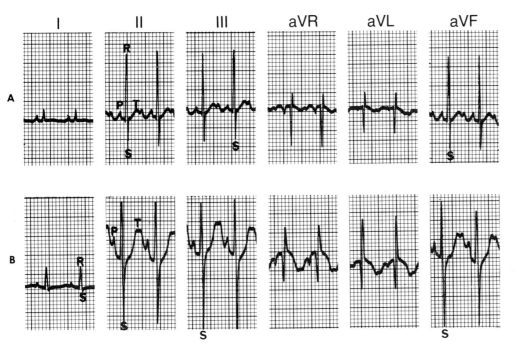

Fig. 4–22. Acute cor pulmonale in a dog with heartworm disease. Paper speed, 25 mm/sec. **A,** Before chemotherapy for the adult heartworms. Right ventricular enlargement is present (large S waves in leads *II, III,* and *aVF*). The mean electrical axis is +75°. **B,** Three days after chemotherapy, coughing was present from pulmonary embolism. The sudden pulmonary hypertension results in right ventricular dilatation. An S wave has formed in lead *I;* and S waves are now larger in leads *II, III,* and *aVF*. Note also the increased height of the P waves and the T waves. The electrical axis is markedly deviated.

Left ventricular enlargement

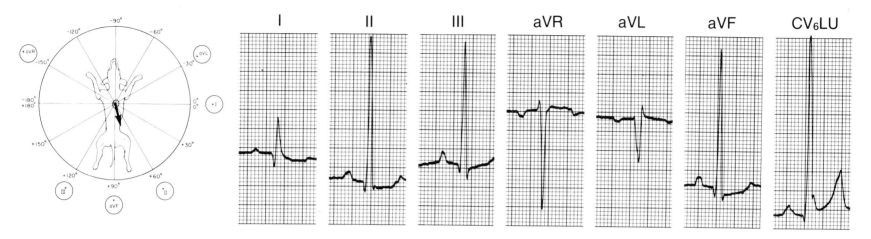

| I | II | III | aVR | aVL | aVF | CV₆LU |

Fig. 4–23. Left ventricular enlargement (dilatation) in an 8-year-old Poodle with mitral insufficiency. There are tall R waves in leads *II, III, aVF,* and *CV₆LU*. The QRS duration is wide (0.06 sec, or 3 boxes). The electrical axis is normal (+75°).

Left ventricular enlargement may indicate dilatation and/or hypertrophy. The left ventricle hypertrophies in three basic patterns: (1) concentric, a response to a systolic or pressure overload (resistance to outflow from ventricle), (2) eccentric, a response to a diastolic or volume overload of the ventricle, and (3) mixed pattern, involving the first two.

The main determinant of electrocardiographic voltage measurements is not ventricular wall thickness but muscle mass. In compensated pressure overload, cavity enlargement does not occur, and wall thickness is the main dimension contributing to ventricular mass. In volume overload, both wall thickness and cavity size increase; wall thickness may be only moderately increased, but it is cavity size that is the main dimension contributing to ventricular muscle mass. Voltage measurement is greater in animals with volume overload than in those with pressure overload.[10,23]

Due to the increased muscle mass in hypertrophy, the height of the R wave is increased, the QRS complex is delayed or altered in conduction, the S-T segment is depressed (endocardial ischemic change), and the T wave or repolarization process is changed.[2,16]

The increased voltage changes in left ventricular enlargement are due primarily to two factors: (1) with heart enlargement, the heart is closer to the chest wall so the voltage recorded (especially in the precordial leads) is greater and (2) an enlarged ventricle with an increased surface area and thickened wall produces greater potentials than does a normal ventricle.[14]

Prolongation of the QRS complexes occurs only with severe left ventricular enlargement. With left ventricular hypertrophy, the activation process in a thickened ventricle takes longer than in a normal left ventricle. Conduction disturbances also should be considered when there is a prolongation of the QRS complex.

An abnormal left axis deviation, another electrocardiographic feature of left ventricular enlargement, is not diagnostic alone for left ventricular enlargement. An abnormal left axis supports the diagnosis of left ventricular enlargement only when the voltage changes are present.

Because the electrocardiographic diagnosis of left ventricular enlargement is based primarily on increased QRS voltages, it should be understood that the voltage criteria can have some inaccuracy. The inaccuracy is related to the fact that limb, and especially precordial, lead voltage is influenced by the distance between the electrodes and the heart. In young, emaciated, or narrow-chested animals, the criteria for increased voltage are not as valid. Also, conditions such as thoracic effusion, pneumothorax, and obesity may reduce the amplitude of the QRS deflections recorded at the body surface.

Left ventricular enlargement—Cont'd

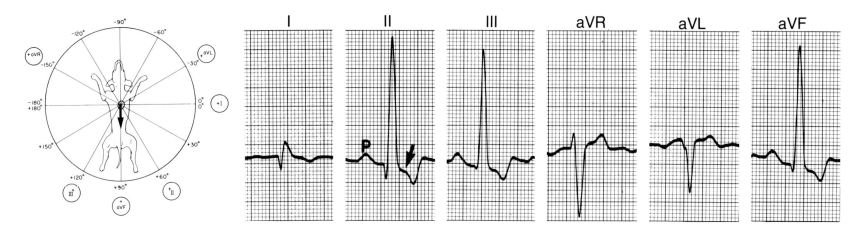

Fig. 4–24. Left ventricular enlargement in a dog with patent ductus arteriosus. The R waves are abnormally high in leads *II, III,* and *aVF*. The QRS duration is wide (0.08 sec, or 4 boxes). Note the S-T segment coving (arrow). The electrical axis is +90°. The P waves are wide (0.08 sec, or 4 boxes), suggesting left atrial enlargement.

Electrocardiographic features[1,2,16,24]

Left bundle branch block and anterior fascicular block must be differentiated from left ventricular enlargement.

1. In dogs under 2 years of age with narrow chest cavities, the R wave of the QRS complex should not be greater than 3.0 mv (30 boxes) in leads II and aVF. In older dogs, the R wave should not exceed 2.5 mv (25 boxes) in leads II, III, and aVF. The R wave should not exceed 3.0 mv (30 boxes) in CV_6LU or 2.5 mv (25 boxes) in CV_6LL.

2. The maximum width of the QRS in small and medium breeds is 0.05 second (2½ boxes); in large breeds, 0.06 second (3 boxes).

3. Displacement of the S-T segment occurs in a direction opposite the main QRS deflection. This causes the S-T segment to sag into the T wave (S-T coving).

4. Repolarization changes cause the T wave to be of increased amplitude (more than 25% larger than the R wave).

5. A mean electrical axis deviation in the frontal plane of less than +40° may be present.

6. Other patterns are characteristic of left ventricular enlargement:
   a. Left atrial enlargement (widened P waves), often seen with left ventricular enlargement
   b. R wave in lead I greater than in leads III and aVF, seen in concentric hypertrophy
   c. Increased amplitude of the R wave in leads I, II, and III, seen in eccentric hypertrophy and dilatation

Associated conditions[12]

1. Eccentric hypertrophy secondary to volume overload, e.g., mitral insufficiency, aortic insufficiency, ventricular septal defect, patent ductus arteriosus

2. Concentric hypertrophy secondary to pressure overload, e.g., aortic stenosis

3. Primary myocardial disease (dilated form of cardiomyopathy)[25]

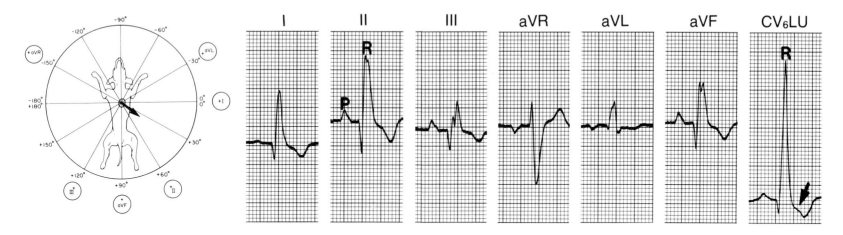

Fig. 4–25. Left ventricular enlargement in a dog with severe aortic stenosis. The QRS complexes are wide (0.08 sec, or 4 boxes) and notched. The R wave is tall (3.7 mv, or 37 boxes) in lead CV_6LU. The mean electrical axis is approximately +35°. Note the S-T coving (arrow).

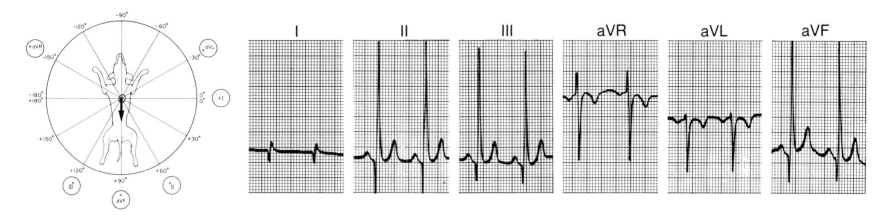

Fig. 4–26. Left ventricular enlargement in a 1-year-old Pomeranian with patent ductus arteriosus. The R waves are tall in leads *II, III,* and *aVF.* The QRS duration is 0.06 second (3 boxes). The electrical axis is normal (+90°). The deep Q waves in leads *II, III,* and *aVF* probably indicate right ventricular enlargement.

Biventricular enlargement

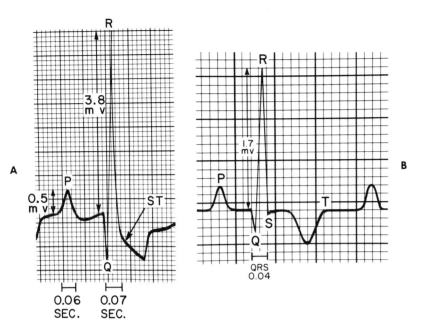

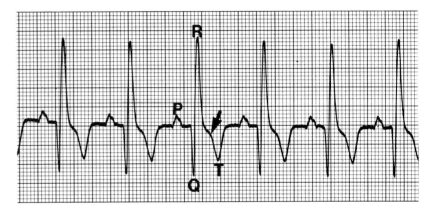

Fig. 4–27. Biventricular enlargement (**A**). A close-up of this lead II P-QRS-T complex reveals a tall and wide QRS, a deep Q wave, and S-T segment coving. Biatrial enlargement also is present (a wide and tall P wave). The P-QRS-T complex in **B** is normal for comparison purposes.

Fig. 4–28. Biventricular enlargement in a dog with primary myocardial disease; 0.5 cm = 1 mv (half sensitivity). There are tall and wide QRS complexes, deep Q waves, and S-T coving (arrow). The P waves are tall and wide.

Simultaneous enlargement of both ventricles is difficult to diagnose accurately by electrocardiography. The diagnosis of left ventricular enlargement is more accurate, whereas the concomitant electrocardiographic diagnosis of right ventricular enlargement is less reliable. This is readily explained by the fact that left ventricular forces can easily counteract any increased forces from an enlarged right ventricle. Also a normal electrocardiogram can be obtained from animals with biventricular enlargement since the potentials from the two hypertrophied ventricles may counterbalance each other.

The most reliable features for biventricular enlargement in man are left ventricular enlargement in the precordial chest leads plus a right axis deviation in the frontal plane.[9]

Electrocardiographic features[2,14]

1. Precordial chest leads show changes for both right (deep S waves in CV_6LL and CV_6LU) and left (tall R waves in CV_6LL and CV_6LU).

2. Left ventricular enlargement is seen on the electrocardiogram along with a right axis deviation (of more than $+103°$).

3. Left ventricular enlargement changes on the electrocardiogram are associated with high-amplitude R waves and increased QRS duration in CV_6LU. Deep Q waves in leads I, II, III, and aVF may indicate septal hypertrophy.

4. A normal electrocardiogram in the presence of severe cardiomegaly on thoracic radiographs may indicate biventricular enlargement (excluding pericardial effusion).

5. Deep Q waves in leads I, II, III, and aVF, along with left ventricular enlargement changes on the electrocardiogram, may indicate biventricular enlargement.

6. Left and right atrial enlargement changes often accompany these electrocardiographic changes.

Associated conditions

1. Mitral and tricuspid valvular insufficiency
2. Certain congenital cardiac defects, e.g., patent ductus arteriosus or mitral insufficiency[12]
3. Primary myocardial disease (dilated form of cardiomyopathy)[25]

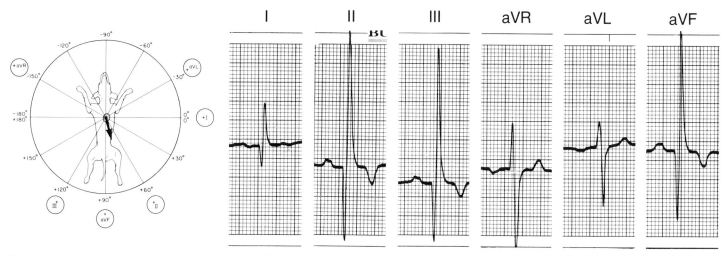

Fig. 4–29. Biventricular enlargement in a dog with patent ductus arteriosus. The QRS complexes are tall and wide with deep Q waves. The electrical axis is normal (+75°).

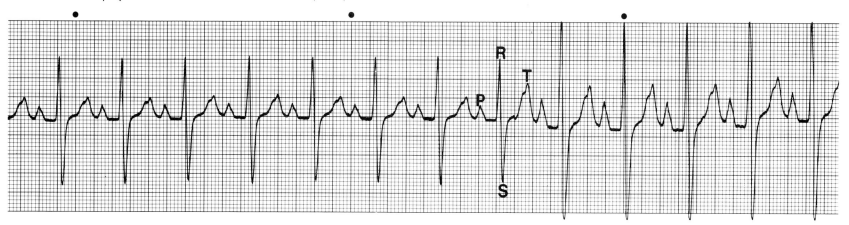

Fig. 4–30. Biventricular enlargement in a 5-year-old dog with patent ductus arteriosus, pulmonary hypertension, and right ventricular enlargement. The latter portion of this lead II strip is at a sensitivity of one (1 cm = 1 mv). The tall R waves (3 mv, or 30 boxes) and the wide QRS complexes (0.07 sec, or 3½ boxes) indicate left ventricular enlargement. The large S waves (present in leads I, III, and aVF) indicate right ventricular enlargement. In addition, note the tall and wide P waves.

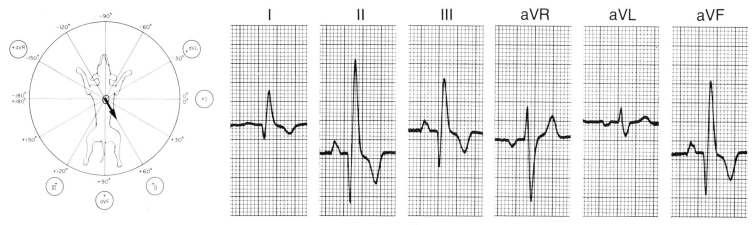

Fig. 4–31. Biventricular enlargement in a dog with chronic mitral and tricuspid insufficiency. The electrical axis is normal (+60°).

INTRAVENTRICULAR CONDUCTION DEFECTS

An intraventricular conduction defect results from a delay or block in one or more of the pathways of the conduction system below the bundle of His. The intraventricular conduction system is composed of three major conduction pathways (Fig. 4–32): (1) the right bundle branch, (2) the anterior fascicle, and (3) the posterior fascicle of the left bundle branch. A block or delay in conduction can occur in one, two, or all three pathways at the same time.

Normally the two ventricles depolarize practically simultaneously. The electrical impulse reaches both bundles at the same time, and the entire ventricular muscle is depolarized. A block or delay in conduction in any of the three major pathways causes the affected side to be depolarized late. This delay in the process of depolarization results in a configuration change of the QRS complex, lengthening the duration of the complex beyond normal limits in left and right bundle branch block. Normally, the early part of the QRS complex represents predominance of the left ventricular events, and the latter part only is of the right ventricular origin. In left bundle branch block, therefore, the changes will be in the whole of the complex, but in right branch block, the changes will be in the latter part of the QRS only.

The major forms of intraventricular block can be classified as follows:[9,26,27]

1. Bundle branch block: right, left (i.e., block in the main left bundle or in each of the two fascicles)
2. Fascicular block: left anterior, left posterior
3. Various combinations of block in the three major conduction pathways, e.g., right bundle branch with anterior or posterior fascicular
4. Block in all three conduction pathways, producing complete heart block

Many experimental studies have been done in dogs for the electrocardiographic analysis of intraventricular conduction defects, and the results have been applied to humans.* In their textbook on fascicular blocks, Rosenbaum and co-workers[27] explained the differences between conduction disturbances in dogs and clinical conduction disturbances in man. The differences are due mainly to the position of the heart within the chest of dogs and in humans. The right septal surface and the right ventricle in the dog are oriented more cranial (superior) than in man. The normal vertical position of the canine heart was made more horizontal in these authors' experiments to approximate that position in humans.

---

*References 27–37.

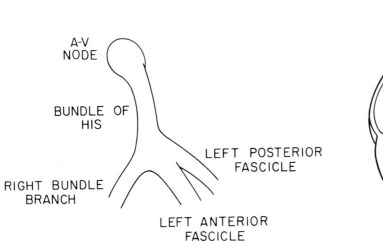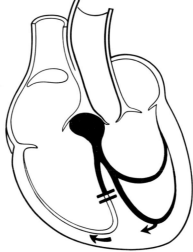

Fig. 4–32. Intraventricular conduction system. A block in the right bundle branch is illustrated, the most frequent form of intraventricular conduction defect in dogs. The right ventricle is stimulated by the impulse, which passes from the left bundle branch to the right side of the septum below the block. It is then activated with delay, causing the QRS complex to become wide and bizarre. (Right illustration from Phillips, R.E., and Feeney, M.K.: *The Cardiac Rhythms.* Philadelphia, W.B. Saunders, 1980, with permission.)

Left bundle branch block

Left bundle branch block is a delay or block of conduction in the left bundle branch, either in the *main branch* or at the level of the anterior and posterior *fascicles*. The two anatomic types cannot be distinguished from each other electrocardiographically. A supraventricular impulse activates the right ventricle first through the right bundle branch. The left ventricle is then activated late, causing the QRS complex to become wide and bizarre (Fig. 4–33).

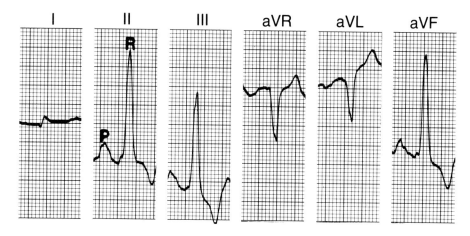

Fig. 4–34. Left bundle branch block and left ventricular hypertrophy in a dog with aortic stenosis diagnosed at necropsy. The QRS complexes are of 0.08 second duration (4 boxes). Left bundle branch block and severe left ventricular hypertrophy can occur simultaneously. No acceptable criteria are available to diagnose the two together.

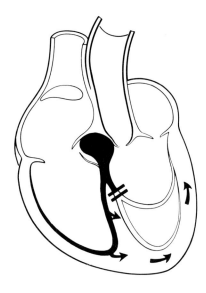

Fig. 4–33. Left bundle branch block located in the main branch. The impulse cannot enter the left bundle system and activate the left septal fibers. Therefore, the septum is initially depolarized from fibers arising from the distal portion of the right bundle branch, resulting in an initial vector oriented to the left. The left ventricle is then activated late, causing the QRS complex to become wide and bizarre. (From Phillips, R.E., and Feeney, M.K.: *The Cardiac Rhythms.* Philadelphia, W.B. Saunders, 1980, with permission.)

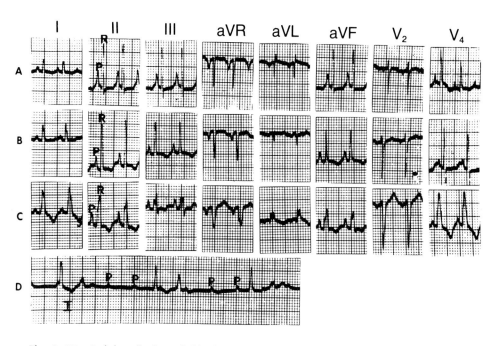

Fig. 4–35. Left bundle branch block and complete heart block in the canine heart. Paper speed, 25 mm/sec. **A,** Control: QRS duration normal. **B,** After cutting the posterior fascicle of the left bundle. **C,** After cutting the anterior fascicle: left bundle branch block; QRS duration now 0.08 second. **D,** After subsequently cutting the right bundle branch: complete heart block. (From Rosenbaum, M., et al.: The hemiblocks. Tampa, Fla., 1970, Tampa Tracings, Inc.; with permission.)

Left bundle branch block—cont'd

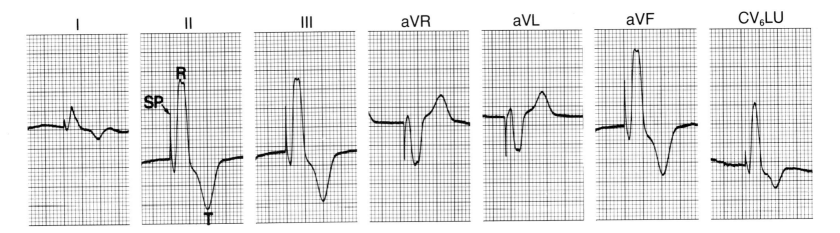

Fig. 4–36. Left bundle branch block pattern in a dog with a transvenous electrode wire in the right ventricle. In right ventricular stimulation, the left ventricle is stimulated with delay. The QRS complex width is increased to 0.10 second (5 boxes) and is positive in leads *I, II, III, aVF,* and *CV₆LU*. The pacemaker spike *(SP)* is the electrical impulse delivered by the artificial pacemaker.

Electrocardiographic features*

1. The QRS complex is of greater than 0.07 second duration in all dogs (0.07 sec or greater in toy breeds).

2. The QRS complex is wide and positive in leads I, II, III, and aVF and in leads over the left precordium (CV₆LL and CV₆LU).

3. The QRS complex is inverted in leads aVR, aVL, and CV₅RL.

4. A small Q wave is often present in lead I and the left precordial leads, even though initial QRS forces are right-to-left rather than normal left-to-right durations. This has also been documented in experimental left bundle branch block in dogs.[27]

5. The presence of first- or second-degree AV block may indicate involvement of the right bundle branch (Fig. 4–38).

6. Left bundle branch block must be differentiated from left ventricular enlargement. The absence of left ventricular enlargement on thoracic radiographs lends support to a diagnosis of isolated left bundle branch block.

7. Intermittent bundle branch block (tachycardia- or bradycardia-dependent) or bundle branch block alternans may be present in serial tracings or the same tracing[14,42,43] (Fig. 4–37).

Associated conditions

1. Severe underlying branch bundle disease (The cardiac lesion in most cases must be large because the left bundle branch is thick and extensive.)

2. Ischemic cardiomyopathy (arteriosclerosis of the coronary arteries,[39] myocardial infarction)

3. Primary myocardial disease (dilated form of cardiomyopathy)

4. Congenital subvalvular aortic stenosis (The lesion involves the septum and accompanying left bundle branch.)

5. Cardiac needle puncture for obtaining blood samples[38]

Treatment

1. Left bundle branch block, in and of itself, does not cause any hemodynamic abnormalities. Treatment is for the underlying condition.

---

*References 2, 27, 38–41.

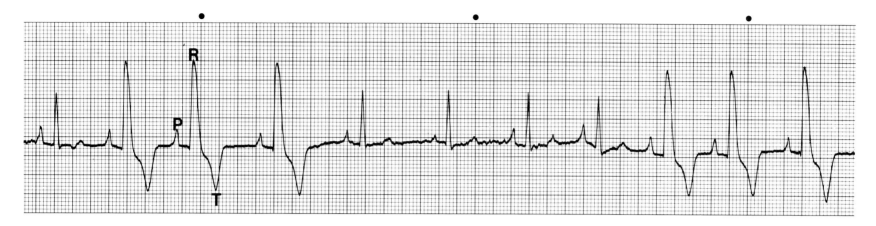

Fig. 4–37. Intermittent left bundle branch block in a Chihuahua. The QRS complexes are wider (0.07 to 0.08 sec) in the second, third, and fourth complexes and in the last three complexes.

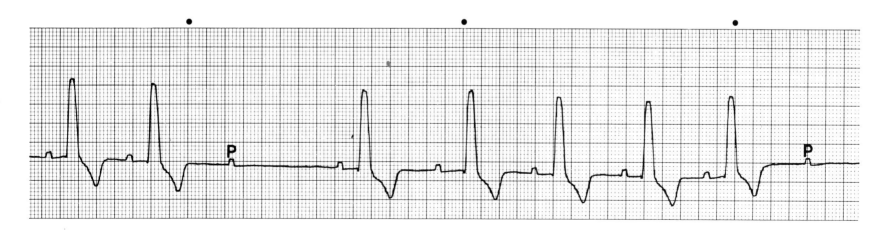

Fig. 4–38. Left bundle branch block and second-degree AV block (marked P waves). The blocked P waves indicate a probable intermittent right bundle branch block. An artificial pacemaker may be needed.

Right bundle branch block

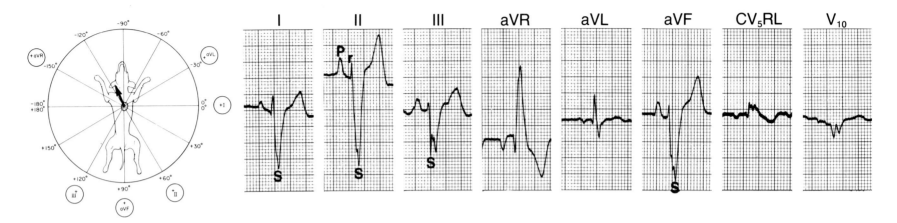

Fig. 4–39. Right bundle branch block in a dog with chronic mitral insufficiency. The QRS duration is 0.09 second (4½ boxes). There are large wide S waves in leads *I, II, III,* and *aVF.* The QRS in CV_5RL has a wide rsR′ pattern (M-shaped). A W-pattern is seen in lead V_{10}. There is a right axis deviation (−110°).

Right bundle branch block is a delay or block of conduction in the right bundle branch. The right ventricle is stimulated by the impulse, which passes from the left bundle branch to the right side of the septum below the block (Fig. 4–32). It is then activated with delay, causing the QRS complex to become wide and bizarre. The block can be located in the *proximal* portion of the right bundle branch (complete block) or more *peripheral* in the right bundle branch (incomplete block).

Electrocardiographic features[2,28,44,45]

1. The QRS complex is of greater than 0.07 second duration in all dogs (0.07 sec or greater in toy breeds) for complete right bundle branch block.
2. A right axis deviation is usually present.
3. The QRS complex is positive in aVR, aVL, and CV_5RL and has a wide RSR′ or rsR′ pattern (often M shaped) in CV_5RL.
4. The QRS complexes have large wide S waves in leads I, II, III, aVF, CV_6LL, and CV_6LU. An S wave or W pattern is usually seen in lead V_{10}.

An incomplete right bundle branch block can be diagnosed when any of features 2 to 4 are observed, but the QRS duration is within the normal limits.

5. Support can be given to the diagnosis of isolated right bundle branch block if diseases causing severe right ventricular enlargement are excluded from laboratory tests. For example, in most cases, the thoracic radiograph can be used to evaluate any right ventricular enlargement.

6. Intermittent bundle branch block (i.e., tachycardia- or bradycardia-dependent) or bundle branch block alternans may be present in serial tracings or in the same tracing[42,44,46] (Fig. 4–41).

7. The presence of first- or second-degree AV block may indicate involvement of the left bundle branch.

Associated conditions

1. Occasionally in normal and healthy dogs[2,39,44]
2. Congenital heart disease[28,39]
3. Chronic valvular fibrosis[39,44]
4. After surgical correction of a cardiac defect[47]
5. Cardiac needle puncture for obtaining blood samples[38]
6. After cardiac arrest[48]
7. Cardiac neoplasia, e.g., hemangiosarcoma or metastatic mammary gland tumor
8. Trauma
9. Incidental electrocardiographic finding with noncardiac conditions[44,45]
10. Incomplete right bundle branch block (This has been found in the Beagle [experimental mating] as a genetically determined localized variation in right ventricular wall thickness;[49] it may also be just focal hypertrophy of the right ventricle.[50])
11. Chronic *Trypanosoma cruzi* infection (Chagas' disease)[51]

Treatment

1. Right bundle branch block, in and of itself, does not cause hemodynamic problems. Therapy should be directed at the primary disease affecting the right ventricle.

2. Many times there is no evidence of a cardiac disease. The right bundle branch is anatomically vulnerable to injury since it is a thin strand of tissue and has a long undivided course.

3. The outcome of right bundle branch block is primarily dependent on whether either of the two fascicles of the left branch becomes involved. Complete heart block can then sometimes be the result and treatment is essential.

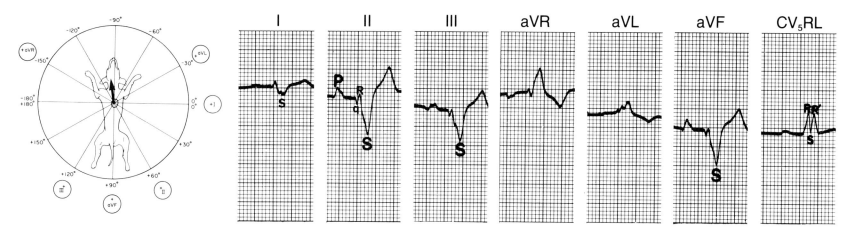

Fig. 4–40. Right bundle branch block in a normal dog. The QRS duration is 0.09 second (4½ boxes). Large and wide S waves are present in leads *I, II, III,* and *aVF*. A wide RSR' pattern is present in *CV₅RL*. There is a right axis deviation (−100°).

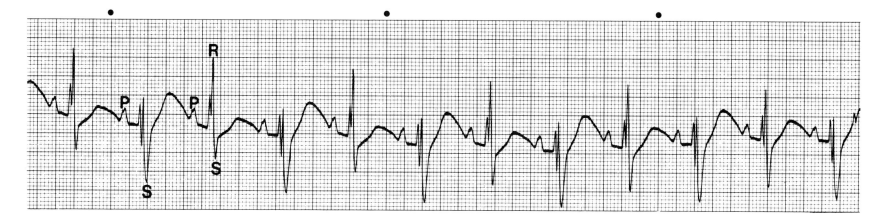

Fig. 4–41. Intermittent right bundle branch block from a dog under anesthesia. A right bundle branch block pattern (second, fourth, sixth, etc. complexes) (0.08 sec, or 4 boxes) alternates with the dog's own normal conduction (0.06 sec, or 3 boxes). This alternation in conduction was present only at certain heart rates.

Fascicular block

As described in Chapter 1, the left bundle branch divides into two interconnected pathways: the *anterior* and the *posterior fascicles*. The interconnection between them over the midseptal area is called the *septal fascicle*. The existence of these midseptal fibers and their possible contribution to fascicular block has been studied.[29,31]

A block in either the anterior or the posterior fascicle of the left bundle causes only a slight prolongation of left ventricular depolarization. The main effect is on the direction of the depolarization. The anterior and posterior fascicles each pass to the base of the corresponding papillary muscle. If the path to one of these papillary muscles is blocked, activation of the left ventricle can begin only at the other papillary muscle. The general direction of left ventricular depolarization is shifted toward the blocked fascicle and corresponding papillary muscle.

Fascicular blocks in the dog have been discussed but briefly in the literature.[2,16,52] Many of the reports of complete heart block in the veterinary literature describe only simultaneous block of the right bundle, anterior and posterior fascicles, and AV node or bundle of His. The uncommon occurrence of fascicular block in the dog can possibly be explained by either of two reasons: First, the normal vertical position of the canine heart produces less dramatic electrocardiographic changes than does the normal horizontal position of the human heart.[26,27] Second, experiments on canine hearts have shown that changes consistent with anterior fascicular block must include lesions in both the anterior and the septal branches.[31] The fascicular block patterns, then, must be related to a very diffuse lesion.

Left posterior fascicular block is the least common intraventricular conduction defect in man. The posterior fascicle is better protected because of its anatomy and greater blood supply. It is shorter and thicker than the anterior fascicle, is not located in the turbulent outflow tract, and has a dual blood supply.[14]

Because definitive clinical data are unavailable, the salient features for the electrocardiographic diagnosis of fascicular block can be only hypothesized. A basis of diagnosis must be extrapolated from reports in man and from experimental studies in dogs.*

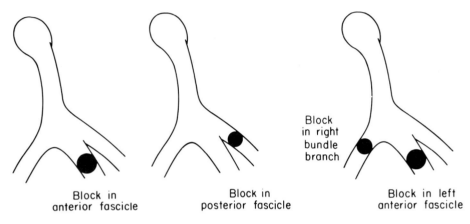

Fig. 4–42. Three forms of fascicular block.

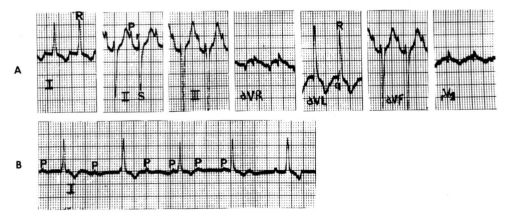

Fig. 4–43. Right bundle branch block with left anterior fascicular block in a dog. **A,** Paper speed, 25 mm/sec. The QRS duration is 0.08 second. Wide S waves are present in leads *II, III,* and *aVF.* An rsR' pattern in *rV₂ (CV₅RL)* completes the features for right bundle branch block. Left anterior fascicular block is illustrated by the marked left axis deviation (−60°), qR pattern in leads *I* and *aVL,* and rS deflections in *II, III,* and *aVF.* The prolonged P-R interval indicates impaired conduction in the posterior fascicle. **B,** After a new cut in the posterior fascicle, complete heart block occurs. (From Rosenbaum, M., et al.: The hemiblocks. Tampa, Fla., 1970, Tampa Tracings, Inc.; reprinted with permission.)

Electrocardiographic features

Left anterior fascicular block (Fig. 4–44). This can be recognized on the basis of the following combination of features:
1. QRS complex of normal duration
2. Marked left axis deviation in the frontal plane
3. Small q wave and tall R wave in leads I and aVL (small q waves may not be required)
4. Deep S waves in leads II, III, and aVF

Other causes of the left anterior fascicular pattern should be excluded, particularly ventricular pre-excitation, hyperkalemia, left ventricular hypertrophy, and an altered position of the heart within the thorax.

In man, new electrocardiographic criteria have been proposed.[53] The use of the proposed criteria requires that the tracings be obtained with three-channel electrocardiographs so that the relation between the QRS complexes in simultaneously recorded limb leads can be inspected. The proposed electrocardiographic criteria are (1) that the QRS complexes in leads aVR and aVL each end in an R wave, and (2) that the peak of the terminal R wave in lead aVR occur later than the peak of the terminal R wave in lead aVL.

Right bundle branch and left anterior fascicular block. This is recognized by the combination of electrocardiographic features given for each block (Fig. 4–43):

---

*References 14, 27, 29, 32, 35–37.

1. QRS complex duration wider than 0.07 second
2. Marked left axis deviation in the frontal plane
3. Wide and deep S waves in leads I, II, III, aVF, and CV_6LU
4. Tall R wave and small q wave in leads I and aVL
5. Wide rsR′ RSR′ pattern (often M shaped) in QRS complex in CV_5RL.

Associated conditions

1. Cardiomyopathy, e.g., hypertrophic cardiomyopathy[52]
2. Causes of left ventricular hypertrophy (left axis deviation not always due to the hypertrophied muscle, since the accompanying subendocardial fibrosis can affect the anterior fascicle)[9]
3. Causes of hyperkalemia[54,55]

4. Ischemic cardiomyopathy (arteriosclerosis of the coronary arteries), myocardial infarction
5. Surgical repair of a cardiac defect, e.g., ventricular septal defect or aortic valvular disease

Treatment[56]

1. Fascicular blocks, in and of themselves, do not cause hemodynamic abnormalities. Therapy should be directed at the underlying primary disease. Right bundle branch block and left anterior fascicular block may eventually develop symptomatic second- or third-degree AV block (Fig. 4–43). Pacemaker insertion is probably advisable, especially when the underlying cause cannot be treated.

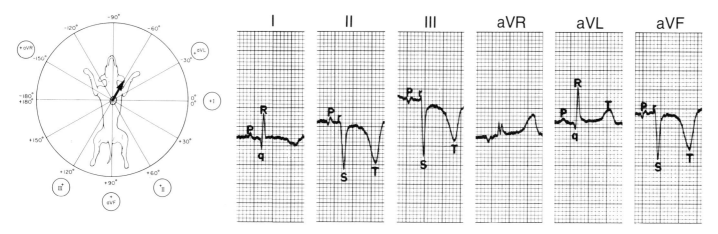

Fig. 4–44. Left anterior fascicular block in a dog with hyperkalemia (serum potassium, 5.3 mEq/L). There is abnormal left axis deviation ($-60°$) with a qR pattern in leads *I* and *aVL* and an rS pattern in leads *II, III,* and *aVF*. The large T waves are compatible with hyperkalemia.

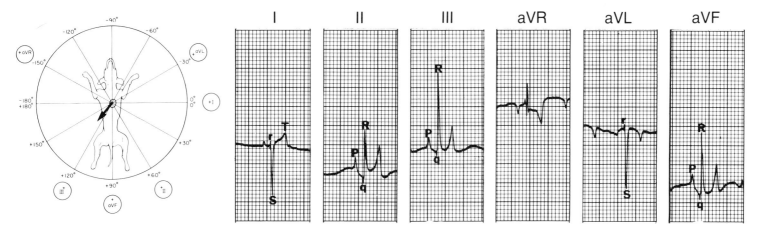

Fig. 4–45. Proposed example of left posterior fascicular block (sudden onset) in a dog with a normal thoracic radiograph. There is abnormal right axis deviation (approximately $+130°$) with an rS pattern in leads *I* and *aVL* and a qR pattern with tall R waves in leads *II, III,* and *aVF*. The diagnosis of left posterior fascicular block is also clinical; with conditions causing right axis deviation excluded, the diagnosis of posterior fascicular block is likely. Paper speed, 25 mm/sec.

Low-voltage QRS complexes (pericardial effusion)

Fig. 4–46. Low-voltage QRS complexes in a dog with pericardial effusion secondary to trauma. The R waves are of less than 0.5 mv (5 boxes) amplitude, and the S-T segment is elevated (arrow).

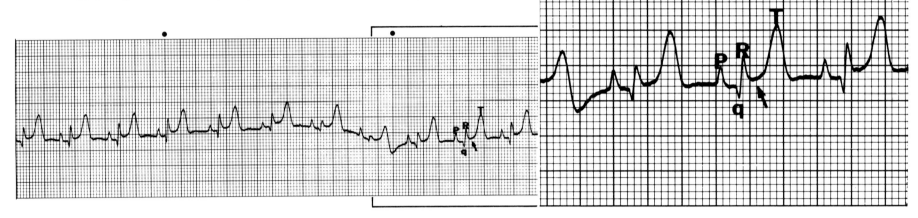

The amplitude or voltage of the QRS complex has wide normal limits depending primarily on the age and breed of the dog. The amplitude of the QRS complex is dependent on many factors besides the effects of cardiovascular diseases. For example, the distance of the heart from the recording electrode leads has a major effect on the amplitude of the QRS. This distance can be influenced by such factors as the size of the chest, thickness of the chest wall (e.g., obesity), and the presence of emphysema or pneumothorax. Pericardial effusion is the cardiovascular disease entity often associated with low-voltage complexes.

Electrocardiographic features

1. R waves are of less amplitude than 0.5 mv (5 boxes) in leads I, II, III, and aVF[2] and should be of low amplitude in all other leads.

2. There is decreased amplitude in the QRS complex on serial electrocardiograms at different time periods.

3. Pericardial effusion occurs[57–59] with the following combination of electrocardiographically observed features:

    a. Generalized low voltage of all QRS complexes due to the short-circuiting action of the pericardial fluid. (The P wave voltage is usually not decreased unless pericardial effusion is severe; several factors can account for the different effects of pericardial fluid on the P wave and QRS complex, e.g., normal QRS complex voltage much greater than P wave voltage, both ventricles completely covered by pericardium while the posterior left atrium not in the pericardial sac.)

    b. S-T segment deviation: elevation in leads I, II, III, and aVF most often seen in acute pericarditis (S-T segment elevation results from compression by fluid and consequent ischemia of subepicardial muscle layers.)

    c. P-R segment depression in leads I, II, III, and aVF (probably representing subepicardial atrial injury)

    d. Electrical alternans[60] (Fig. 6–121): complexes that are regular but that alternate in height or direction (configuration of the complexes remaining the same)

Associated conditions[2,61]

1. Normal variation
2. Incorrect standardization
3. Various causes of pericardial effusion
4. Severe myocardial damage, e.g., myocardial infarction, cardiomyopathy (an infiltrative neoplasm, myocardial fibrosis), or loss of muscle mass
5. Pulmonary diseases, e.g., pulmonary edema, emphysema, or pneumonia
6. Obesity
7. Pneumothorax
8. Pleural effusion
9. Cardiomyopathy after adriamycin chemotherapy

Treatment

1. Treatment should be directed at the underlying disorder, if one is present.

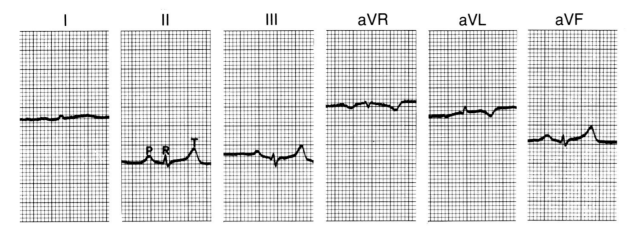

Fig. 4–47. Low-voltage QRS complexes in a large-breed dog with benign pericardial effusion. The R waves are abnormally small in all the leads.

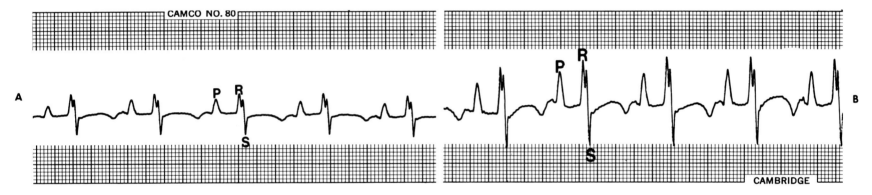

Fig. 4–48. **A,** Low-voltage QRS complexes in a dog with pericardial effusion just before a pericardiocentesis was performed. **B,** After 200 ml of fluid was withdrawn by pericardiocentesis. The amplitude of the complexes is now increased. Note the tall P waves (probable right atrial enlargement). The notch in the R waves may indicate a conduction abnormality, or it may be normal.

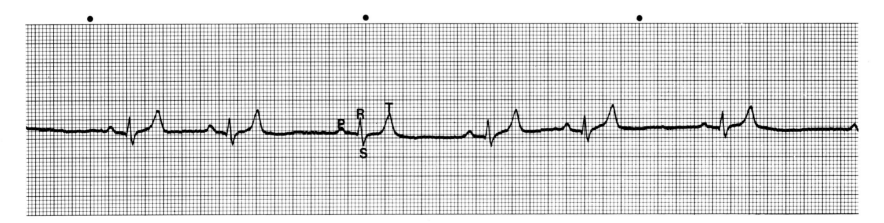

Fig. 4–49. Low-voltage QRS complexes in an obese dog. Thoracic radiographs revealed no cardiac or pulmonary diseases. The electrocardiogram is normal for this dog. Low-voltage QRS complexes are also normal in dogs with large thoracic cavities.

S-T segment abnormalities

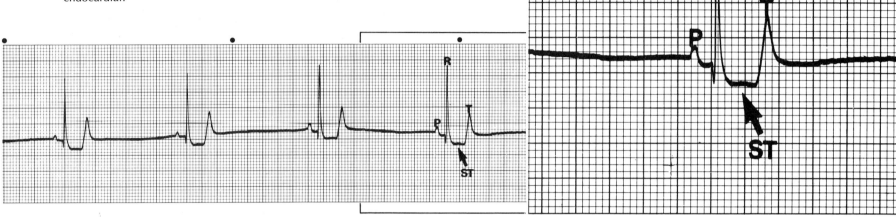

Fig. 4–50. S-T segment depression in a dog struck by an automobile. This horizontal depression of the S-T segment indicates cardiac injury, possibly subendocardial.

The S-T segment represents the time from the end of the QRS interval to the onset of the T wave, i.e., the early phase of ventricular repolarization. It may be above (elevated), at, or below (depressed) the level of the baseline. The baseline or isoelectric line is on the same level as the T-P segment, between the T wave and the P wave. The shape of the S-T segment is significant.

Electrocardiographic features[2,3]

1. Abnormal deviations of the S-T segment are depression of 0.2 mv (2 boxes) or elevation of 0.15 mv (1½ boxes) in leads I through aVF, depression of 0.3 mv (3 boxes) in leads CV_6LL, or elevation of 0.3 mv (3 boxes) in leads CV_6LL and CV_6LU.

2. The S-T segment normally curves gently into the proximal limb of the T wave.

3. It is helpful to compare any S-T segment changes with those seen on previous tracings from that animal.

Associated conditions[2,62,63]

1. Normal variation
2. S-T segment depression in leads II, III, aVF, and CV_6LU or those with dominant R waves:
   a. Myocardial ischemia (inadequate circulation)[14]
   b. Acute myocardial infarction (subendocardial): changes in leads overlying the site of injury[64]
   c. Hyperkalemia,[65] hypokalemia[66,67]
   d. Digitalis: a "sagging" effect to the S-T segment[68]
   e. Trauma to the heart[69]
3. S-T segment elevation in leads II, III, aVF, and CV_6LU or those with dominant R waves:
   a. Myocardial infarction (transmural, i.e., entire thickness of the left ventricle): changes in leads overlying the infarction[70]
   b. Pericarditis[59]
   c. Myocardial hypoxia (oxygen deficiency)[65]
4. Secondary S-T segment changes following abnormalities of QRS complex, e.g., hypertrophy, bundle branch block, and ventricular premature complexes (The displacement is in a direction opposite that of the main ventricular deflection.)
5. Artifact, e.g., wandering baseline
6. Pseudodepression of the S-T segment, due to a prominent T_a wave (atrial repolarization) in tachycardia or atrial changes

Treatment

1. Treatment should be directed at the underlying disorder, if one is present.

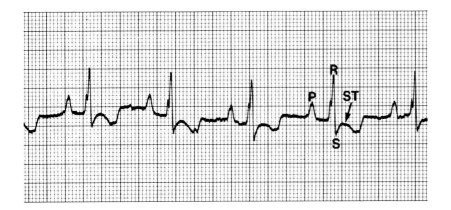

Fig. 4–51. S-T segment depression of less than 2 boxes (0.2 mv) in a normal dog. This small amount of S-T segment depression is within normal limits.

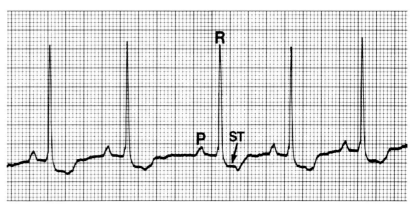

Fig. 4–52. S-T segment depression in a dog with aortic stenosis. The reduced coronary blood flow can lead to myocardial ischemia.

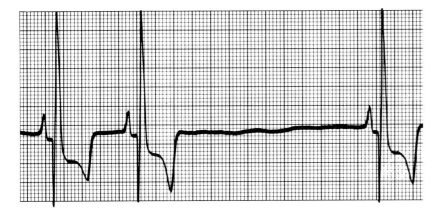

Fig. 4–53. S-T segment depression in a dog with severe left ventricular enlargement. This marked S-T segment depression (also called S-T coving) reflects the repolarization process of the large left ventricle. Deep Q waves probably indicate right ventricular enlargement.

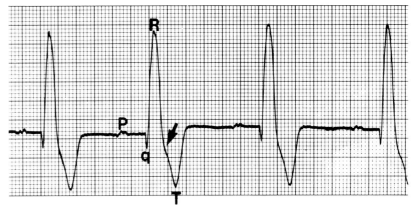

Fig. 4–54. A displaced S-T segment, or S-T segment coving (arrow), in a dog with left bundle branch block.

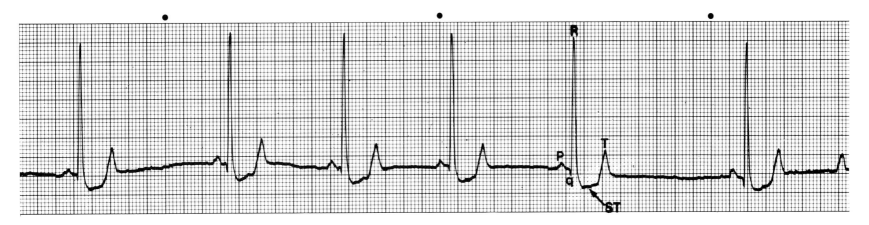

Fig. 4–55. S-T segment depression in a dog with hypokalemia (serum potassium, 3.3 mEq/L) secondary to a respiratory alkalosis.

S-T segment abnormalities—Cont'd

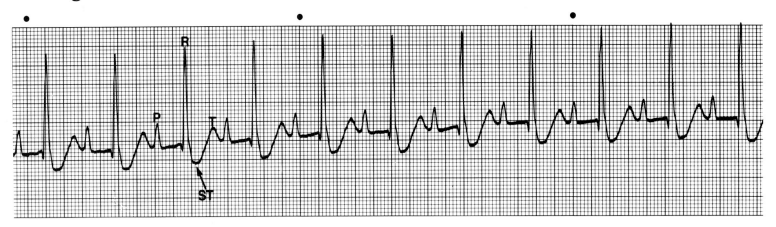

Fig. 4–56. "Sagging" type of S-T segment depression in a dog with digitalis toxicity. This concavity to the S-T segment is most often correlated with digitalis. The long P-R interval is also compatible with digitalis toxicity.

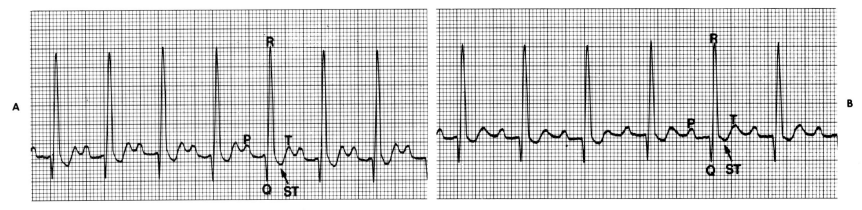

Fig. 4–57. **A,** False depression of the S-T segment in a dog with sinus tachycardia due to a depression of the P-R segment (baseline following the P wave). **B,** After a reduction in the heart rate. The pseudodepression of the S-T segment is no longer present.

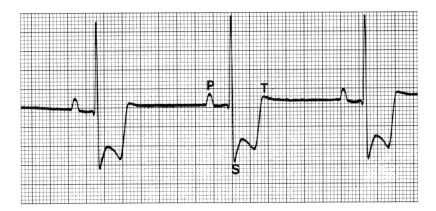

Fig. 4–58. Sudden onset of severe S-T segment depression in a dog with an acute myocardial infarction due to emboli from a generalized septicemia.

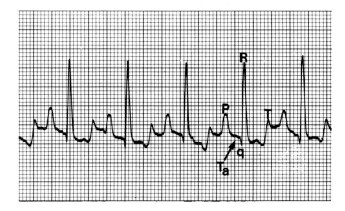

Fig. 4–59. Pseudodepression of the S-T segment due to a prominent T_a wave secondary to right atrial enlargement. The P wave is of increased amplitude. This type of S-T segment depression should not be regarded as abnormal.

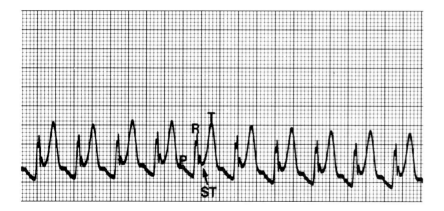

Fig. 4–60. S-T segment elevation in a dog with pericardial effusion. Note also the small amplitude of the P and R waves. The large T waves may indicate hypoxia.

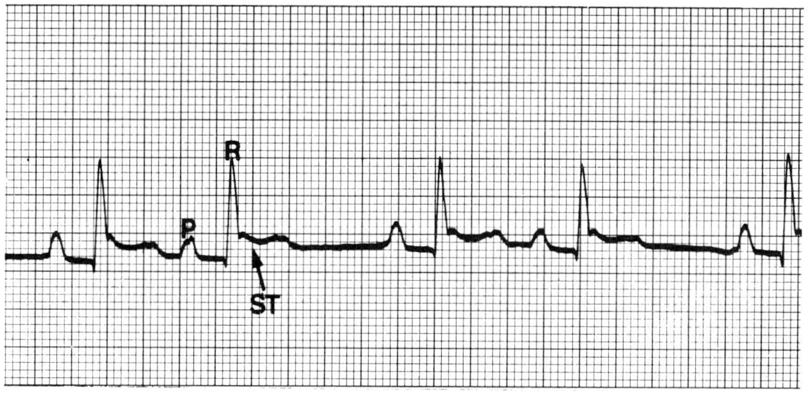

Fig. 4–61. S-T segment elevation from myocardial hypoxia in a dog during surgery. The S-T segment returned to normal after the level of anesthesia was reduced and oxygen increased.

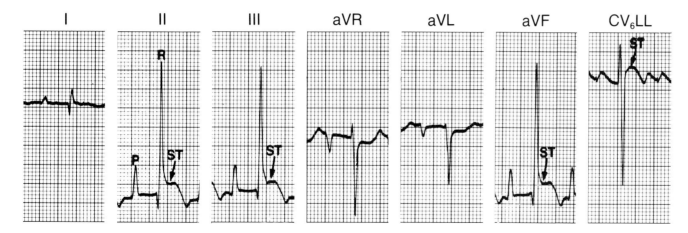

Fig. 4–62. Severe S-T segment elevation (arrows) (leads *II, III, aVF,* and *CV₆LL*) in a dog during a respiratory crisis secondary to a collapsed trachea. There is probable severe myocardial hypoxia. The tall P waves indicate right atrial enlargement.

Fig. 4–63. Sudden onset of S-T segment elevation in a dog with a myocardial infarction secondary to coronary arteriosclerosis.

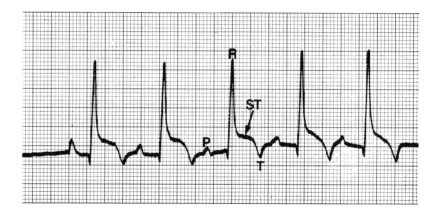

Q-T interval abnormalities

Fig. 4–64. Prolonged Q-T interval (0.48 sec, or 24 boxes) in a dog with severe ethylene glycol poisoning (metabolite oxalic acid binds calcium). Severe hypocalcemia (serum calcium, 2.2 mg/100 ml in this case) and renal failure are the result. The approximate heart rate of 50 beats/min can be within normal range for this size dog. Using tables from various electrocardiographic textbooks in man, the Q-T interval is prolonged despite the low normal rate for this large-breed dog.

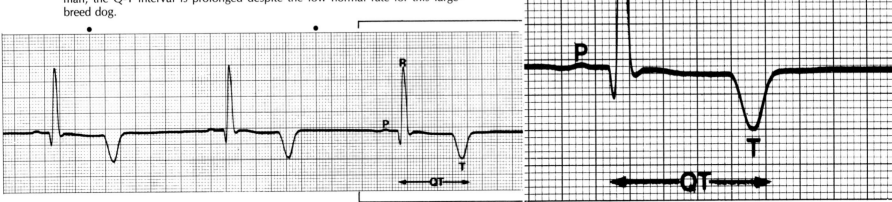

The Q-T interval is measured from the onset of the Q wave to the end of the T wave. It is the summation of ventricular depolarization and repolarization and represents electrical systole. The longest interval found in any lead is regarded as the most nearly correct.

The Q-T interval varies inversely with the heart rate, the faster the heart rate the shorter the interval. Various formulas and tables define the relationship of the Q-T interval to heart rate, age, and sex in humans.[14] In veterinary medicine the Q-T interval alone is not helpful in diagnosis.

Drugs that affect the autonomic nervous system can influence the Q-T interval directly or by changing the heart rate. It has been shown in man that atropine and propranolol shorten the Q-T interval independent of rate, demonstrating a direct vagal effect on the Q-T interval.[71] The deviation of the Q-T interval is chiefly determined by an interplay of autonomic influences. Recent findings suggest that the heart rate and Q-T interval are governed separately by different sympathetic neurons that may or may not be activated together.[71a] Corrections of the Q-T interval for heart rate appear to be applicable under circumstances such as exercise. During neurally mediated cardiovascular adjustments that do not involve exercise, the Q-T interval is maintained within narrow limits.[71a]

Electrocardiographic features

1. The normal range is 0.15 to 0.25 second (7½ to 12½ boxes).
2. A sometimes useful rule is that the Q-T interval should be less than half the preceding R-R interval for normal sinus heart rates (70 to 160 beats/min in the adult dog, not faster than 220 in puppies).

Associated conditions

1. Prolonged Q-T interval[1,2,14,66,72,73]
   a. Hypocalcemia, due to hypoparathyroidism, renal failure with phosphorus retention, eclampsia in the lactating bitch, alkalosis, or pancreatitis
   b. Hypokalemia, due to metabolic and respiratory alkalosis, Cushing's syndrome, diuretics, or insulin-glucose therapy
   c. Quinidine
   d. Intraventricular conduction defects or left ventricular hypertrophy with prolonged QRS complex
   e. Ethylene glycol poisoning
   f. Strenuous exercise[74]
   g. Hypothermia
   h. Clinically, hyperkalemia and hypocalcemia often coexist, especially in animals with advanced renal failure.
   i. Central nervous system disorders
2. Shortened Q-T interval[2,14,66,75]
   a. Hypercalcemia, due to primary hyperparathyroidism, pseudohyperparathyroidism with lymphomas, multiple myeloma, or intravenous calcium
   b. Digitalis
   c. Hyperkalemia

Treatment

1. Therapy should be directed at the underlying disorder. The significance of a prolonged Q-T interval is greater than a shortened one because of the effect of prolonging the relative refractory period. The relative refractory period includes the T wave, which is the vulnerable period of the ventricles. If a ventricular premature complex falls within that period, ventricular fibrillation can result.

2. For hypocalcemia, calcium gluconate infusion and oral supplements are indicated if clinical signs exist. For acute ethylene glycol poisoning, ethanol and sodium bicarbonate along with intravenous fluids are usually indicated.

3. For hypercalcemia, corticosteroids are administered followed by rehydration with saline infusion and diuretics for severely elevated levels.

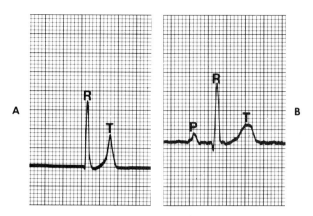

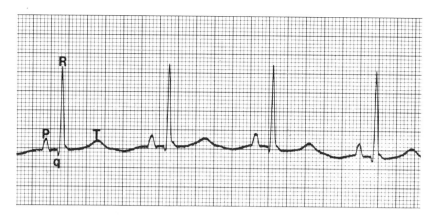

Fig. 4–65. **A,** Shortened Q-T interval in a dog with a high serum potassium level from adrenal insufficiency (Addison's disease). Note the lack of a P wave and the tall peaked T waves. **B,** After therapy. The Q-T interval is now longer compared with that in strip **A,** the P wave is present, and the T wave is smaller.

Fig. 4–66. Prolonged Q-T interval (0.28 sec, or 14 boxes) in a dog with chronic renal failure associated with retention of phosphorus and subsequent hypocalcemia.

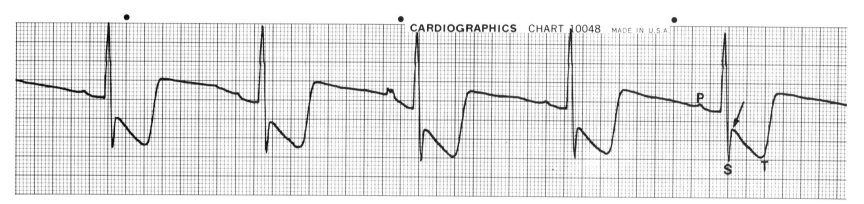

Fig. 4–67. Hypothermia during surgery. As the temperature decreased (to 25° C) in this dog, there was a progressive slowing of the heart rate, a change in direction of the T wave, the appearance of a terminal positive deflection (also called the "J point," arrow) in the QRS, and a prolongation of the P-R, QRS, and Q-T intervals.

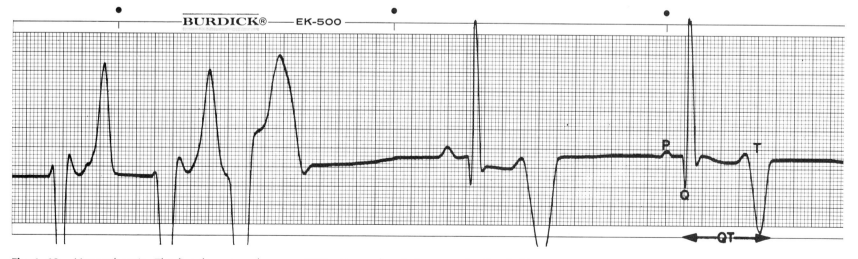

Fig. 4–68. Hypocalcemia. The first three complexes are VPCs. Hypocalcemia increases the threshold potential and thereby the rate of automatic discharge in the rest of the heart. The Q-T intervals are prolonged in the two sinus complexes.

Myocardial infarction

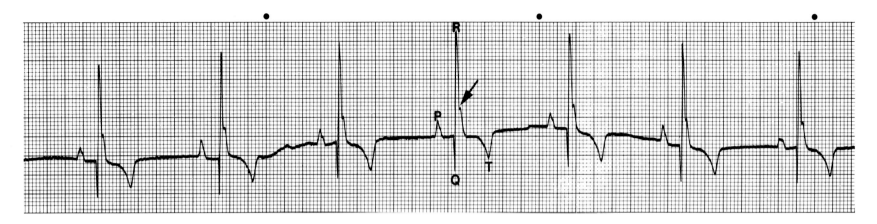

Fig. 4–69. The "notched" R wave descent (arrow) in this old dog may indicate a microscopic intramural myocardial infarction (MIMI).

Dogs have been commonly used for experimental infarction.[70,76,77] As a naturally occurring disease, however, myocardial infarction is infrequent in the dog.[2,64,78–80] Most cases of myocardial infarction reported have involved the left ventricle. Infarctions of the left ventricle will be discussed in this section.

Microscopic intramural myocardial infarctions (MIMI) and focal areas of myocardial fibrosis are common findings in dogs with acquired cardiovascular diseases.[81,82] Although the electrocardiographic changes associated with the naturally occurring diseases have been described,[64,78] consistent electrocardiographic signs for the diagnosis of spontaneous myocardial infarction and precise locations are still unavailable.

Electrocardiographic features[14,25,64,83]

1. If serial tracings with QRS and ST-T wave changes are present, the diagnosis and location of myocardial infarction can be established with a higher degree of accuracy. The localization is based on QRS changes in transmural infarction (i.e., infarction of the entire thickness of the myocardium as well as the epicardium) and on ST-T changes in subendocardial infarction (endocardial half of the ventricle). The zone of ischemia that surrounds the infarcted region accounts for the S-T segment and T wave abnormalities.

2. Some possible indications of infarction that may be seen include the following:

a. Sudden deviation of the S-T segment
b. Tall peaked T waves (first few hours)
c. Sudden development of Q waves or a change in direction of the T wave
d. Axis shift in the frontal plane
e. Low-voltage QRS complexes
f. Sudden development of bundle branch block or heart block
g. Sudden onset of ventricular arrhythmias, due to ischemic effects on the ventricular muscle
h. Ventricular arrhythmias 12 to 24 hours later due to ischemic effects on the subendocardial Purkinje system[84]

3. A "sloppy" R wave descent may be associated with MIMI.[24,82]

Associated conditions

1. Emboli from foci of bacterial endocarditis, from neoplasms, or in association with generalized septicemia[61]
2. Intramural coronary arteriosclerosis in older dogs,[79,85] subvalvular aortic stenosis

Treatment

1. Treatment should be directed at the underlying disorder, as should symptomatic therapy (e.g., congestive heart failure often seen with macroscopic myocardial infarction). Identification and immediate treatment of life-threatening arrhythmias are imperative.

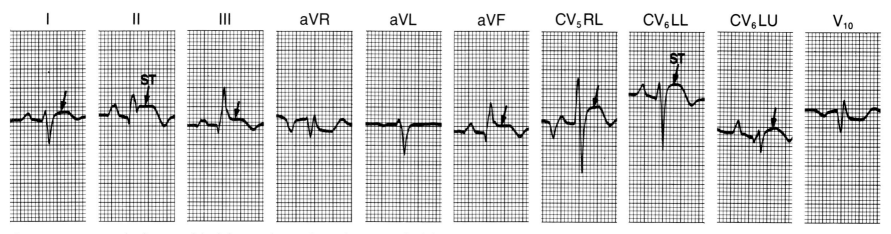

Fig. 4–70. Transmural infarction of the left ventricle in a dog with injury to the left coronary artery after open chest cardiac massage during a cardiac arrest. Infarction changes include S-T segment elevation (arrows), decreased voltage of the QRS complexes, and a right axis deviation (+120°) (possibly consistent with a posterior fascicular block). These changes persisted for 2 days.

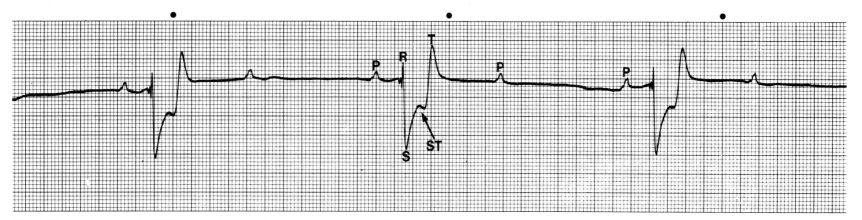

Fig. 4–71. Sudden onset of S-T segment depression and second-degree AV block in a dog with a myocardial infarction and disseminated intravascular coagulation (hemorrhagic pancreatitis was the primary disease). An intraventricular conduction defect also is present.

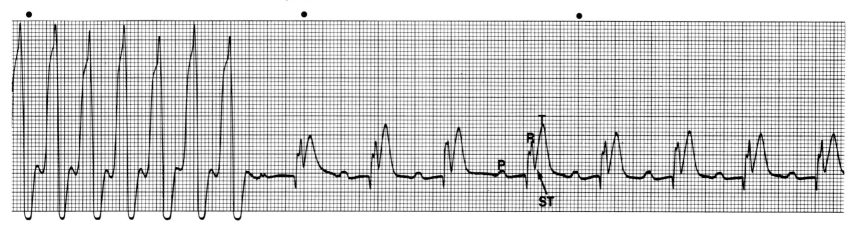

Fig. 4–72. Transmural infarction of the left ventricle in a dog with arteriosclerosis and hypothyroidism. The first seven rapid successive complexes represent a ventricular tachycardia. The sinus rhythm that follows illustrates small complexes, marked elevation of the S-T segment, and first-degree AV block (prolonged P-R interval).

T wave abnormalities

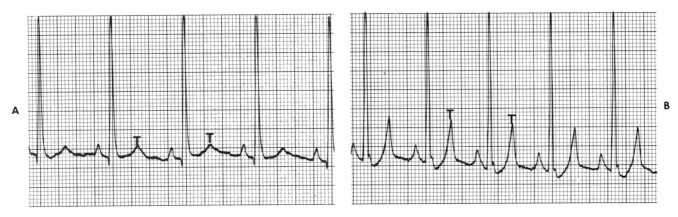

Fig. 4–73. **A,** Normal T waves in a dog during clinical evaluation for a pyometra. **B,** Large peaked T waves after the pyometra ruptured. The T waves slowly returned to normal after surgical correction.

The T wave is the first major deflection following the QRS complex. It represents the recovery period or repolarization of the ventricles and may be positive, notched, negative, or biphasic. In the dog, it is most accurately analyzed when compared with T waves on previous tracings from the same dog or during anesthesia.

The T wave may be of abnormal amplitude, shape, or direction (polarity). Abnormalities can be classified into two general types:[14] (1) primary, changes independent of depolarization, and (2) secondary, changes directly dependent on the depolarization process.

In man, alterations in the sequence of ventricular activation (for example, left bundle block) may alter ventricular repolarization and apparently cause primary T wave abnormalities. The T wave changes may persist for days or weeks after the change in activation sequence (the left bundle branch block) is discontinued. The polarity of the abnormal T wave is the same as the polarity of the major QRS deflection in the same lead. These transient T wave abnormalities can be indicative of myocardial disease, but can also occur in the absence of clinically detectable heart disease.[86]

Electrocardiographic features

1. The T wave generally should not be greater than 25% of the R wave (Q wave if larger).[2]

2. The T wave is normally slightly asymmetric. T waves that are sharply pointed or notched may indicate an underlying abnormality such as electrolyte imbalances. A marked change in the shape of the T wave on serial electrocardiograms is usually abnormal.

3. Polarity of secondary T wave changes is not always equal to that of the QRS complex, as is common in man. The T wave should be positive in leads CV_5RL in dogs over 2 months of age. It can normally be biphasic. It should be negative in lead V_{10} in all breeds except the Chihuahua.[87] Reversal in polarity of the T wave on serial electrocardiograms is most often abnormal.

4. Isolated T wave alternans can occur (Fig. 4–78). This phenom-enon consists of the rhythmic alteration of the configuration of the T wave without any concomitant change in the QRS complex.[88,89]

Associated conditions

1. Myocardial hypoxia (oxygen deficiency),[65] due to anesthetic complications or hyperventilation in heat stroke and in animals with heart disease during bradycardia (T waves larger), myocardial infarction (T waves larger with a change in polarity.[1,64]) (These changes represent a primary abnormality independent of depolarization.)

2. Intraventricular conduction defects: right or left bundle branch block, ventricular enlargement (T waves become larger secondary to QRS change.)

3. Electrolyte imbalances (T waves become larger and spiked with hyperkalemia, smaller and biphasic with hypokalemia.[65,66])

4. Metabolic diseases, e.g., anemia, shock, uremia, ketoacidosis, hypoglycemia, and fever (T wave changes are nonspecific.)

5. Drug toxicity, e.g., digitalis, quinidine, and procainamide (T wave changes are nonspecific.)

6. Certain physiologic factors, e.g., respiratory abnormalities and autonomic neural control (T wave abnormalities can also be seen in normal animals.)

7. T wave alternans: associated with occlusion of a coronary artery, increases in circulatory catecholamines, hypocalcemia, and acute increases in sympathetic discharge ("long Q-T" syndrome)[88,89]

Treatment

1. Treatment should be directed at the underlying disorder if one is present.

2. The disappearance of the T wave changes after administration of the proper drugs (e.g., glucose in hypoglycemia, atropine in a sinus bradycardia, or oxygen in an anesthetic complication) is strong evidence that the T wave abnormality is physiologic.

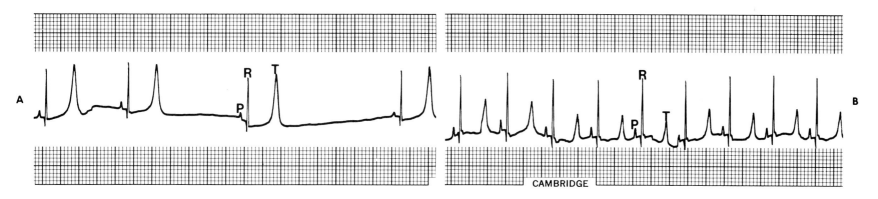

Fig. 4–74. **A,** Tall T waves and a slow heart rate in a dog with probable myocardial hypoxia during surgery. **B,** After the anesthesia was stopped and oxygen given, the T waves became smaller and the heart rate increased. A cardiac arrest was probably averted.

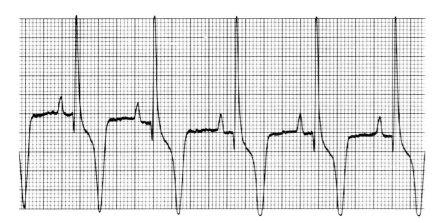

Fig. 4–75. Large negative T waves in a Poodle with left-sided congestive heart failure. Myocardial hypoxia as well as left ventricular enlargement (tall R waves) may have combined to cause this marked change in the T wave.

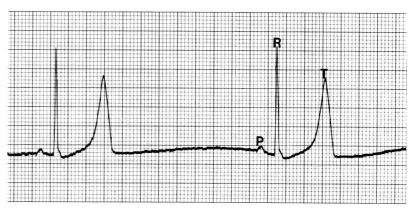

Fig. 4–76. The characteristic tall, narrow, and pointed T waves of hyperkalemia (serum potassium, 6.2 mEq/L) in a dog. Note also the small amplitude of the P waves.

Fig. 4–77. Large negative T waves and S-T segment elevation in a dog with an acute myocardial infarction.

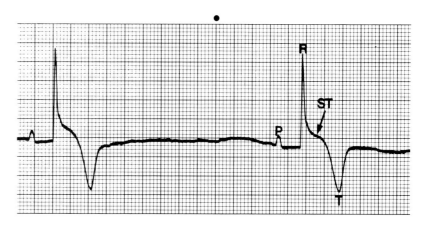

T wave abnormalities—cont'd

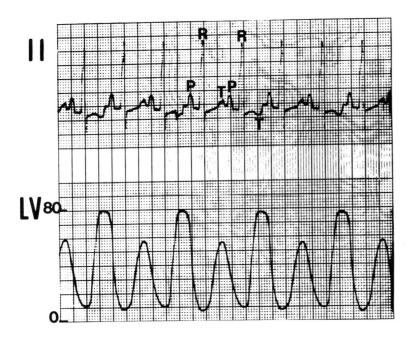

Fig. 4–78. Sequential lead II and left ventricular (LV) pressure during T wave electrical alternans in a dog with EDTA infusion (to induce hypocalcemia). Note the mechanical alternans as revealed by the presence of alternans in the LV pressure. This is consistent with intracellular studies in which contractile tension changes are associated with changes in duration of the action potentials (repolarization). (From Navarro-Lopez, F., et al.: Isolated T wave alternans elicited by hypocalcemia in dogs. J. Electrocardiol., *11*:103, 1978, with permission.)

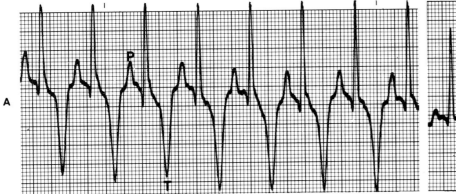
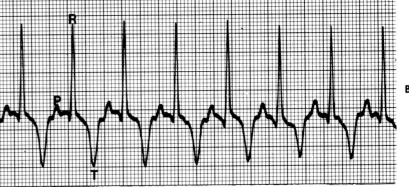

Fig. 4–79. **A,** Large negative T waves in a dog with right- and left-sided congestive heart failure. Both left ventricular enlargement (tall R waves) and myocardial hypoxia likely caused this T wave abnormality. **B,** Same pattern but at half the sensitivity (0.5 cm = 1 mv), so the complexes are not off the paper as in **A.**

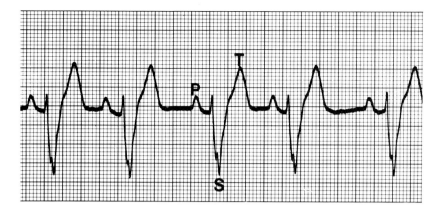

Fig. 4–80. Right bundle branch block with large T waves secondary to the altered QRS deflections.

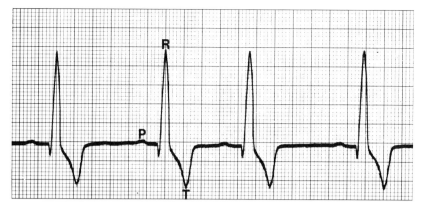

Fig. 4–81. Large negative T waves in a dog with left ventricular enlargement. This secondary T wave abnormality is also seen in left bundle branch block; 0.5 cm = 1 mv.

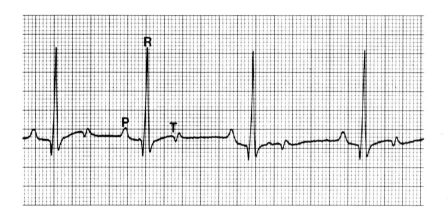

Fig. 4–82. The T wave became biphasic and flattened in this dog with severe vomiting as the serum potassium (2.8 mEq/L) decreased. The Q-T interval is at the upper limits of normal (0.24 sec). A biphasic T wave can also be a normal finding and should not be confused with a U wave (seen in man with hypokalemia), a small deflection that follows the T wave.

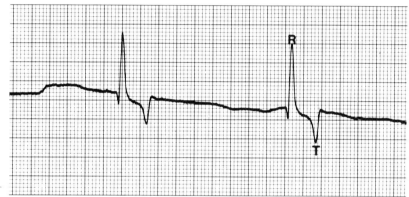

Fig. 4–83. Hyperkalemia (serum potassium, 6.5 mEq/L) in a dog with Addison's disease. Note the slow heart rate, the absence of P waves, and the large abnormally shaped T waves. The changing baseline is due to respiratory movements.

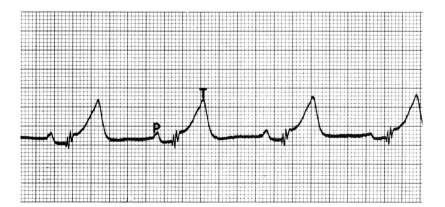

Fig. 4–84. Large positive T waves, S-T segment elevation, and small QRS complexes in a dog with pericardial effusion. The T wave changes are probably due to an epicardial inflammation.

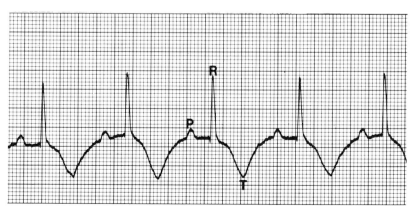

Fig. 4–85. Deep, broad, and negative T waves in a dog with cerebral disease. Note also the prolonged Q-T interval. These two findings are often seen with subarachnoid hemorrhage in humans.

Use of the precordial chest leads

The precordial chest leads are exploring electrodes that can record electrical activity from the dorsal and ventral surfaces of the heart. When the lead selector is set at the V position, the electrocardiograph connects the RA, LA, and LL electrodes together. The machine can then measure the voltage from the heart to the selected location of the chest electrodes. The chest electrode is the positive pole of each unipolar precordial lead. The clip for the V lead (C) is attached at the various positions for each of the unipolar chest leads.

To keep the nomenclature consistent with that for human medicine, the following terminology for precordial chest leads is recommended:[3,90] $rV_2 = CV_5RL$, $V_2 = CV_6LL$, $V_4 = CV_6LU$, and V_{10}. The unipolar chest leads are not well established in canine and feline electrocardiography. The precordial chest leads are most valuable for*

1. Detecting right and left ventricular enlargement
2. Diagnosing bundle branch block
3. Diagnosing myocardial infarction
4. Diagnosing cardiac arrhythmias, since P waves are often better visualized in the precordial leads
5. Confirming data obtained from the three standard bipolar and three augmented unipolar limb leads

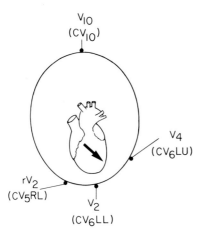

Fig. 4–86. Various positions of the unipolar precordial chest leads in a cross section of the thoracic cavity.

---

*References 2, 5, 16, 17, 24, 30, 39, 87, 90.

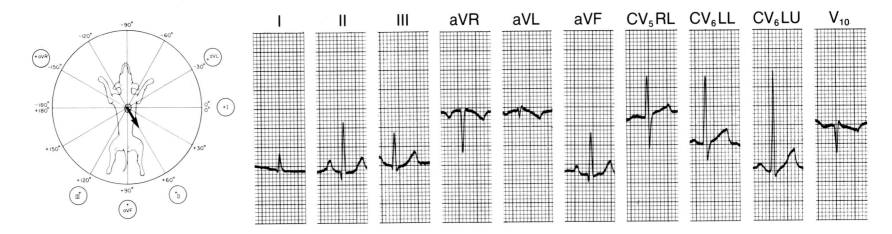

Fig. 4–87. Normal canine electrocardiogram illustrating the unipolar precordial chest leads: CV_5RL, CV_6LL, CV_6LU, and V_{10}.

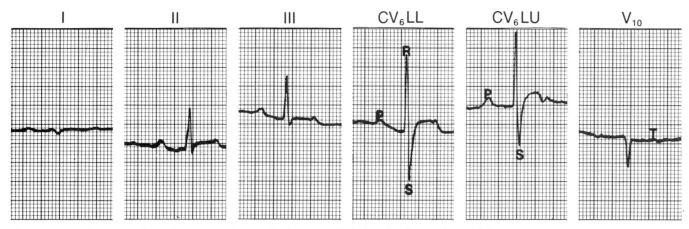

Fig. 4–88. Right ventricular enlargement changes in the precordial chest leads in a dog with heartworm disease. There are deep S waves present in CV_6LL (greater than 0.8 mv, or 8 boxes) and CV_6LU (greater than 0.7 mv, or 7 boxes) and a small positive T wave in lead V_{10}. The three bipolar limb leads do not show right ventricular enlargement.

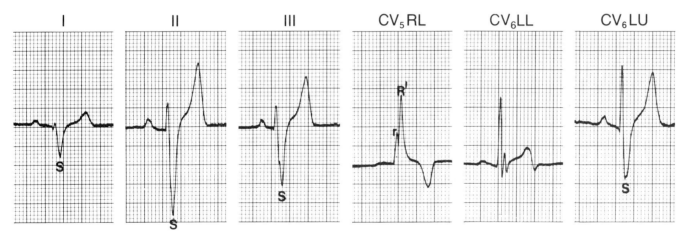

Fig. 4–89. Right bundle branch block in a dog. The wide rR′ pattern of CV_6RL, along with the large wide S waves in leads *I, II, III,* and CV_6LU, are important features in right bundle branch block.

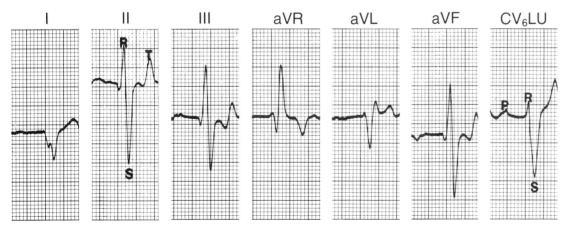

Fig. 4–90. The P waves in the six basic limb leads of this dog are essentially impossible to distinguish. Use of the precordial chest lead CV_6LU allowed the P wave to be easily seen. Severe right ventricular enlargement changes are also present as a result of this dog's pulmonic stenosis.

REFERENCES

1. Bolton, G.R.: *Handbook of Canine Electrocardiography.* Philadelphia, W.B. Saunders, 1975.
2. Ettinger, S.J., and Suter, P.F.: *Canine Cardiology.* Philadelphia, W.B. Saunders, 1970.
3. Hahn, A.W. (chairman), Hamlin, R.L., and Patterson, D.F.: Standards for canine electrocardiography. The Academy of Veterinary Cardiology Committee Report, 1977.
4. Hill, J.D.: The electrocardiogram in dogs with standardized body and limb positions. J. Electrocardiol., *1*:175, 1968.
5. Lannek, N.: A clinical and experimental study of the electrocardiogram in dogs. Thesis, Stockholm, 1949.
6. Eckenfels, A., and Trieb, G.: The normal electrocardiogram of the conscious Beagle dog. Toxicol. Appl. Pharmacol., *47*:567, 1979.
6a. Bonagura, J.D.: M-mode echocardiography: basic principles. Vet. Clin. North Am., *13*:299, 1983.
7. Simonson, E.: *Differentiation between Normal and Abnormal in Electrocardiography.* St. Louis, C.V. Mosby, 1961.
8. Surawicz, B. (chairman), et al.: Task Force 1: Standardization of terminology and interpretation. Am. J. Cardiol., *41*:130, 1978.
9. Goldman, M.J.: *Principles of Clinical Electrocardiography.* 11th Edition. Los Altos, Calif., Lange Medical Publications, 1982.
10. Johnson, J.C., Horan, L.G., and Flowers, N.C.: Diagnostic accuracy of the electrocardiogram. In *Clinical-electrocardiographic Correlations.* Edited by A.N. Brest. Philadelphia, F.A. Davis, 1979.
11. Tranchesi, J., Adelardi, V., and deOliveira, J.M.: Atrial repolarization—its importance in clinical electrocardiography. Circulation, *22*:635, 1960.
12. Edwards, N.J., and Tilley, L.P.: Congenital heart defects. In *Pathophysiology of Small Animal Surgery.* Edited by M.J. Bojrab. Philadelphia, Lea & Febiger, 1981.
13. Liu, S.-K., and Tilley, L.P.: Dysplasia of the tricuspid valve in the dog and cat. J. Am. Vet. Med. Assoc., *169*:623, 1976.
13a. Scott, C.S., et al.: The effect of left atrial histology and dimension on P wave morphology. J. Electrocardiol., *16*:363, 1983.
14. Friedman, H.H.: *Diagnostic Electrocardiography and Vectorcardiography.* 2nd Edition. New York, McGraw-Hill, 1977.
15. Brown, F.K., Brown, W.J., Ellison, R.G., and Hamilton, W.F.: Electrocardiographic changes during development of right ventricular hypertrophy in the dog. Am. J. Cardiol., *21*:223, 1968.
16. Hamlin, R.L.: Electrocardiographic detection of ventricular enlargement in the dog. J. Am. Vet. Med. Assoc., *153*:1461, 1968.
17. Hill, J.D.: Electrocardiographic diagnosis of right ventricular enlargement in dogs. J. Electrocardiol., *4*:347, 1971.
18. Knight, D.H.: Heartworm heart disease. Adv. Vet. Sci. Comp. Med., *21*:107, 1977.
19. Rawlings, C.A., and Lewis, R.E.: Right ventricular enlargement in heartworm disease. Am. J. Vet. Res., *38*:1801, 1977.
20. Pyle, R.L., et al.: Patent ductus arteriosus with pulmonary hypertension in the dog. J. Am. Vet. Med. Assoc., *178*:565, 1981.
20a. Lombard, C.W., and Buergelt, C.D.: Echocardiographic and clinical findings in dogs with heartworm-induced cor pulmonale. Compend. Contin. Educ. Small Anim. Pract., *12*:971, 1984.
21. Harpster, N.K.: Pulmonary vascular disease in the dog. In *Current Veterinary Therapy: Small Animal Practice.* Volume 6. Edited by R.W. Kirk. Philadelphia, W.B. Saunders, 1977.
22. Slauson, D.O., and Gribble, D.H.: Thrombosis complicating renal amyloidosis in dogs. Vet. Pathol., *8*:352, 1971.
23. Battler, A., et al.: Effects of changes in ventricular size on regional and surface QRS amplitudes in the conscious dog. Circulation, *62*:174, 1980.
24. Harpster, N.K.: Chronic valvular myocardial heart disease in dogs. In *Current Veterinary Therapy: Small Animal Practice.* Volume 5. Edited by R.W. Kirk. Philadelphia, W.B. Saunders, 1974.
25. Tilley, L.P., Liu, S.-K., Fox, P.R.: Myocardial disease. In *Textbook of Veterinary Internal Medicine.* Edited by S.J. Ettinger. 2nd Edition. Philadelphia, W.B. Saunders, 1983.
26. Rosenbaum, M.B.: The hemiblocks: diagnostic criteria and clinical significance. Mod. Concepts Cardiovasc. Dis., *39*:141, 1970.
27. Rosenbaum, M.B., Elizari, M.V., and Lazzari, J.O.: The hemiblocks. Oldsmar, Fla., Tampa Tracings, 1970.
28. Hill, J.D., Moore, E.N., and Patterson, D.F.: Ventricular epicardial activation studies in experimental and spontaneous right bundle branch block in the dog. Am. J. Cardiol., *21*:232, 1968.
29. Kulbertus, H.E., and DeMoulin, J.C.: Pathological basis of concept of left hemiblock. In *The Conduction System of the Heart.* Edited by H.J.J. Wellens, K.I. Lie, and M.J. Janse. Philadelphia, Lea & Febiger, 1976.
30. Moore, E.N., Hoffman, D.F., Patterson, D.F., and Stuckey, J.H.: Electrocardiographic changes due to delayed activation of the wall of the right ventricle. Am. Heart J., *68*:347, 1964.
31. Myerberg, R.J., Nilsson, K., and Gelband, H.: Physiology of canine intraventricular conduction and endocardial excitation. Circ. Res., *30*:217, 1972.
32. Okuma, K.: ECG and VCG changes in experimental hemiblock and bifascicular block. Am. Heart J., *92*:473, 1976.
33. Pruitt, R.D., and Watt, T.B.: Experimental intraventricular block. Bull. N.Y. Acad. Med., *47*:931, 1971.
34. Van Dam, R.T.: Ventricular activation in human and canine bundle branch block. In *The Conduction System of the Heart.* Edited by H.J.J. Wellens, K.I. Lie, and M.J. Janse. Philadelphia, Lea & Febiger, 1976.
35. Watt, T.B.: Features of fascicular block imposed upon existing right bundle branch block in the dog and baboon. Am. J. Cardiol., *39*:1000, 1977.
36. Watt, T.B., et al.: Left anterior arborization block combined with right bundle branch block in canine and primate hearts. Circ. Res., *22*:57, 1968.
37. Watt, T.B., and Pruitt, R.D.: Electrocardiographic findings associated with experimental arborization block in dogs. Am. Heart J., *69*:642, 1965.
38. Buchanan, J.W., and Botts, R.P.: Clinical effects of repeated cardiac punctures in dogs. J. Am. Vet. Med. Assoc., *161*:814, 1972.
39. Patterson, D.F., Detweiler, D.K., Hubben, K., and Botts, R.P.: Spontaneous abnormal cardiac arrhythmias and conduction disturbances in the dog (a clinical and pathological study of 3000 dogs). Am. J. Vet. Res., *22*:355, 1961.
40. Romagnoli, A.: Su di un caso di Blocco di Branca nel Cane. An. Fac. Med. Vet. Pisa, *6*:3, 1953.
41. Tilley, L.P.: Feline cardiology. In *Katzen Krankheiten, Klinik und Therapie.* Edited by W.K. Herausgeger and U.M. Durr. Hannover, Germany, Verlag M. & H. Schaper, 1978.
42. Cohen, H.C., et al.: Tachycardia- and bradycardia-dependent bundle branch block alternans. Circulation, *55*:242, 1977.
43. Elizari, M.V., Lazzari, J.O., and Rosenbaum, M.B.: Phase-3 and phase-4 intermittent left bundle branch block occurring spontaneously in a dog. Eur. J. Cardiol., *1*:95, 1973.
44. Bolton, G.R., and Ettinger, S.J.: Right bundle branch block in the dog. J. Am. Vet. Med. Assoc., *160*:1104, 1972.
45. Zannetti, G.: Clinical aspects of RBBB in a dog. Clinica Vet., *97*:313, 1974.
46. Rosenbaum, M.B., and Elizari, M.V.: Mechanism of intermittent bundle-branch block and paroxysmal atrioventricular block. Postgrad. Med., *53*(5):87, 1973.
47. Breznock, E.M., Hilwig, R.W., Vasko, J.S., and Hamlin, R.L.: Surgical correction of an interventricular septal defect in the dog. J. Am. Vet. Med. Assoc., *157*:1343, 1970.
48. Silber, E.N., and Katz, L.N.: *Heart Disease.* New York, Macmillan, 1975.
49. Patterson, D.F.: Congenital defects of the cardiovascular system of dogs: studies in comparative cardiology. Adv. Vet. Sci. Comp. Med., *20*:1, 1976.
50. Moore, E.N., Boineau, J.P., and Patterson, D.F.: Incomplete right bundle branch block: an electrocardiographic enigma and possible misnomer. Circulation, *44*:678, 1971.
51. Andrade, Z.A., et al.: Experimental Chagas' disease in dogs. Arch. Pathol. Lab. Med., *105*:460, 1981.
52. Liu, S.-K., Maron, B.J., and Tilley, L.P.: Canine hypertrophic cardiomyopathy. J. Am. Vet. Med. Assoc., *174*:708, 1979.
53. Warner, R.A., Hill, N.E., Mookherjee, S., and Smulyan, H.: Improved electrocardiographic criteria for the diagnosis of left anterior hemiblock. Am. J. Cardiol., *51*:723, 1983.
54. Bashour, T., et al.: Atrioventricular and intraventricular conduction in hyperkalemia. Am. J. Cardiol., *35*:199, 1975.
55. Ewy, G.A., Karliner, J., and Bednyer, J.: Electrocardiographic QRS axis as a manifestation of hyperkalemia. JAMA, *215*:429, 1971.
56. Merideth, J., and Pruitt, R.D.: Symposium on cardiac arrhythmias. Disturbances in cardiac conduction and their management. Circulation, *47*:1098, 1973.

57. Friedman, H.S., et al.: Electrocardiographic features of experimental cardiac tamponade in closed-chest dogs. Eur. J. Cardiol., 6:311, 1977.
58. Suarwicz, B., and Lasseter, K.C.: Electrocardiogram in pericarditis. Am. J. Cardiol., 26:471, 1970.
59. Tilley, L.P., and Wilkins, R.J.: Pericardial disease. In Current Veterinary Therapy: Small Animal Practice. Volume 5. Edited by R.W. Kirk. Philadelphia, W.B. Saunders, 1974.
60. Sbarbaro, J.A., and Brooks, H.L.: Pericardial effusion and electrical alternans, echocardiographic assessment. Postgrad. Med., 63(3):105, 1978.
61. Marriott, H.J.L.: Practical Electrocardiography. 6th Edition. Baltimore, Williams & Wilkins, 1977.
62. Goldberger, E.: Textbook of Clinical Cardiology. St. Louis, C.V. Mosby, 1983.
63. Rothfeld, E.L.: The itinerant ST-T segment. Heart Lung, 6:857, 1977.
64. Fregin, G.F., Luginbuhl, H., and Guarda, F.: Myocardial infarction in a dog with bacterial endocarditis. J. Am. Vet. Med. Assoc., 160:956, 1972.
65. Coulter, D.B., Duncan, R.J., and Sander, P.D.: Effects of asphyxia and potassium on canine and feline electrocardiograms. Can. J. Comp. Med., 39:442, 1975.
66. Feldman, E.C., and Ettinger, S.J.: Electrocardiographic changes associated with electrolyte disturbances. Vet. Clin. North Am., 7:487, 1977.
67. Ono, I., Hukuoka, T., and Onodera, I.: The effects of varying dietary potassium on the electrocardiogram and blood electrolytes in young dogs. Jpn. Heart J., 5:272, 1964.
68. Hahn, A.W.: Digitalis glycosides in canine medicine. In Current Veterinary Therapy: Small Animal Practice. Volume 5. Edited by R.W. Kirk. Philadelphia, W.B. Saunders, 1974.
69. Alexander, J.W., Bolton, G.R., and Koslow, G.L.: Electrocardiographic changes in nonpenetrating trauma to the chest. J. Am. Anim. Hosp. Assoc., 11:160, 1975.
70. Irvin, R.G., and Cobb, F.R.: Relationship between epicardial ST-segment elevation, regional myocardial blood flow, and extent of myocardial infarction in awake dogs. Circulation, 55:825, 1977.
71. Browne, K.F., et al.: Influence of the autonomic nervous system on the Q-T interval in man. Am. J. Cardiol., 50:1099. 1982.
71a. Davidowski, T.A., and Wolf, S.: The QT interval during reflex cardiovascular adaptation. Circulation, 69:22, 1984.
72. Musselman, E.E., and Hartsfield, S.M.: Complete atrioventricular heart block due to hypokalemia following ovariohysterectomy. Vet. Med. Small Anim. Clin., 71:155, 1976.
73. Vincent, M.G., Abildskov, J.A., and Burgess, J.J.: Q-T interval syndromes. Prog. Cardiovasc. Dis., 16:523, 1974.
74. Schwartz, P.J., Periti, M., and Malliani, A.: The long Q-T syndrome. Am. Heart J., 89:378, 1975.
75. Drazner, F.H.: Hypercalcemia in the dog and cat. J. Am. Vet. Med. Assoc., 178:1252, 1981.
76. Harris, A.S.: Delayed development of ventricular ectopic rhythms following experimental coronary occlusion. Circulation, 1:1318, 1950.
77. Langer, P.H., DeMott, T., and Hussey, M.: High fidelity electrocardiography: effects of induced localized myocardial injury in the dog. Am. Heart J., 71:790, 1966.
78. Jaffe, K.R., and Bolton, G.R.: Myocardial infarction in a dog with complete heart block. Vet. Med. Small Anim. Clin., 69:197, 1974.
79. Luginbuhl, J., and Detweiler, D.K.: Cardiovascular lesions in dogs. Ann. N.Y. Acad. Sci., 127:517, 1965.
80. Wierich, W.E., Bisgard, G.E., Will, I.A., and Rowe, G.G.: Myocardial infarction and pulmonic stenosis in a dog. J. Am. Vet. Med. Assoc., 159:315, 1971.
81. Detweiler, D.K., et al.: Diseases of the cardiovascular system. In Canine Medicine. Edited by E.J. Catcott. Santa Barbara, Calif., American Veterinary Publications, 1968.
82. Ogburn, P.N.: Myocardial diseases in the dog. In Current Veterinary Therapy: Small Animal Practice. Volume 6. Edited by R.W. Kirk. Philadelphia, W.B. Saunders, 1977.
83. Pietsch, G.E.: ECG of the month. J. Am. Vet. Med. Assoc., 172:1394, 1978.
84. Wit, A.L., and Bigger, T.J.: Possible electrophysiological mechanisms for lethal arrhythmias accompanying myocardial ischemia and infarction. Circulation, 52(Suppl. III):96, 1975.
85. Lindsay, S., Chaikoff, I.L., and Dilmore, J.W.: Arteriosclerosis in the dog. I. Spontaneous lesions in the aorta and the coronary arteries. Arch. Pathol., 53:281, 1952.
86. Rosenbaum, M.B., et al.: Electronic modulation of the T wave and cardiac memory. Am. J. Cardiol., 50:213, 1982.
87. Detweiler, D.K., and Patterson, D.F.: The prevalence and types of heart disease in dogs. Ann. N.Y. Acad. Sci., 127:481, 1965.
88. Navarro-Lopez, F., et al.: Isolated T wave alternans elicited by hypocalcemia in dogs. J. Electrocardiol., 11:103, 1978.
89. Schwartz, P.J., and Malliani, A.: Electrical alternation of the T-wave: Clinical and experimental evidence of its relationship with the sympathetic nervous system and with the long Q-T syndrome. Am. Heart J., 89:45, 1975.
90. Hellerstein, H.K., and Hamlin, R.: QRS component of the spatial vectorcardiogram and of the spatial magnitude and velocity of electrocardiograms of the normal dog. Am. J. Cardiol., 6:1049, 1960.

5 Analysis of feline P-QRS-T deflections

NORMAL FELINE ELECTROCARDIOGRAM

If the electrocardiogram is interpreted systematically as presented in Chapter 3, the values obtained are then compared with the normal values. The determination of the normal electrocardiographic limits should be based on three prerequisites: (1) adequate sample size, (2) composition of the sample representative of the average healthy population, and (3) adequate statistical evaluation.[1,2] In most of the literature on the subject, at least one of these principles has been disregarded. The electrocardiographic values reported in the literature are frequently on anesthetized cats.[3–5]

Following is a summary of the essential criteria for determining the normal limits in nonanesthetized cats.[6–10] The normal values are based primarily on studies by Gompf and myself:[6,8]

These data were obtained from 48 unanesthetized normal cats of various breeds, ages, and sexes. Each cat was determined to have a normal heart from history, physical examination, and thoracic radiographs.

The literature available presents primarily deflections and intervals in terms of the minimum, maximum, and mean. This is the poorest method for establishing normal limits because an excessive overlap with the abnormal often results. The use of standard deviations does give a better evaluation of the data if the values follow a "normal" (or Gaussian) distribution. A reliable method for establishing normal limits may be by a percentile distribution, especially if the data are not distributed normally. The values established in the foregoing outline used standard deviations since the data in this study followed a normal distribution.[6]

The electrocardiographic studies by Gompf and me[6,8] also evaluate the normal electrocardiogram in lateral recumbency and sternal recumbency. No marked differences have been found between values determined for the two positions. For sternal recumbency, the values are the same as for right lateral recumbency except that the height of the P wave is 0.3 mv, the height of the QRS is 1.0 mv, and the axis is −10° to +150°. The sternal position would appear, at the present time, to be the position of choice for accuracy in recording as well as for ease of restraint (cats tolerate it well). Further studies are necessary to firmly establish it as the standard, however. The normal values and the electrocardiographic examples presented in this textbook are all primarily from a position of right lateral recumbency.

The determination of the normal electrocardiographic limits in the cat is essential for the accurate evaluation of feline cardiac disease. It is hoped that the values outlined will serve as a strong basis toward this goal. I am continuing to evaluate the normal feline electrocardiogram using these standards.[1]

Rate

Range: 160 to 240 beats/min
Mean: 197 beats/min

Rhythm

Normal sinus rhythm
Sinus tachycardia (physiologic reaction to excitement)

Measurements (lead II, 50 mm/sec, 1 cm = 1 mv)*

P wave
    Width: maximum, 0.04 second (2 boxes wide)
    Height: maximum, 0.2 mv (2 boxes tall)

P-R interval
    Width: 0.05 to 0.09 second (2½ to 4½ boxes)

QRS complex
    Width: maximum, 0.04 second (2 boxes)
    Height of R wave: maximum, 0.9 mv (9 boxes)

S-T segment
    No marked depression or elevation

T wave
    Can be positive, negative, or biphasic; most often positive
Maximum amplitude: 0.3 mv (3 boxes)

Q-T interval
    Width: 0.12 to 0.18 second (6 to 9 boxes) at normal heart rate (range 0.07 to 0.20 sec, 3½ to 10 boxes); varies with heart rate (faster rates, shorter Q-T intervals; and vice versa)

Electrical axis (front plane)

0 to +160°

Precordial chest leads

No well-established normal values to date
CV_6LU (V_4): R wave not greater than 1.0 mv (10 boxes)

---

*From The Animal Medical Center.[6] Computed by adding and subtracting 1.96 times the standard deviation from the mean for the axis (P < 0.05 or 95% of the observations) and 1.645 times the standard deviation for widths and heights of waves and intervals (P < 0.10 or 90% of the observations). Numbers are rounded off to the nearest whole.

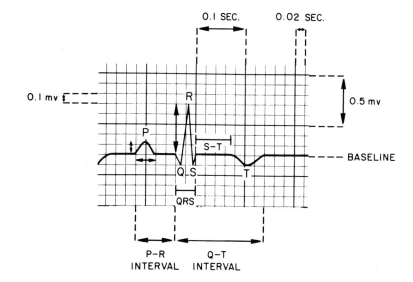

Fig. 5–1. Close-up of a normal feline lead II P-QRS-T complex with labels and intervals.

Abnormalities in cardiac enlargement that are detected on the electrocardiogram require further definition with thoracic radiography or angiocardiography. Echocardiography in veterinary medicine recently has been proved useful in the noninvasive assessment of structure and function of such intracardiac structures as the ventricular chambers, left atrium, right and left atrioventricular valves, and aortic valves.[8a]

As stated in Chapter 4, the primary purpose of this textbook is to present the clinician with features that are essential to electrocardiographic diagnosis. Associations with cardiac diseases and appropriate therapy are also discussed for each electrocardiographic entity. Based on the numerous publications on electrocardiography (see "References") and my experience with a large case load, the electrocardiographic features, associated causes, and therapy outlined for each entity are considered. These factors outlined for each electrocardiographic entity are discussed only when there is a significant basis for diagnostic experience.

Electrocardiography has proved to be an important laboratory test in the diagnosis and management of feline cardiac disease.* The general principles already discussed for canine electrocardiography can easily be applied to the cat.[4]

---

*References 8, 11–17.

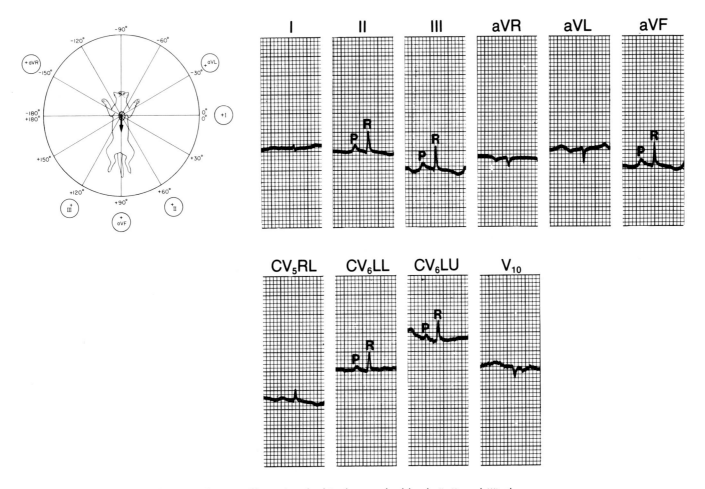

Fig. 5–2. Normal feline electrocardiogram illustrating the bipolar standard leads *(I, II, and III)*, the augmented unipolar limb leads *(aVR, aVL, and aVF)*, and the unipolar precordial chest leads *(CV₅RL, CV₆LL, CV₆LU, and V₁₀)*. Mean electrical axis, +90° (isoelectric lead is I). Note the normal small amplitudes of complexes in all leads.

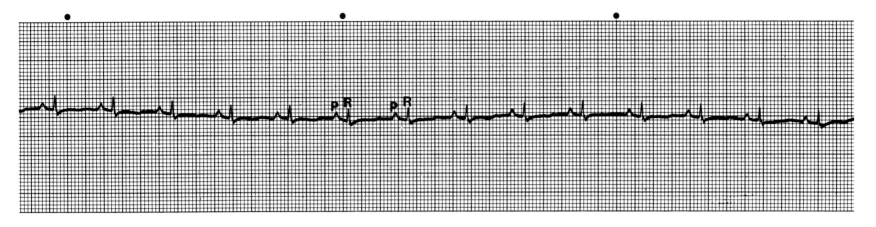

Fig. 5–3. Normal sinus rhythm (lead II) at a rate of 188 beats/min. The heart rate is normally accelerated in cats because of excitement, which influences the sympathetic system.

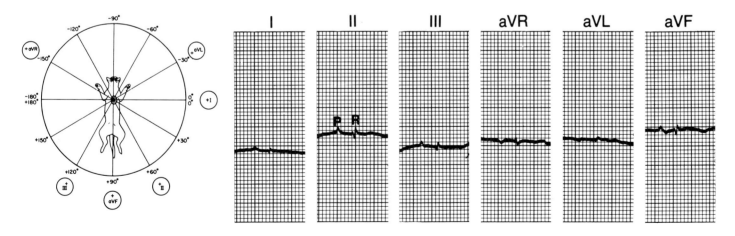

Fig. 5–4. Normal standard bipolar and augmented unipolar leads. The complexes are small, and all leads are essentially isoelectric. The electrical axis cannot be calculated when this happens.

Atrial enlargement

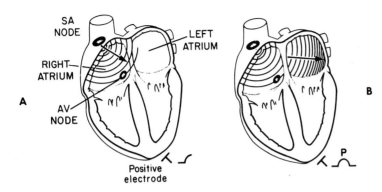

Fig. 5–5. **A,** As depolarization waves spread from the SA node through the right atrium, the P wave begins. The P wave is positive since the activation force is directed toward the positive electrode. **B,** The P wave is completed with depolarization of the left atrium.

The P wave represents atrial depolarization. The first portion of the P wave is produced primarily by the right atrium (Fig. 5–5); the latter portion, primarily by the left atrium. In right atrial enlargement, the P wave is of increased amplitude in leads II, III, and aVF; in left atrial enlargement, it is of increased duration; and in biatrial enlargement, it is of increased amplitude and duration. The term *enlargement* is used in conditions causing atrial hypertrophy and/or dilatation.

The diagnosis of atrial enlargement from the electrocardiogram is not always accurate. There is considerable normal variation in the voltage, duration, morphology, and direction of the P wave. Intra-atrial or interatrial conduction defects can cause changes in the P wave. The term *abnormality* may be more correct to indicate changes in P wave morphology.[18]

In man, P wave morphology has been correlated with left atrial appendage cell size, atrial fibrosis and echocardiographic measurement of left atrial size. Mitral valve disease leads to a hemodynamic insult to the left atrium that injures and destroys some cells. The increased pressure and/or volume load leads to cellular hypertrophy and atrial dilatation which results in death of some atrial cells with replacement fibrosis. The percent fibrosis is roughly correlated with the length of the P wave.[18a]

Electrocardiographic features

Right atrial enlargement (Fig. 5–6)
1. The P wave is greater than 0.2 mv (2 boxes) and usually slender and peaked.
2. A T_a wave is sometimes present. This slight depression of the baseline following the P wave represents atrial repolarization.

Left atrial enlargement (Fig. 5–7)
1. The duration of the P wave is greater than 0.04 second (2 boxes) Notching of the P wave is abnormal when the wave is also wide.

Biatrial enlargement (Fig. 5–8)
1. The P wave is greater than 0.2 mv (2 boxes) and wider than 0.04 second (2 boxes)

Associated conditions[11–13,16,19,20]

1. Right atrial enlargement: severe chronic respiratory disease, tricuspid dysplasia,[21] occasionally hypertrophic cardiomyopathy
2. Left atrial enlargement: cardiomyopathy (both hypertrophic and dilated), various congenital heart defects (e.g., mitral valvular insufficiency, aortic stenosis, ventricular septal defect, and patent ductus arteriosus), acquired mitral valvular insufficiency
3. Biatrial enlargement: most often seen with chronic hypertrophic cardiomyopathy (The possible mechanisms for the P wave abnormalities are [a] elevated end diastolic pressure with resistance to atrial emptying, [b] distortion of the AV valves by the hypertrophied ventricular septum, and [c] diffuse myocardial fibrosis causing intra-atrial conduction abnormalities. The presence of biatrial enlargement in cats with hypertrophic cardiomyopathy usually indicates the advanced stage of the disease. Other causes of biatrial enlargement include common AV canal, dilated form of cardiomyopathy, and ventricular septal defect.)

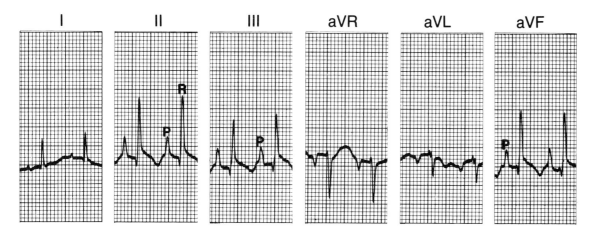

Fig. 5–6. Right atrial enlargement in a cat with hypertrophic cardiomyopathy. P waves are tall in leads *II, III,* and *aVF*.

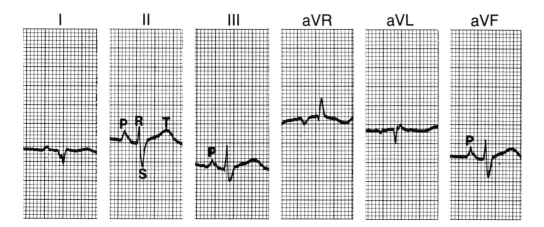

Fig. 5–7. Left atrial enlargement. P waves are wide (0.05 sec, or 2½ boxes) in leads *II, III,* and *aVF*. A distinct notch is present in the P waves of leads *III* and *aVF*.

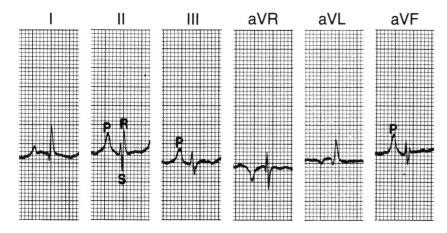

Fig. 5–8. Biatrial enlargement in a kitten with a common AV canal (septal defect). The P waves are both abnormally wide and abnormally tall in leads *II, III,* and *aVF*.

Right ventricular enlargement

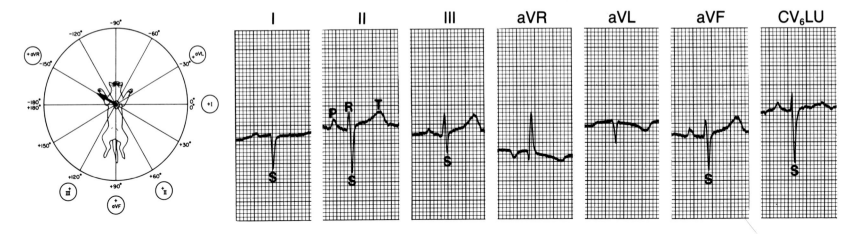

Fig. 5–9. Severe right ventricular enlargement in a cat with pulmonic stenosis. There is a right axis deviation of approximately −150°. Note the large S waves in leads *I, II, III, aVF,* and *CV₆LU.*

It is usually not possible to distinguish between ventricular hypertrophy and ventricular dilatation on the electrocardiogram, so the term *enlargement* is preferred. The heart is composed mainly of left ventricle. Because of the order of depolarization and the dominance of the left ventricle, the right ventricle must be markedly enlarged to cause changes on the electrocardiogram. Right ventricular enlargement therefore is often not detectable by electrocardiography. Prolongation of the QRS complex does not occur in right ventricular enlargement without conduction delay in the right bundle branch. The activation of even a very large right ventricle takes no longer than the normal activation of the left ventricle.[18]

Electrocardiographic features[8,12]

1. The electrocardiographic criteria for right ventricular enlargement in the cat have not been well established. Severe right ventricular enlargement produces some of the same electrocardiographic features observed in the dog. The most frequently observed electrocardiographic signs include the following:

   a. S waves in leads I, II, III, and aVF (usually 0.5 mv [5 boxes] or greater)
   b. Mean electrical axis of the QRS complex in the frontal plane greater than +160° and clockwise, especially when serial electrocardiograms on the same animal are compared

   c. Large S waves in leads CV_6LL and CV_6LU (usually greater than 0.7 mv or 7 boxes)
   d. Positive T wave in lead V_{10}
   e. Right atrial enlargement (tall P waves)

2. Right bundle branch block is often difficult to differentiate from right ventricular enlargement. The exclusion of diseases and radiographic signs of right ventricular enlargement supports the diagnosis of a conduction defect.

Associated conditions

1. Certain congenital cardiac defects, e.g., pulmonic stenosis, tetralogy of Fallot, patent ductus arteriosus with pulmonary hypertension, and common AV canal[11,19,20,22,23]
2. Heartworm disease[24]

Right ventricular enlargement is uncommon in cats with cardiomyopathy. In man electrocardiographic changes for right ventricular enlargement are commonly observed with the restrictive form of cardiomyopathy.[25] In a series of 28 cats with restrictive cardiomyopathy at The Animal Medical Center, electrocardiographic evidence of right ventricular enlargement was seen in only two cats. A more accurate clinical picture will be established as more cases of this type are seen.

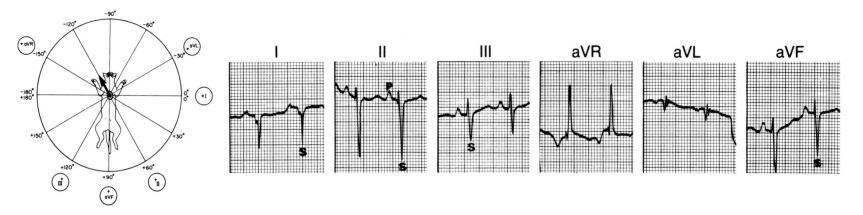

Fig. 5–10. Severe right ventricular enlargement in a cat with tetralogy of Fallot. There is abnormal right axis deviation (−120°). The S waves are large in leads *I, II, III,* and *aVF.*

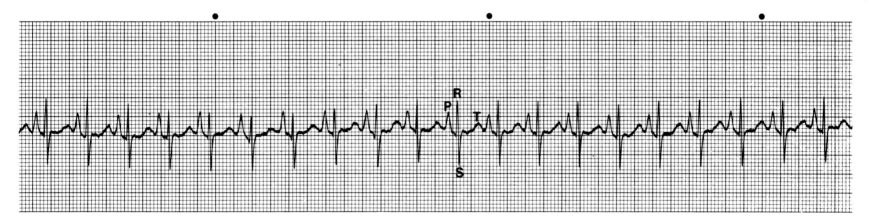

Fig. 5–11. Right ventricular enlargement (large S waves) and right atrial enlargement (tall and peaked P waves) in a cat with a ventricular septal defect. All these changes were also present in leads III and aVF.

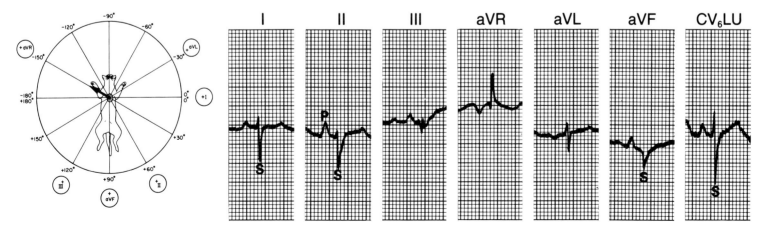

Fig. 5–12. Right ventricular enlargement in a cat with the restrictive form of cardiomyopathy. There is a right axis deviation of −150°. The S waves are large in leads *I, II, aVF,* and *CV₆LU.*

Left ventricular enlargement

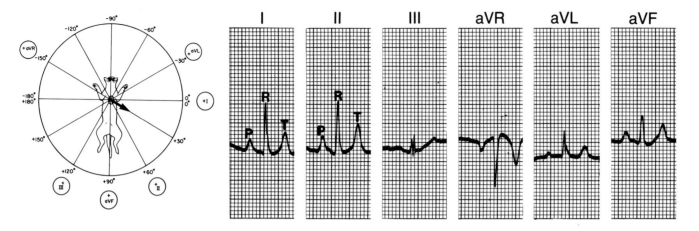

Fig. 5–13. Left ventricular enlargement in a cat with aortic stenosis. The R waves are abnormally high (1.3 mv, or 13 boxes) in leads *I* and *II*. The electrical axis is + 30°. The increased amplitude of the T waves (secondary changes) is often present when the R waves are tall.

Left ventricular enlargement may indicate dilatation and/or hypertrophy. The electrocardiographic evidence is common in cats with cardiomyopathy, especially the hypertrophic form. In one study, 17 of 59 cats (29%) with cardiomyopathy had features of left ventricular enlargement on the electrocardiogram.[11]

Due to the increased muscle mass in hypertrophy, the height of the R wave is increased, the QRS complex is delayed or altered in conduction, the S-T segment is depressed, and the T wave or repolarization process is changed. The diagnosis of left ventricular enlargement is based primarily on increased voltage of the QRS deflections (lead II and left precordial leads). An enlarged ventricle with thickened walls and increased surface area produces larger potentials than does a normal ventricle. An enlarged ventricle also brings the heart closer to the chest wall, so voltages recorded by the precordial leads are greater.[18]

Electrocardiographic features

1. The R wave of the QRS complex exceed 0.9 mv (9 boxes) in lead II. The R wave should not exceed 1.0 mv or 10 boxes in CV_6LU.

2. The maximum width of the QRS is 0.04 second (2 boxes).

3. Displacement of the S-T segment occurs in a direction opposite the main QRS deflection. This causes the S-T segment to sag into the T wave (S-T coving).

4. Repolarization changes cause the T wave to be of increased amplitude (usually greater than 0.3 mv or 3 boxes in lead II).

5. A mean electrical axis deviation in the frontal plane of less than 0° may be present.

6. Other patterns are characteristically seen with left ventricular enlargement:

   a. Left atrial enlargement (widened P waves) and/or right atrial enlargement (often with hypertrophic cardiomyopathy)[26]

   b. Intraventricular conduction defects (The occurrence of these may invalidate the electrocardiographic features of left ventricular enlargement. For example, subendocardial fibrosis often occurs with left ventricular hypertrophy in hypertrophic cardiomyopathy. The anterior fascicle is frequently affected at the same time.)

   c. Deep Q waves in leads I and aVL (normal values not established, but usually greater than 0.5 mv) (This may suggest an asymmetric hypertrophy of the septum [Fig. 5–15]. Abnormal Q waves are probably the result of an abnormal depolarization vector of the thickened septum.[27,28])

Associated conditions

1. Certain congenital cardiac defects, e.g., aortic stenosis, patent ductus arteriosus, and ventricular septal defect[11,20,29]

2. Primary myocardial disease: both hypertrophic and dilated forms of cardiomyopathy[16,17,30]

3. Chronic anemia, chronic renal disease due possibly to systemic hypertension[31]

4. Hyperthyroidism due to functional thyroid adenomas in 22 of 45 cats.[32] In 131 cases from The Animal Medical Center, 29% had increased R-wave amplitude and 23% had prolonged QRS duration.[32a]

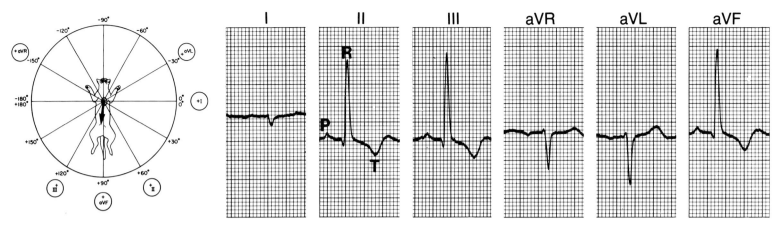

Fig. 5–14. Left ventricular enlargement in a 16-year-old cat with chronic renal disease. A positive relationship probably exists between renal disease and hypertension; secondary left ventricular hypertrophy is the result. The R waves are strikingly tall in leads *II, III,* and *aVF.* The QRS duration is wide (0.06 sec, or 3 boxes). The electrical axis is normal (+100°).

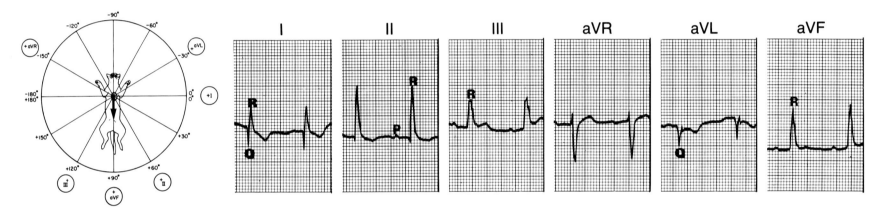

Fig. 5–15. Left ventricular enlargement. Note the increased width and amplitude of the QRS complexes in leads *II* and *aVF.* Note also the deep Q waves in leads *I* and *aVL.* A diagnosis of asymmetric septal hypertrophy with severe obstruction of the left ventricular outflow tract was found at necropsy. (From Tilley, L.P., et al.: Am. J. Pathol., *87:*493, 1977; with permission.)

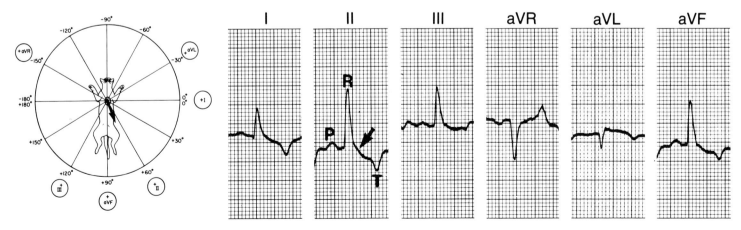

Fig. 5–16. Left ventricular enlargement in a cat with hypertrophic cardiomyopathy. The R waves are abnormally high in leads *II, III,* and *aVF.* The QRS duration is wide (0.05 sec, or 2½ boxes). The S-T segment coving (arrow) adds support to the diagnosis of left ventricular enlargement. Left atrial enlargement is also present (0.06 sec, or 3 boxes in width).

Intraventricular conduction defects

An intraventricular conduction defect results from a delay or block in one or more of the pathways of the conduction system below the bundle of His. The intraventricular system is composed of three major conduction pathways (Fig. 5–17): (1) the right bundle branch and (2) the anterior and (3) posterior fascicles of the left bundle branch. A block or delay in conduction can occur in one, two, or all three pathways at the same time.

Intraventricular conduction defects are frequently observed in cats with cardiomyopathy, especially the hypertrophic form. In one report conduction disturbances occurred in 5 of 27 cats with hypertrophic cardiomyopathy (4 with left anterior hemiblock and 1 with left bundle branch block).[28] Degeneration or fibrosis of the AV node and its bundle branches, associated with endocardial and myocardial fibrosis and organized endomyocarditis, was consistently observed in the hearts of 63 cats with cardiomyopathy.[33] Lesions occurred in the left bundle branch in 54 cats; the right bundle branch was involved in 20 cats. Lesions were absent in 10 hearts of normal adult cats used as controls.

The major forms of intraventricular block occurring in cats can be classified as follows:[34–36]

1. Bundle branch block: right, left, (i.e., block in the main left bundle or in each of the two fascicles)
2. Fascicular block: left anterior, left posterior
3. Various combinations of block in all three major conduction pathways, e.g., right bundle branch with anterior or posterior fascicular
4. Block in all three conduction pathways, producing complete heart block

A block or delay in conduction in any of the three major pathways causes the affected side to be depolarized late (Figs. 5–18 and 5–19). In right and left bundle branch block, the duration of the QRS complex is lengthened. The duration of the QRS complex in bundle branch block is not well established in man, dogs, and cats.

Many physiologic and pathologic factors are involved in establishing the criteria for bundle branch block. For example, the end of the QRS complex is not readily identified. The QRS complex widens as the heart size increases during growth of the kitten and during advanced age because of physiologic aging of the conduction system.[37] Also, the duration of the QRS complex depends on the cardiac mass and therefore on the sex, weight, and breed. A prolonged QRS complex can be normal in some cats. An intraventricular conduction defect should not be diagnosed just on the basis of a wide QRS complex. Intraventricular conduction defects can also occur in animals without evidence of heart disease.

Unless criteria for diagnosing and classifying different types of intraventricular conduction defects are well established, the word *pattern* may be more appropriate than *block*.[38] Because definitive data regarding the genesis of the QRS complex in cats are not available, the salient features for the electrocardiographic diagnosis of intraventricular conduction defects can be only proposed. A basis of diagnosis must be extrapolated from criteria established in both man and the dog.[18]

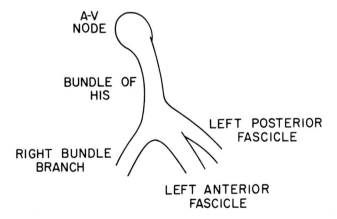

Fig. 5–17. The intraventricular conduction system.

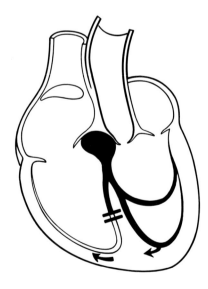

Fig. 5–18. Right bundle branch block. The right ventricle is stimulated by the impulse, which passes from the left bundle branch to the right side of the septum below the block. It is then activated with delay, causing the QRS complex to become wide and bizarre. (From Phillips, R.E., and Feeney, M.K.: *The Cardiac Rhythms*. Philadelphia, W.B. Saunders, 1980, with permission.)

Left bundle branch block

Left bundle branch block is a delay or block of conduction in the left bundle branch, whether in the *main branch* (Fig. 5–19) or at the level of the anterior and posterior *fascicles*. The two anatomic types cannot be distinguished electrocardiographically. A supraventricular impulse activates the right ventricle first through the right bundle branch. The left ventricle is then activated late, causing the QRS complex to become wide and bizarre.

Left bundle branch block is an uncommon intraventricular conduction defect in cats. Because of the extensive network of the left bundle (anterior fascicle, posterior fascicle, and septal interconnections), the lesion must be large to cause a block.

Electrocardiographic features

1. The QRS complex is of 0.06 second (3 boxes) or greater duration. This value may be subject to change in the future. Bundle branch block has been defined as greater than 0.07 second.[12]
2. The QRS complex is wide and positive in leads I, II, III, and aVF and in leads over the left precordium (CV$_6$LL and CV$_6$LU).
3. The QRS complex is inverted in leads aVR and CV$_5$RL.
4. When the left branch is blocked, the normal initial activation of the septum is disturbed and the first part of the QRS is altered. The Q wave is often absent in leads that definitely record septal activity in the right-to-left axis, e.g., leads I and CV$_6$LU. For example, distinct Q waves are normally present in close to 60% of normal cats.[6]

5. The presence of first- or second-degree AV block may indicate involvement of the right bundle branch (Fig. 5–20).
6. Left bundle branch block must be differentiated from left ventricular enlargement. The absence of left ventricular enlargement on thoracic radiographs lends support to a diagnosis of isolated left bundle branch block. Both left ventricular hypertrophy and left bundle branch block may occur simultaneously. Subendocardial fibrosis often accompanies hypertrophied muscle.[33]
7. Intermittent left bundle branch block (tachycardia- or bradycardia-dependent) or bundle branch block alternans may be present in serial tracings or on the same tracing.[18,39,40]

Associated conditions

1. Underlying severe cardiac disease. (The cardiac lesion must be large because the left bundle branch is so thick and extensive.)
2. Primary myocardial disease. (Left bundle branch block has been seen with the hypertrophic form of cardiomyopathy.[28])

Treatment

1. Left bundle branch block, in and of itself, does not cause any severe hemodynamic abnormalities. If the right bundle branch becomes involved, complete heart block can result (Fig. 5–20); then treatment is essential.

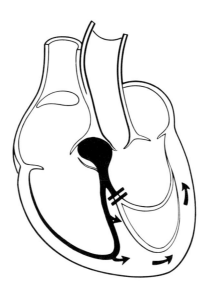

Fig. 5–19. Left bundle branch block in the main left bundle branch. Block can also occur at the level of the anterior and posterior fascicles. The impulse cannot enter the left bundle system and activate the left septal fibers. Therefore, the septum is initially depolarized from fibers arising from the distal portion of the right bundle branch, resulting in an initial vector oriented to the left. The left ventricle is then activated late, causing the QRS complex to become wide and bizarre. (From Phillips, R.E., and Feeney, M.K.: *The Cardiac Rhythms*. Philadelphia, W.B. Saunders, 1980, with permission.)

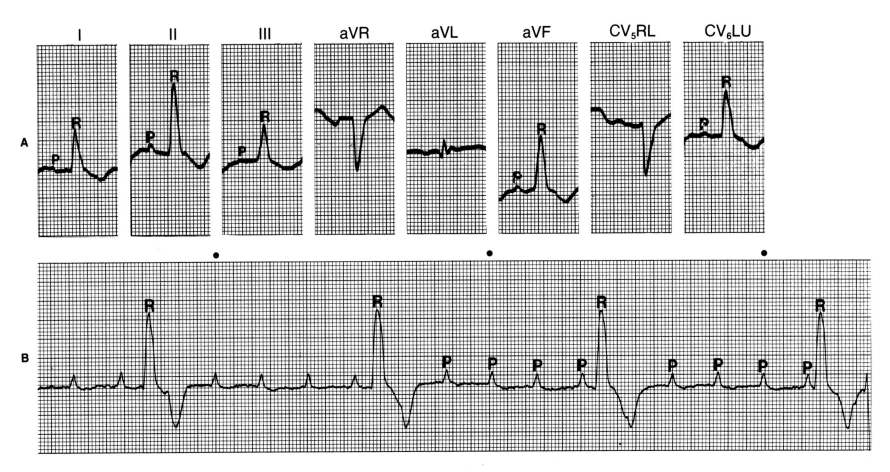

Fig. 5–20. Left bundle branch block and AV block. **A,** Left bundle branch block in a cat with severe hypertrophic cardiomyopathy. The QRS complex is of 0.07 second (3½ boxes) duration and is positive in leads *I, II, III, aVF,* and *CV₆LU*. Neither a Q wave nor an S wave is present in these leads. The QRS complex is inverted in leads *aVR* and *CV₅RL*. The prolonged P-R interval of 0.12 second (6 boxes) may indicate involvement of the right bundle branch or the AV junction. **B,** Complete heart block in a cat with hypertrophic cardiomyopathy. The P waves are totally independent of the R waves. The QRS configuration is of a left bundle branch block. The QRS complex width is increased to 0.08 second (4 boxes) and is positive. Involvement of the right bundle branch is probably also present since a sinus rhythm with first-degree AV block and left bundle branch block was observed 2 weeks prior to this strip. The ventricular pacemaker is located in the His-Purkinje system. An artificial pacemaker is needed.

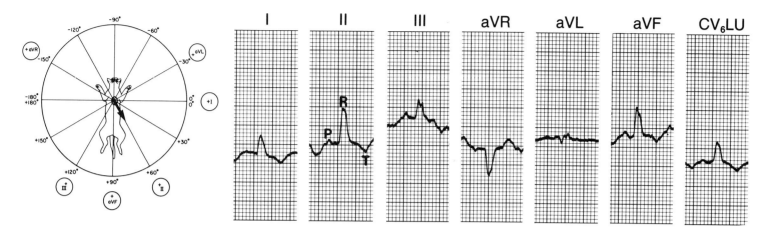

Fig. 5–21. Left bundle branch block in a cat with hypertrophic cardiomyopathy. The QRS complexes are of 0.06 second (3 boxes) duration. The lack of Q waves gives support to this diagnosis. The mean electrical axis is +60°.

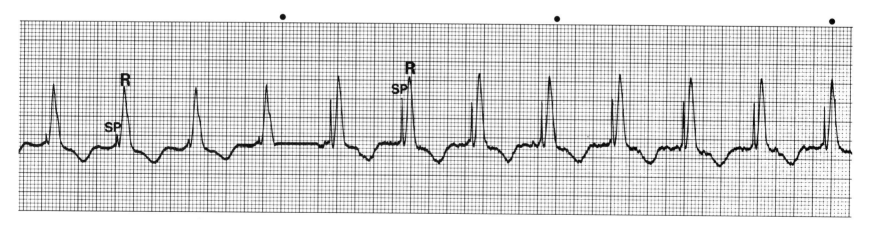

Fig. 5–22. Left bundle branch block pattern in a cat with a transvenous electrode wire in the right ventricle. In right ventricular stimulation, the left ventricle is activated late. The QRS complex width is increased to 0.06 second (3 boxes) and is positive. The first four complexes are lead I; the rest of the strip is lead II. *SP*, Pacemaker spike, electrical impulse delivered by the artificial pacemaker.

Right bundle branch block

Right bundle branch block refers to a delay or block of conduction in the right bundle branch (Fig. 5–18). The right ventricle is stimulated by the impulse, which passes from the left bundle branch to the right side of the septum below the block. It is then activated with delay, causing the QRS complex to become wide and bizarre.

Electrocardiographic features[8,11]

1. The QRS complex is of 0.06 second (3 boxes) or greater duration.
2. A right axis deviation is usually present.
3. The QRS complex is positive in aVR and CV₅RL and has a wide rsR' or RSR' pattern (often M shaped) in CV_5RL.
4. The QRS complexes have large wide S waves in leads I, II, III, aVF, CV_6LL, and CV_6LU. An S wave or W pattern may be seen in lead V_{10}.
5. Support can be given to the diagnosis of isolated right bundle branch block if diseases causing severe right ventricular enlargement are excluded from laboratory tests. For example, the thoracic radiograph can be used to evaluate any right ventricular enlargement.
6. Intermittent bundle branch block (dependent on tachycardia or bradycardia) or bundle branch block alternans may be present in serial tracings or in the same tracing.[41]
7. The presence of first- or second-degree AV block may indicate involvement of the left bundle branch (see Fig. 5–29).

Associated conditions

1. Occasionally in normal and healthy cats
2. Congenital heart disease, e.g., persistent common AV canal[11,19]
3. Cardiac neoplasia, e.g., lymphosarcoma or metastatic mammary gland tumor[43]
4. Primary myocardial disease. Right bundle branch block has been seen in three cats with dilated cardiomyopathy, in five cats with hypertrophic cardiomyopathy and in six cats with restrictive cardiomyopathy (form with excessive moderator bands).[16,42] Right bundle branch block is not as frequent as left anterior fascicular block. The difference is probably due to the fact that the endomyocardial fibrosis predominately affects the left ventricle.[17,33]
5. Causes of hyperkalemia, especially feline urethral obstruction[8] (Fig. 5–25)

Treatment

1. Right bundle branch block, in and of itself, does not cause any hemodynamic problems. Therapy should be directed at the primary disease affecting the right ventricle.
2. The outcome of right bundle branch block is primarily dependent on whether either of the two fascicles of the left branch becomes involved. Complete heart block can then sometimes be the result, and treatment is essential.

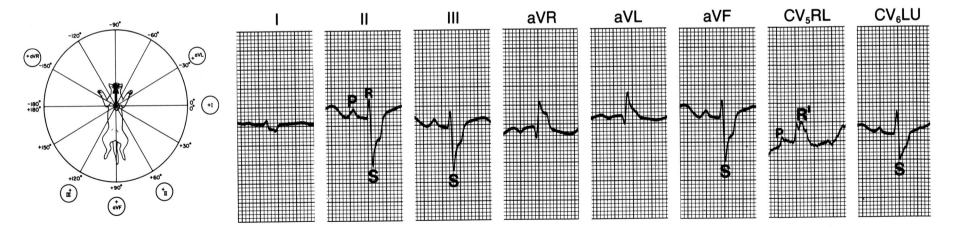

Fig. 5–23. Right bundle branch block in a cat with the dilated form of cardiomyopathy. The QRS duration is 0.08 sec (4 boxes). Large and wide S waves are present in leads *I, II, III, aVF,* and *CV₆LU*. The QRS in *CV₅RL* has a wide R wave (M-shaped). There is a marked axis deviation (approximately −90°).

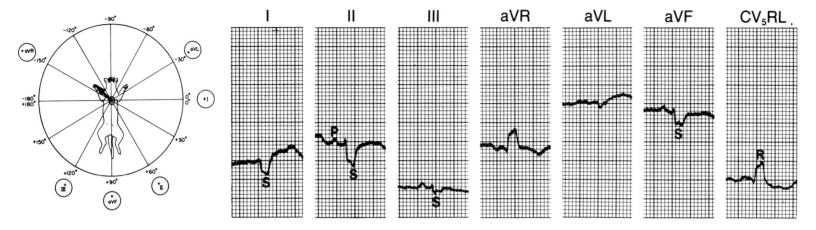

Fig. 5–24. Right bundle branch block in a cat with a common AV canal. The QRS duration is 0.07 second (3½ boxes). Large and wide S waves are present in leads *I, II, III,* and *aVF*. A wide and positive R wave is present in *CV₅RL*. There is a right axis deviation (−135°).

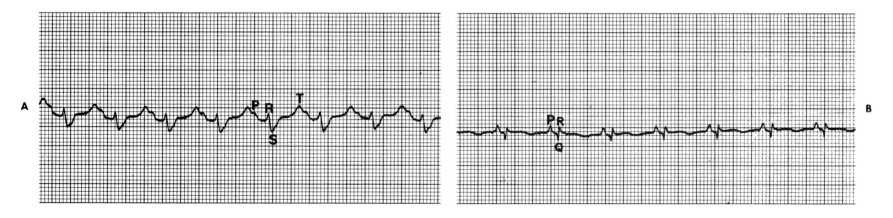

Fig. 5–25. **A,** Right bundle branch block in a cat with hyperkalemia (serum potassium, 7.5 mEq/L) due to a urethral obstruction. The QRS duration is 0.07 second with a large S wave (also present in leads I, III, and aVF, not shown). The P wave is superimposed on the previous T wave, and the P-R interval is 0.08 second. **B,** Five hours after therapy, the conduction defect has disappeared and AV conduction is normalized. The QRS-T complexes are now normal.

Fascicular block

As described in Chapter 1, the left main bundle divides into the anterior and posterior fascicles and the septal fascicle (the last an interconnection of the first two with distribution over the mid-septal area).

A block in either the anterior or the posterior fascicle of the left bundle (Fig. 5–26) causes only a slight prolongation of left ventricular depolarization. The main effect is on the direction of the depolarization. The general direction of depolarization is shifted toward the blocked fascicle.

Fascicular blocks in the cat have been described frequently in the literature.[8,12,16,28,44] Anterior fascicular block is a common intraventricular conduction defect in cats. The electrocardiographic pattern of anterior fascicular block has been shown to be commonly associated with hypertrophic cardiomyopathy.[28,45] This pattern in hypertrophic cardiomyopathy is compatible with an actual conduction defect and/or left ventricular hypertrophy. Based on studies by Rosenbaum,[35] the anterior fascicle is more vulnerable because (1) it has a different blood supply (in man, the anterior fascicle has only a single blood supply), (2) it is longer and thinner, and (3) it is located in the turbulent outflow tract of the left ventricle. Both myocardial fibrosis and left ventricular outflow disturbances occur in feline hypertrophic cardiomyopathy.

Electrocardiographic features

Left anterior fascicular block (Fig. 5–27). This can be recognized by the following combination of observed features:

1. QRS complex duration usually within normal limits (If widening occurs, it does not reach 0.06 sec.)
2. Marked left axis deviation in the frontal plane, or a shift to the left when compared with the electrocardiogram before the block. (The axis is usually around −60° [aVR being isoelectric].)
3. Small q wave and tall R wave in leads I and aVL (One report in man indicates that small q waves may not be required.[46])
4. Deep S waves in leads II, III, and aVF exceeding the r wave

Other causes of the left anterior fascicular pattern should be excluded, particularly hyperkalemia, left ventricular hypertrophy, and an altered position of the heart within the thorax.

In man, new electrocardiographic criteria have been proposed.[47] The use of the proposed criteria requires that the tracings be obtained with three-channel electrocardiographs so that the relation between the QRS complexes in simultaneously recorded limb leads can be inspected. The proposed electrocardiographic criteria are: (1) that the QRS complexes in leads aVR and aVL each end in an R wave, and (2) that the peak of the terminal R wave in lead aVR occurs later than the peak of the terminal R wave in lead aVL.

Right bundle branch and left anterior fascicular block. This is recognized by the combination of electrocardiographic features for each block[8,44] (Fig. 5–28):

1. QRS complex duration 0.06 second (3 boxes) or greater
2. Marked left axis deviation in the frontal plane (usually greater than −60°)
3. Wide and deep S waves in leads I, II, III, aVF, and CV_6LU
4. Tall R wave and small q wave in leads I and aVL
5. QRS complex in CV_5RL with a wide rsR′ or RSR′ pattern (often M shaped)

Associated conditions

1. Hypertrophic cardiomyopathy[26,28,44,48]
2. Restrictive cardiomyopathy[16,42]
3. Causes of left ventricular hypertrophy, e.g., aortic stenosis[19]
4. Causes of hyperkalemia[49,50]

Treatment

1. Fascicular blocks, in and of themselves, do not cause hemodynamic abnormalities. Therapy should be directed at the underlying primary disease (e.g., drugs to lower the serum potassium in hyperkalemia).

2. Right bundle branch block and left anterior fascicular block may develop symptomatic second- or third-degree AV block, making treatment essential (Fig. 5–29).

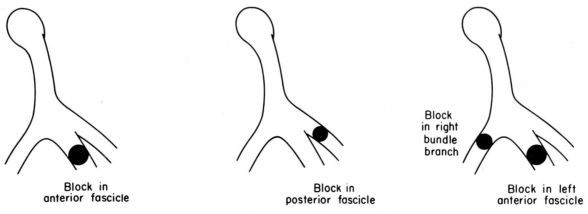

Fig. 5–26. Three forms of fascicular block.

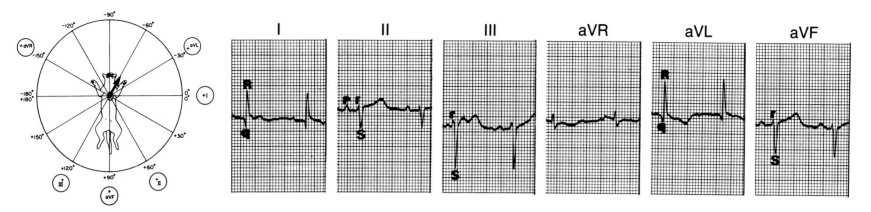

Fig. 5–27. Left anterior fascicular block in a cat with hypertrophic cardiomyopathy. There is a severe left axis deviation (−60°) with a qR pattern in leads *I* and *aVL* and an rS pattern in leads *II, III,* and *aVF*. The QRS complexes are of normal duration. (From Tilley, L.P.: Vet. Clin. North Am., 7:257, 1977; with permission.)

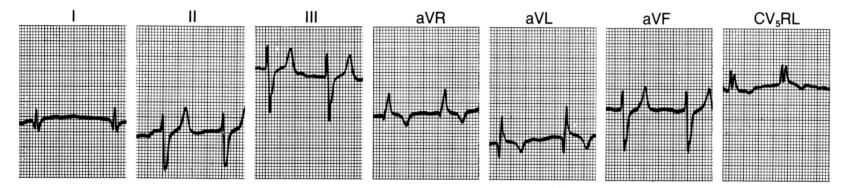

Fig. 5–28. Right bundle branch block with left anterior fascicular block in a cat with hypertrophic cardiomyopathy. Combination of criteria for each type of block: wide QRS complex (0.06 sec); large S waves in leads *I, II, III,* and *aVF;* small q and large R in leads *I* and *aVL;* and a marked left axis deviation (−90°). A wide M-shaped complex (RsR') is present in *CV₅RL* to complete the criteria. Atrial fibrillation is also present, explaining the lack of P waves.

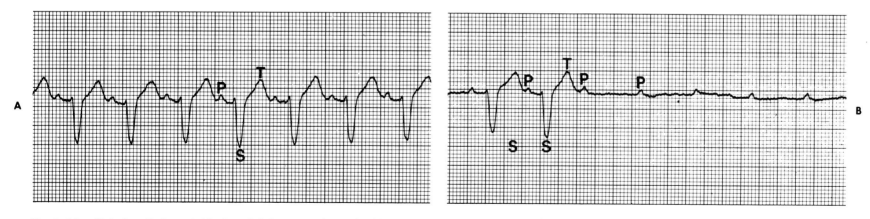

Fig. 5–29. Right bundle branch block with left anterior fascicular block and intermittent AV block in a cat with hypertrophic cardiomyopathy. **A,** Normal sinus rhythm with QRS duration of 0.07 second and large S waves. The other leads (not shown) documented the two conduction defects. **B,** Minutes later a period of blocked P waves (advanced AV block) after two sinus complexes. The AV block is probably caused by an added conduction block in the posterior fascicle.

S-T segment abnormalities

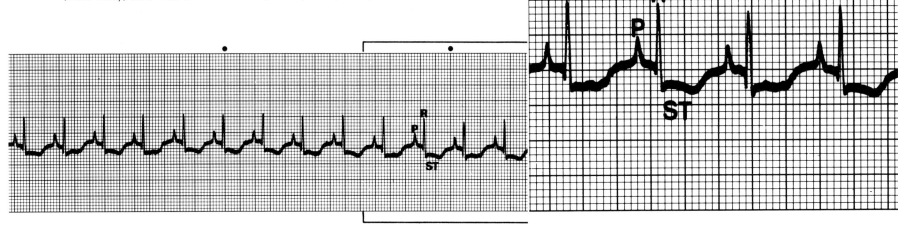

Fig. 5–30. S-T segment depression in a cat with hypertrophic obstructive cardiomyopathy. Reduced coronary blood flow can produce myocardial ischemia. (From Tilley, L.P.: Vet. Clin. North Am., 7:273, 1977; with permission.)

The S-T segment represents the time from the end of the QRS interval to the onset of the T wave, i.e., the early phase of ventricular repolarization. It may be above (elevated), at, or below (depressed) the level of the baseline. The baseline or isoelectric line is on the same level as the T-P segment, between the T wave and the P wave.

Electrocardiographic features[8,12]

1. Deviations of the S-T segment are usually marked, i.e., of at least ±0.1 mv (1 box) or more.
2. The S-T segment normally curves gently into the proximal limb of the T wave.
3. It is helpful to compare any S-T segment changes with those seen on previous tracings from that animal.

Associated conditions

1. Normal variation
2. S-T segment depression in leads II, III, aVF, and CV_6LU or those with dominant R waves:
   a. Myocardial ischemia (inadequate circulation)[12]
   b. Hyperkalemia[51,52]
   c. Hypokalemia[51]
   d. Digitalis: a "sagging" effect to the S-T segment
3. S-T segment elevation in leads II, III, aVF, and CV_6LU or those with dominant R waves:
   a. Myocardial infarction (transmural, entire thickness of the left ventricle): changes in leads overlying the infarction[53]
   b. Pericarditis[54,55]
   c. Myocardial hypoxia (oxygen deficiency)[51]
   d. An electrocardiographic indication for digoxin toxicosis is S-T segment elevation[56]
4. Secondary S-T segment changes from abnormalities of the QRS complex, e.g., hypertrophy, bundle branch block, and VPCs. (The displacement is in a direction opposite that of the main ventricular deflection.)
5. Artifact, e.g., wandering baseline
6. Pseudodepression of the S-T segment, due to a prominent T_a wave (atrial repolarization) in tachycardia or atrial changes

Treatment

1. Treatment should be directed at the underlying disorder, if one is present.

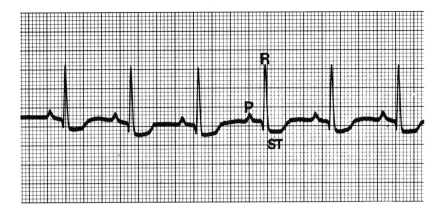

Fig. 5–31. "Sagging" type S-T segment depression in a cat with digoxin toxicity. The concavity of the S-T segment disappeared after digoxin was stopped. The tall R waves represent left ventricular enlargement, from dilated cardiomyopathy.

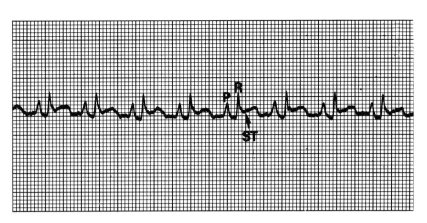

Fig. 5–32. S-T segment elevation in a cat with pericardial effusion. The amplitude of the R wave increased (not shown) after pericardiocentesis. The P-R segment depression could represent subepicardial atrial injury.

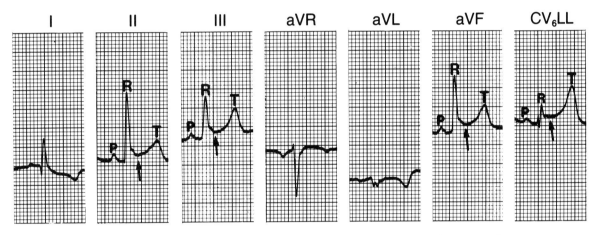

Fig. 5–33. S-T segment elevation (arrows) (leads *II, III, aVF,* and *CV₆LL*) in a cat with severe pulmonary edema secondary to hypertrophic cardiomyopathy. There is probable severe myocardial hypoxia. The S-T segment elevation and the large T waves disappeared after treatment (not shown).

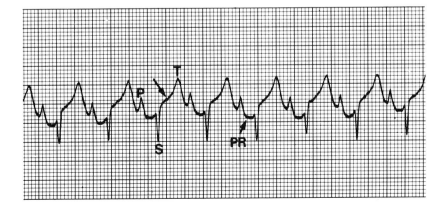

Fig. 5–34. S-T segment elevation (upper arrow) in a cat with right ventricular enlargement (large S waves also present in leads I, II, III, and aVF). The S-T segment elevation reflects the repolarization process of the large right ventricle. Note also the depressed P-R segment, secondary to the tall P wave and/or sinus tachycardia.

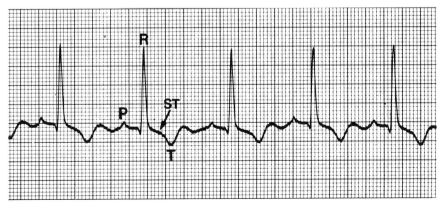

Fig. 5–35. S-T segment depression in a cat with severe left ventricular enlargement. This S-T segment depression (S-T coving) is a secondary change due to the high amplitude of the R wave.

117

T wave abnormalities

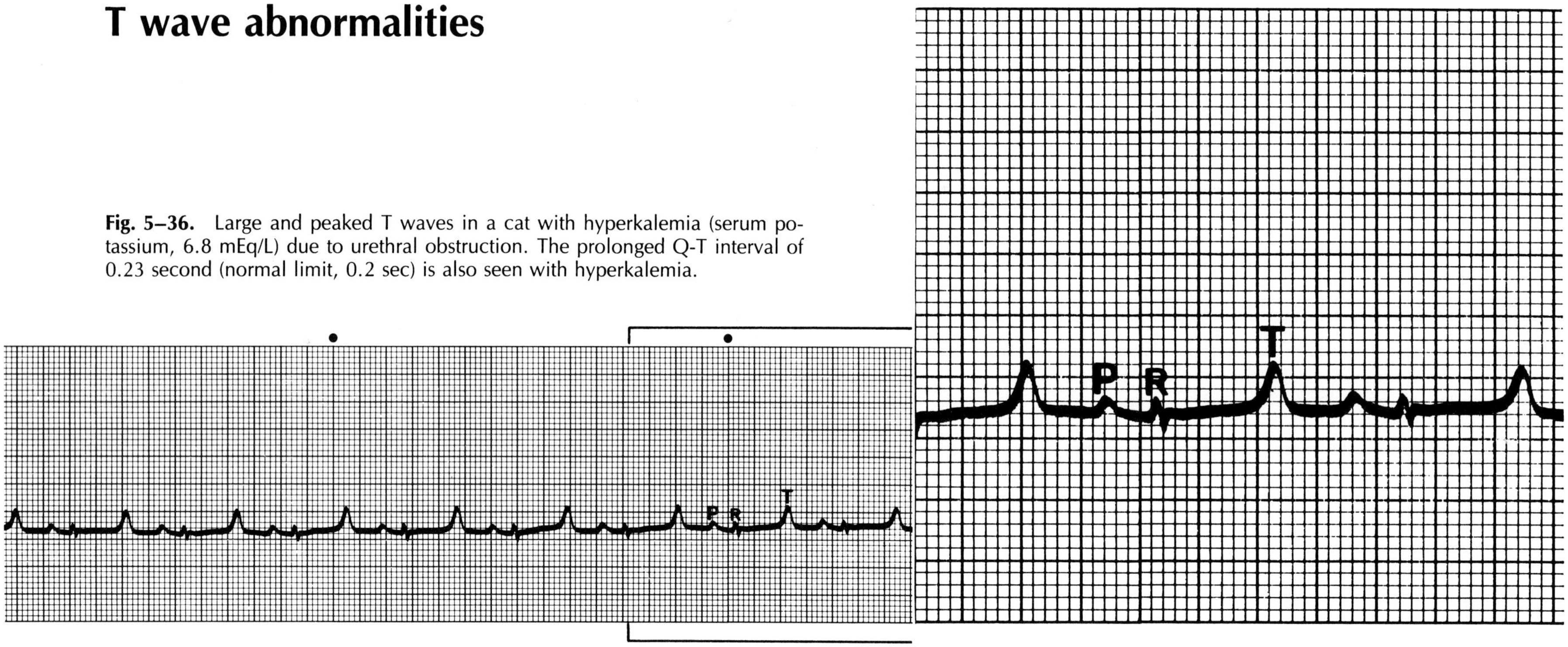

Fig. 5–36. Large and peaked T waves in a cat with hyperkalemia (serum potassium, 6.8 mEq/L) due to urethral obstruction. The prolonged Q-T interval of 0.23 second (normal limit, 0.2 sec) is also seen with hyperkalemia.

The T wave is the first major deflection following the QRS complex. It represents the recovery period or repolarization of the ventricles and may be positive, notched, negative, or biphasic. In the cat it is most accurately analyzed when compared with T waves on previous tracings from the same animal or during anesthesia.

The T wave may be of abnormal amplitude, shape, or direction (polarity). Abnormalities can be classified into two general types:[18] (1) primary, changes independent of depolarization, and (2) secondary, changes directly dependent on the depolarization process.

In man, alterations in the sequence of ventricular activation (for example, left bundle branch block) may alter ventricular repolarization and apparently cause primary T wave abnormalities. The T wave changes may persist for days or weeks after the change in activation sequence (the left bundle branch block) is discontinued. The polarity of the abnormal T wave is the same as the polarity of the major QRS deflection in the same lead. These transient T wave abnormalities can be indicative of myocardial disease, but can also occur in the absence of clinically detectable heart disease.[57]

Electrocardiographic features

1. The T wave rarely exceeds 0.3 mv (3 boxes).[12] Accuracy as to diagnosis is improved if serial electrocardiograms are compared.

2. The T wave is normally slightly asymmetric. T waves that are sharply pointed or notched may indicate an underlying abnormality such as electrolyte imbalances. A marked change in the shape of the T waves on serial electrocardiogram is usually abnormal.

3. The polarity of secondary T wave change is usually not the same as that of the QRS complex. Reversal of T wave polarity on serial electrocardiograms is most often abnormal.

4. Isolated T wave alternans can occur (Fig. 5–40). This phenomenon consists of the rhythmic alternation of the configuration of the T wave without any concomitant change in the QRS complex.[58]

Associated conditions

1. Myocardial hypoxia (oxygen deficiency),[51] due to anesthetic complications and in animals with heart disease during bradycardia (T waves larger), myocardial infarction (T waves larger with a change in polarity[53]) (These changes represent a primary abnormality independent of depolarization.)

2. Intraventricular conduction defects: ventricular enlargement and VPCs (T waves become larger secondary to the altered course of the QRS deflections. The direction of the T wave is usually opposite that of the main QRS deflection.)

3. Electrolyte imbalances (T waves become larger and spiked with hyperkalemia.[51,52])

4. Metabolic diseases, e.g., anemia, shock, uremia, ketoacidosis, hypoglycemia, and fever (T wave changes are nonspecific. Other abnormalities appear when compared with previous tracings.)

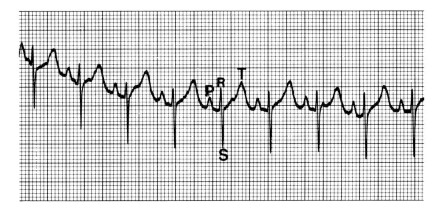

Fig. 5–37. Anterior fascicular block (remaining criteria confirmed on other leads) with secondary large positive T waves due to the altered QRS deflections.

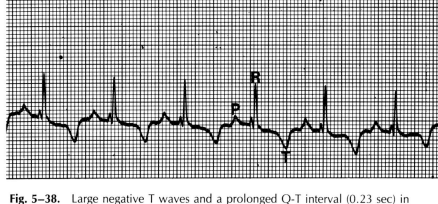

Fig. 5–38. Large negative T waves and a prolonged Q-T interval (0.23 sec) in a cat with chronic renal failure and subsequent hypocalcemia and hyperkalemia.

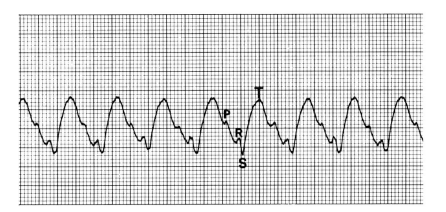

Fig. 5–39. Large positive T waves in a cat with pleural effusion from right-sided congestive heart failure. The rapid heart rate of 230 beats/min and tall T waves are probably secondary to myocardial hypoxia. An artifact from respiratory movements should be considered but was not present in this case.

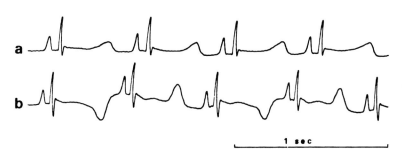

Fig. 5–40. Anesthetized cat. **a,** control; **b,** 5 seconds after the cessation of a 30-second electrical stimulation of both stellate ganglia. Alternation in polarity of the T wave is evident. (From Schwartz, P.J., and Malliani, A.: Electrical alternation of the T-wave. Am. Heart J., *89:*45, 1975, with permission.)

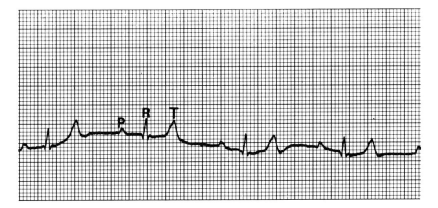

Fig. 5–41. Hyperkalemia (serum potassium, 6.5 mEq/L) in a cat with urethral obstruction. T waves are tall and pointed, and the P-R interval is prolonged (0.12 sec).

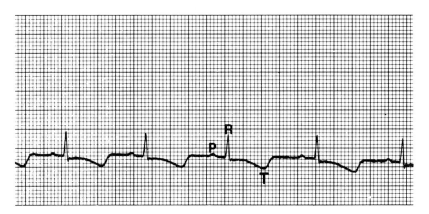

Fig. 5–42. Large negative T waves in a cat with dilated cardiomyopathy. The slow heart rate of 120 beats/min in conjunction with the heart disease has possibly caused myocardial hypoxia. T waves decreased in size as the heart rate increased.

5. Drug toxicity, e.g., digitalis and propranolol (T wave changes are nonspecific.)
6. Certain physiologic factors, e.g., respiratory abnormalities and autonomic neural control[59] (T wave abnormalities can also be seen in normal animals.)
7. T wave alternans: increases in circulatory catecholamines, hypocalcemia, and acute increases in sympathetic discharge[58]

Treatment

1. Treatment should be directed at the underlying disorder if one is present.

REFERENCES

1. Simonson, E.: *Differentiation between Normal and Abnormal in Electrocardiography*. St. Louis, C.V. Mosby, 1961.
2. Tilley, L.P. (chairman), Gompf, R.E., Bolton, G., and Harpster, N.: Criteria for the normal feline electrocardiogram. The Academy of Veterinary Cardiology Committee Report, 1977.
3. Blok, J., and Boeles, J.T.F.: The electrocardiogram of the normal cat. Acta Physiol. Pharmacol., *6*:95, 1957.
4. Hamlin, R.L., Smetzer, D.L., and Smith, C.R.: The electrocardiogram, phonocardiogram and derived ventricular activation process of domestic cats. Am. J. Vet. Res., *24*:792, 1963.
5. Rogers, W.A., and Bishop, S.P.: Electrocardiographic parameters of the normal domestic cat. A comparison of standard limb leads and an orthogonal system. J. Electrocardiol., *4*:315, 1971.
6. Gompf, R.E., and Tilley, L.P.: Comparison of lateral and sternal recumbent position for electrocardiography of the cat. Am. J. Vet. Res., *40*:1483, 1979.
7. Robertson, B.T., Figg, F.A., and Ewell, W.M.: Normal values for the electrocardiogram in the cat. Feline Pract., *2*:20, 1976.
8. Tilley, L.P., and Gompf, R.E.: Feline electrocardiography. Vet. Clin. North Am., *7*:257, 1977.
8a. Soderberg, S.F., et al.: M-mode echocardiography as a diagnostic aid for feline cardiomyopathy. Vet. Radiol., *24*:66, 1983.
9. Rousselot, J.F.: The normal electrocardiogram in the cat. Rec. Med. Vet., *156*:439, 1980.
10. Coulter, D.B., and Calvert, C.A.: Orientation and configuration of vectorcardiographic QRS loops from normal cats. Am. J. Vet. Res., *42*:282, 1981.
11. Harpster, N.K.: Cardiovascular diseases of the cat. Adv. Vet. Sci. Comp. Med., *21*:39, 1977.
12. Harris, S.G., and Ogburn, P.N.: The cardiovascular system. In *Feline Medicine and Surgery*. Edited by E.J. Catcott. 2nd Edition. Santa Barbara, Calif., American Veterinary Publications, 1975.
13. Tilley, L.P.: Feline cardiology. Proc. Am. Anim. Hosp. Assoc., *43*:79, 1976.
14. Tilley, L.P.: Feline cardiac arrhythmias. Vet. Clin. North Am., *7*:273, 1977.
15. Tilley, L.P.: Feline cardiology. In *Katzen Krankheiten, Klinik und Therapie*. Edited by W.K. Herausgeber and U.M. Durr. Hannover, Germany, Verlag M. & H. Schaper, 1978.
16. Tilley, L.P., Liu, S.-K., and Fox, P.R.: Myocardial disease. In *Textbook of Veterinary Internal Medicine*. Edited by S.J. Ettinger. 2nd Edition. Philadelphia, W.B. Saunders, 1983.
17. Bond, B., and Tilley, L.P.: Cardiomyopathy in the dog and cat. In *Current Veterinary Therapy VII. Small Animal Practice*. Edited by R.W. Kirk. Philadelphia, W.B. Saunders, 1980.
18. Friedman, H.H.: *Diagnostic Electrocardiography and Vectorcardiography*. 2nd Edition. New York, McGraw-Hill, 1977.
18a. Scott, C.S., et al.: The effect of left atrial histology and dimension on P-wave morphology. J. Electrocardiol., *16*:363, 1983.
19. Bolton, G.R., and Liu, S.-K.: Congenital heart diseases of the cat. Vet. Clin. North Am., *7*:341, 1977.
20. Edwards, N.J., and Tilley, L.P.: Congenital heart defects. In *Pathophysiology of Small Animal Surgery*. Edited by M.J. Bojrab. Philadelphia, Lea & Febiger, 1981.
21. Liu, S.-K., and Tilley, L.P.: Dysplasia of the tricuspid valve in the dog and cat. J. Am. Vet. Med. Assoc., *169*:623, 1976.
22. Bolton, G.R., Ettinger, S.J., and Liu, S.-K.: Tetralogy of Fallot in three cats. J. Am. Vet. Med. Assoc., *160*:1622, 1972.
23. Jeraj, K., Ogburn, P., Lord, P.F., and Wilson, J.W.: Patent ductus arteriosus with pulmonary hypertension in a cat. J. Am. Vet. Med. Assoc., *172*:1432, 1978.
24. Calvert, C.A., Mandell, C.P.: Diagnosis and management of feline heartworm disease. J. Am. Vet. Med. Assoc., *180*:550, 1982.
25. Hollister, R.M., and Goodwin, J.F.: The electrocardiogram in cardiomyopathy. Br. Heart J., *25*:357, 1963.
26. Savage, D.D., et al.: Electrocardiographic findings in patients with obstructive and nonobstructive hypertrophic cardiomyopathy. Circulation, *58*:402, 1978.
27. Spodick, D.H.: Hypertrophic obstructive cardiomyopathy of the left ventricle (idiopathic hypertrophic subaortic stenosis). Cardiovasc. Clin., *4*:133, 1972.
28. Tilley, L.P., et al.: Primary myocardial disease in the cat. Am. J. Pathol., *87*:493, 1977.
29. Cohen, J.S., Tilley, L.P., Liu, S.-K., and DeHoff, W.D.: Patent ductus arteriosus in five cats. J. Am. Anim. Hosp. Assoc., *11*:95, 1975.
30. Liu, S.-K., and Tilley, L.P.: Animal models of primary myocardial disease. Yale J. Biol. Med., *53*:191, 1980.
31. Harpster, N.K.: Feline cardiomyopathy. Vet. Clin. North Am., *7*:355, 1977.
32. Peterson, M.E., et al.: Electrocardiographic findings in 45 cats with hyperthyroidism. J. Am. Vet. Med. Assoc., *180*:934, 1982.
32a. Peterson, M.E., et al.: Feline hyperthyroidism: pretreatment clinical and laboratory evaluation of 131 cases. J. Am. Vet. Med. Assoc., *183*:103, 1983.
33. Liu, S.-K., Tilley, L.P., and Tashjian, R.J.: Lesions of the conduction system in the cat with cardiomyopathy. Recent Adv. Stud. Cardiac Struct. Metab., *10*:681, 1975.
34. Goldman, M.J.: *Principles of Clinical Electrocardiography*. 11th Edition. Los Altos, Calif., Lange Medical Publications, 1982.
35. Rosenbaum, M.B.: The hemiblocks: diagnostic criteria and clinical significance. Mod. Concepts Cardiovasc. Dis., *39*:141, 1970.
36. Rosenbaum, M.B., Elizari, M.V., and Lazzari, J.O.: *The Hemiblocks*. Oldsmar, Fla., Tampa Tracings, 1970.
37. Lepeschkin, E., and Surawicz, B.: The measurement of the duration of the QRS interval. Am. Heart J., *44*:80, 1952.
38. Sung, R.J., Castellanos, A., and Gelband, H.: ECG criteria for BBB (Letters to the editor). Circulation, *56*:127, 1977.
39. Cohen, H.C., et al.: Tachycardia and bradycardia-dependent bundle branch block alternans. Circulation, *55*:242, 1977.
40. Elizari, M.V., Lazzari, J.O., and Rosenbaum, M.B.: Phase-3 and phase-4 intermittent left bundle branch block occurring spontaneously in a dog. Eur. J. Cardiol., *1*:95, 1973.
41. Rosenbaum, M.B., and Elizari, M.V.: Mechanism of intermittent bundle branch block and paroxysmal atrioventricular block. Postgrad. Med., *53*(5):87, 1973.
42. Liu, S.-K., Fox, P.R., and Tilley, L.P.: Excessive moderator bands in the left ventricle of 21 cats. J. Am. Vet. Med. Assoc., *180*:1215, 1981.
43. Tilley, L.P., Bond, B., Patnaik, A.K., and Liu, S.-K.: Cardiovascular tumors in the cat. J. Am. Anim. Hosp. Assoc., *17*:1009, 1981.
44. Reinhard, D.W., and Bolton, G.R.: ECG of the month. J. Am. Vet. Med. Assoc., *172*:142, 1978.
45. Tilley, L.P.: Feline cardiomyopathy. In *Current Veterinary Therapy VI. Small Animal Practice*. Edited by R.W. Kirk. Philadelphia, W.B. Saunders, 1977.
46. Jacobsen, L.B., La Folette, L., and Cohn, K.: An appraisal of initial QRS forces in left anterior fascicular block. Am. Heart J., *94*:407, 1977.
47. Warner, R.A., Hill, N.E., Mookherjee, S., and Smulyan, H.: Improved electrocardiographic criteria for the diagnosis of left anterior hemiblock. Am. J. Cardiol., *51*:723, 1983.
48. Hamby, R.I., and Raia, F.: Electrocardiographic aspects of primary myocardial disease in 60 patients. Am. Heart J., *76*:316, 1968.
49. Ewy, G.A., Karliner, J., and Bednyer, J.: Electrocardiographic QRS axis as a manifestation of hyperkalemia. JAMA, *215*:429, 1971.
50. Schaer, M.: Hyperkalemia in cats with urethral obstruction: electrocardiographic abnormalities and treatment. Vet. Clin. North Am., *7*:407, 1977.
51. Coulter, D.B., Duncan, R.J., and Sander, P.D.: Effects of asphyxia and potassium on canine and feline electrocardiograms. Can. J. Comp. Med., *39*:442, 1975.
52. Parks, J.: Electrocardiographic abnormalities from serum electrolyte imbalance due to feline urethral obstruction. J. Am. Anim. Hosp. Assoc., *11*:102, 1975.

53. Colcolough, H.L.: A comparative study of acute myocardial infarction in the rabbit, cat and man. Comp. Biochem. Physiol., *49A*:121, 1974.
54. Owens, J.M.: Pericardial effusion in the cat. Vet. Clin. North Am., 7:373, 1977.
55. Tilley, L.P., Owens, J.M., Wilkins, R.J., and Patnaik, A.K.: Pericardial mesothelioma with effusion in a cat. J. Am. Anim. Hosp. Assoc., *11*:60, 1975.
56. Bolton, G.R., and Powell, A.A.: Plasma kinetics of digoxin in the cat. Am. J. Vet. Res., *43*:1994, 1982.
57. Rosenbaum, M.B., et al.: Electronic modulation of the T wave and cardiac memory. Am. J. Cardiol., *50*:213, 1982.
58. Schwartz, P.J., and Malliani, A.: Electrical alternation of the T-wave: clinical and experimental evidence of its relationship with the sympathetic nervous system and with the long Q-T syndrome. Am. Heart J., *89*:45, 1975.
59. Corr, P.B., Witkowski, F.X., and Sobel, B.E.: Mechanisms contributing to malignant dysrhythmias induced by ischemia in the cat. J. Clin. Invest., *61*:109, 1978.

Section Three

Interpretation of Common Cardiac Arrhythmias

6 Analysis of common canine cardiac arrhythmias

An arrhythmia can be defined as (1) an abnormality in the rate, regularity, or site of origin of the cardiac impulse and/or (2) a disturbance in conduction of the impulse such that the normal sequence of activation of the atria and ventricles is altered.[1] During normal sinus rhythm the cardiac impulse originates in the sinoatrial (SA) node and spreads in an orderly fashion throughout the atria, through the AV node and His-Purkinje system, and throughout the ventricles.

Abnormalities of impulse formation or impulse conduction are the basic mechanisms that underlie the arrhythmias and give a basis for the following classification. Arrhythmias, from the viewpoint of the electrophysiologist, arise also from alterations in either automaticity or conductivity, or both. Table 9-1 in Chapter 9 shows the current classification of the mechanisms of arrhythmias. These fundamental mechanisms are also explained in Chapter 9.

Sinus rhythm
Normal sinus rhythm
Sinus tachycardia
Sinus bradycardia
Sinus arrhythmia
Wandering sinus pacemaker

Abnormalities of impulse formation
Supraventricular
Sinus arrest
Atrial premature complexes (APCs)
Atrial tachycardia
Atrial flutter
Atrial fibrillation
Atrioventricular (AV) junction
AV junctional premature complexes
AV junctional tachycardia
AV junctional escape rhythm (secondary arrhythmia)
Ventricular
Ventricular premature complexes (VPCs)
Ventricular tachycardia
Ventricular flutter, fibrillation
Ventricular asystole
Ventricular escape rhythm (secondary arrhythmia)

Abnormalities of impulse conduction
Sinoatrial (SA) block
Persistent atrial standstill ("silent" atrium)
Atrial standstill (hyperkalemia)
AV block
First degree
Second degree
Third degree (complete heart block)

Abnormalities of both impulse formation and impulse conduction
Pre-excitation (Wolff-Parkinson-White syndrome), reciprocal rhythm (re-entry)
Parasystole
Other complex rhythms (Chapter 12)

In this book, the definition and criteria of terms related to cardiac rhythm are discussed on the basis of two recent reports dealing with standardization of terminology published by the World Health Organization and International Society of Cardiology Task Force.[2,3] Acceptable terms were selected according to their scientific accuracy, understandability, simplicity, and current use (in that order of priority). This textbook attempts to comply with these standardizations. With the increasing use of electrocardiography in veterinary medicine, there is a need for a common language.

The frequency of arrhythmias and conduction disturbances in 3000 dogs which were brought to one veterinary clinic during an 18-month period is summarized in Table 6–1.[4] In 115 dogs with gastric dilation studied at one veterinary school, cardiac arrhythmias were diagnosed in 48 dogs (42%). Of the 48 dogs, 33 had ventricular arrhythmias.[5] At another veterinary school, in 19 male Doberman Pinschers with congestive cardiomyopathy, atrial fibrillation was found as the primary arrhythmia in 4 dogs, while 15 dogs had ventricular arrhythmias.[6] The incidence of all the various arrhythmias has not been studied in detail at The Animal Medical Center. One study from this institution, however, provides a good indication of the number of arrhythmias being observed.[7] During the 3 years from September 1972 to September 1975, 148 dogs were diagnosed as having atrial fibrillation. The inpatient case load for that time period was approximately 17,000 dogs.

Table 6–1. Frequency of spontaneous arrhythmias in 95 dogs from a sample of 3000

Arrhythmia	Number
Ventricular premature complexes (VPCs)	43
Atrial premature complexes (APCs)	14
Atrial fibrillation	13
First-degree AV block	12
Second-degree AV block	12
Ventricular tachycardia	8
Atrial tachycardia	3
AV junctional premature complexes	3
AV dissociation	3
Atrial flutter	2
Complete heart block (third degree)	2
Wolff-Parkinson-White syndrome	1

From Patterson, D.F., et al.: Am. J. Vet. Res., 22:355, 1961.

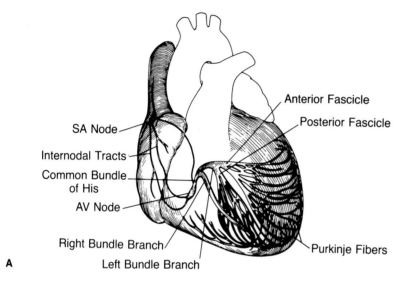

SA Node

Internodal Tracts

Common Bundle
of His

AV Node

Right Bundle Branch

Left Bundle Branch

Anterior Fascicle

Posterior Fascicle

Purkinje Fibers

A

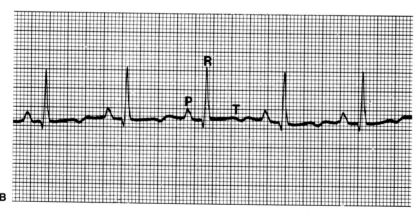

B

Fig. 6–1. **A,** Impulse-forming and impulse-conducting system of the heart. (From DeSanctis, R.W.: Disturbances of cardiac rhythm and conduction. In *SCIENTIFIC AMERICAN MEDICINE.* Edited by E. Rubenstein. New York, Scientific American, 1982, with permission.) **B,** The normal lead II electrocardiogram shows a normal cardiac rhythm, termed sinoatrial or sinus rhythm.

One of my studies reviews the diagnosis of cardiac arrhythmias and conduction disturbances in 2000 dogs by means of transtelephonic electrocardiography.[8] The 2000 electrocardiograms were transmitted transtelephonically to New York from 42 states in the United States as well as from two other countries (England, 2 transmissions; Canada, 32 transmissions). The electrocardiograms were transmitted for the following reasons: as part of a routine evaluation of the cardiovascular system, for the evaluation of antiarrhythmic therapy, and for the confirmation of suspected arrhythmias.

Eighteen different arrhythmias were documented in 396 dogs (20%). Twenty electrocardiograms showed evidence of more than one arrhythmia. Atrial arrhythmias, the most common arrhythmia in the dog, were recorded in 190 dogs (9.6%). The atrial arrhythmias included atrial premature complexes (113 dogs), atrial tachycardia (13 dogs), atrial fibrillation (63 dogs), and atrial flutter (1 dog). Ventricular arrhythmias were found in 114 dogs (5.75%) and included ventricular premature complexes (101 dogs), ventricular tachycardia (11 dogs), and ventricular fibrillation (2 dogs). Abnormality of impulse conduction was found in 72 dogs (3.65%) and included first-degree AV block (30 dogs), second-degree AV block (35 dogs), and third-degree AV block (5 dogs). Sinus arrest and/or sinoatrial block was found in 27 dogs (1.3%). One case each was found with persistent atrial standstill, sinoatrial standstill, and Wolff-Parkinson-White syndrome. The high percent of abnormalities in this study is not significant since the majority of the electrocardiograms transmitted were for suspected arrhythmias.

A knowledge of the anatomic and physiologic properties of the unique impulse-forming and impulse-conducting system of the atria, the AV junction, and the ventricles is essential for the accurate analysis of cardiac arrhythmias (Fig. 6–1).

Activation of heart muscle results from spontaneous discharge in a pacemaker and conduction of this impulse from cell to cell. The physiologic pacemaker is located in the SA node. The rate and rhythm of the heart are controlled by the SA node; hence the normal cardiac rhythm is termed *sinoatrial* or sinus rhythm (Fig. 6–1). The impulse originating there is propagated through the atria via internodal tracts leading from the AV node. After a delay at the AV node, the impulse travels down the bundle of His, the bundle branches and their subsidiaries, and the Purkinje fiber system (which eventually comes in contact with ventricular myocardium). The heart has many potential pacemaking cells. The SA node has the fastest inherent discharge rate, whereas the cells in the rest of the conduction system exhibit a slower rate of impulse formation. The more distal a potential pacemaker is from the SA node, the slower is its inherent discharge rate. The normal pacemaker is under the influence of the autonomic nervous system. Its rate is constantly adjusted by autonomic impulses according to need.

RECOGNITION OF ARRHYTHMIAS—a systematic approach

With the foregoing general knowledge of the normal anatomic and physiologic properties of the impulse-forming and impulse-conducting system of the heart (Fig. 6–1) and the use of a systematic approach to the electrocardiographic strip, the accurate diagnosis of arrhythmias can be greatly simplified. A systematic method for an accurate electrocardiographic analysis of a rhythm strip (usually lead II) for arrhythmias includes the steps detailed next.[9–11]

Step 1. General inspection of the electrocardiogram. A determination should be made as to whether the arrhythmia is occasional, frequent, or continuous; regular or irregular; and repetitive or occurring with various combinations—in other words, whether the rhythm is a normal sinus rhythm or is characteristic of a type of cardiac arrhythmia. The heart rate should also be classified as rapid (tachycardia), slow (bradycardia), or normal.

Step 2. Identification of P waves. This should include a determination of whether the atrial activity is uniform or regular. The lead (usually lead II) should be carefully selected to illustrate discrete P waves. The precordial chest leads often demonstrate P waves that are easy to see. The crucial part of the electrocardiographic examination is identification and analysis of the P waves. Doubling the standardization may be helpful in magnifying the P waves. The direction and shape of the P wave can also help to analyze an arrhythmia. A normal P wave (positive and rounded, as in lead II) in most cases indicates that the impulse is originating in the SA node. A P wave that differs in shape and is upright may represent an ectopic pacemaker in the atrium. P waves that are inverted in leads I, II, III, and aVF most often indicate formation of the impulse in or near the AV junction. The absence of P waves usually signifies atrial fibrillation, atrial standstill, atrial activity of low voltage in the respective lead, or buried P waves in QRS complexes of AV junctional rhythms. In various supraventricular tachycardias the P wave can be superimposed on a portion of the QRS complex, S-T segment, or T wave of the preceding cardiac cycle.

Step 3. Recognition of QRS complexes. The QRS complexes should be characterized as to their morphology, uniformity, and regularity. A QRS complex of normal width and morphology and also identical to those recorded before an arrhythmia indicates a probable normal activation of the ventricles. Such complexes may be the result of an impulse formed in the SA node or an abnormal impulse originating anywhere above the bundle of His. Normal-appearing QRS complexes can be categorized as "supraventricular." Wide QRS complexes with various configurations may indicate an ectopic pacemaker below the bundle of His (ventricular) or a lesion in the intraventricular conduction system.

Two other conditions giving abnormal QRS complexes are *aberration* and *fusion* complexes. Aberration is a condition in which the impulse traveling from above the bundle of His finds a part of the ventricular conducting system still in a refractory phase. A common example of a fusion complex is the simultaneous activation of the ventricles that results when one impulse arrives from the SA node at the same time another arrives from a ventricular ectopic pacemaker. These conditions are illustrated later in this chapter as well as in Chapter 12.

Step 4. Relationship between P waves and QRS complexes. The time from the onset of the P wave to the onset of the QRS complex is called the P-R interval and is a measure of atrioventricular (AV) conduction. The P-R intervals are essentially constant in normal sinus rhythm. P waves may precede normal QRS complexes by different time spans. An abnormally long P-R interval usually indicates an AV conduction delay or first-degree heart block.

An abnormally short P-R interval may be seen in conditions such as accessory conduction around the AV node or in AV junctional rhythms in which the P wave is positioned close to the QRS complex. When all P waves are not followed by QRS complexes, an AV block (also termed second-degree heart block) has occurred. The P-R interval also can lengthen gradually until the P wave occurs without a succeeding QRS complex (called Wenckebach atrioventricular block). When the P-R interval varies, the relationship of the atria and ventricles in the cardiac cycle should be determined. Complete heart block, a form of AV dissociation, represents an interrupted connection between the atria and the ventricles. One impulse formation site is the SA node; the other is an independent ventricular escape rhythm.

By establishing the relationship of the P wave and QRS complex, the clinician can determine the dominant rhythm. As previously discussed (Chapter 1, Table 1–1), the four major sites of the heart having pacemaker cells from which impulses may arise are the SA node, the atrial conduction tissue, the AV junction (AV node—His bundle region), and the ventricular conduction tissue (bundle branches and Purkinje fibers).

At each of these sites, impulses may originate at rates faster than, slower than, or the same as the normal sinus rate. Arrhythmias with rates slower than the sinus rate usually occur because of SA nodal depression, allowing "escape" of other pacemakers from its influences. These slow cardiac rhythms are called passive or escape rhythms. By contrast, a normal-functioning SA node may not be able to act as the pacemaker because other pacemakers are abnormally forming impulses at a faster rate. These arrhythmias are then "active." Both types of abnormal impulse formation may be intermittent or persistent, repetitive, or occurring in varying combinations.

Step 5. Summary of findings and final classification of the arrhythmia. By following the preceding four steps, the clinician can determine the final interpretation of the arrhythmia.

a. What is the predominant rhythm? The dominant rhythm in most simple common arrhythmias is sinus, normal impulses from the SA node. An ectopic rhythm may also be dominant, such as in atrial tachycardia. Occasionally the dominant rhythm will change from the SA node to an ectopic focus (atrial, AV junction, or ventricular) on the same strip. It is also not unusual to see the dominant rhythm change from one ectopic to another ectopic rhythm on the same strip (e.g., from atrial fibrillation to ventricular tachycardia).

b. Is the arrhythmia an abnormality of impulse formation or of impulse conduction or both? If either or both, what is the site of the abnormality?

When these basic questions are answered, the final classification of the arrhythmia can be made.[12] The terminology for each arrhythmia is basically the same. Terms used for abnormalities of impulse formation usually state the first word as the site of the dominant rhythm (sinus, atrial, AV junction, or ventricular), with the following word indicating the rhythm or rate (e.g., "atrial tachycardia"). Terms used for abnormalities of impulse conduction commonly state the first word as the site of the conduction defect, with the following word indicating the conduction defect (e.g., "sinoatrial block").

Each of the arrhythmias will be discussed in this chapter using the systematic method just described, outlined as follows. This outline will be used on one page to present and discuss the respective arrhythmia, and representative examples will be arranged on the facing page:

Electrocardiographic features

General inspection: heart rate and rhythm
P waves: present or absent; if present, morphology, uniformity, and regularity
QRS complexes: morphology, uniformity, and regularity
P and QRS relationship: measurement of P-R interval, dominant rhythm

Associated conditions

Treatment

The pathophysiologic basis of cardiac arrhythmias will be discussed in Chapter 8. A detailed discussion of the use of antiarrhythmic drugs in the dog and cat can be found in Chapter 10 by Dr. John D. Bonagura and Dr. William W. Muir. *Tables 10–10 and 10–12 list drugs used in the therapy of cardiac arrhythmias.* Special methods for analyzing and treating arrhythmias are discussed in Chapter 11. *Table 11–2 lists drugs used in the management of cardiac resuscitation.*

Based on the proper electrocardiographic diagnosis and the establishment of the cause, the majority of cardiac arrhythmias can be managed with the drugs discussed in Chapter 10. It is important, however, to determine whether the animal has been on cardiac drugs, especially digitalis. Digitalis can cause almost every arrhythmia reported. The specific antiarrhythmic drugs are often more effective when the underlying cause of the arrhythmia is treated. For example, the correction of hypoxia or acid-base and/or electrolyte imbalance alone may eliminate the arrhythmia or make the specific antiarrhythmic drug effective. The treatment of congestive heart failure by the usual methods will often terminate the existing arrhythmia. The central nervous system drugs such as phenytoin (diphenylhydantoin) and diazepam can be useful for digitalis- and excitement-induced arrhythmias.[13] Propranolol has been advised for preventing neurogenic arrhythmias secondary to increased sympathetic activity during naturally elicited emotional behavior.[14]

Normal sinus rhythm

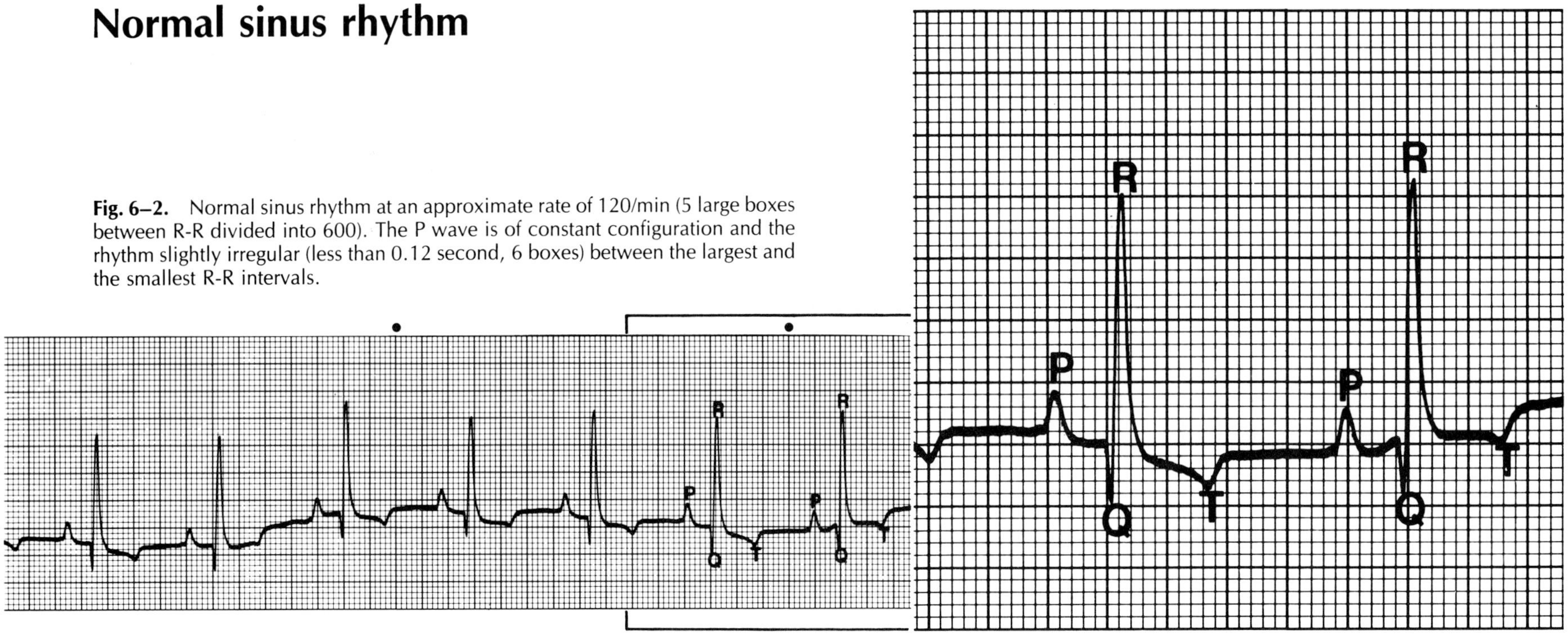

Fig. 6–2. Normal sinus rhythm at an approximate rate of 120/min (5 large boxes between R-R divided into 600). The P wave is of constant configuration and the rhythm slightly irregular (less than 0.12 second, 6 boxes) between the largest and the smallest R-R intervals.

Sinus rhythm is the normal mechanism for initiating cardiac systole. The normal cardiac impulse originates in the SA node and spreads to the atria, the AV node, and the ventricles. The SA node normally has an inherent pacemaker rate of 70 to 160 beats/min in the adult dog. The rates can become as high as 180 in toy breeds and up to 220 in puppies. The normal heart rate can be regular or irregular. A regular sinus rhythm below the normal heart rate range is a sinus bradycardia, whereas above the normal heart rate is a sinus tachycardia. An irregular sinus rhythm is called sinus arrhythmia.

Electrocardiographic features

1. The rhythm is regular at 70 to 160 beats/min (up to 220 in toy breeds and puppies). The difference between the largest and smallest R-R intervals is less than 0.12 second (6 boxes), or less than 10% variation in the R-R intervals.[15]

2. P waves are positive in lead II (except in dextrocardia) with a constant configuration.[16]

3. The QRS complexes are normal, or they may be wide and bizarre if an intraventricular conduction defect is present.

4. The P-QRS complex is normal with a constant P-R interval (0.06 to 0.13 sec).

Failure of the rhythm to meet any of these criteria indicates the possibility of some *abnormality of impulse formation and/or impulse conduction*, i.e., an arrhythmia.

Associated conditions

1. Sinus rhythm, the normal rhythm of the heart, usually varying with respiration (Exercise causes an increase in the sinus rate; vagal stimulation causes a decrease.)

Treatment

1. No specific therapy is required.

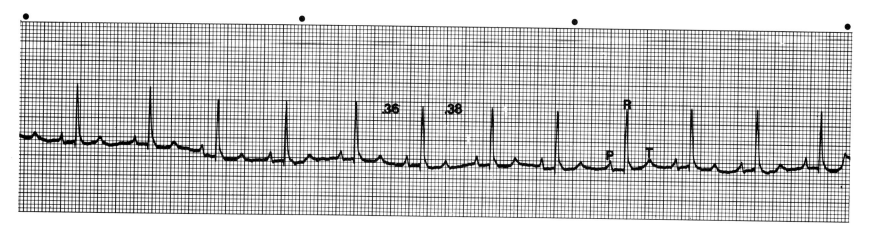

Fig. 6–3. Regular normal sinus rhythm at 160/min. Rhythm irregularity is only minimal (0.02 sec).

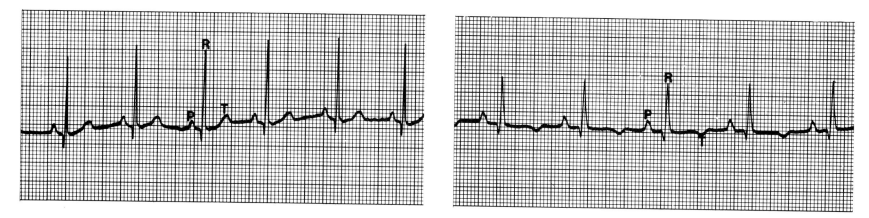

Fig. 6–4. Regular normal sinus rhythm at 160/min.

Fig. 6–5. Regular normal sinus rhythm at 130/min. The rhythm is regular with essentially no variance in the R-R intervals.

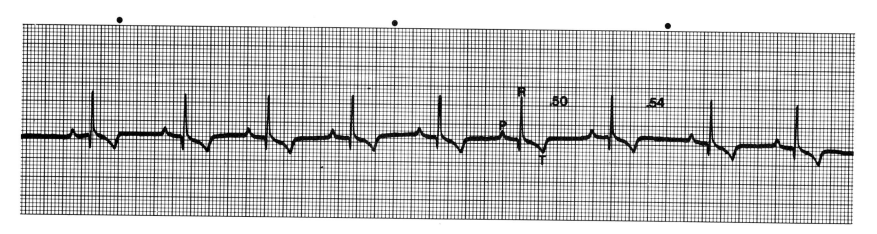

Fig. 6–6. Normal sinus rhythm at 120/min. All the P waves are of normal configuration.

Sinus rhythms at various rates

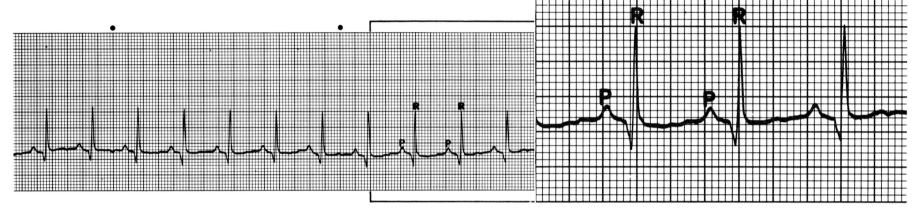

Fig. 6–7. Sinus tachycardia at a rate of 200/min (3 large boxes between R-R divided into 600) in an adult dog. The P waves are of constant configuration, and the rhythm is regular.

SINUS TACHYCARDIA

Sinus tachycardia is a regular sinus rhythm, with a heart rate above 160 beats/min (above 180 in toy breeds and above 220 in puppies). It is the *most common arrhythmia* in dogs.

Electrocardiographic features

1. All criteria of a normal sinus rhythm are met except that the heart rate is above 160 beats/min (above 180 in toy breeds and above 220 in puppies).
2. The rhythm is regular with a slight variation in R-R intervals and the presence of constant P-R intervals. Ocular pressure produces only a gradual transient slowing of the heart rate, if any change at all.

Associated conditions

1. Physiologic: exercise, pain, or restraint procedures (such as during the electrocardiographic recording)
2. Pathologic: fever, hyperthyroidism, shock, anemia, infection, congestive heart failure, hypoxia
3. Drugs: atropine, epinephrine, vasodilators (hypotension)
4. Hexachlorophene poisoning, electrical cord shock[17]

Treatment

1. The treatment of a sinus tachycardia is a common mistake. Treatment consists of simply identifying and controlling the causes. For example, if the tachycardia is due to excitement, a tranquilizer will slow the heart rate; if it is due to congestive heart failure, digoxin for the underlying cardiac insufficiency is indicated.

SINUS BRADYCARDIA

Sinus bradycardia is a regular sinus rhythm, with a heart rate less than 70 beats/min (less than 60 in giant breeds).

Electrocardiographic features

1. All criteria of normal sinus rhythm are met, except that the heart rate is less than 70.
2. The rhythm is usually regular with a slight variation in the R-R intervals; the P-R interval is constant.

Associated conditions

1. Physiologic: an increased vagal tone due to carotid sinus pressure, eyeball pressure, or elevated intracranial pressure; hypothermia, hypothyroidism
2. Pathologic: systemic disease with toxicity (e.g., renal failure), cardiac arrest (Sinus bradycardia can be a warning of an impending cardiac arrest during surgery.)
3. Drugs: tranquilizers (especially the phenothiazines), propranolol, digitalis, quinidine, morphine, anesthesia
4. Central nervous system lesions

The bradycardia may be a normal variation. Many large breeds can normally have heart rates of 60 to 70 beats/min.

Treatment

1. Treatment is rarely required.
2. If clinical signs exist (weakness or collapse), atropine or glycopyrrolate should be administered intravenously followed by continuous intravenous infusion of isoproterenol if atropine is not helpful.
3. Right atrial pacing with a transvenous pacing catheter is effective.[18]

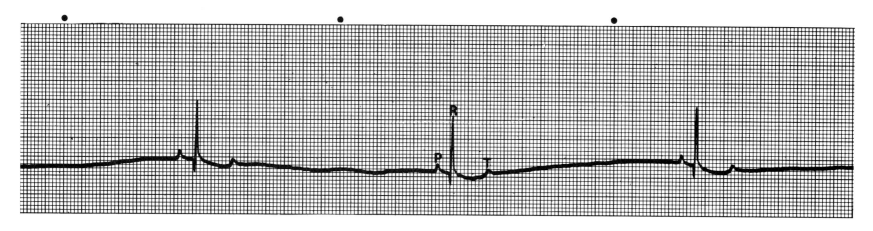

Fig. 6–8. Sinus bradycardia at a rate of 40/min in a dog with acute renal failure. The rhythm is regular with only a slight variation in the R-R intervals.

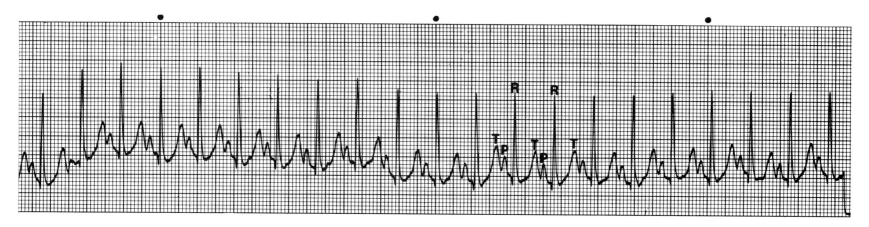

Fig. 6–9. Sinus tachycardia at a rate of 272/min in a dog in shock. The rhythm is sinus since the P waves are normal, the P-R relationship is normal, and the rhythm regular. The P wave is touching the T wave of the preceding complex.

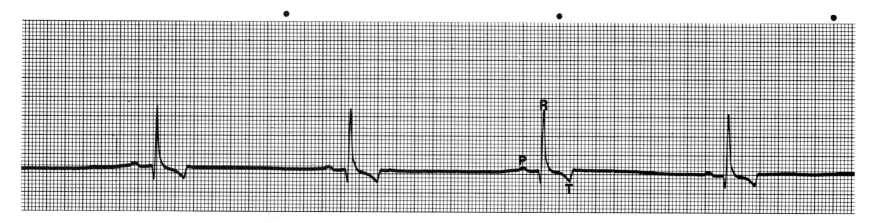

Fig. 6–10. Sinus bradycardia at an approximate rate of 60/min in a dog during surgery. Close monitoring as well as atropine is indicated to prevent any complications.

Sinus arrhythmia

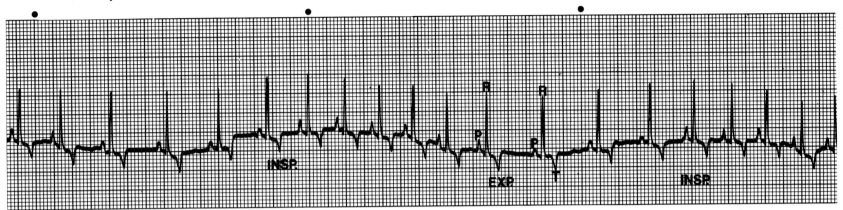

Fig. 6–11. Respiratory sinus arrhythmia with an average rate of 120/min (paper speed, 25 mm/sec; 6 complexes between one set of time lines × 20). The rate increases during inspiration *(INSP)* and decreases during expiration *(EXP)*. The fluctuation of the baseline correlates with the movement of the electrodes by the thoracic cavity.

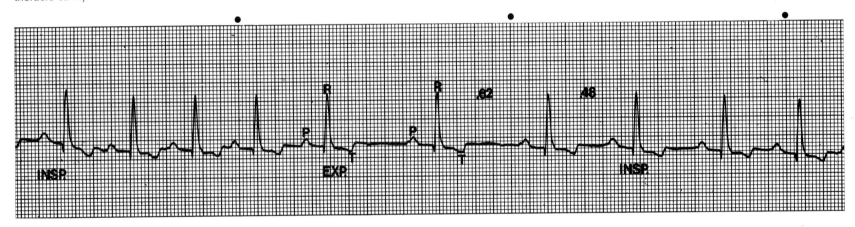

Fig. 6–12. Respiratory sinus arrhythmia with an average rate of 120/min. The R-R intervals vary more than 0.12 second as the rate changes with inspiration *(INSP)* and expiration *(EXP)*.

Sinus arrhythmia is an irregular sinus rhythm originating in the SA node. It is represented by alternating periods of slower and more rapid heart rates usually related to respiration (respiratory sinus arrhythmia), the heart rate increasing with inspiration and decreasing with expiration. A nonrespiratory sinus arrhythmia has no relationship to the phases of respiration. Respiratory sinus arrhythmia is a frequent normal finding in the dog. The use of the term sinus arrhythmia is controversial, since "arrhythmia" should not be used as a synonym for irregular impulse formation.

Electrocardiographic features

1. All criteria of normal sinus rhythm are met, except that a variability of 0.12 second or more exists between successive P waves (or variation of R-R intervals greater than ± 10%).[15] The heart rate increases during inspiration and decreases during expiration in respiratory sinus arrhythmia.

2. The P wave, QRS complexes, and P-R impulses are normal.

3. A wandering pacemaker (P waves varying in configuration), a variant of sinus arrhythmia, is often present.

Associated condition

1. Respiratory sinus arrhythmia, a normal finding in dogs (A respiratory sinus arrhythmia is often seen in brachycephalic breeds, in which vagal tone is increased by upper airway obstruction. Sinus arrhythmia is accentuated by vagotonic procedures: carotid sinus and eyeball pressure and administration of digitalis. Atropine eliminates it, indicating that its origin is vagal in nature. A sinus arrhythmia associated with sinus bradycardia can be an indication of digitalis toxicity.)

It is important to differentiate sinus arrhythmia from the other dangerous arrhythmias.

Treatment

1. No specific therapy is required.

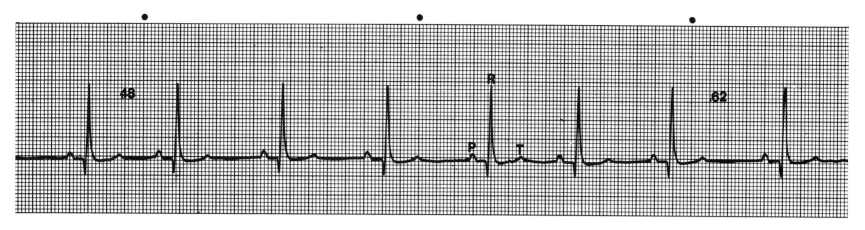

Fig. 6–13. Sinus arrhythmia in which the rhythm is much less irregular than in Figures 6–11 and 6–12.

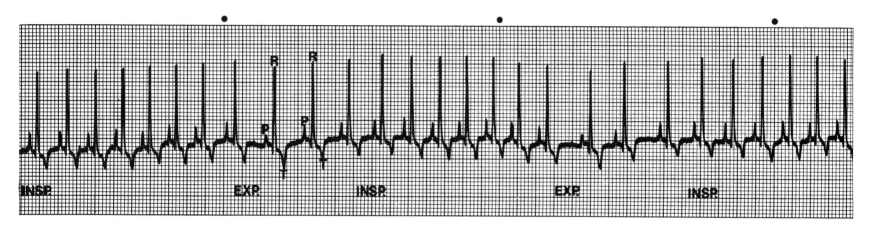

Fig. 6–14. Respiratory sinus arrhythmia with an average rate of 180/min. The configuration of the P waves during expiration is different from that during inspiration. This wandering pacemaker within the SA node is often present (paper speed, 25 mm/sec).

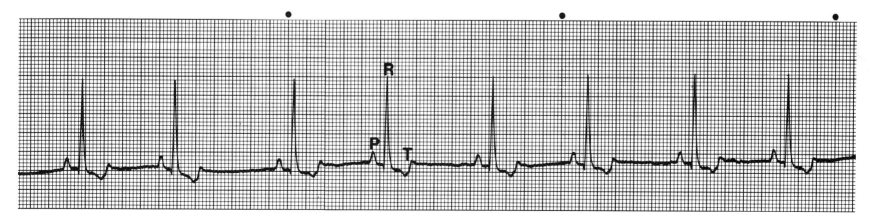

Fig. 6–15. Sinus arrhythmia in which the rhythm is not so irregular. The effects of respiration on vagal tone are not pronounced.

Wandering sinus pacemaker

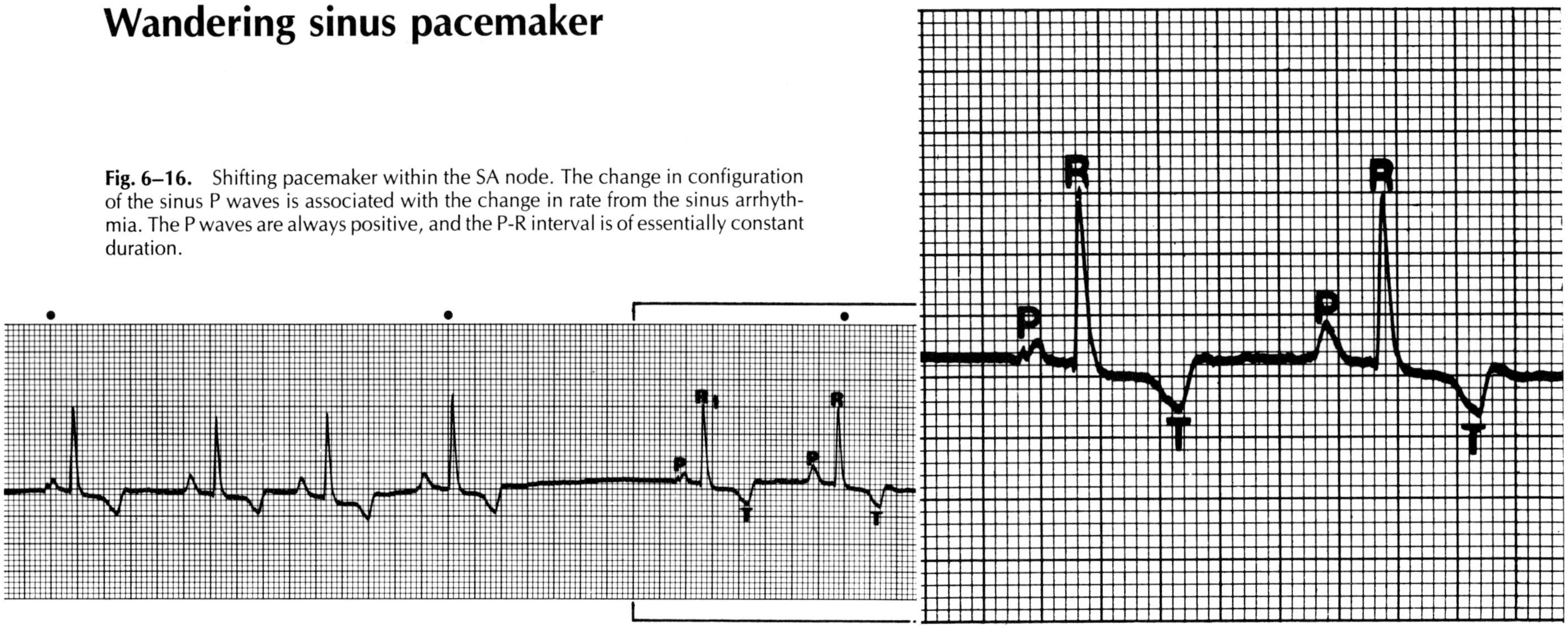

Fig. 6–16. Shifting pacemaker within the SA node. The change in configuration of the sinus P waves is associated with the change in rate from the sinus arrhythmia. The P waves are always positive, and the P-R interval is of essentially constant duration.

Wandering sinus pacemaker, a variant of sinus arrhythmia, is a shift of the pacemaker from within the SA node or from the SA to the AV node. This is a frequent normal finding in dogs.

The term *wandering* is controversial since it implies a mechanism that is not readily known. A wandering pacemaker is an irregular, multiform, supraventricular rhythm with changing P wave morphology.

Electrocardiographic features

1. Shifting of the pacemaker within the SA node causes a gradual change in configuration of the P wave without it becoming negative. The P-R interval is basically constant, never of short duration (below 0.06 sec). The QRS complexes are the same as in a sinus rhythm.

2. Shifting of the pacemaker between the SA node and AV junction (often cyclical) causes a gradual change in the configuration of the P wave, which becomes positive, biphasic, isoelectric, and negative. The changes are temporary. The P-R intervals vary from short to normal duration. The P waves may precede, occur within, or follow the QRS complex. The QRS complexes are the same as in a sinus rhythm. It is important to recognize that the P waves in leads II, III, and aVF are not always negative when the atria are activated from sites low in the right atrium; they can be biphasic or positive. The diagnosis of atrial arrhythmias should not always be dependent on the polarity of the P wave. Studies in both dogs and man[19,20] indicate that the specialized atrial pathways (internodal tracts) determine the sequence of atrial activation. An impulse can rapidly spread upward (retrograde) through one of the internodal tracts (including Bachmann's bundle, a connection to the left atrium) to the SA node and from there depolarize the atria in a sequence similar to a normal sinus rhythm.

Associated conditions

1. Wandering sinus pacemaker (frequent in the dog)
2. Sinus arrhythmia

It is important to differentiate a wandering sinus pacemaker from other dangerous arrhythmias such as atrial premature complexes (APCs) and AV junctional rhythms.

Treatment

1. No specific therapy is required.

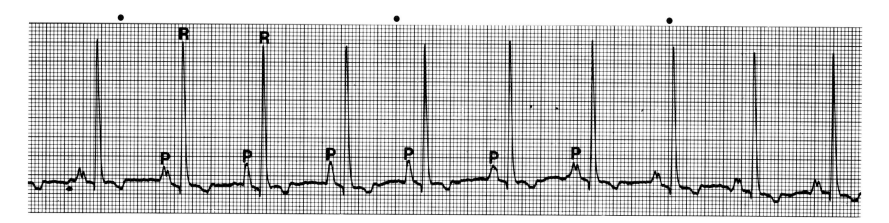

Fig. 6–17. Shifting of the pacemaker within the SA node. Note the gradual and temporary change in the configuration of the P waves. The P waves are also tall and wide, suggesting biatrial enlargement.

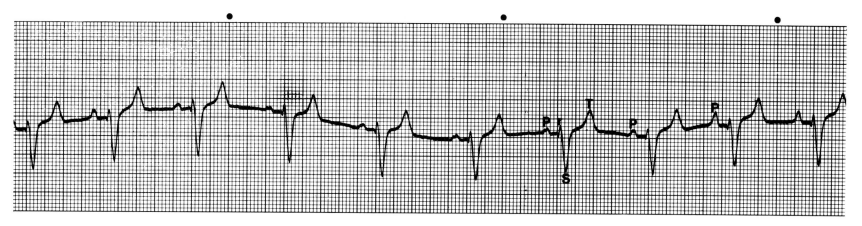

Fig. 6–18. Wandering pacemaker within the SA node in a dog with right bundle branch block (wide S waves). The sinus P waves gradually change configuration.

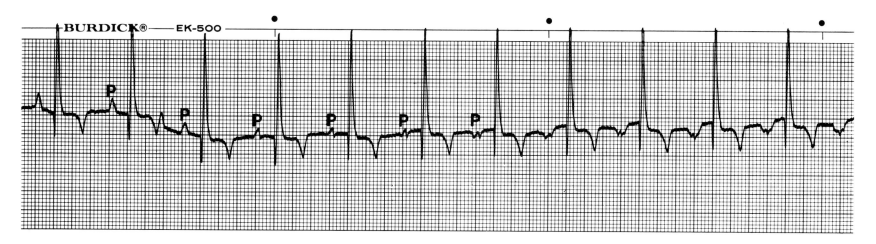

Fig. 6–19. Shifting pacemaker probably from the SA node to (and from) the AV node. The P wave configuration gradually changes from positive to negative.

Atrial premature complexes

Fig. 6–20. Atrial premature complex (APC). The P′ represents the premature complex. The premature QRS resembles the basic QRS. The upright P′ wave is superimposed on the T wave of the preceding complex.

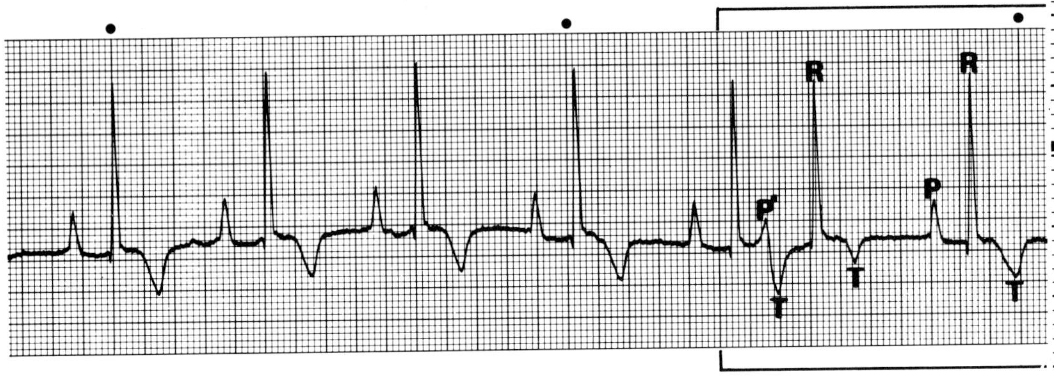

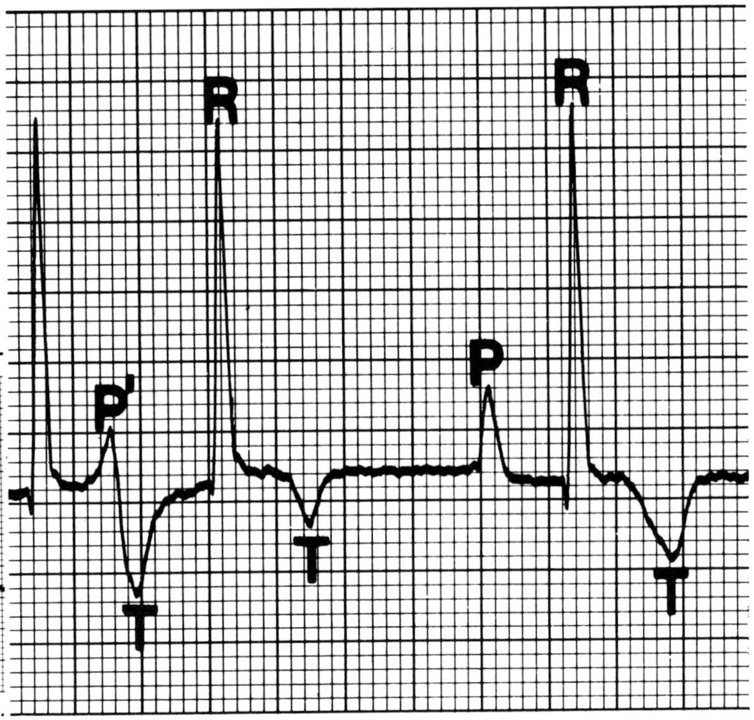

Atrial premature complexes (APCs) (also known as atrial extrasystoles, atrial premature contractions, and atrial premature impulses) arise from ectopic foci in the atria. They are frequently caused by cardiac disease and may lead to atrial tachycardia, atrial flutter, or atrial fibrillation. Atrial premature complexes can be of normal variation in very aged dogs. The impulses spread through the atria to the AV node, and they may or may not reach the ventricles.

Electrocardiographic features

1. The heart rate is usually normal, and the rhythm is irregular due to the premature P wave (called a P′ wave) that disrupts the normal P wave rhythm.
2. The ectopic P′ wave is premature, and its configuration is different from that of the sinus P waves. It may be negative, positive, biphasic, or superimposed on the previous T wave. The polarity of the P′ wave is not always predictive of the site of origin, as discussed for wandering sinus pacemaker.
3. The QRS complex is premature, and its configuration is usually normal (same as that of the sinus complexes). It is absent when the P′ wave occurs too early. The AV node is not completely recovered (refractory), so ventricular conduction does not occur (a nonconducted P′ wave). If there is partial recovery in the AV node or the intraventricular conduction system, the P′ wave is conducted with a long P′-R interval or is conducted with a change in the normal QRS configuration (aberrant conduction). The more premature the complex happens to be, the more marked will be the aberration.

4. The P′-R interval is usually as long as or longer than the sinus P-R interval.
5. A noncompensatory pause, i.e., when the R-R interval of the two normal sinus complexes enclosing the premature atrial complex is less than the R-R intervals of three consecutive sinus complexes, usually follows an APC. The ectopic atrial impulse discharges the SA node and resets its cycle. The R-R intervals in sinus arrhythmia may be difficult to determine accurately.

Associated conditions

1. Atrial enlargement secondary to chronic AV valvular insufficiency[21]
2. Any atrial disease: right atrial hemangiosarcoma, congenital cardiac defects (e.g., tricuspid dysplasia, mitral insufficiency, or patent ductus arteriosus)[22,23]
3. Drugs: digitalis toxicity, general anesthesia, diuretics (hypokalemia)

Treatment (See Chapter 10)

1. Digoxin is the treatment of choice for APCs and is also indicated for the cardiac decompensation that is usually present. Propranolol is at least equally valuable but should be used only when the heart is well compensated.
2. Treat the underlying condition.

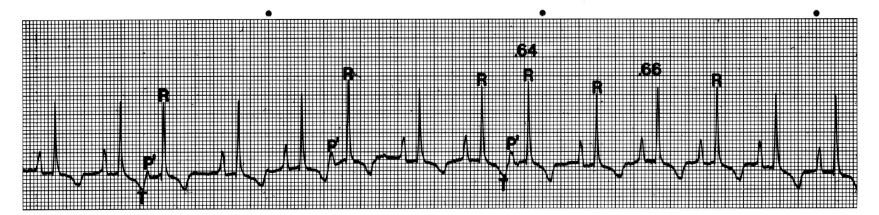

Fig. 6–21. Atrial premature complexes (APCs). The upright premature P′ waves are superimposed on the T waves of the preceding complexes. The pause following each premature complex is noncompensatory. The R-R interval of three sinus complexes (0.66 sec) is greater than the R-R interval of the two sinus complexes enclosing the premature complex (0.64 sec).

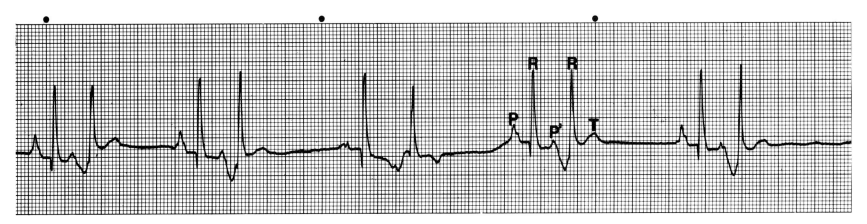

Fig. 6–22. Atrial premature complexes (APCs) in bigeminy in a dog with digoxin toxicity. The second complex of each pair is an APC, whereas the first complex is sinus.

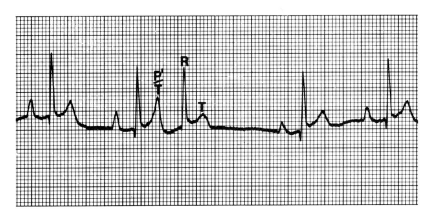

Fig. 6–23. Atrial premature complex (APC) in a dog with a right atrial hemangiosarcoma. The upright P wave is superimposed on the previous T wave. The T wave is more pointed and peaked than the others.

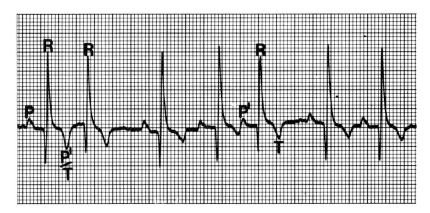

Fig. 6–24. Two supraventricular premature complexes, the second and fifth complexes. A positive premature ectopic P′ wave can be seen in the fifth complex, an indication that the ectopic focus is atrial. The second complex can only be termed a supraventricular premature complex since the premature P′ wave is hidden in the T wave. (The premature complex could be from the AV junction.)

139

Atrial tachycardia

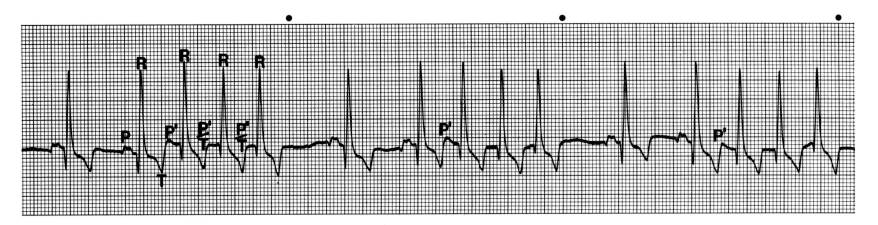

Fig. 6–25. Paroxysms of atrial tachycardia in a dog with severe left atrial enlargement from mitral valvular insufficiency. A hint of a P′ wave can be seen in the previous T wave at the start of each brief period of tachycardia. The other premature P′ waves (P′/T) are hidden in the previous T waves.

Atrial tachycardia is a rapid regular rhythm originating from a focus in the atria away from the SA node. Three or more consecutive APCs are considered to be atrial tachycardia. Recent studies have established two mechanisms for atrial tachycardia: (1) an enhanced automaticity of an ectopic focus and (2) re-entry.[24,25] (See Chapters 9 and 12 for a detailed explanation.)

Electrocardiographic features

1. The heart rate is rapid, above 160 beats/min (above 180 in toy breeds). Rhythm is perfectly regular in most cases, but may be slightly irregular. The atrial tachycardia can be either intermittent (paroxysmal) or continuous.

2. P′ waves are usually positive in lead II, with the P′-P′ intervals regular. They may not be easily seen because of the fast ventricular rate or a prolonged P′-R′ interval. Configuration of the P′ waves is generally somewhat different from that of the sinus P waves. If the atrial rhythm is irregular and the P′ waves are of varying configurations, the term multifocal atrial tachycardia is used. The ectopic rhythm is due to the rapid firing of two or more ectopic atrial foci.

3. The QRS configuration is usually normal (same as for the sinus complexes) or wide and bizarre due to bundle branch block, aberrant ventricular conduction, or ventricular pre-excitation.

4. The P′-R interval of the P-QRS is usually constant (1:1 AV conduction). At extremely high heart rates, varying degrees of AV block can occur (2:1, i.e., ventricular rate half the atrial rate; 3:1; 4:1; etc.).

Associated conditions

1. Same conditions that caused APCs, those causing atrial enlargement being the most common

2. Ventricular pre-excitation (Wolff-Parkinson-White syndrome)

3. Atrial tachycardia with AV block, often due to digitalis toxicity[26]

Treatment *(See Chapter 10 and Fig. 10–9)*

1. It is very important to distinguish atrial tachycardia from sinus tachycardia. Atrial tachycardia is usually terminated immediately with ocular pressure. P′ waves are different from sinus P waves and generally occur with underlying cardiac disease.[26]

2. Digoxin is the drug of choice for atrial tachycardia.

3. The following steps should be taken: (1) carotid sinus or ocular pressure during a lead II recording, (b) rapid intravenous digitalization with ocular pressure during regulation if no conversion, (c) electrical cardioversion (after digoxin has been stopped) or intracardiac pacing (especially if the animal is critical) (small doses of electrical energy should be used first), (d) intravenous propranolol may be effective.

4. If these methods fail, edrophonium chloride (for its vagal effects) may be given intravenously with caution.

5. A thump on the chest can often correct an atrial tachycardia, especially in an emergency when resuscitative drugs and equipment are not available.[27] *(See Chapter 11.)*

6. Other antiarrhythmic drugs: lidocaine and procainamide are occasionally successful. Calcium-blocking agents in man are commonly used and are very effective. Studies are now being done in the dog.[28,29]

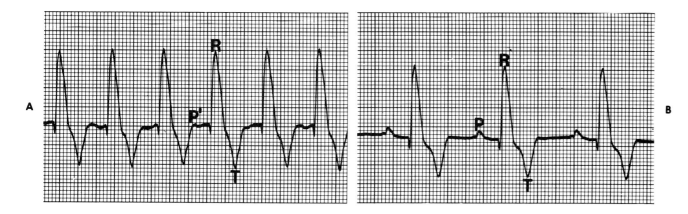

Fig. 6–26. **A,** The focus of origin cannot be identified with accuracy in this strip. **B,** After ocular pressure the tachycardia has been terminated. The configuration of these sinus QRS complexes is the same as in strip **A.** A supraventricular tachycardia, probably atrial tachycardia, is demonstrated in **A.**

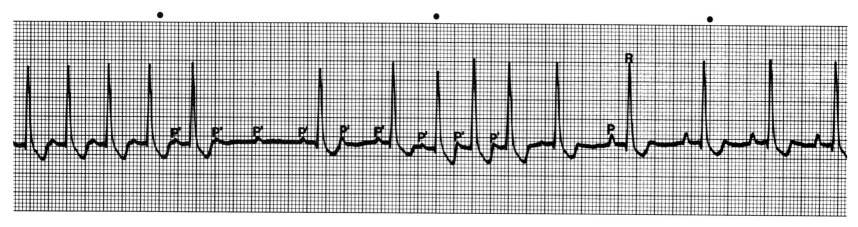

Fig. 6–27. Atrial paroxysmal tachycardia with varying degrees of AV block in a dog with digoxin toxicity. The last four complexes are normal sinus in origin. The atrial rate (P′) averages 280 beats/min with P′ waves different in configuration from the sinus P waves.

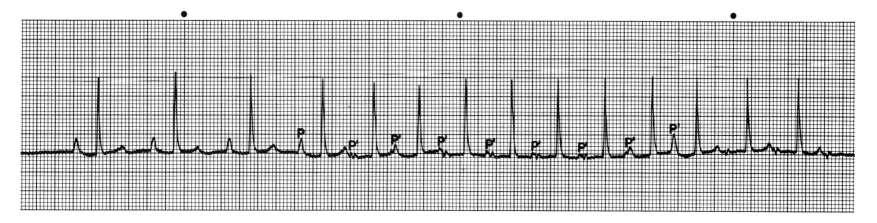

Fig. 6–28. Multifocal atrial tachycardia with an average atrial rate of 230/min in a dog with digitalis toxicity. The first four complexes are normal sinus in origin. Note the irregular atrial rhythm, the varying configuration of the P′ waves, and the varying P′-R intervals.

Atrial flutter

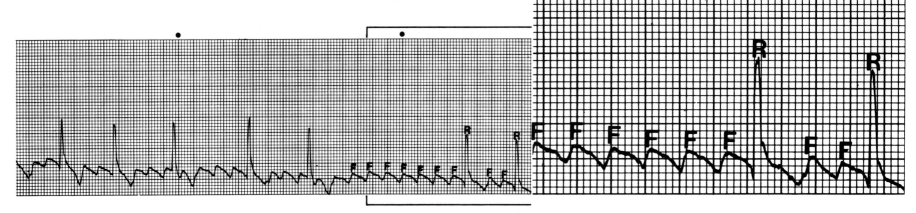

Fig. 6–29. Atrial flutter (F waves) at a rate of over 450/min with varying degrees of conduction to the ventricles. The ventricular rate averages only 120/min.

Atrial flutter is a rapid and regular atrial rhythm at a rate varying usually from 300 to 500 beats/min. Typical and atypical forms can be present. The typical variety is regular, with the P waves being replaced by sawtooth waves (called F waves). The sawtooth flutter waves are not seen in the atypical form, making it difficult to distinguish atrial flutter from atrial tachycardia. Varying degrees of AV conduction are usually present.[21,30] Four possible mechanisms for atrial flutter include: (1) a circus movement of electrical impulses in a ring of tissue between the two venae cavae, (2) unifocal atrial impulse formation, (3) multiple re-entry, and (4) multifocal atrial impulse formation.[11,31] One or a combination of these may be responsible for initiating atrial flutter.

Electrocardiographic features

1. The atrial rhythm (F waves) is regular with a rate usually above 300 beats/min. The ventricular rhythm and rate depend on the atrial rate and the state of AV conduction (same as the atrial rate, 1:1 conduction; half the atrial rate, 2:1; 3:1; 4:1; etc.).

2. Normal P waves are replaced by sawtooth flutter waves (F waves), a combination of ectopic and pronounced atrial repolarization waves (T_a waves). The isoelectric line cannot be distinguished between the flutter waves. The flutter waves are best seen in leads II and CV_5RL. In some leads the flutter waves are absent.

3. The QRS configuration is normal (same as for the sinus complexes) or wide and bizarre due to bundle branch block, aberrant ventricular conduction, or ventricular pre-excitation.

4. When conduction through the atrioventricular node is constant, the interval between the QRS complex and the F wave is of constant duration. This interval varies in duration based on the changing sec-

ond-degree AV block. All the atrial impulses cannot be conducted to the ventricles.

Associated conditions

1. Same conditions that cause the other atrial arrhythmias, those producing atrial enlargement being the most common
2. Others: ruptured chordae tendineae,[21] quinidine therapy for atrial fibrillation, atrial septal defect,[22] tricuspid dyplasia, chronic mitral valvular fibrosis,[21] ventricular pre-excitation (Wolff-Parkinson-White syndrome)[22]

Atrial flutter is common in cardiac catheterization procedures in dogs with a large right atrium.

Treatment[31] (See Chapter 10 and Fig. 10–9)

1. The urgency of therapy depends on the ventricular rate, since fast ventricular rates usually cause heart failure. Digoxin is usually the drug of choice for atrial flutter.

2. Ocular or carotid sinus pressure slows the ventricular rate by decreasing the number of conducted flutter waves into the ventricles.

3. Low-energy precordial shock usually converts atrial flutter. Cardioversion should be attempted if digoxin is not effective and if the animal is in critical condition. Digoxin should be stopped 24 hours before the procedure. Quinidine may be helpful in cardioversion but should be given only after digoxin has been used. If the patient is critical, propranolol or verapamil may be effective.

4. A thump on the chest, especially in an emergency situation, may be effective (Fig. 12–17).

5. Following the conversion, quinidine and/or propranolol may be effective in preventing recurrences.

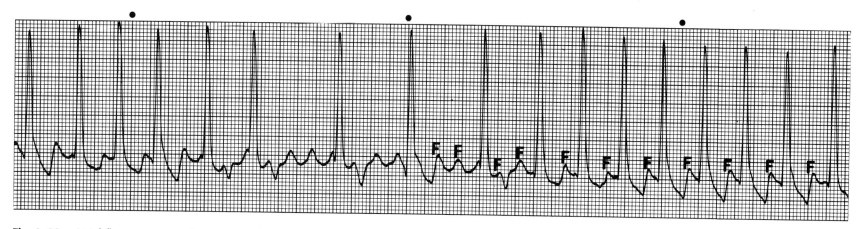

Fig. 6–30. Atrial flutter at a rate of 500/min with varying degrees of conduction to the ventricles. For example, the last eight complexes represent 2:1 conduction (one F wave is hidden within each QRS). This dog had tricuspid dysplasia and right atrial enlargement.

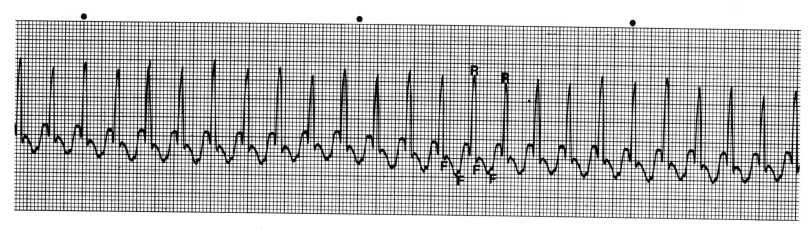

Fig. 6–31. Atrial flutter with 2:1 conduction at a ventricular rate of 330/min in a dog with an atrial septal defect. This supraventricular tachycardia was associated with a Wolff-Parkinson-White pattern.

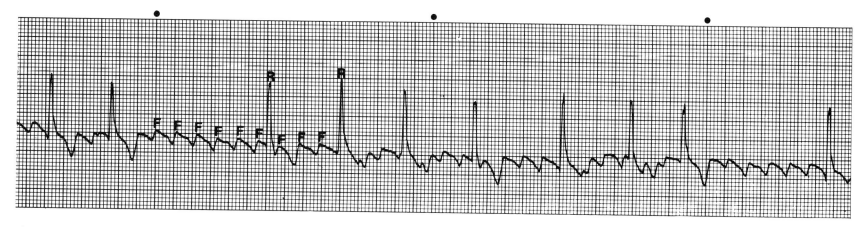

Fig. 6–32. Atrial flutter at a rate of over 450/min with varying degrees of conduction to the ventricles. This high degree of AV block occurred after digoxin was used to treat a rapid ventricular rate.

Atrial fibrillation

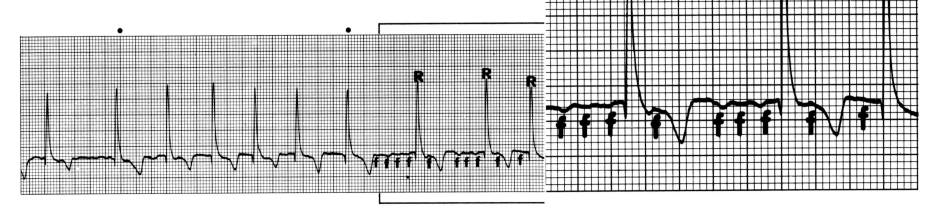

Fig. 6–33. "Fine" atrial fibrillation with an average ventricular rate of 200/min in a dog with severe mitral valvular insufficiency. Note the total irregularity of the R waves and the f waves.

The possible mechanisms discussed for atrial flutter apply to atrial fibrillation.[11] Atrial fibrillation is common in the dog, most often associated with severe underlying heart disease. It can be paroxysmal.[32] The loss of the "atrial kick," combined with the rapid heart rate, may substantially reduce cardiac output and cause congestive heart failure.

Electrocardiographic features

1. Atrial and ventricular rates are rapid and totally irregular. At very rapid ventricular rates, however, ventricular rhythm appears less irregular.

2. In coarse atrial fibrillation, large oscillations (f waves) of varying amplitude replace the normal sinus P waves. Sometimes these prominent f waves resemble atrial flutter. The term atrial flutter fibrillation is then used.[33] In fine atrial fibrillation, small f waves take the place of the sinus P waves.

3. The QRS configuration is normal (same as for the sinus complexes) or wide and bizarre owing to bundle branch block or ventricular pre-excitation. Normal QRS complexes sometimes vary in amplitude, especially during fast heart rates. Numerous supraventricular impulses arrive so early that parts of the ventricle are not yet completely recovered.

4. The ventricular rate is totally irregular because the atrioventricular junction allows only a limited number of fibrillatory waves to be conducted to the ventricles. Digoxin and propranolol prolong the refractory period in the AV node, allowing even fewer fibrillatory waves to reach the ventricle.

Associated conditions

1. Same conditions that cause the other atrial arrhythmias, those causing marked atrial enlargement being the most common. In our series of dogs,[7] the arrhythmia was usually associated with chronic AV valvular insufficiency. The dilated form of cardiomyopathy was nearly equal in prevalence, especially in the large breeds.[34–36]

2. Congenital heart defects: patent ductus arteriosus, mitral insufficiency, tricuspid dysplasia, pulmonic stenosis, double-chambered right ventricle, and ventricular septal defects*

3. Miscellaneous: digitalis toxicity, anesthesia, heartworm disease, cardiac trauma, hypertrophic cardiomyopathy[37,39]

Atrial fibrillation may occur in the absence of cardiac disease, without any clinical signs.[7,17]

Treatment *(See Chapter 10 and Fig. 10–12)*

1. The animal usually succumbs within 3 months to a year.

2. To reduce the heart rate to less than 160 beats/min, digoxin may be administered followed by propranolol or verapamil if additional slowing of the ventricular rate is necessary.[40,41] Digoxin should be given first and then propranolol because of the negative inotropic effects of the latter. Electrical cardioversion with precordial shock is indicated only when a rapid ventricular rate is unresponsive to drugs and when clinical signs exist.[42] Quinidine has been used for conversion to normal sinus rhythm in animals with atrial fibrillation of recent onset and that do not exhibit other signs of heart disease.

3. The congenital defect should be corrected if possible. For example, patent ductus arteriosus with atrial fibrillation will sometimes convert to sinus rhythm after surgery.

---

*References 7, 17, 22, 23, 37, 38.

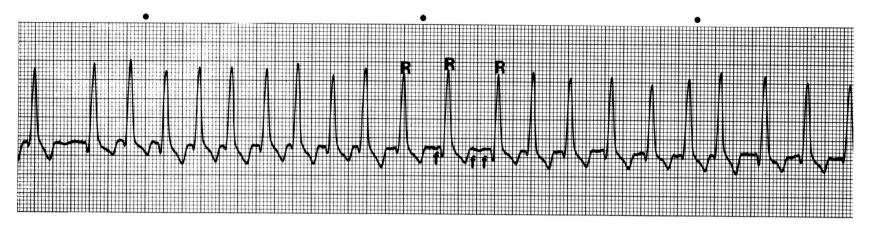

Fig. 6–34. Atrial fibrillation with a rapid ventricular rate averaging 300/min in a dog with the dilated form of cardiomyopathy. The irregular ventricular rhythm is less obvious in certain portions of the strip.

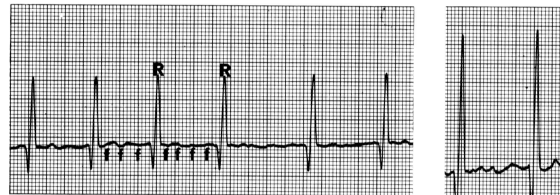

Fig. 6–35. "Fine" atrial fibrillation in a dog with chronic mitral valvular insufficiency. Note the irregular ventricular rhythm and the lack of P waves.

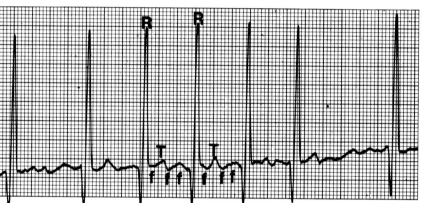

Fig. 6–36. "Coarse" atrial fibrillation in a dog with patent ductus arteriosus. The f waves are prominent.

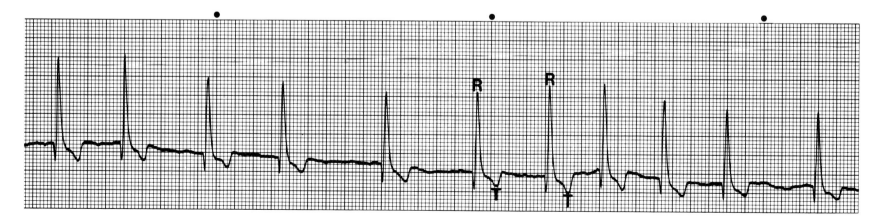

Fig. 6–37. "Fine" atrial fibrillation in a large-breed dog with the dilated form of cardiomyopathy. The heart rate has been reduced to an average ventricular rate of 160/min with the use of digoxin.

Atrioventricular junctional premature complexes

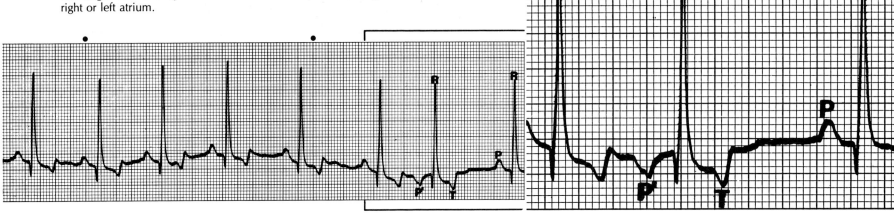

Fig. 6–38. AV junctional premature complex in a dog with mitral valvular insufficiency. The P′ wave is inverted and precedes the premature QRS complex. The origin of this ectopic focus is either the AV junctional region or the lower right or left atrium.

AV junctional premature complexes, also termed AV nodal premature contractions and AV nodal extrasystoles, are caused by the premature firing of an ectopic AV junctional focus. The impulse spreads backward (retrograde) to the atria as well as forward (anterograde) to the ventricles. The AV junction is actually a network of fibers, with no pacemaker cells in the main body.[43] The term *junctional* is more accurate for describing rhythms that arise in the region extending from the atrial fibers approaching the AV junction to the bifurcation of the bundle of His. The earlier, historic term, A-V nodal is now being reconsidered. The restoration of A-V nodal, without clinical subdivision into upper, middle, and lower A-V node has been recently recommended as the preferred term for rhythms from the A-V node.[43a]

Electrocardiographic features

1. The heart rate is usually normal. The rhythm is irregular due to the premature P′ waves that disrupt normal P wave rhythm.

2. The P′ wave is almost always negative in lead II. As discussed for wandering atrial pacemaker, however, the direction of the P wave is not always a reliable criterion for the diagnosis of AV junctional complexes.

3. The QRS complex is premature. Its configuration is usually normal (same as for the sinus complexes) or wide and bizarre due to

bundle branch block, aberrant ventricular conduction, or ventricular pre-excitation.

4. The P′ wave may precede, be superimposed on, or follow the QRS depending on the location of the ectopic focus and on the conduction velocity above and below the atrioventricular junctional focus. For example, the negative P′ wave precedes the QRS when conduction of the impulse retrograde is faster than anterograde conduction. A high AV junctional premature complex may have a normal or short P′-R interval and cannot be distinguished from a low atrial ectopic focus. The term *supraventricular premature complex* should be used.

5. A noncompensatory pause is usually present; in other words, the R-R interval between two normal complexes on each side of the premature complex is less than twice the normal R-R interval.

Associated conditions

1. Digitalis toxicity
2. Same conditions that cause APCs

Treatment *(See Chapter 10)*

1. If digitalis toxicity exists, discontinue the digitalis.
2. Treatment is the same as for APCs (digitalis), especially if cardiac decompensation is present. Propranolol may also be effective.

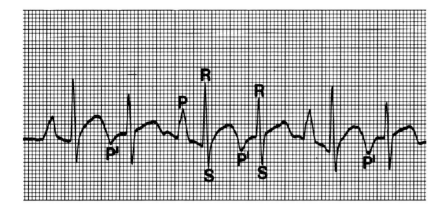

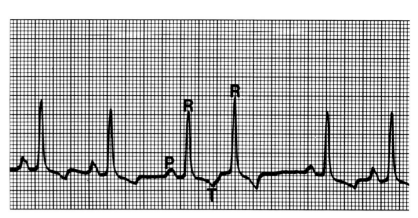

Fig. 6–39. Three supraventricular premature complexes in a dog with digitalis toxicity. The configuration of the second, fourth, and sixth premature QRS complexes is approximately the same as that of the sinus QRS complexes. The premature P' waves are negative and precede the QRS complexes. The ectopic focus is probably in the junctional region. The sinus P waves are tall and wide, indicating biatrial enlargement.

Fig. 6–40. Sinus rhythm with a supraventricular premature complex (fourth QRS complex); the P' wave is hidden within the QRS-T complex. A noncompensatory pause is present.

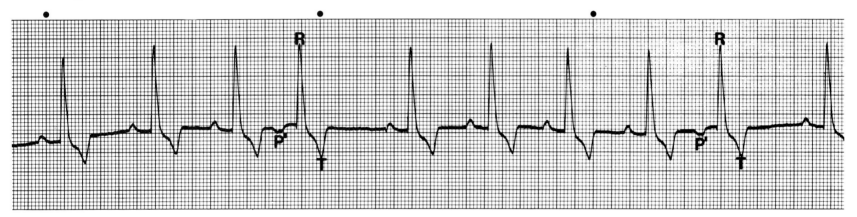

Fig. 6–41. Two supraventricular premature complexes (fourth and ninth complexes) possibly arising from within the AV junctional region. The atrium is activated in a retrograde fashion prior to activation of the ventricle. This produces a normal P'-R interval. These complexes cannot be distinguished from an atrial ectopic complex arising from a low atrial focus and therefore are best referred to as supraventricular or AV junctional premature complexes.

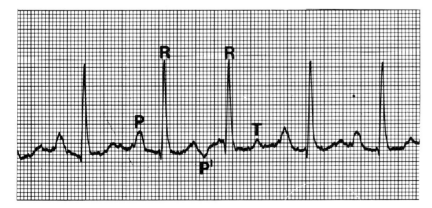

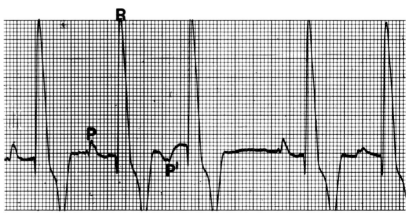

Fig. 6–42. One probable junctional premature complex (third complex) in a dog with chronic mitral valvular insufficiency. The duration of the P'-R interval is long, indicating a possible conduction delay below the junctional focus.

Fig. 6–43. Junctional premature complex (third complex) in a dog with digoxin toxicity. The predominantly negative P' wave precedes the QRS complex.

Atrioventricular junctional tachycardia

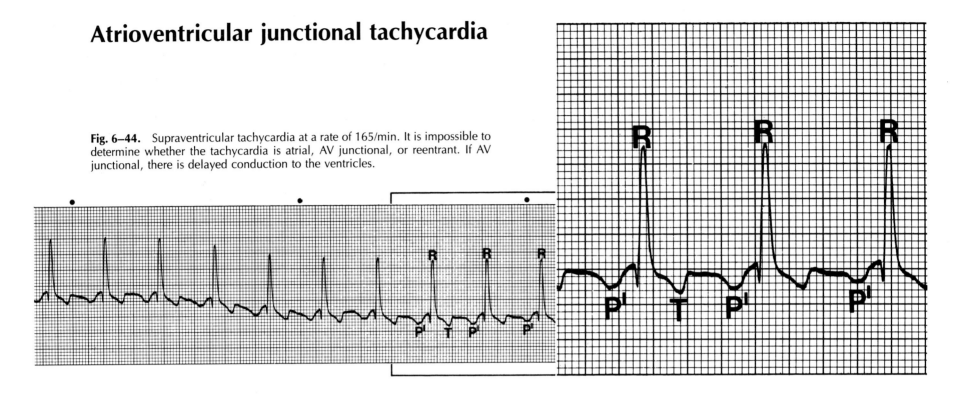

Fig. 6–44. Supraventricular tachycardia at a rate of 165/min. It is impossible to determine whether the tachycardia is atrial, AV junctional, or reentrant. If AV junctional, there is delayed conduction to the ventricles.

In AV junctional tachycardia the ectopic focus in the AV junction acts as the primary pacemaker. The heart rate is faster than the AV junctional inherent rate of 40 to 60 beats/min, indicating a tachycardia. The term *enhanced AV junctional rhythm* is used for rates above 60 but less than 100. The mechanism for junctional tachycardia, like that for atrial tachycardia, is most often re-entry.[24,25] (See Chapters 9 and 12 for a detailed explanation.)

It is usually impossible to differentiate atrial tachycardia from an AV junctional tachycardia since the inverted P waves are superimposed on the QRS-T complexes. Because the two arrhythmias are essentially the same, with similar mechanisms, the term *supraventricular tachycardia* can be used for both atrial tachycardia and AV junctional tachycardia.

Electrocardiographic features

1. The heart rate is over 60 beats/min. The rhythm is usually regular. Junctional tachycardia can be either paroxysmal or continuous.

2. P' waves are negative in lead II and may precede, be superimposed on, or follow the QRS complex.

3. The configuration of the QRS complex is usually normal (same as for the sinus complexes) or can be wide and bizarre as a result of bundle branch block, aberrant ventricular conduction, or ventricular pre-excitation.

4. The P'-R interval is constant (1:1 atrioventricular conduction). The P'-R interval for a high AV junctional focus is normal (less than 0.13 sec) or longer when there is conduction delay below the AV junctional focus. At higher rates, varying degrees of AV block can occur (2:1, ventricular rate half the atrial rate; 3:1; 4:1; etc.). The R-P' interval is variable depending on the conduction delay above the focus.

Associated conditions

1. Digitalis toxicity (The rate usually is less than 160 beats/min, has a gradual onset and termination, and can be temporarily slowed by carotid sinus or ocular pressure.[44])

2. AV junctional tachycardia at a faster heart rate (greater than 160) that is of sudden onset and terminated by carotid sinus or ocular pressure.[44] (This is usually associated with cardiac disease.)

Treatment *(See Chapter 10 and Fig. 10–9)*

1. If the animal is being treated with digitalis, stop the digitalis. Give intravenous potassium if serum potassium is low. Phenytoin (diphenylhydantoin) may be useful in restoring normal sinus rhythm. Atropine can sometimes be used to accelerate the SA pacemaker to overdrive a junctional focus. Once the rhythm is controlled, maintenance doses of digitalis should be reduced.

2. Carotid sinus or ocular pressure sometimes terminates an AV junctional tachycardia not due to digitalis toxicity. Digitalis is the drug of choice, especially if the tachycardia results from a reentry mechanism. Digitalis alters the conduction through the pathways of the AV junction. Propranolol also affects the conduction pathways and can be used if digitalis is ineffective.[31]

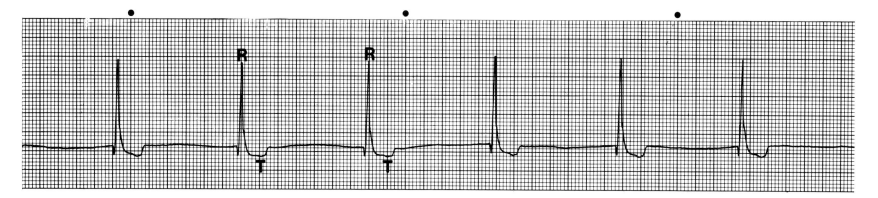

Fig. 6–45. Enhanced AV junctional rhythm at a rate of 85/min in a dog with digitalis toxicity. The P' waves are hidden within the QRS complexes.

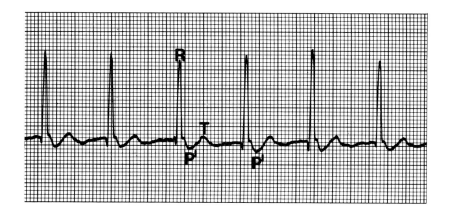

Fig. 6–46. AV junctional tachycardia at a rate of 165/min. The inverted P' waves appear to immediately follow the QRS complexes. The inverted P' waves on later strips (not shown) preceded the QRS complexes.

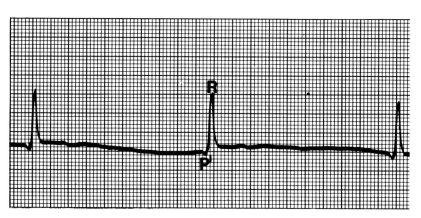

Fig. 6–47. AV junctional rhythm at a rate of 60/min (the approximate AV junctional inherent rate). The SA node is *not* functioning; the AV junction is pacing the heart.

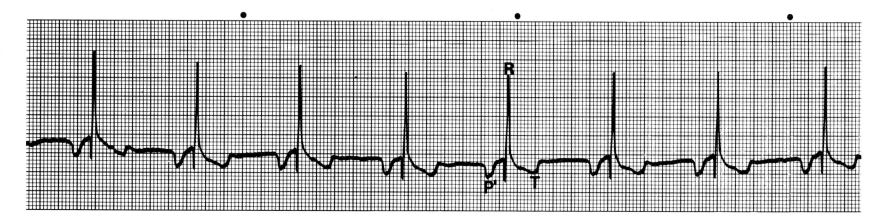

Fig. 6–48. AV junctional tachycardia at a rate of 100/min in a dog with digitalis toxicity.

Escape rhythms

Fig. 6–49. An escape rhythm in a dog with complete AV block due to digitalis toxicity. The last escape complex is ventricular, whereas the others are probably located below the area of AV block.

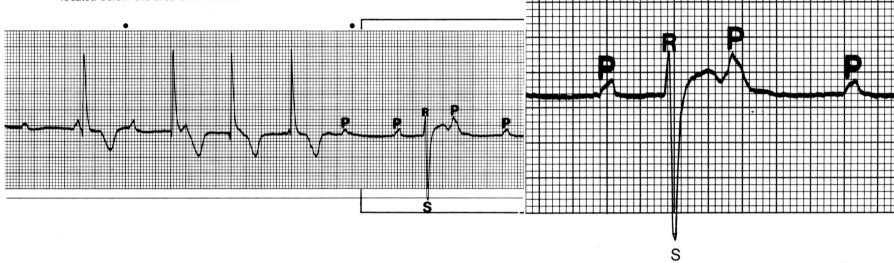

The escape rhythms occur when the pacemaker with the highest automaticity (usually the SA node) either slows down or stops. The intrinsic pacemaker activity of the lower regions of the heart (usually the AV junction of the ventricles) rescues the heart rhythm after a pause in the dominant rhythm. A single spontaneous impulse from a slower subsidiary pacemaker appearing after a pause is called an escape complex. If the subsidiary pacemaker temporarily takes over the role of the cardiac pacemaker, the rhythm is known as an escape rhythm (three or more consecutive escapes).[26] Escape complexes are most often of AV junctional or ventricular origin. When ventricular escape impulses control the rhythm, the term *idioventricular rhythm* is used instead of ventricular escape rhythm.

Electrocardiographic features

Junctional escape rhythms

1. The heart rate is usually slow. Escape complexes follow a pause longer than the normal cycle length (R-R interval). Rhythm is regular when the AV junction persists as the dominant pacemaker. The inherent rate of the AV junction is frequently less than 60 beats/min. The more rapid junctional rhythms are called enhanced junctional rhythms.
2. The P wave is usually negative.
3. The QRS configuration is usually normal.
4. The P waves may precede, be superimposed on, or follow the QRS.

Ventricular escape rhythm (idioventricular rhythm)

1. The heart rate is usually slow. Escape complexes follow a pause longer than the normal sinus cycle length. An idioventricular rhythm (a series of ventricular escape complexes) is generally regular, with the rate less than 40 beats/min.
2. P waves are usually not present, unless complete AV block or a severe second-degree AV block exists (a common cause of ventricular escape rhythm). The P waves will then be unrelated and precede, be hidden within, or follow the ectopic QRS complexes.
3. The QRS configuration is wide and bizarre, similar to that of ventricular premature complexes.
4. No relationship exists between the P wave and the QRS complex.

Associated conditions

Escapes are never a primary diagnosis. They are always secondary to an abnormality of impulse formation or conduction; therefore

1. All the causes of sinus bradycardia, sinus arrest (block), and AV block (Complete AV block is the most common cause since no impulses can originate from the junctional region.)
2. Digitalis toxicity, increased vagal tone, sick sinus syndrome[15]

Treatment *(See Chapter 10 and Fig. 10–18)*

1. Treat the underlying cause of the arrhythmia, since the escape rhythm is a secondary phenomenon. The actual escape complex or rhythm should *not* be suppressed (e.g., quinidine for ventricular escape complexes). The escape rhythm is a safety mechanism for maintaining cardiac output.
2. Atropine, glycopyrrolate, or isoproterenol is often indicated. Artificial pacing is used if the arrhythmia is resistant to drug treatment.

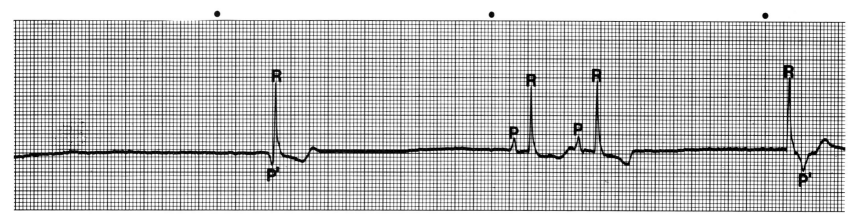

Fig. 6–50. AV junctional escape complexes with severe sinus bradycardia and SA arrest in a dog with digitalis toxicity. An inverted P' wave precedes the first escape complex, whereas an inverted P' wave follows the QRS complex (last complex) in the other escape complex.

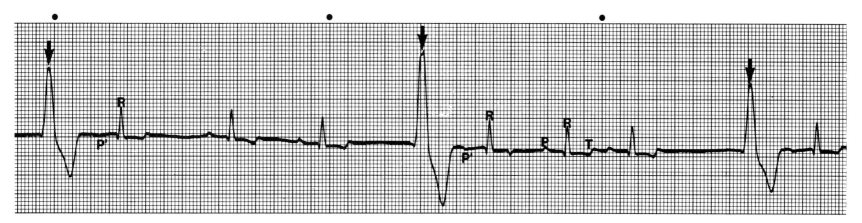

Fig. 6–51. Ventricular escape complexes (arrows) during various phases in the dominant sinus rhythm in a dog during anesthesia. AV junctional escape complexes appear to follow each ventricular escape complex. The inverted P' waves precede the QRS complexes. The sinus rate increased (not shown) after the anesthesia was stopped; ½ cm = 1 mv.

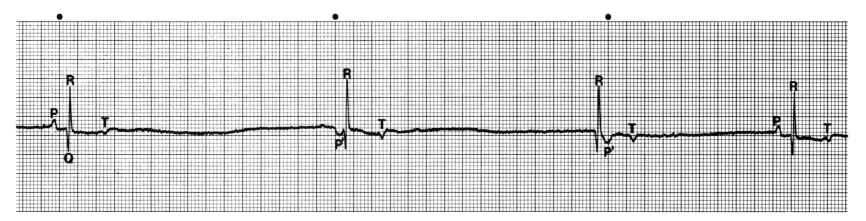

Fig. 6–52. AV junctional escape complexes in a dog with a severe sinus bradycardia. The inverted P' waves precede and follow the QRS complexes. Atropine later eliminated the sinus bradycardia as well as the secondary AV junctional escape impulses.

151

Ventricular premature complexes

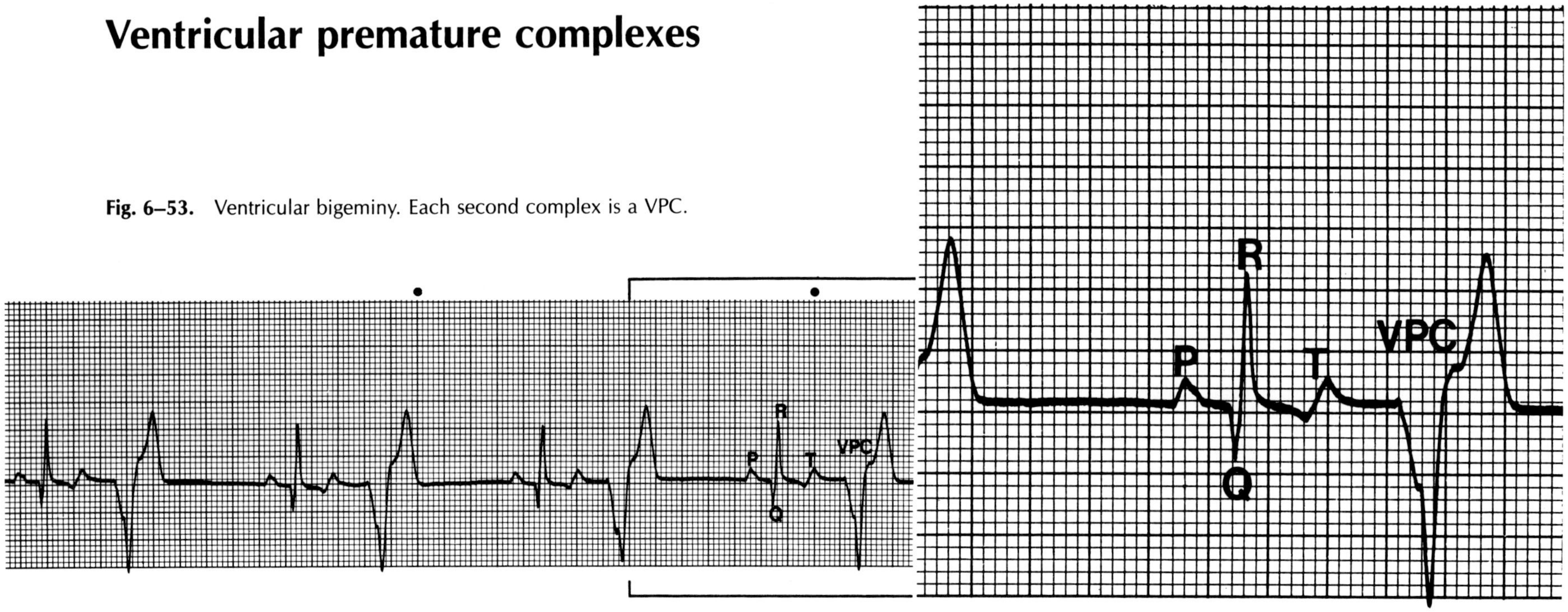

Fig. 6–53. Ventricular bigeminy. Each second complex is a VPC.

Ventricular premature complexes (VPCs) (also called ventricular premature contractions) are impulses that arise from an ectopic focus in the ventricles. They do not travel through the specialized conduction system but through ordinary muscle, spreading through both ventricles with delay and causing a bizarre widened QRS complex. VPCs are the most frequent type of abnormal rhythm in dogs.

Electrocardiographic features

1. The heart rate is usually normal. The rhythm is irregular due to the premature QRS complex that disrupts the normal ventricular rhythm.
2. P waves that can be seen are of normal configuration.
3. The QRS complex is premature, bizarre, and often of large amplitude. The T wave is directed opposite the QRS.

The origin of the VPCs can usually be determined as either the left or the right ventricle: if the major QRS deflection is negative in lead II, the ectopic focus is in the left ventricle; the reverse is true for right VPCs. VPCs with narrow QRS complexes arise from one of the proximal intraventricular conduction branches. QRS complexes of identical shape are called *unifocal VPCs*. Premature complexes that are of variable shape are termed *multiform*. The coupling interval (i.e., the time between the beginning of the VPC and the beginning of the preceding complex) is identical in unifocal VPCs and variable in multiform VPCs.

4. VPCs are not associated with the P wave. The independent normal P wave may precede, be within, or follow the VPC.
5. A compensatory pause usually follows a VPC. The ectopic impulse generally cannot penetrate through the AV junction and disturb the normal SA rhythm. The sinus rhythm continues undisturbed; the next sinus impulse after the VPC occurs on time.

Associated conditions[40]

There are numerous causes of VPCs (the cause of the myocarditis often not found): primary cardiac diseases, secondary cardiac diseases, and drugs. In a number of dogs, VPCs may occur in normal hearts with no apparent cause.

1. Cardiac: congestive heart failure, myocardial infarction, neoplasia, pericarditis, cardiomyopathy, traumatic myocarditis, idiopathic myocarditis in Boxers (in 63 Boxers in one study, 45 had occasional to frequent VPCs),[40a] and Doberman Pinschers[6]
2. Secondary: changes in autonomic tone (excitement), hypoxia, anemia, uremia, pyometra, gastric dilatation–volvulus, pancreatitis, parvovirus[47]
3. Drugs: digitalis, epinephrine, anesthetic agents, atropine[36,46]

Treatment[31,40,41,48] (See Chapter 10)

1. Treat the underlying condition
2. Indications for aggressive treatment (intravenous antiarrhythmics) are more than 16 VPCs per minute, runs of two or more VPCs, multiform VPCs (varying configuration), and R-on-T phenomena (R wave of the VPC at the peak of the preceding T wave, the "vulnerable" period). The R-on-T phenomenon may induce ventricular tachycardia (Fig. 6–66) or ventricular fibrillation (Fig. 6–68) and also a deteriorating hemodynamic status.
3. Lidocaine should be used first because it is most effective and safest. Digoxin may eliminate VPCs when cardiac failure exists. Other drugs are procainamide, quinidine, propranolol, diazepam, phenytoin, aprindine, and disopyramide phosphate (Norpace).[49]
4. Supportive measures are important; acid-base and electrolyte abnormalities should be corrected.

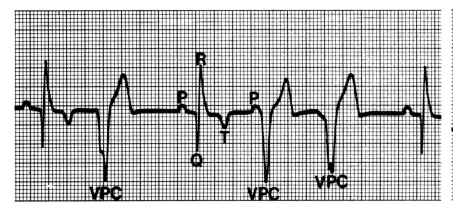

Fig. 6–54. Multiform VPCs; the second, fourth, and fifth complexes are of variable shape. This constitutes a serious condition. A sinus P wave happens to just precede the second VPC.

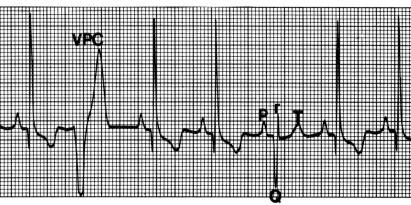

Fig. 6–55. VPC and a fusion complex (fifth complex) in a dog with myocarditis from a pancreatitis. A fusion complex is the simultaneous activation of the ventricle by impulses coming from the SA node and the ventricular ectopic foci. The QRS complex is intermediate in form.

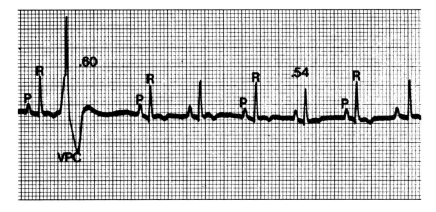

Fig. 6–56. VPC that probably originates in the right ventricle. A compensatory pause is present. The R-R interval (0.60 sec, or 30 boxes) between the two sinus complexes enclosing the VPC is slightly greater than the R-R interval (0.54 sec, or 27 boxes) between three sinus complexes.

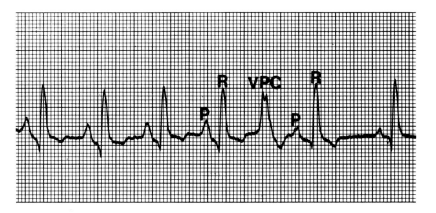

Fig. 6–57. Interpolated VPC from the right ventricle. The VPC occurs between two normal sinus complexes without disturbing the basic rhythm. The P-R interval following the VPC is slightly prolonged; the VPC has traveled retrograde into part of the AV junction.

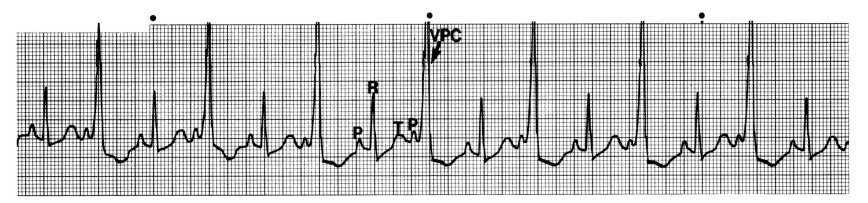

Fig. 6–58. Ventricular bigeminy in a dog under anesthesia with a thiobarbiturate. The rhythm alternates between a normal sinus complex and a VPC. The coupling interval is constant. The normal independent sinus P waves just happen to precede each VPC. They are not the cause of the ventricular activity.

Ventricular tachycardia

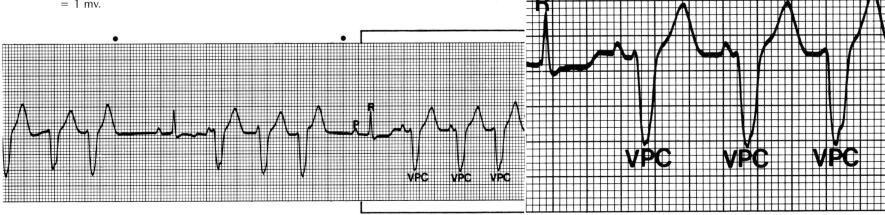

Fig. 6–59. Intermittent ventricular tachycardia, three or more ventricular VPCs in a row. The rhythm is interrupted by conducted sinus complexes; 0.5 cm = 1 mv.

Ventricular tachycardia can be thought of as a continuous series of VPCs resulting from stimulation of an ectopic ventricular focus. It may be intermittent (three or more VPCs in a row) or persistent (all complexes originating in the ventricles). Ventricular tachycardia is generally considered the most serious of all tachyarrhythmias. It is often associated with serious underlying cardiac disease. Dogs with ventricular tachycardia often present with concomitant hypotension and congestive heart failure.

Electrocardiographic features[21,40]

1. The ventricular rate is usually above 100 beats/min with a regular rhythm. Ventricular tachycardia between 60 and 100 is termed *idioventricular tachycardia* (also called an enhanced ventricular rhythm).
2. P waves that can be seen are of normal configuration.
3. QRS complexes are wide and bizarre. Ventricular fusion and capture complexes occur commonly in ventricular tachycardia.
4. There is no relationship between the QRS complexes and the P waves; the P waves may precede, be hidden within, or follow the QRS complexes.

Associated conditions[50]

1. Same conditions causing VPCs (Ventricular tachycardia is usually a manifestation of significant organic heart disease.)

Clinical data indicate that ventricular ectopic activity often does not occur until 12 to 36 hours after the myocardial ischemic event (e.g., gastric dilatation—volvulus, myocardial infarction, or traumatic myocarditis).[39,48,50,51]

Treatment[31,41,48] *(See Chapter 10 and Fig. 10–16)*

1. Treatment should begin as soon as possible.
2. Supportive measures are important; acid-base and electrolyte abnormalities should be corrected.
3. The treatment of choice is lidocaine administered intravenously, first as a bolus and then as a constant intravenous infusion. Procainamide is also effective as a bolus injection and constant infusion. Other drugs include quinidine, propranolol, and digitalis (in congestive heart failure). Phenytoin (diphenylhydantoin) or propranolol may be used in ventricular tachycardia caused by digitalis toxicity.
4. Electrical cardioversion, starting at low watt-seconds, is indicated when the animal is in a hemodynamic crisis and when lidocaine fails. *(See Chapter 11.)*
5. A thump delivered to the precordium with a clenched fist can be used, especially in an emergency when resuscitative drugs and equipment are unavailable. *(See Chapter 11.)*
6. When conventional antiarrhythmic drugs are unsuccessful, the experimental drug aprindine can be effective.[50] Side effects can occur because of aprindine's narrow toxic-therapeutic ratio.

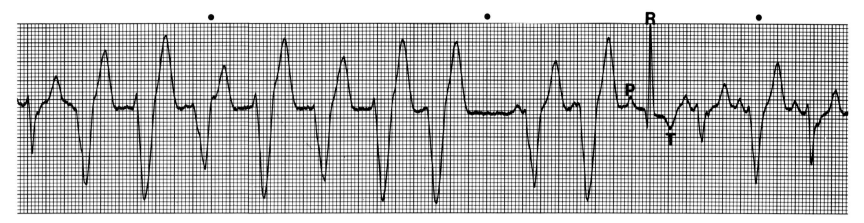

Fig. 6-60. Multiform (varying configuration of ventricular ectopic complexes) ventricular tachycardia at an average of 180/min in a dog with a gastric dilatation. The fourth complex from the end of the strip is a capture complex. A normal sinus impulse has reached the AV junction in a recovered state, capturing the ventricles for one complex. The last three complexes represent different degrees of fusion: simultaneous activation of the ventricles by a sinus impulse (the P wave just preceding) and a ventricular ectopic focus.

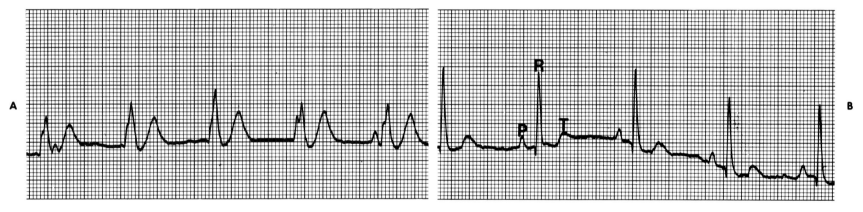

Fig. 6-61. **A,** Ventricular tachycardia (complexes positive, probably of right ventricular origin) in a dog hit by a car. **B,** Normal sinus rhythm only minutes after an intravenous bolus of lidocaine.

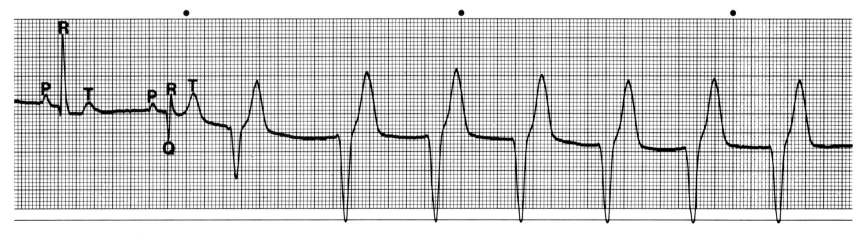

Fig. 6-62. Ventricular tachycardia at a rate of 125/min following one normal sinus complex in a dog with a toxic myocarditis from a pyometra. The second complex represents a fusion complex, which results from the simultaneous activation of the ventricles by a sinus impulse (the second P wave) and a ventricular ectopic focus (a late diastolic extrasystole). The QRS complex is of intermediate shape.

155

Ventricular tachycardia—cont'd

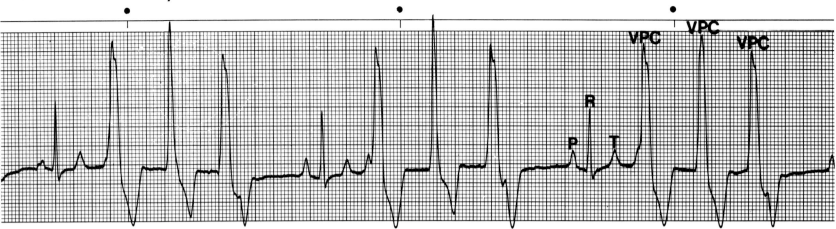

Fig. 6–63. Intermittent ventricular tachycardia, three VPCs in a row with a normal sinus complex capturing the rhythm every fourth complex. This dog has a mammary tumor with metastases to the myocardium.

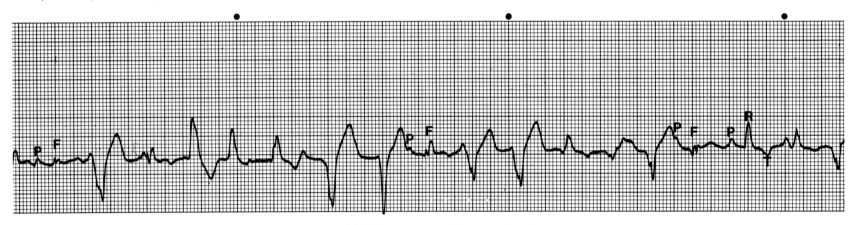

Fig. 6–64. Multiform ventricular tachycardia at an average rate of 220/min in a dog with severe digitalis toxicity. The rhythm is interrupted toward the end of the strip by a conducted sinus complex, which captures the ventricle. Numerous ventricular fusion complexes (F) also are present, a simultaneous activation of the ventricle.

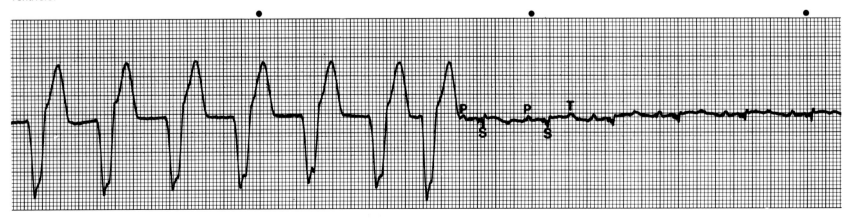

Fig. 6–65. Ventricular tachycardia at a rate of 155/min in a dog with pericardial effusion. Note the small P-QRS-T sinus complexes that eventually dominate the rhythm.

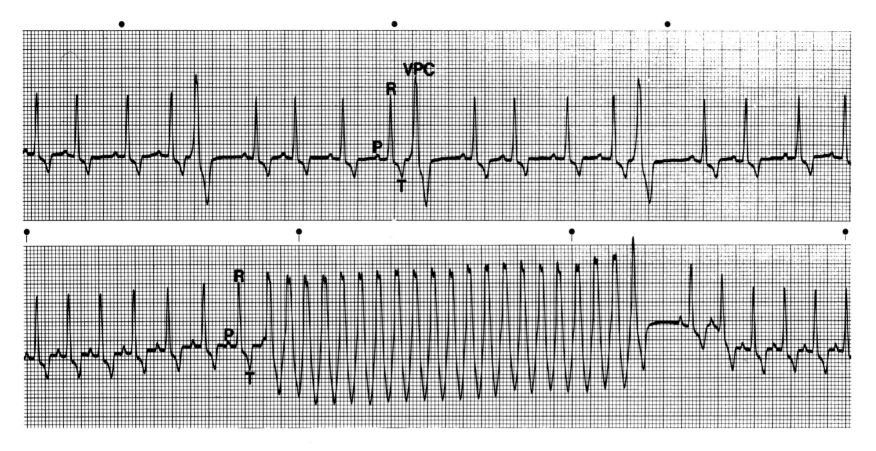

Fig. 6–66. Two separate strips 1 hour apart in a dog with episodes of fainting. The top strip reveals VPCs that represent the R-on-T phenomenon. The R wave of the VPC is near the peak of the preceding T wave, the vulnerable period. VPCs during the vulnerable period may result in ventricular tachycardia (as observed later on the bottom strip) or ventricular fibrillation. Paper speed, 25 mm/sec.

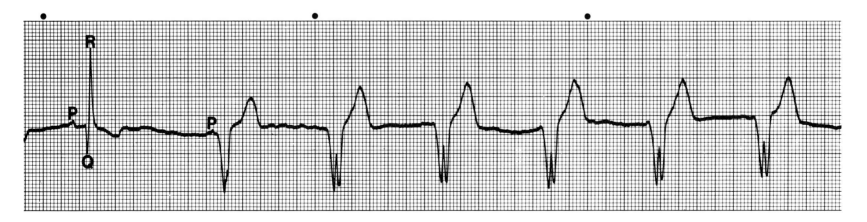

Fig. 6–67. Enhanced idioventricular rhythm at a rate of 103/min. The rhythm results from a late diastolic ventricular ectopic focus (first complex after the second sinus P wave) when the sinus pacemaker slows. This first abnormal complex could also be termed a ventricular escape complex.

157

Ventricular fibrillation

Fig. 6–68. Ventricular fibrillation. Following the third sinus complex, a ventricular ectopic complex occurs within the T wave or in the vulnerable period. This starts a coarse ventricular fibrillation.

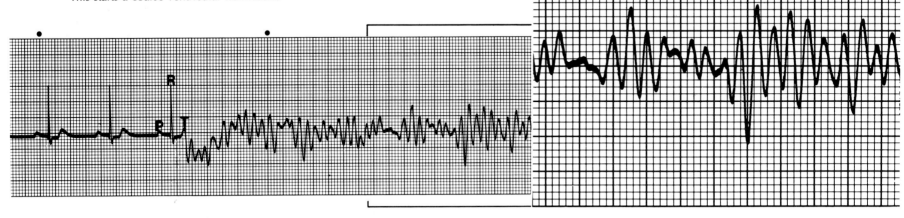

Ventricular fibrillation causes cardiac arrest and is often a terminal event. The contractions of the ventricles are weak and uncoordinated; cardiac output is essentially zero. The electrocardiogram shows completely irregular, chaotic, and deformed deflections of varying amplitude, width, and shape. There are two types of ventricular fibrillation: one with large (*coarse*) oscillations and one with small (*fine*) oscillations.

Electrocardiographic features

1. The heart rate is rapid with irregular, chaotic, and bizarre waves.
2. P waves cannot be recognized.
3. The QRS and T deflections cannot be recognized.
4. There are two types of fibrillation: one whose oscillations are large and coarse, the other with small (fine) oscillations.

Associated conditions

1. Shock
2. Anoxia
3. Myocardial damage: trauma, myocardial infarction
4. Electrolyte and acid-base imbalances: hypokalemia, hypocalcemia, alkalosis
5. Aortic stenosis
6. Drug reactions[52,53]: anesthetic agents, particularly halothane or ultrashort-acting barbiturates, digitalis toxicity
7. Cardiac surgery
8. Electrical shock
9. Autonomic effects, especially enhanced sympathetic neural tone or catecholamine administration[54]
10. Myocarditis, VPCs (during the apex of the T wave of the preceding complex)
11. Hypothermia[55]

Treatment[31,52] (See Chapter 11, Fig. 11–50, and Table 11–2)

1. Initiate the "A-B-C-D-E" of cardiac resuscitation.
2. Defibrillate with direct-current shock. Repeat twice if ineffective.
3. If fine fibrillations are occurring, intracardiac epinephrine or calcium chloride may produce coarse fibrillations (and permit successful defibrillation).
4. Lidocaine and sodium bicarbonate should be tried if fibrillations are still present. Then defibrillate again.
5. If successful, evaluate serum electrolytes and blood gases; search for and treat the basic cause of the arrest.
6. Chemical cardioversion of ventricular fibrillation has recently been shown to be effective: a mixture of 1.0 mEq potassium/kg body weight and 6.0 mg acetylcholine/kg body weight by intracardiac injection.[56]

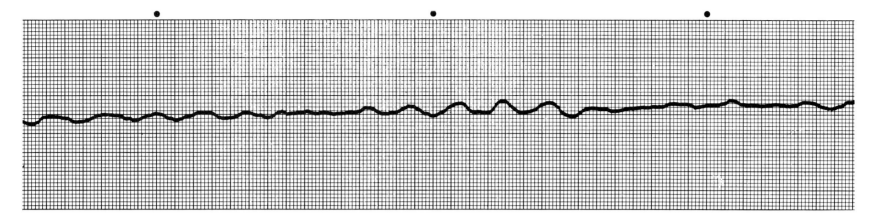

Fig. 6–69. Fine ventricular fibrillation.

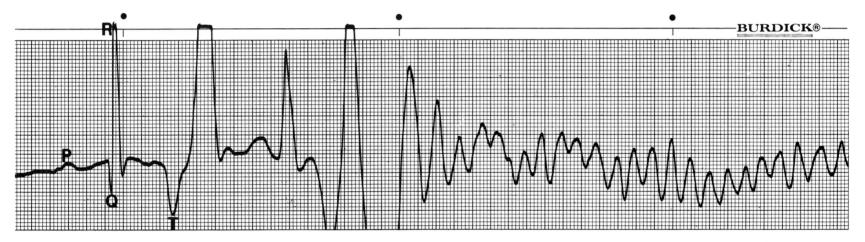

Fig. 6–70. Ventricular flutter-fibrillation in a dog with hypocalcemia. Note the long Q-T. Following the sinus complex (first complex), a ventricular ectopic complex occurs within the vulnerable period of the T wave. Ventricular flutter next occurs for a very brief period. The complexes are wide, bizarre, tall, and rapid. Ventricular flutter is essentially a very rapid ventricular tachycardia. A coarse ventricular fibrillation immediately follows. Torsades de pointes should also be considered (see Chapter 12), especially if sinus complexes return.

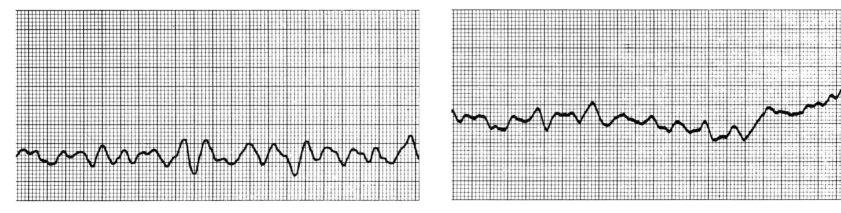

Fig. 6–71. Coarse ventricular fibrillation.

Fig. 6–72. Coarse ventricular fibrillation.

Ventricular asystole

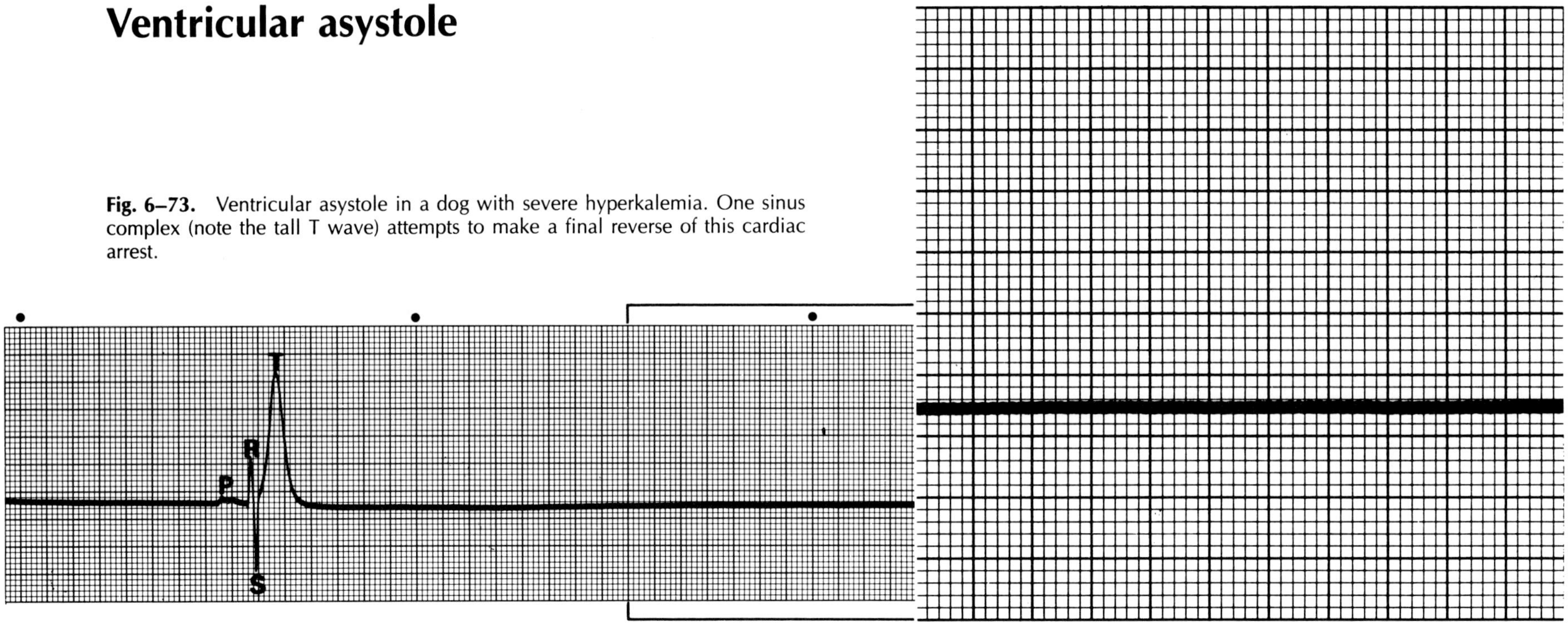

Fig. 6–73. Ventricular asystole in a dog with severe hyperkalemia. One sinus complex (note the tall T wave) attempts to make a final reverse of this cardiac arrest.

Ventricular asystole is the absence of any ventricular complexes. As does ventricular fibrillation, it represents *cardiac arrest.* If the ventricular rhythm is not restored in 3 to 4 minutes, irreversible brain damage can occur. Cardiac arrest can also be detected by the dissociation between a recordable electrocardiogram and no effective cardiac output. This "pump failure" is termed *electrical-mechanical dissociation.*

Clinically, a peripheral pulse cannot be palpated with the three types of cardiac arrest: ventricular fibrillation, ventricular asystole, and electrical-mechanical dissociation. An electrocardiogram is needed to differentiate the types.

Electrocardiographic features

Ventricular asystole may be caused by severe SA block or sinus arrest or by severe third-degree AV block (without a junctional or ventricular escape rhythm).

1. There is no ventricular rhythm. P waves are present at a regular rhythm if complete AV block exists. With severe SA block or arrest, the faster the original rate the longer is the period of asystole.[45,57]

2. P waves are of normal configuration with severe complete AV block.

3. No QRS complexes are seen.

Electrical-mechanical dissociation is diagnosed by the absence of a palpable femoral pulse or a readable systemic blood pressure with a cardiac rhythm (P-QRS-T complexes) on the electrocardiographic monitor.

Associated conditions

Ventricular asystole has a grave prognosis. The electrocardiogram represents a dying heart with *final* cardiac arrest unless cardiac resuscitation is successful.

1. Ventricular fibrillation and complete AV block
2. Severe underlying electrolyte and acid-base imbalance (e.g., severe acidosis and hyperkalemia) (Electrical-mechanical dissociation is often present after defibrillation to sinus rhythm.)

Treatment[31] *(See Chapter 11, Fig. 11–50, and Table 11–2)*

1. Initiate the "A-B-C-D-E" of cardiac resuscitation.

2. Specific drugs of importance include intracardiac epinephrine, sodium bicarbonate, and intravenous or intracardiac calcium chloride (repeat if indicated). The basic cause of cardiac arrest should be treated, and serum electrolytes and blood gases evaluated.

3. With severe sinus bradycardia (long periods of SA block or arrest) or bradycardia with AV block, atropine sulfate intravenously or an intravenous drip of isoproterenol is indicated.

4. A transvenous pacemaker may be needed for artificial pacing but requires a mechanically responsive myocardium.

5. With electrical-mechanical dissociation, dopamine hydrochloride can be quite effective.

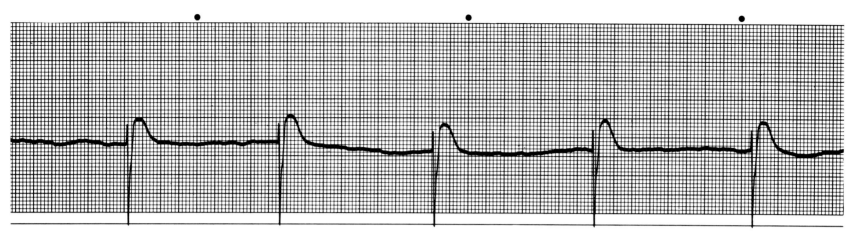

Fig. 6–74. Electrical-mechanical dissociation, dissociation between a recordable electrocardiogram and no effective cardiac output. The femoral pulse, the blood pressure, or the exposed heart needs to be monitored to diagnose this "pump failure."

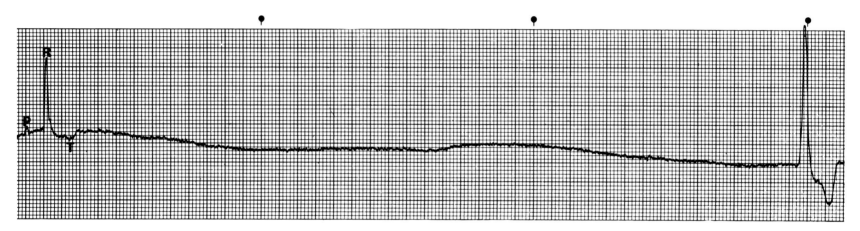

Fig. 6–75. Ventricular asystole caused by severe SA arrest in a dog with SA node disease. No P waves or QRS complexes are seen for 4.5 seconds after the sinus complex. A ventricular escape complex at the end attempts to rescue the heart.

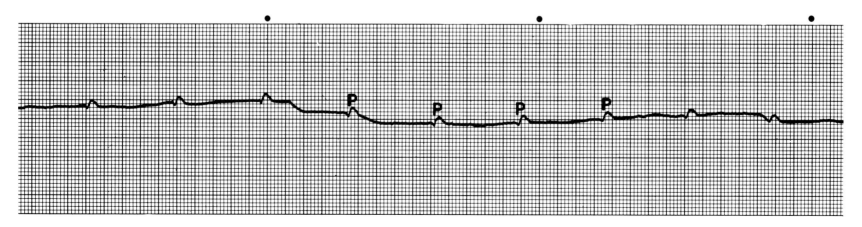

Fig. 6–76. Ventricular asystole in a dog with severe complete AV block. Only P waves (atrial activity) are present; there is no ventricular activity.

Sinoatrial block (sinus arrest)

Fig. 6–77. SA block or arrest in a dog with digoxin toxicity. After the fourth sinus complex, P-QRS-T complexes fail to occur for 1.5 seconds, causing a pause.

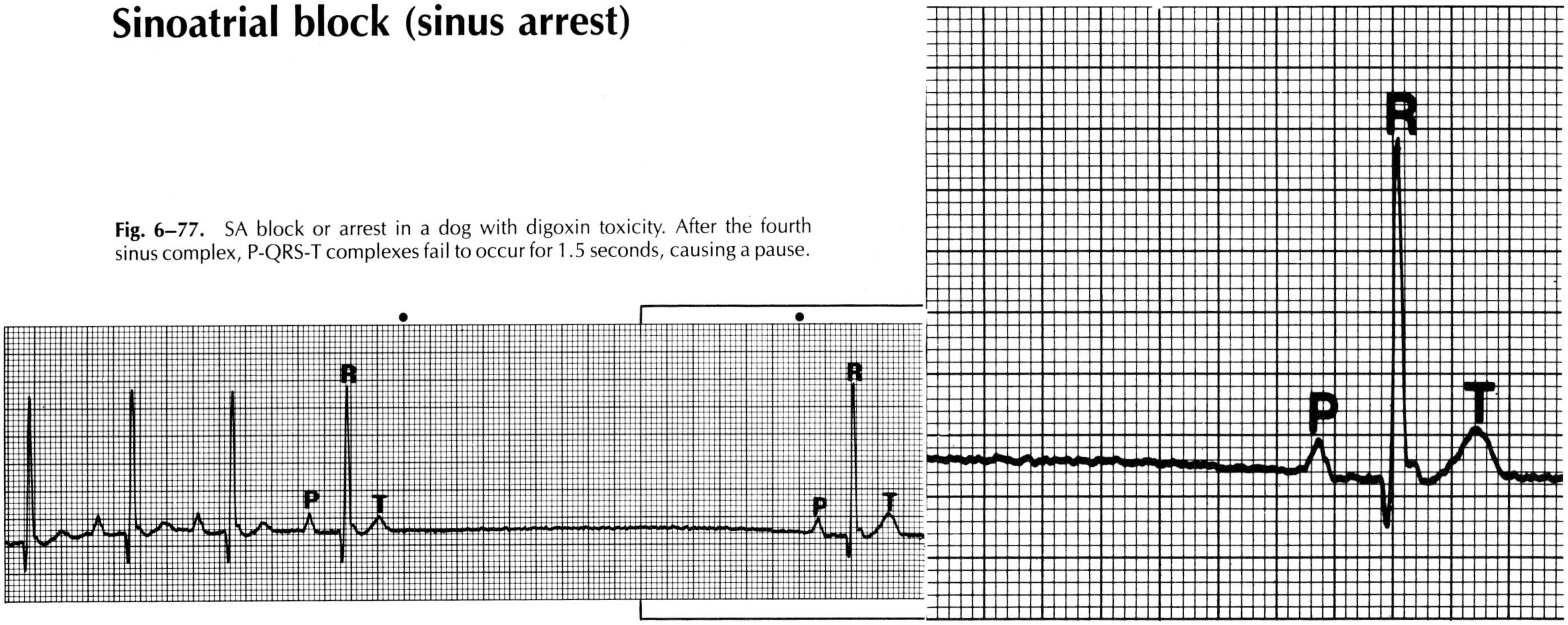

Sinus arrest is the failure of impulses to be formed within the SA node owing to a depression of automaticity in the node. SA block, with the same electrocardiographic pattern, is a disturbance of conduction from a regularly fired SA node. Differentiating between the two is usually difficult. The failure of the SA node to fire on time can cause fainting or even sudden death (ventricular asystole), especially if a lower focus fails to take over the control of the heart.[58]

Electrocardiographic features

1. The heart rate can be variable, depending on the underlying mechanism. The rhythm is regularly irregular (an exaggerated sinus arrhythmia) or irregular with pauses demonstrating a lack of P-QRS-T complexes. The pauses are twice or greater than twice the normal R-R interval. If pauses are exact series of normal R-R intervals, an SA block is suggested; and if long enough, junctional or ventricular escape complexes may occur.

2. P waves are usually of normal configuration but may vary in shape if a wandering pacemaker is present.

3. The QRS configuration is normal unless an intraventricular conduction defect exists.

4. The P-R interval is essentially constant.

Associated conditions

Intermittent sinus arrest can be a normal incidental finding in brachycephalic breeds. Inspiration in these breeds causes a reflex increase in vagal tone, which leads to an exaggerated sinus arrhythmia. Ocular or carotid sinus pressure often produces a sinus arrest.

1. Irritation of the vagus nerve, e.g., surgical manipulation, thoracic neoplasms, or cervical neoplasms (carotid body tumors, thyroid carcinoma)[59,60]
2. Pathologic conditions of the atria: dilatation, fibrosis, cardiomyopathy, hemangiosarcoma; drug toxicity (quinidine, propranolol, and especially digitalis); electrolyte imbalances
3. Sick sinus syndrome[45] (There are two recognized causes for the SA block: [a] failure of the SA node to discharge impulses without the occurrence of a junctional ectopic rhythm and [b] a preceding tachycardia that depresses the SA node.)

A line of purebred Pugs with stenosis of the bundle of His and episodes of syncope associated with long periods of sinus arrest has been described.[61,62] The AV junction was suggested as a possible component of a stabilizing mechanism for the SA node.[63] In patched Dalmatian coach hounds that are born deaf, the SA node and multiple atrial arteries are often abnormal, with SA block possible.[64]

Treatment[41,65] (See Chapter 10)

1. Asymptomatic sinus arrest or SA block does not require therapy. If it is symptomatic, the underlying cause should be treated, the causative drug removed, and atropine, glycopyrrolate, or isoproterenol administered. Time-release Darbazine or Combid capsules containing isopropamide (Darbid) may be effective.[40]

2. An artificial-demand pacemaker may be needed in selected cases; permanent pacemakers are being used in chronic cases and those not responsive to therapy. (See Chapter 11.)

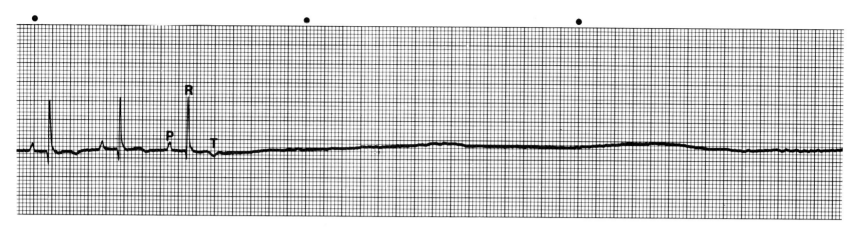

Fig. 6–78. Severe SA block or sinus arrest in a dog with disease of the SA node and AV junction. After three normal sinus complexes, a period of at least 3.5 seconds (ventricular asystole) occurs with failure of a lower focus to pace the heart.

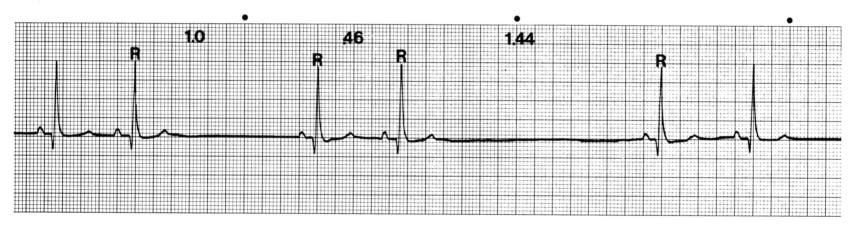

Fig. 6–79. Intermittent sinus arrest in a brachycephalic breed with an upper respiratory disorder and episodes of fainting. The pauses (1 and 1.44 sec) are greater than twice the normal R-R interval (0.46).

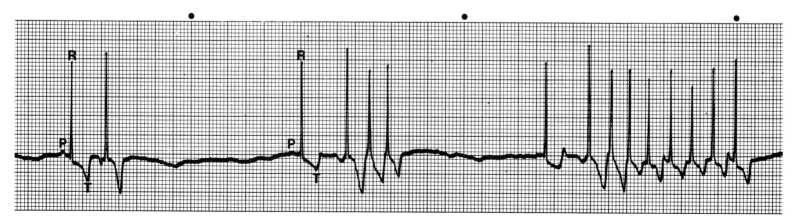

Fig. 6–80. SA block in a female Miniature Schnauzer with numerous episodes of syncope. Note the long pauses between QRS complexes and the periods of supraventricular tachycardia (atrial and/or junctional). Paper speed, 25 mm/sec.

163

Persistent atrial standstill ("silent atrium")

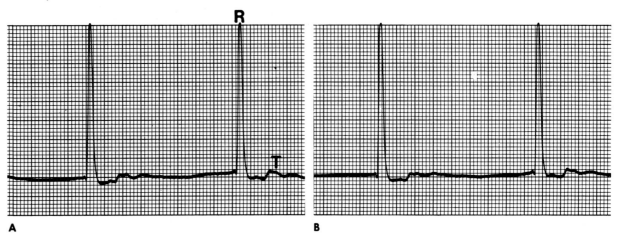

Fig. 6–81. Persistent atrial standstill in an English Springer Spaniel, serum potassium normal. **A,** No P waves present, heart rate 70/min, and QRS complexes of a probable junctional focus. **B,** After atropine the heart rate is still close to 70/min with no P waves.

Atrial standstill is characterized by an absence of P waves and by a regular escape rhythm with a supraventricular-type QRS. It may be temporary, terminal, or persistent.[66] Temporary atrial standstill occurs with digitalis toxicity and hyperkalemia. Terminal atrial standstill is associated with a dying heart or with severe hyperkalemia.

The disorder occurs in man along with various types of muscular dystrophy (often involving the facioscapulohumeral muscles), amyloidosis, familial heart disease, coronary heart disease and long-standing cardiac disease.[67]

Three of the four dogs (two English Springer Spaniels and a Shih Tzu) reported at The Animal Medical Center had the facioscapulohumeral type of muscular dystrophy that is seen in man.[68] An Old English Sheepdog had persistent standstill of only the left atrium with no skeletal muscle involvement. Clinical signs included weakness, fainting, and congestive heart failure.

Since the first edition was published, the author has recognized another 16 dogs (12 English Springer Spaniels and 4 Mixed).[68a] Two Springer Spaniels have also been reported by other authors.[69,69a]

Electrocardiographic features[66,67]

1. The heart rate is slow, usually 60 beats/min or less, and the rhythm is regular.

2. No P waves are observed in any lead, including intracardiac electrograms. Extremely small P waves were found in the Old English Sheepdog with persistent standstill of the left atrium.

3. The QRS is of nearly normal configuration with supraventricular-type escape QRS complexes or of increased duration in bundle branch block.

4. There is no increase in heart rate, nor are P waves evident after injection of atropine sulfate or exercise.

5. An "a" wave component on the right atrial pressure tracing is missing.

6. The atria are immobile at fluoroscopy, and they cannot be stimulated electrically or mechanically.

7. Serum electrolytes are normal.

Associated conditions

1. Underlying heart disease (In three of our four cases, a condition similar to facioscapulohumeral-type muscular dystrophy was diagnosed. The three dogs had marked muscle wasting of the upper forearms and scapula. A biopsy specimen was examined from the three dogs.[68] At necropsy, greatly enlarged and paper-thin atria were observed [one dog had only left atrial and atrial septal involvement]. Such atria also were observed in the fourth dog during thoracic surgery for permanent pacemaker implantation. At microscopic examination, little atrial myocardium was present. The dam of the Shih Tzu in this study was checked and found to have persistent atrial standstill on the electrocardiogram. Muscular dystrophy in the dog has been described.[71] Facioscapulohumeral-type muscular dystrophy is a hereditary disease in man.[70] Hypoplasia of the atrial parenchyma has previously been reported in a dog.[72]

2. Neuromuscular diseases that are associated with cardiomyopathy in man[67]: Duchenne muscular dystrophy, myasthenia gravis

Persistent atrial standstill may also be acquired. Diffuse involvement of the atria (from the increased load due to hemodynamic dysfunction in mitral valvular disease or from an inflammatory disorder) can result in fibrous replacement of normal atrial muscle cells.[73] Systemic lupus erythematosus can involve the skeletal muscles as well as cardiac muscle.

Treatment (See Chapter 10)

1. A permanent ventricular pacemaker should be implanted if the animal is symptomatic. (See Chapter 11.) The complications of heart failure should be treated.

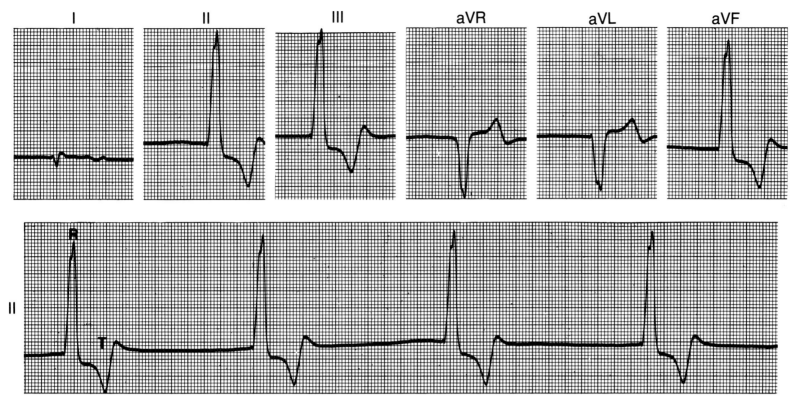

Fig. 6–82. Persistent atrial standstill in another English Springer Spaniel. No P waves are present on any of the leads (also including chest leads and intracardiac electrocardiograms, not shown here). The regular bradycardia is either junctional in origin, with pathologic involvement of the left bundle branch block (wide positive QRS complexes), or ventricular.

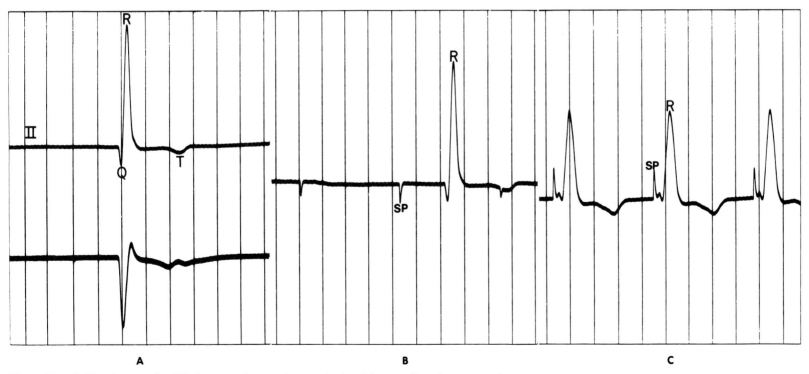

Fig. 6–83. **A,** Simultaneous lead II electrocardiogram (top tracing) and intracardiac electrogram (bottom tracing). Lack of P waves is confirmed by the electrogram; the electrode catheter is located in the right atrium. **B,** Electrical pacing at high milliamperes from the right atrium at multiple sites under fluoroscopy elicited neither an atrial nor a ventricular response. *SP,* Pacemaker spike, electrical impulse from the pacemaker. **C,** In contrast to **B,** electrical pacing from within the right ventricle easily produced ventricular activation.

First-degree atrioventricular block

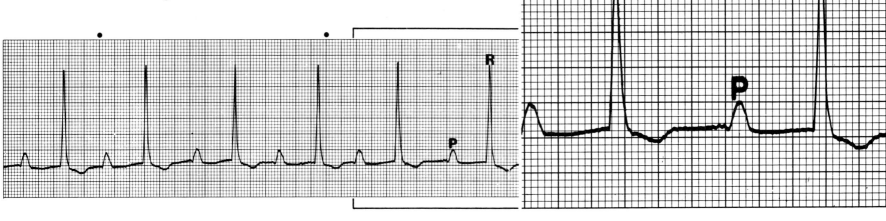

Fig. 6–84. First-degree AV block in a dog with mitral insufficiency and digoxin toxicity. The P-R interval is 0.26 second (13 boxes). The wide P wave also contributes to the long P-R interval.

A delay or interruption in conduction of a supraventricular impulse through the AV junction and bundle of His is called AV block. The term block should not be used if delay or failure of conduction occurs because the supraventricular impulse has reached the AV junction or bundle of His too early; then the AV junction or bundle of His has not recovered from its normal refractory period. The term *nonconducted* is more accurate for this situation. *Block* implies a pathologic event. The term block is often used for both situations, however.

There are three types or degrees of AV block: (1) first degree, a delay in conduction, (2) second degree, intermittent interruptions of conduction, and (3) third degree, complete or permanent interruption of conduction.

Electrocardiographic features[17]

1. The rate and rhythm depend on the presence of other arrhythmias, but the rate is usually normal.
2. The P wave is normal.
3. The configuration of the QRS is usually normal. If bundle branch block is present, the first-degree AV block may be caused by the conduction delay in the other bundle branch rather than in the AV junction.
4. The P-R interval (actually a misnomer; it is, in fact, the P-Q interval except when the QRS begins with R) is longer than 0.13 second. This is true only in the presence of a regular sinus rhythm. The long P-R interval with an APC is not called a first-degree AV block.

Associated conditions

First-degree AV block may occur in dogs that are clinically normal and healthy. Commonly, a prolonged P-R interval is the result of degenerative changes in the AV conduction system caused by aging (common in Cocker Spaniels and Dachshunds). The P-R interval tends to lengthen with age and shorten with rapid heart rates.

1. Moderate to severe digitalis intoxication (Lengthening of the P-R interval should not be used as an indicator of the degree of "digitalization"; an increase in the P-R interval was seen in only 50% of digitalized dogs in one study.[74])
2. Propranolol, quinidine, procainamide, all causes of hyperkalemia and hypokalemia

Low doses of intravenous atropine initially will prolong the P-R interval after the initial increase in heart rate.[46] Reflex vagal stimulation associated with respiratory sinus arrhythmia or with conditions affecting the vagus nerve can cause a cyclic increase in P-R interval.[75] The interval may be prolonged in chronic mitral insufficiency (due to the wide P wave from left atrial enlargement). Delay in AV conduction can occur with protozoal myocarditis; trypanosomiasis.[76]

Treatment

1. Treat the underlying condition.
2. First-degree AV block with bundle branch block merits observation for the signs of progression to higher degrees of AV block.[77]

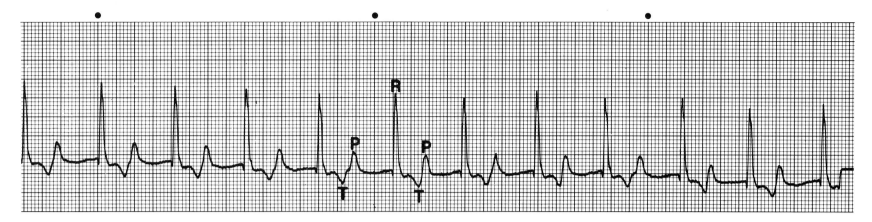

Fig. 6–85. First-degree AV block in a dog with digoxin toxicity. The P-R interval is 0.22 second (11 boxes). The P wave is superimposed on the preceding T wave. The QRS complex is normal, indicating that the conduction delay is probably above the bifurcation of the bundle of His.

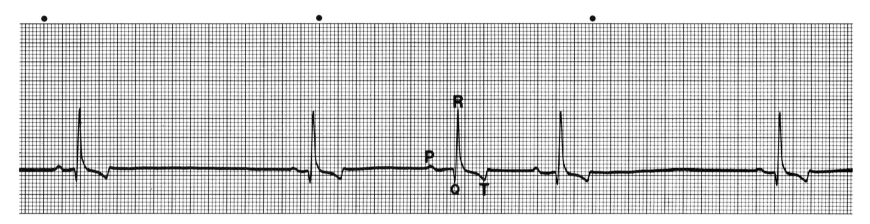

Fig. 6–86. Pronounced sinus arrhythmia (sinus arrest) associated with respiration, from reflex vagal stimulation. The P-R interval is variable, being prolonged (0.14 sec) in the third P-QRS complex. Changes in P-R intervals with fluctuations in vagal tone are usually normal findings.

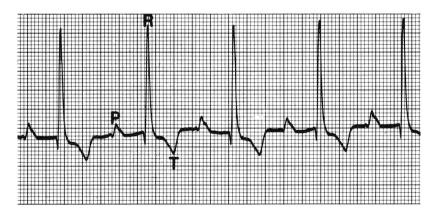

Fig. 6–87. First-degree AV block; the P-R interval is 0.18 second (9 boxes). The P wave is also wide and notched. This dog had left atrial enlargement. On auscultation, a soft first heart sound is often heard.

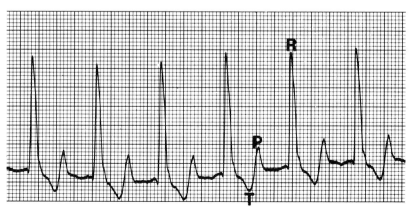

Fig. 6–88. First-degree AV block. The P-R interval is approximately 0.18 second (9 boxes). The P wave is superimposed on the preceding T wave owing to the long P-R interval and rapid heart rate.

Second-degree AV block

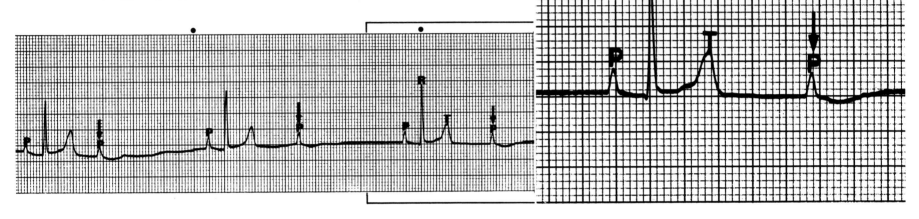

Fig. 6–89. Second-degree AV block, 2:1 block. Every other atrial impulse (P wave) is conducted. Arrows indicate blocked P waves. The QRS complexes are normal, suggesting a type A block.

Second-degree AV block is characterized by an intermittent failure or disturbance of AV conduction. One or more P waves are not followed by QRS-T complexes. Second-degree AV block can be classified into two types: Mobitz type I (Wenckebach phenomenon) and Mobitz type II. A new proposed classification takes into consideration the width of the QRS complexes:[78] type A block, with a normal QRS duration, and type B, with a wide QRS. In the type A block the site of conduction failure is assumed to be above the bifurcation of the His bundle (mostly within the AV node). In type B the site of blockage is assumed to be below the bifurcation. The recording of His bundle electrograms is needed to document these types in the dog. I have tentatively found this classification to be clinically useful.

Electrocardiographic features

Mobitz type I (Wenckebach phenomenon), usually type A

1. The ventricular rate is slower than the atrial rate because of blocked P waves. The rhythm is regularly irregular in the typical form of Wenckebach. The R-R interval becomes progressively shorter as the P-R interval becomes longer until a P wave is blocked.

2. The P wave is usually of normal configuration.

3. The QRS is usually normal, an indication that the bundle branches also are normal.

4. In the typical Wenckebach phenomenon, there may be a progressive prolongation of the P-R interval with successive beats until a P wave is blocked. Most cases of Mobitz type I, however, do not follow this pattern. Sometimes the longest P-R interval is seen only with the last conducted P wave. The P-R interval is often variable, especially in sinus arrhythmia in dogs.[75]

Mobitz type II, usually type B

1. The ventricular rate is slower than the atrial rate because of blocked P waves. The rhythm is broken by the absence of one or more QRS complexes.

2. The P wave is usually normal.

3. The QRS complexes are often of abnormal configuration, an indication that the conduction defect involves the bundle of His or proximal bundle branches.[62] In our cases Mobitz type II AV block (type B) often has progressed to higher degrees of AV block.

4. There is a fixed relationship between the atria and the ventricles of 2:1 (two P waves to one QRS), 3:1, 4:1, etc. The P-R interval is always constant but may be either normal or longer than normal.

Associated conditions

Recent work indicates that second-degree AV block may be a normal finding in dogs, especially young ones.[75] It is often associated with sinus arrhythmia and other causes of increased vagal tone.

1. Supraventricular tachycardia, e.g., atrial tachycardia or atrial flutter (The block is physiologic.)
2. Microscopic idiopathic fibrosis (in older dogs, especially Cocker Spaniels and Dachshunds)
3. Hereditary stenosis of the bundle of His in Pugs[62]
4. Digitalis toxicity, low doses of intravenous atropine, xylazine as an anesthetic,[21,79] quinidine toxicity, electrolyte imbalances

Treatment (See Chapter 10 and Fig. 10–18)

1. For Mobitz type I (type A), treatment is usually not necessary. This condition is often a normal finding. If digitalis toxicity is the cause, the drug should be stopped.
2. If wide QRS complexes coexist with second-degree AV block (type B), treatment may be necessary. These cases often have the tendency to develop third-degree AV block and accompanying clinical signs. Treatment may include atropine, glycopyrrolate, isoproterenol, or artificial pacing. (See Chapter 11.)

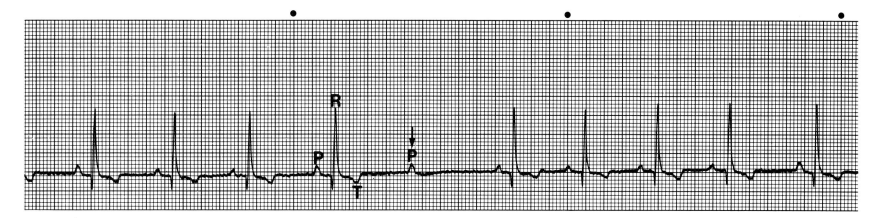

Fig. 6–90. Second-degree AV block and sinus arrhythmia (varying R-R intervals) in normal dog. At one point a P wave (arrow) is not conducted to the ventricles. The P-R intervals in preceding complexes are the same.

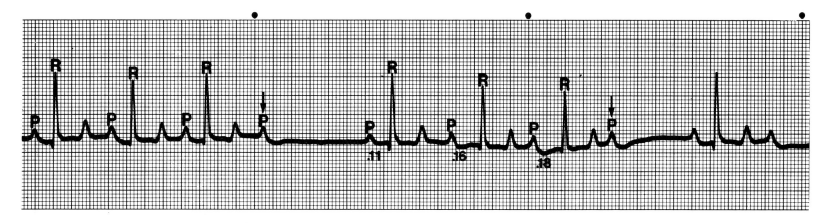

Fig. 6–91. Mobitz type I AV block (typical Wenckebach phenomenon) in a dog with digoxin toxicity. Note the progressive lengthening of P-R interval from the first sinus complex to the third complex. The P wave (arrow) that follows is blocked. The R-R interval becomes shorter.

Second degree AV block—cont'd

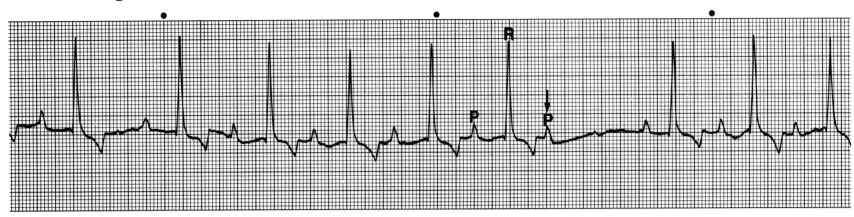

Fig. 6–92. Second-degree AV block (nonconducted P wave) and first-degree AV block (prolonged P-R interval of 0.2 sec) in a dog with digoxin toxicity. The P-R interval is constant except for the last three complexes.

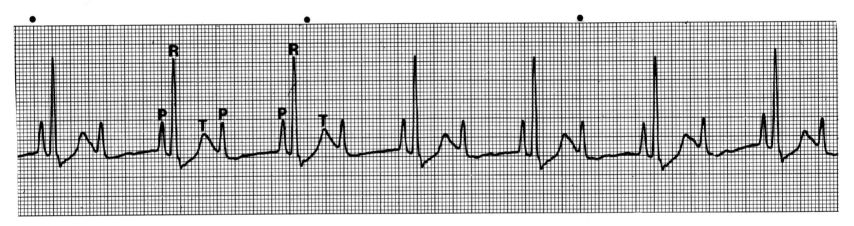

Fig. 6–93. Second-degree 2:1 AV block (Mobitz type II), as well as probable right atrial enlargement (P waves, 0.8 mv or 8 boxes). Because the QRS complexes are normal, the conduction failure is probably within the AV node.

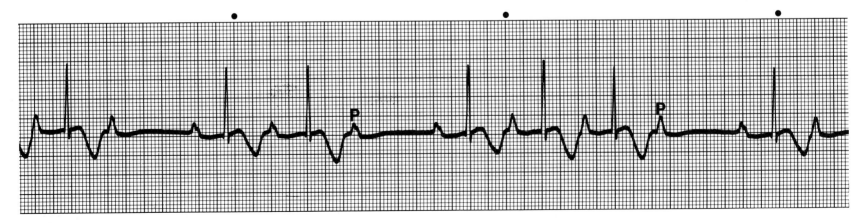

Fig. 6–94. Typical Wenckebach phenomenon (Mobitz type I) for the first labeled nonconducted P wave. The longest P-R interval precedes this nonconducted P wave. The P-R intervals preceding the second labeled nonconducted P wave are variable, an atypical form of Mobitz type I.

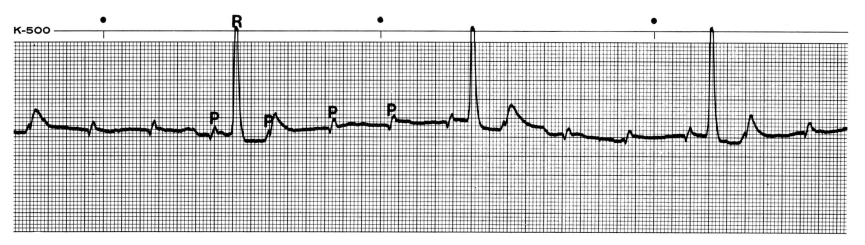

Fig. 6–95. Advanced AV block in a dog with infiltrative cardiomyopathy secondary to a metastatic mammary gland tumor. Advanced AV block is characterized by two or more consecutive blocked P waves, with a constant P-R interval on the conducted complexes. The increased duration of the QRS complex may indicate involvement of the left bundle branch or AV conduction failure below the bundle of His (type B). Complete heart block did occur the following day.

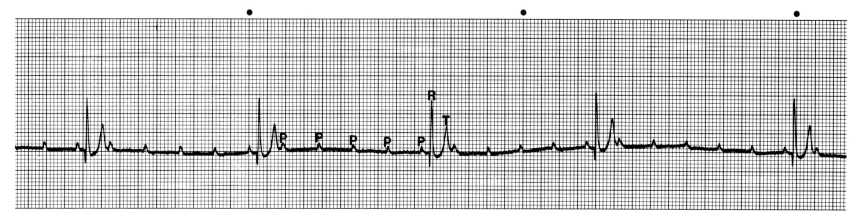

Fig. 6–96. Advanced AV block at an atrial rate of 160/min (paper speed, 25 mm/sec). The P-R interval is constant on conducted P-QRS complexes. The normal QRS duration indicates that the conduction failure is most likely in the AV node.

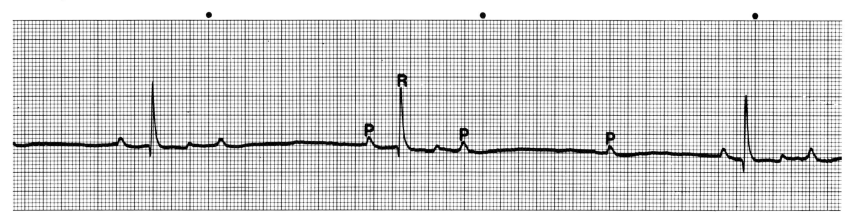

Fig. 6–97. Second-degree AV block (first-degree at times). The varying P-R interval of conducted complexes and the varying P-P intervals are probably the result of a pronounced sinus arrhythmia. Intravenous atropine was later effective in restoring normal conduction.

Third-degree AV block (complete block)

Fig. 6–98. Complete heart block with an idioventricular escape rhythm. The P waves occur regularly at a rate of 200/min, being totally independent of the ventricular rate of 55. The apparently constant P-R interval is coincidental.

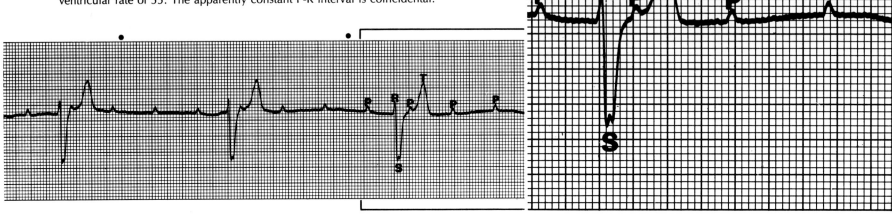

Complete AV block occurs when there is no AV conduction and the ventricles are under the control of pacemakers below the area of the block. The atria are thus activated by one pacemaker, usually the SA node, and the ventricles by another. No relationship exists between the P waves and the QRS complexes.

The clinical signs associated with complete heart block are syncope and, occasionally, congestive heart failure. The fainting episodes are caused by either sudden asystole or the development of ventricular tachyarrhythmias leading to circulatory arrest. If adequate cerebral perfusion is restored promptly, the animal recovers consciousness rapidly and is almost immediately oriented. This response contrasts with the disoriented state that follows a seizure of central nervous system origin. Physical examination will reveal variation in the intensity of the first heart sound, intermittent cannon waves in the jugular venous pulses, and variable third and fourth heart sounds. The venous pressure is elevated with characteristic "cannon waves" observed in the neck occurring when the P wave falls between the QRS and T wave (e.g., when the right atrium contracts against a closed tricuspid valve).[11]

Electrocardiographic features

1. The ventricular rate is slower than the atrial rate (more P waves than QRS complexes). The ventricular escape rhythm (idioventricular) usually has a rate below 40 beats/min, whereas in a junctional escape rhythm (idiojunctional), the rate is between 40 and 60.
2. P waves are usually a normal configuration.
3. The QRS is wide and bizarre when the rescuing pacemaker is located in either the ventricle or the lower AV junction with bundle branch block. It is normal when the escape pacemaker is located in the lower AV junction (above the bifurcation of the bundle of His) without bundle branch block. In congenital complete AV block in man, the site of the block is always in the AV node, and the bundle branch system is not involved.[78]
4. There is no conduction between the atria and the ventricles. The P waves bear no constant relationship to the QRS complexes. The P-P and R-R intervals are relatively constant (except with a sinus arrhythmia).

Associated conditions

A review of 38 cases with complete AV block from The Animal Medical Center disclosed the following causes:*

1. Isolated congenital AV block
2. Other congenital defects: aortic stenosis, ventricular septal defect
3. Severe digitalis toxicity (usually underlying cardiac pathology)
4. Infiltrative cardiomyopathy: amyloidosis, neoplasia
5. Idiopathic fibrosis, in older dogs, especially Cocker Spaniels
6. Hypertrophic cardiomyopathy
7. Bacterial endocarditis
8. Myocardial infarction
9. Hyperkalemia

---

*References 4, 17, 77, 80–89.

Other reported conditions include arteriosclerosis,[72] repeated cardiac punctures,[90] hypokalemia,[91] hyperkalemia, and aortic body tumor.[4]

Syncope and sudden death have been associated with AV conduction defects: lesions actually in the bundle of His in Doberman Pinschers[92] and in Pugs.[62] Numerous other breeds (5 of 12 dogs being Doberman Pinschers) in a recent report from The Animal Medical Center also had AV bundle lesions with sudden death.[93] Electrocardiograms were not obtained on some of these dogs. AV bundle lesions were assumed to be the cause of the syncope and sudden death. In complete heart block in man, ventricular arrhythmias are often the cause of syncope and sudden death.[44]

Treatment[17,41,83] *(See Chapter 10 and Fig. 10–18)*

1. Treatment with drugs is usually of no value. These drugs include atropine, time-release isoproterenol, and corticosteroids (if inflammation is suspected). Artificial pacing is usually necessary, especially in symptomatic animals.[80,94] In dogs who have a very slow ventricular rate, sympathomimetic drugs (isoproterenol or epinephrine) can be given until pacing can be established.

2. Long-term treatment of symptomatic AV block is a permanent cardiac pacemaker. *(See Chapter 11.)*

3. Ventricular antiarrhythmic agents are contraindicated unless an electrical pacemaker is in place. These drugs are extremely dangerous because they tend to suppress lower escape foci.

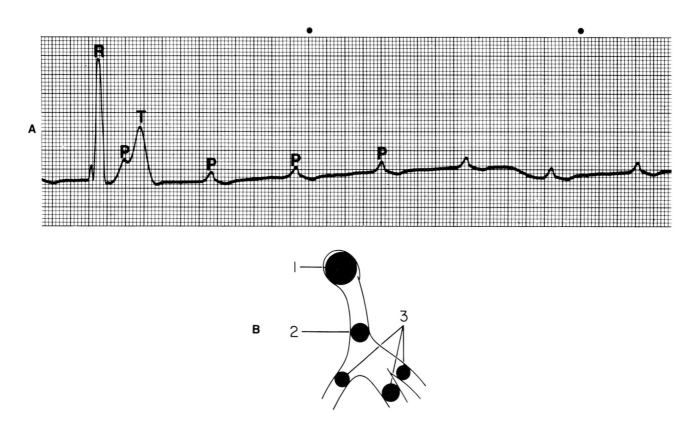

Fig. 6–99. A, Complete heart block with a failing ventricular pacemaker, resulting in ventricular asystole. The one wide and bizarre QRS complex is from a focus below the branching of the bundle of His. **B,** The three possible sites of lesions in complete heart block. *1,* AV node or junction; *2,* bundle of His; *3,* right bundle branch and two fascicles of the left bundle branch.

Third-degree AV block (complete block)—cont'd

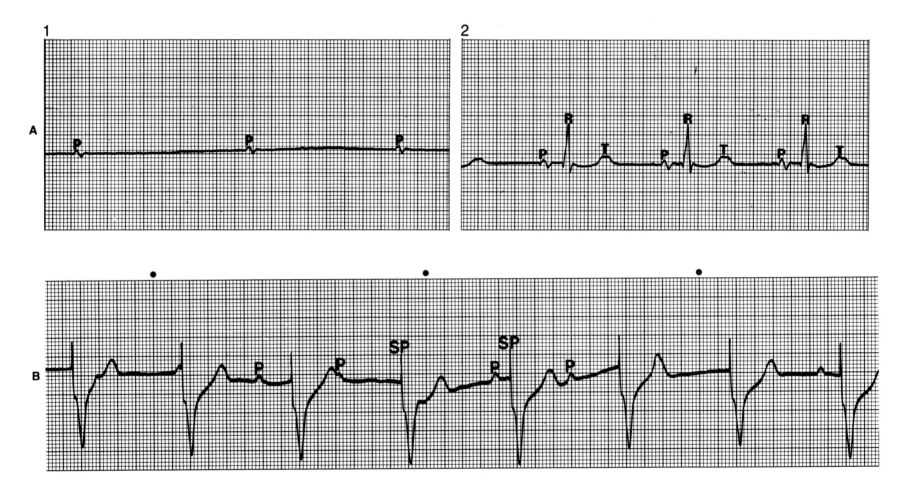

Fig. 6–100. Two forms of treatment of complete heart block, **A,** Use of drugs. **1,** Complete heart block with a failing ventricular pacemaker, resulting in ventricular asystole. **2,** Effect of an isoproterenol intravenous drip, resulting in a normal sinus rhythm. A normal QRS complex now follows each P wave. Such drugs as atropine and corticosteroids also may have been effective. The major disadvantage of drugs is the uncertainty of their dependability in life-threatening situations. In this case, isoproterenol was effective as an emergency form of therapy. The main problem with isoproterenol is its inability to maintain an uninterrupted effect. The chronic use of isoproterenol at home usually is not suitable for cases of complete heart block. **B,** Fixed-rate artificial pacemaker rhythm with the electrode attached to the left ventricle in a dog with complete heart block. The blocked P waves can still be seen. When the ventricular rate was increased with the pacemaker, this dog's fainting episodes were eliminated. *SP,* Pacemaker spike or electrical impulse from the artificial pacemaker. A wide and bizarre QRS complex follows each spike, representing ventricular activation.

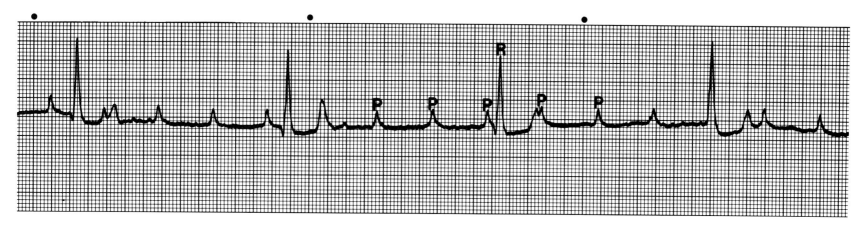

Fig. 6–101. Complete heart block in a dog with congenital AV block. The P waves occur regularly at a rate of 200/min, totally independent of the ventricular rate of 50. Because the QRS complex is of normal configuration, the ventricular pacemaker is probably above the bifurcation of the bundle of His.

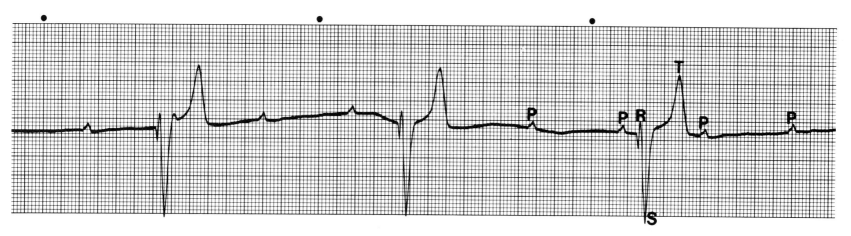

Fig. 6–102. Complete heart block. The P waves occur at a rate of 120, independent of the ventricular rate of 50. The QRS configuration is a right bundle branch block pattern. The regular rate and stable QRS indicate that the rescuing focus is probably near the AV junction.

Ventricular pre-excitation and the Wolff-Parkinson-White syndrome

ATRIUM

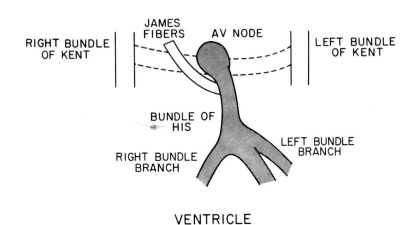

Fig. 6–103. Various accessory conduction pathways that are probably responsible for ventricular pre-excitation.

Ventricular pre-excitation occurs when impulses originating in the SA node or atrium activate a portion of the ventricles prematurely through an accessory pathway. SA impulses are able to reach the ventricles initially without going through the AV node. The Wolff-Parkinson-White syndrome (WPW) consists of ventricular pre-excitation with episodes of paroxysmal supraventricular tachycardia.[44]

The anatomic basis of ventricular pre-excitation is controversial. Three accessory conduction pathways are postulated: bundles of Kent (accessory AV connections), James fibers (A-V nodal bypass tracts), and Mahaim fibers (nodoventricular tracts). The bundles of Kent are the most important, being documented in one dog by epicardial mapping.[95,96]

The sinus or atrial impulses conducted via the accessory pathway activate a portion of the ventricle without passing through the bundle of His; the rest of the ventricle is activated via the normal AV pathway. The accessory pathway may go to the left ventricle (left type or type A) or to the right ventricle (right type or type B).[97] This classification is an arbitrary one, because some cases cannot be classified clearly into either type A or B. The pre-excitation shortens the P-R interval because the entire impulse is not slowed by normal conduction delay in the AV junction. The QRS complex has a slurred upstroke (delta wave) and is wide because the pre-excitation impulse is conducted through ordinary myocardium without the aid of the specialized conduction system. If the atrial impulse is conducted over the James bypass fibers, a short P-R interval with a QRS complex of normal duration will result (Lown-Ganong-Levine syndrome).[98]

The paroxysmal tachycardias associated with ventricular pre-excitation (WPW syndrome) can be explained by the *re-entry* mechanism (Chapters 9 and 12). An impulse traveling to the ventricles through the AV junction may turn around and re-enter the atria through the accessory pathway. A reciprocal rhythm or "electrical circuit" is thus established.[99]

Electrocardiographic features[44,96,99,100]

1. Heart rate and rhythm are normal in ventricular pre-excitation. In the WPW syndrome the heart rate is extremely rapid, often greater than 300 beats/min.

2. Sinus P waves are normal in ventricular pre-excitation but difficult to recognize in the WPW syndrome.

3. The QRS in ventricular pre-excitation is widened with slurring or notching of the upstroke of the R wave (delta wave). The left type (type A) has predominantly positive QRS complexes in CV_5RL, whereas the right type (type B) has predominantly negative QRS complexes in CV_5RL. In the WPW syndrome, the configuration of the QRS complexes can be normal, wide with a delta wave, or very wide and bizarre.

4. The P-R interval of the P-QRS in ventricular pre-excitation is short. In the WPW syndrome there is usually 1:1 conduction (P wave for every QRS complex).

Associated conditions[4,21,96]

1. Congenital, no organic heart disease present
2. Congenital and acquired cardiac defects: one dog with atrial septal defect, one dog with mitral valvular fibrosis, and one dog with tricuspid valvular dysplasia from The Animal Medical Center clinical files

Alternating pre-excitation should not be confused with ventricular bigeminy, often seen during anesthesia with thiobarbiturates and/or atropine.[46,101,102]

Treatment[103,103a,b] *(See Chapters 10 and 12)*

1. Ventricular pre-excitation without tachycardia does not require therapy.

2. The WPW syndrome (atrial tachycardia, atrial flutter, or atrial fibrillation) requires conversion by (a) ocular or carotid sinus pressure, (b) propranolol, (c) other drugs, including quinidine, digitalis, and lidocaine or (d) direct-current shock, the most effective treatment. The first drug of choice is lidocaine, followed by procainamide. Calcium blocking agents can be effective.[29] Digitalis can dangerously accelerate anterograde conduction and is best avoided with pre-excitation. Encainide, a new cardiac drug may be effective.[103a]

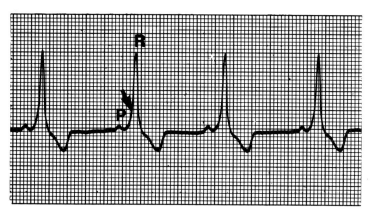

Fig. 6–104. Ventricular pre-excitation. The sinus impulse is conducted through the bundle of Kent without delay but is delayed physiologically in the AV node. The portion of the ventricle adjacent to the Kent bundle is prematurely activated and causes a delta wave (arrow) on the electrocardiogram. The remainder of the ventricle is then activated from both the normal and the accessory pathways. The existence of an accessory pathway is not always evident from the ECG. The location of the accessory pathway, the intra-atrial conduction time, and the times required to traverse the AV node-His bundle branch pathway (James fibers) and the accessory pathway determine the configuration of the electrocardiogram in the WPW syndrome.

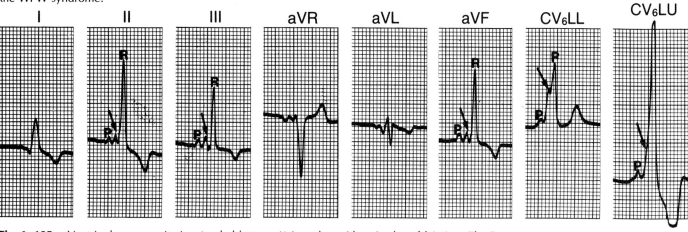

Fig. 6–105. Ventricular pre-excitation (probably type A) in a dog with episodes of fainting. The P waves are normal, the P-R interval is short, the QRS complex is wide, and delta waves (arrows) are present.

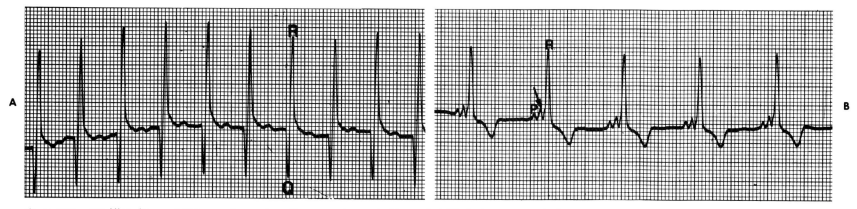

Fig. 6–106. Wolff-Parkinson-White syndrome from the same dog as in Figure 6–105. **A,** A supraventricular tachycardia (probably atrial tachycardia) at a rate of 260 beats/min. **B,** Temporary conversion to a sinus rhythm with ocular pressure; ventricular pre-excitation is now present. The configuration of the QRS complexes is markedly different from that of the QRS complexes in strip **A.** The QRS complexes in the WPW syndrome can sometimes mimic those in ventricular tachycardia.

Hyperkalemia (atrial standstill)

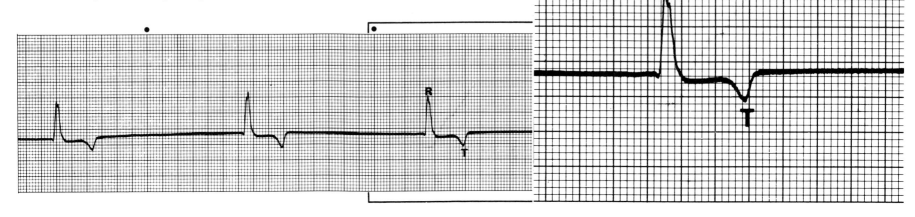

Fig. 6–107. Atrial standstill. Hyperkalemia in a dog with Addison's disease. The heart rate is slow (45/min), and P waves are absent; the duration of the QRS and the Q-T interval is prolonged. The serum potassium was 8.6 mEq/L.

Hyperkalemia, an increase in the serum potassium level, is not an uncommon clinical problem in dogs. The effects of hyperkalemia on cardiac rhythm are severe and often lethal. Defects in the specialized intraventricular conduction are common.[104] The wide and bizarre QRS complexes simulate an idioventricular rhythm. Experimental studies indicate, however, that the SA node continues to fire and its impulses are transmitted via the internodal pathways to the AV junction and ventricles. The rhythm should be termed *sinoventricular*. No P wave is recorded because the atrial myocardium is not activated.[26] Electrocardiographic changes may not be expected to develop consistently until serum potassium concentrations are greatly elevated.[105]

Electrocardiographic features[106–108]

The following sequential electrocardiographic changes are observed:

1. Serum potassium greater than 5.5 mEq/L (earliest change with hyperkalemia: increased amplitude of the T waves, which become thin and peaked)
2. Serum potassium greater than 6.5 mEq/L (decreased amplitude of the R wave, prolongation of the QRS and P-R intervals, and S-T segment depression)
3. Serum potassium greater than 7 mEq/L (decreased amplitude of the P wave with increased duration, longer QRS and P-R intervals, and prolongation of the Q-T interval)
4. Serum potassium greater than 8.5 mEq/L (disappearance of the P wave with a slow sinoventricular rhythm, usually below 40 beats/min; atrial standstill is the result)
5. Serum potassium greater than 10.0 mEq/L (increased widening of the QRS complex, with eventual replacement by a smooth biphasic curve; final stage is ventricular flutter, ventricular fibrillation, or ventricular asystole)

Associated conditions[107]

1. Addison's disease (adrenocortical insufficiency), renal insufficiency (usually from oliguric renal failure or obstructive uropathy)
2. Other conditions: untreated diabetic ketoacidosis, transfusion of stored blood, excessive potassium infusion, shock, administration of potassium-sparing diuretics, metabolic acidosis

Treatment[109]

1. First, lower the serum potassium, especially if greater than 8 mEq/L. The Na:K ratio may be less than 25:1 (normal, 33:1) in Addison's disease. Then, treat the underlying cause; e.g., Addison's disease requires administration of a mineralocorticoid (deoxycorticosterone acetate).

2. Lowering the serum potassium includes fluid therapy (saline for Addison's disease), sodium bicarbonate (1 to 2 mEq/kg body weight), soluble intravenous glucocorticoids (hydrocortisone), regular insulin for emergency treatment (0.5 to 1 unit/kg body weight with 2 g dextrose/unit insulin), and mineralocorticoid; fludrocortisone (Florinef), 0.1 to 0.6 mg every 24 hours for Addison's disease. Calcium gluconate (0.5 ml/kg of body weight) antagonizes the cardiotoxic effects of potassium.

3. The electrocardiogram should be monitored throughout treatment. Ideally, electrolytes are assayed every 4 to 8 hours.

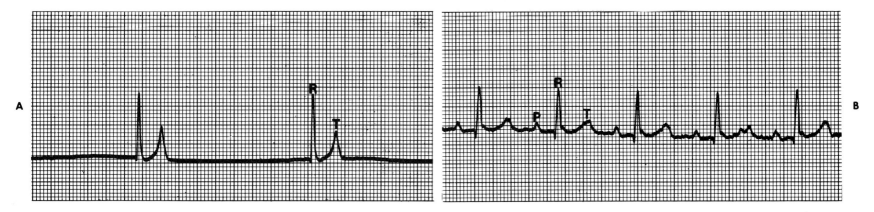

Fig. 6–108. **A,** Hyperkalemia in a dog presenting with hypovolemic shock, consistent with an addisonian crisis. P waves are absent, and T waves are tall and peaked. Serum potassium was 8.4 mEq/L. **B,** After institution of therapy. P waves are now present, and the QRS-T complex is of smaller amplitude. Serum potassium is now 4.8 mEq/L.

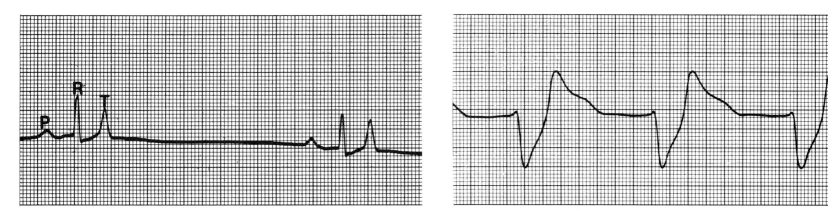

Fig. 6–109. Early changes of hyperkalemia (serum potassium, 6.0 mEq/L) in a dog with renal insufficiency. Changes include increased duration of the P wave, prolonged P-R interval, small QRS, S-T segment depression, and a tall peaked T wave.

Fig. 6–110. Severe hyperkalemia (serum potassium, 9.9 mEq/L). No P waves are present. The QRS complexes are widened markedly. The rhythm is sinoventricular.

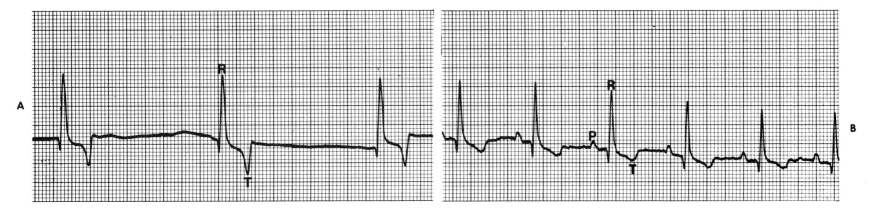

Fig. 6–111. **A,** Hyperkalemia in a dog with an addisonian crisis (serum potassium, 8.6 mEq/L). Atrial standstill is present (no P waves). The T waves are of large amplitude and negative deflection. **B,** After therapy. The dog is now ambulatory and alert.

Sick sinus syndrome

Sick sinus syndrome is a term given to a number of electrocardiographic abnormalities of the SA node, including (in both dog and man) severe sinus bradycardia and severe SA block and/or sinus arrest. Many cases with these electrocardiographic abnormalities have recurrent episodes of supraventricular tachycardias in addition to the underlying slow SA rhythm. This pattern of sick sinus syndrome is called the "bradycardia-tachycardia syndrome."[110]

The majority of dogs with the sick sinus syndrome also have coexisting abnormalities of the AV junction and/or bundle branches. During the long periods of SA block, the latent AV junctional pacemaker fails to pace the heart; the result is cardiac standstill.[45,111] Under normal circumstances, the occurrence of a junctional escape mechanism should prevent these long pauses. The term *sick escape pacemaker syndrome* has sometimes been used.[112] The SA node disorder is the primary problem, however. With a normal SA node, delayed junctional complexes would not be present.

The clinical manifestations of the sick sinus syndrome are quite variable. Heart rates may be so slow as to reduce cardiac output and cause cardiac failure, or so rapid as to preclude adequate filling. More often, the clinical signs result from hypoperfusion of vital organs. The most common clinical signs are syncope and weakness.

Electrocardiographic features[45,111,113,114,114a,b]

1. Severe and persisting sinus bradycardia not induced by drugs.
2. Short or long pauses of SA block occur with or without escape rhythms.
3. The sinus rhythm fails to begin after electrical cardioversion of a tachycardia (caused by organic disease or electrical pacing).
4. Atrial fibrillation with a slow ventricular rate in the absence of drugs is usually due to accompanying disease of the AV junction.
5. In the bradycardia-tachycardia syndrome, there are periods of severe sinus bradycardia alternating with ectopic supraventricular tachycardias (atrial tachycardia, atrial fibrillation, or atrial flutter).
6. Long pause following an atrial premature complex.
7. AV junctional escape rhythm (with or without slow and unstable sinus activity).
8. Any combination of these.

Tests for sinoatrial node dysfunction[110,111,113,115]

1. Ocular or carotid sinus massage may cause periods of sinus arrest longer than 3 seconds. An increased vagal tone may partially be responsible for this syndrome.
2. Atropine intravenously (0.015 mg/kg body weight) fails to cause a marked increase in heart rate (normal is at least a 50% increase), indicating that the SA node dysfunction is not due to excessive vagal tone. Also, exercise usually does not increase the rate.
3. Simultaneous automatic monitoring with radiotelemetry and time-lapse videorecordings have been used in dogs to correlate syncope with the electrocardiogram.[61]
4. After rapid right atrial pacing the atrium can fail to depolarize for as long as 15 seconds following the pacing (normal in the dog is 1.5 sec).[116]

Associated conditions

My own experience includes 42 dogs with the sick sinus syndrome, diagnosis of which was based on the preceding electrocardiographic features. Prognosis for most of these dogs has been quite favorable; some have been followed for more than 6 years. All but two of the dogs were Miniature Schnauzers (two were Dachshunds), all were female and at least 6 years of age, and all had a history of syncope. Causes included the following:

1. Possibility of disease affecting the SA node artery
2. Replacement of the SA node with fibrous tissue (sometimes involving the rest of the conduction system), possibly a form of cardiomyopathy
3. Good possibility of genetic inheritance (as frequently occurs with female Miniature Schnauzers)

Digitalis toxicity can cause changes consistent with the sick sinus syndrome.

Treatment[114a] *(See Chapter 10 and Fig. 10–7)*

1. If the animal is asymptomatic or has only minimal clinical signs, treatment is not necessary. Treatment should be considered with far-advanced sick sinus syndrome documented by the electrocardiogram and/or electrophysiologic study, even if there are no significant signs.
2. Drug therapy (e.g., atropine and digitalis) alone is usually unsuccessful because: (a) the drug for treatment of the tachyarrhythmia component is harmful for or aggravates the bradyarrhythmia component and vice versa; (b) there is a lack of long-term therapeutic effects of pharmacologic agents (e.g., atropine or isoproterenol) for bradyarrhythmias; (c) there may be significant side effects of the drug used.
3. The treatment of choice is a permanent artificial pacemaker (ventricular-demand unit). *(See Chapter 11.)* After implantation of the pacemaker, antiarrhythmic agents can be safely used (Fig. 6–118). The drugs indicated are similar to the recommendations for the various tachyarrhythmias not associated with sick sinus syndrome.

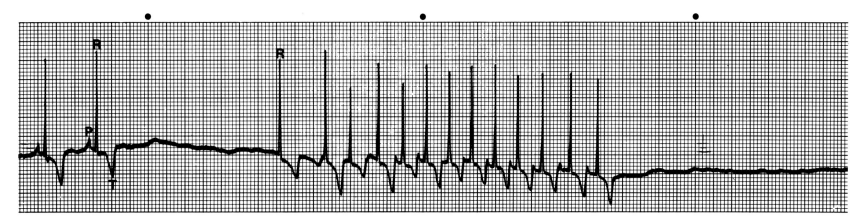

Fig. 6–112. Sick sinus syndrome (paper speed, 25 mm/sec), a bradycardia-tachycardia pattern. Note the two long periods of SA block. The first period is followed by a junctional escape complex and a rapid supraventricular tachycardia. The continuous bombardment of the SA node by these impulses suppresses its automaticity, causing another long pause.

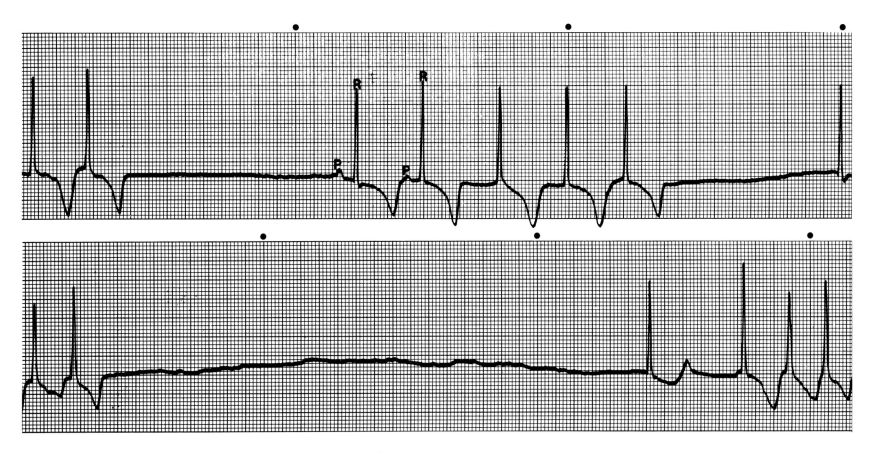

Fig. 6–113. Short and long pauses of SA block followed by junctional escape complexes in two continuous tracings. One period of SA block (ventricular asystole) in the bottom strip lasted up to 3 seconds. Two sinus complexes terminate the first pause in the top strip.

Sick sinus syndrome—cont'd

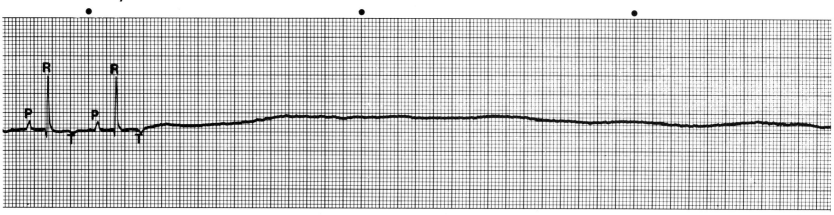

Fig. 6–114. Severe sinus arrest of over 5 seconds after ocular pressure in a dog with sick sinus syndrome. An AV junctional escape complex or rhythm should normally occur after such a long pause. This may suggest a disturbance of impulse formation in the AV junction. Both the SA node and the AV junction are then abnormal.

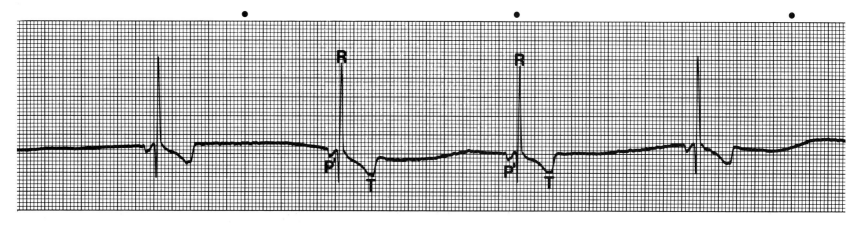

Fig. 6–115. This junctional rhythm from high in the AV junction persisted for days in a dog with the sick sinus syndrome. Fibrotic changes were found in the SA node and atrial tissue at necropsy.

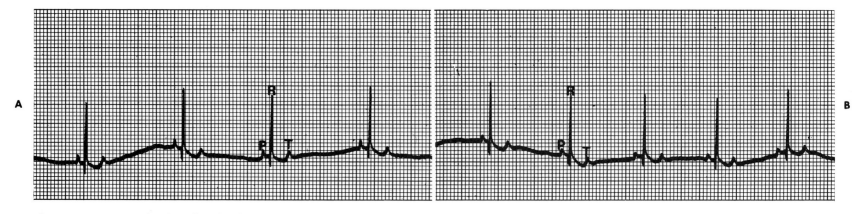

Fig. 6–116. **A,** Sinus bradycardia of 55 beats/min in a dog with sick sinus syndrome. **B,** After intravenous atropine, a marked sinus tachycardia failed to develop. The heart rate increased only to 68/min. Also, the sinus rate did not increase significantly with exercise. Paper speed, 25 mm/sec.

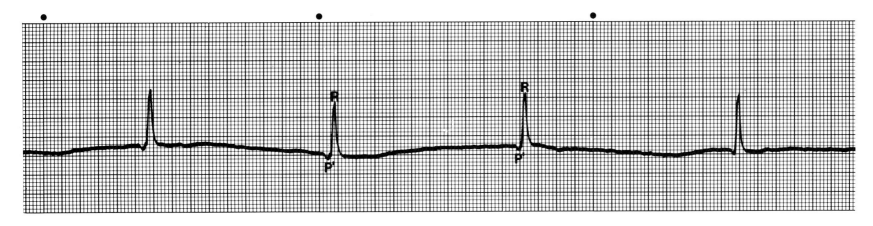

Fig. 6–117. Junctional escape rhythm of 50/min from an AV junctional focus. This persisted for several minutes in a Miniature Schnauzer with a history of weakness. Atropine had no effect on the rhythm.

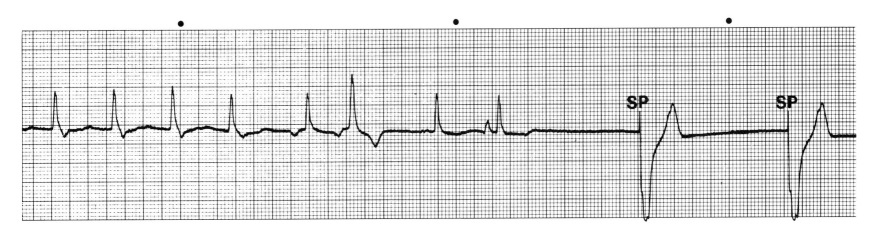

Fig. 6–118. An artificial pacemaker (ventricular demand unit) in a dog with sick sinus syndrome. The supraventricular tachycardia and junctional escape complexes at the beginning of the strip temporarily inhibit the artificial pacemaker's electrical output. The unit operates only on demand, firing when the heart rate is below a predetermined level. The episodes of fainting during periods of SA block were thus eliminated. Digoxin was later given for the paroxysms of tachycardia. *SP*, Pacemaker spike, electrical impulse generated by the pacemaker.

Electrical alternans

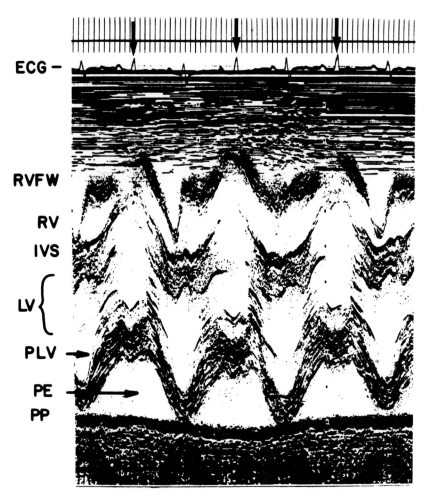

Fig. 6–119. Echocardiogram at the ventricular (apical) level, showing electrical alternans, pericardial effusion, and dramatic abnormal motion (swinging) of the heart. The frequency (vertical arrows) of abnormal cardiac motion (time needed for the heart to swing away from and back to its original position) is exactly one half the heart rate. Every other cardiac cycle occurs during maximal cranioventral cardiac displacement. *RVFW* = right ventricular free wall; *RV* = right ventricle; *IVS* = interventricular septum; *LV* = left ventricle; *PLV* = posterior wall of left ventricle; *PE* = pericardial effusion; *PP* = posterior portion of pericardium. (From Bonagura, J.D.: Electrical alternans associated with pericardial effusion in the dog. J. Am. Vet. Med. Assoc., *178*:574, 1981, with permission.)

Electrical alternans is diagnosed when the P, QRS, or T complexes (or any combination) alter their configuration on every other complex, every third complex, every fourth complex, etc.; each complex, however, must originate from the same focus.[117,118] The most common alternating ratio is every other complex (2:1 electrical alternans). Electrical alternans usually involves the QRS complex alone.

Two theories have been proposed to explain the mechanism of electrical alternans: the actual anatomic motion of the whole heart or the alternating conduction within the myocardium.[117,118] Cardiac motion is accepted as essentially the source of electrical alternans in pericardial effusion.[119] By means of echocardiography, the heart was seen to shift position in the pericardium during every other beat. The anatomic relationship of the heart to any given electrode then alternates. This theory is demonstrated echocardiographically in Figure 6–119, which shows a large pericardial effusion and abnormal cardiac motion in a dog. At very fast heart rates or in certain types of bundle branch block, electrical alternans results from the differences in recovery rate of the individual fibers; the refractory phase of the heart can also become prolonged on an alternating basis. The heart rate often is the dependent factor for electrical alternans.[120,121] In man, the presence of QRS alternation during sustained narrow QRS supraventricular tachycardia is highly indicative of a retrograde accessory AV pathway in the tachycardia circuit.[121a]

Electrocardiographic features

The three causes of electrical alternans that I have recognized are pericardial effusion, alternating bundle branch block, and supraventricular tachycardia. True electrical alternans should not be confused with ventricular bigeminy or the effects of respiration.

1. The heart rate is usually normal in pericardial effusion. Electrical alternans has been reported in four dogs after administration of atropine when large pericardial volumes were present.[122]

2. The P waves may be of alternating amplitude and hidden in supraventricular tachycardia.

3. The QRS may show alternating amplitudes and configurations.

4. The P waves are always related to the QRS complexes; all complexes must be from the same pacemaker. A constant interval exists between alternating complexes.

Associated conditions[10,117,121,122]

I have evaluated 38 dogs with electrical alternans. The majority of cases resulted from pericardial effusion.

1. Causes of pericardial effusion:[123] neoplasia (heart base tumors, metastatic carcinoma), right-sided heart failure, benign idiopathic pericardial effusion

2. Causes of bundle branch block and supraventricular tachycardia

In one study, 7 of 11 dogs (64%) with pericardial effusion had electrical alternans.[124] Severe hypocalcemia can cause isolated T wave alternans in experimental canine preparations.[125]

Treatment

1. Electrical alternans in pericardial effusion usually indicates a large effusion with possible cardiac tamponade. A physical examination and chest radiograph are needed for confirmation. Pericardiocentesis is often indicated.

2. Electrical alternans in bundle branch block and in supraventricular tachycardia is usually of no added significance.

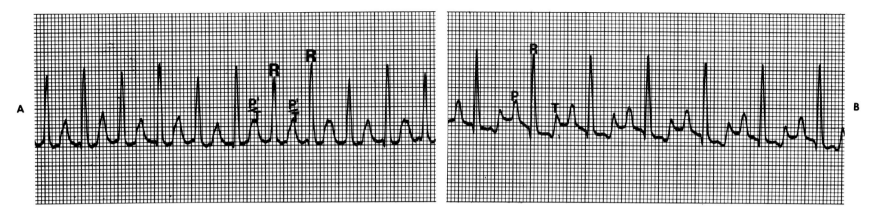

Fig. 6–120. **A,** Atrial tachycardia with alternating amplitude of the R waves due to differences in recovery rate of the individual fibers (aberrant ventricular conduction). **B,** After ocular pressure, the tachycardia and electrical alternans are terminated.

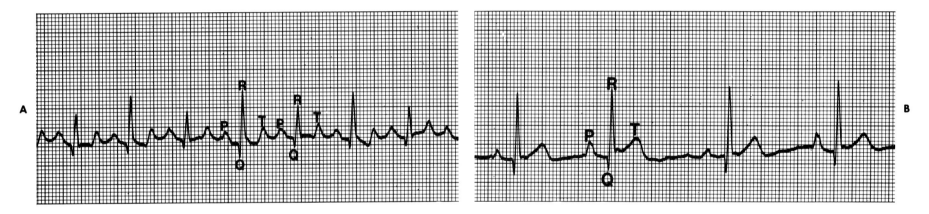

Fig. 6–121. **A,** Electrical alternans in a dog with pericardial effusion. **B,** After pericardiocentesis, the complexes are now larger, and there is no electrical alternans.

| I | II | III | aVR | aVL | aVF |

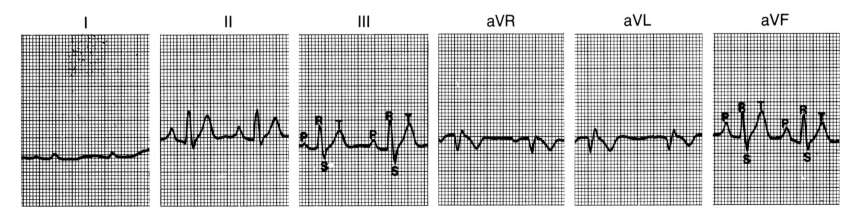

Fig. 6–122. Electrical alternans in a dog with pericardial effusion, easily seen in leads *III* and *aVF*.

Drug-induced arrhythmias

The secondary effects of drugs on the heart may or may not be of clinical significance. Some of the more commonly used drugs with their undesirable arrhythmias are summarized in this section. The effects of these drugs on the electrocardiogram have been reviewed in the literature.[21,44,79,126–128] The toxic signs of the various antiarrhythmic drugs are discussed in detail in Chapter 10.

Because of the increased frequency of surgical procedures performed on older dogs, the importance of arrhythmias in the anesthetized animal should be emphasized even more. Alterations in vagal and sympathetic tone as well as electrolyte and acid-base disturbances that occur during anesthesia and surgery are a major factor. The anesthetic agents themselves, intubation, and surgical manipulations can also promote arrhythmias. Pre-existing cardiac and respiratory diseases can also affect the frequency of arrhythmias during surgery. Intraoperative arrhythmias can be frequent, but the majority are usually clinically insignificant.[11] Arrhythmias are also frequent during recovery from general anesthesia; 15 of 50 dogs (30%) in one study.[129]

For successful nonarrhythmogenic anesthesia, the following principles should be applied: minimal stress of induction, proper ventilation of the patient, light plane of anesthesia, gentle surgical manipulation, proper fluid and electrolyte balance during surgery, and maintenance of a normal body temperature. If arrhythmias occur during anesthesia, the anesthetic concentration should first be lowered and the patient ventilated with higher oxygen concentration. Most arrhythmias can be eliminated by implementing these simple steps.

The common preanesthesia medications, intravenous anesthetics, and inhalation anesthetics will first be reviewed,[127,128] before discussing the other drug-induced arrhythmias.

Acetylpromazine. The phenothiazine derivatives all possess alpha-adrenergic blocking activity; sinus bradycardia is often seen (Fig. 6–126). The drug also can depress myocardial contractility and excitability and slow impulse conduction. In one study, it was suggested that acetylpromazine has a protective effect on epinephrine-induced arrhythmias.[53]

Xylazine (Rompun). Xylazine causes an increase in vagal tone and interferes with cardiac conductivity. It can cause sinus bradycardia, SA block, and varying degrees of AV block (Fig. 6–123).[130] An anticholinergic such as atropine or glycopyrrolate should be used. Xylazine also may induce a variety of ventricular arrhythmias in the presence of epinephrine and halothane. Both blood pressure and sympathetic tone can be altered.

Ketamine. Ketamine, an analogue of phencyclidine, causes an increase in the heart rate, cardiac output, and arterial blood pressure. The drug also appears to have an antiarrhythmic quality. Ketamine has been shown to abolish epinephrine-induced ventricular arrhythmias in dogs anesthetized with halothane.[131]

Atropine. Atropine given intravenously in dosages greater than 0.015 mg/kg of body weight gives a bradycardia followed by a tachycardia. Lower doses (less than 0.015 mg/kg of body weight) may produce APCs or VPCs, second-degree AV block, and, eventually, sinus tachycardia (Fig. 6–125).[46] It is recommended to give atropine to dogs with preanesthesia heart rates below 140 beats/min. This will usually prevent potentially dangerous sinus tachycardia and other arrhythmias that occur during the anesthetic induction and early maintenance periods.

Glycopyrrolate (Robinul-V). This anticholinergic has some advantages over atropine. It has a longer vagal blocking effect, and ventricular premature complexes occur less frequently following its use.[132]

Barbiturates and Thiobarbiturates. These include thiopental, thiamylal, methohexital, and pentobarbital. Ventricular arrhythmias may persist into the anesthetic period with thiobarbiturates. Ventricular bigeminy is common with thiamylal and thiopental, with treatment usually not necessary unless the heart rate is below 70 beats/min (Fig. 6–124). The arrhythmia is usually transient.[102,126] The cause has been related to increased arterial pressure and an imbalance between parasympathetic and sympathetic tone. Thiopental combined with lidocaine causes no arrhythmias and resulted in less cardiopulmonary depression than thiopental alone.[133]

Inhalation anesthetics. These include halothane, methoxyflurane, isoflurane, and nitrous oxide. Halothane and methoxyflurane cause a dose-related depression of sinus node automaticity.[128] Halothane sensitizes the myocardium to catecholamines, causing severe ventricular arrhythmias. This is usually of no significance unless a cardiac emergency develops in which epinephrine is used. Great care should be used to minimize palpation of the adrenal glands and in the use of epinephrine as a hemostatic agent.[134] Acetylpromazine as a preanesthetic agent can help prevent these arrhythmias.[53] Cardiac arrhythmias are rare with methoxyflurane, and sensitivity to catecholamine-induced changes is lower than the sensitivity caused by halothane. Isoflurane should be considered when there is a need for reducing anticipated arrhythmias during general anesthesia.[134a] Arrhythmias associated with inhalation anesthesia are dose related; most can be controlled by decreasing the concentration of anesthetic delivered to the animal. Nitrous oxide rarely produces arrhythmias.

Norepinephrine and isoproterenol. These sympathomimetic drugs are able to stimulate the beta receptors, causing an increased ventricular excitability and an increase in pacemaker automaticity (e.g., sinus tachycardia or atrial tachycardia).

Doxorubicin. This drug is a potent, broad-spectrum antineoplastic agent. Cardiomyopathy will be consistently produced at doses in excess of 240 mg/m^2.[135] Doxorubicin may exert its arrhythmogenic effect by enhancing automaticity of latent pacemaker cells of the His-Purkinje system, altering refractoriness of Purkinje cells, inducing reentrant conduction, and reducing myocardial function.[136,137] Arrhythmias and conduction disturbances include atrial premature complexes, atrial fibrillation, ventricular premature complexes, ventricular tachycardia, and AV block.[138]

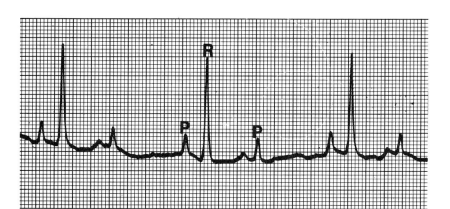

Fig. 6–123. Second-degree 2:1 AV block after xylazine (Rompun) was given for tranquilization. If atropine or glycopyrrolate had been given with this drug, the arrhythmia might have been prevented.

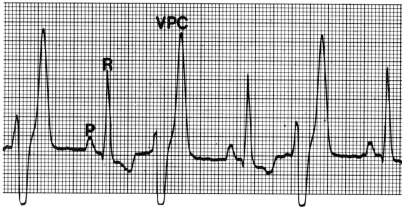

Fig. 6–124. Ventricular bigeminy just after the intravenous use of the barbiturate thiamylal. VPCs alternate with sinus complexes.

Drug-induced arrhythmias—cont'd

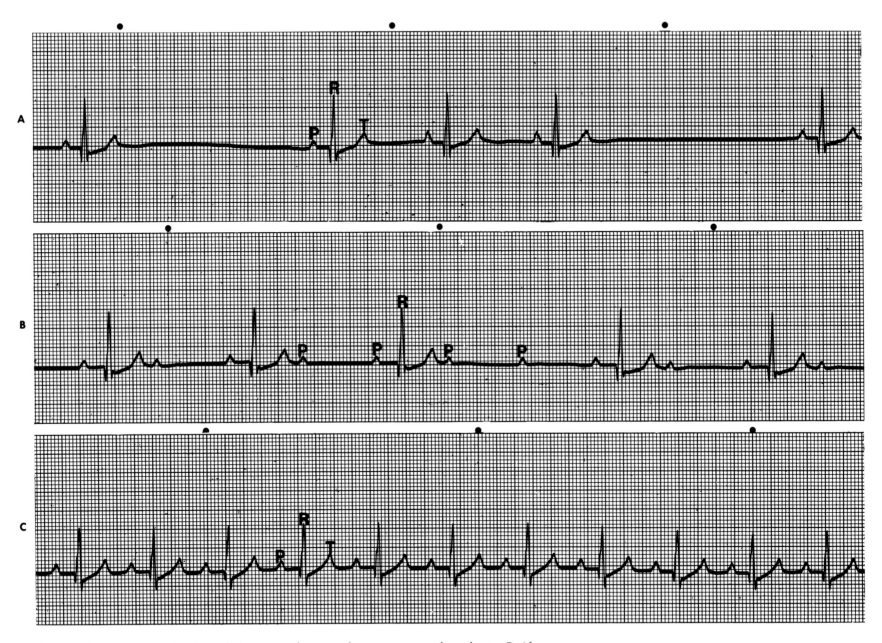

Fig. 6–125. **A,** Sinus arrest and wandering pacemaker secondary to pronounced vagal tone. **B,** After intravenous atropine, second-degree AV block has developed. VPCs are often also seen at this time. **C,** Within 5 minutes a faster heart rate of 150/min is the result. Atropine prior to anesthetic induction is probably not advisable in all surgical cases.

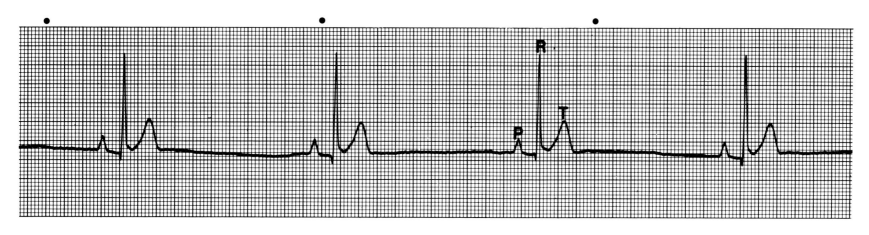

Fig. 6–126. Sinus bradycardia of 55/min after acetylpromazine had been given. The S-T segment elevation and large T waves probably represent myocardial hypoxia. Phenothiazine derivatives can depress myocardial contractility and excitability and slow impulse conduction. Animals with heart disease or a history of ventricular arrhythmias may receive protection from catecholamine-induced ventricular arrhythmias.

Digitalis-induced arrhythmias

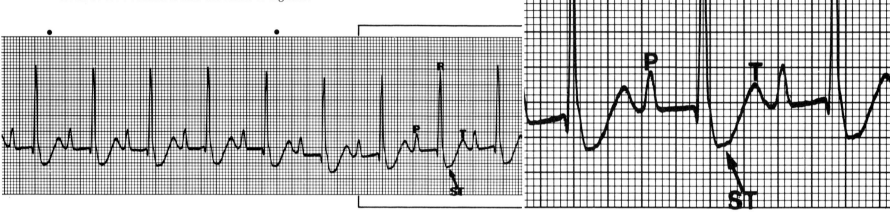

Fig. 6–127. Digitalis toxicity. The "sagging" effect to the S-T segment (also termed "hammock shaped") is characteristic of digitalis. The prolonged P-R interval of 0.14 second is also the result of digitalis.

Digitalis toxicity occurs frequently in clinical practice.[139] The clinician should understand the pharmacokinetics of the drug, the proper dosage, and the conditions that predispose to digitalis sensitivity.[140] Digitalis acts directly on the myocardium, vagus nerve, and AV junction. The toxic signs of digitalis are discussed in Chapter 10.

The manifestations of digitalis toxicity are usually either gastrointestinal or cardiac. The gastrointestinal signs (which usually occur before the cardiac signs) include anorexia, vomiting, and diarrhea. These effects outside the heart are troublesome but not life threatening. The lethal effects of digitalis toxicity are due to its cardiac effects, the formation of arrhythmias. *Digitalis can cause any cardiac arrhythmia.*[141]

The arrhythmias that strongly suggest digitalis toxicity are as follows:

1. Abnormalities of impulse formation: enhanced junctional escape rhythms, VPCs, ventricular tachycardia, sinus bradycardia, sinus arrest

2. Abnormalities of impulse conduction (depression of pacemaker cells in the SA node and AV junction): sinus block, first-degree AV block, severe slowing of heart rate in atrial fibrillation, complete heart block

3. Combination of both mechanisms: AV dissociation, paroxysmal atrial tachycardia with block

4. Atrial fibrillation with a slow, regular ventricular rhythm and/or ventricular bigeminy indicates almost a 100% chance of digitalis toxicity.

These digitalis-induced arrhythmias are often created by the misconception that the P-R interval must be lengthened for proper digitalization. It has been well documented that the P-R interval is often not increased in therapeutic digitalization.[74] In fact, prolongation of the P-R interval can be a borderline sign of toxicity.

Treatment[17,140]

1. *Stop the digitalis,* even if there is some question in your mind.

2. An electrocardiogram should be obtained at least three or four times a day during the toxicity, for the arrhythmias are often intermittent.

3. Diuretics should be stopped since their lowering of the extracellular potassium can aggravate digitalis toxicity. This also pertains to intravenous dextrose solutions, which likewise can lower extracellular potassium.

4. If digitoxin was being used, the liver function tests should be evaluated. Renal function tests should be evaluated with digoxin usage. These organs affect the excretion of digitalis and are often the underlying cause for digitalis toxicity.

5. For life-threatening arrhythmias, specific therapy can include intravenous potassium, lidocaine (drug of choice for ventricular arrhythmias), propranolol, phenytoin, and a temporary transvenous pacemaker or atropine for symptomatic bradycardia.

6. Following are some helpful suggestions that may aid the clinician who is using digitalis:[142]

   a. Generic cardiac glycosides should probably be avoided since a wide variation in generic equivalence or bioavailability exists. Branded cardiac glycosides (e.g., Lanoxin [digoxin] and Foxalin [digitoxin]) are advisable. Kinetic studies on other glycoside preparations need to be conducted.

   b. The dose of digoxin should be calculated on the basis of lean body weight (usually 10% to 15% of body weight). Dogs that are obese or that have excessive fluid (e.g., ascites) should have actual weight adjusted accordingly.

   c. The *minimum dosage* for the maximum possible therapeutic effects should be used.

   d. In renal disease, the digoxin dosage should be reduced (often by 50%) and the total daily dose given more frequently (e.g., three times per day).

   e. Maintenance digitalization should be used in all nonemergency situations. The slow oral maintenance use of digoxin is preferred, without administering a loading dose.

   f. New formulas for the maintenance digitalization daily dosage have been developed by the Burroughs-Wellcome Co., of North Carolina. The following formulas apply to digoxin (Lanoxin) only:

     Elixir. 75% × Total body weight × 0.01 mg = Total dose
     Tablet. 85% × Total body weight × 0.01 mg = Total dose

The elixir form has more bioavailability than the tablet form, the reason for an additional 10% reduction in the lean body weight dosage.[143] The doses for larger dogs should be proportionately less than for smaller dogs on a milligram per kilogram body weight basis (an excess of 0.75 to 1 mg of digoxin per day is rarely needed).

   g. Digoxin dosage should be reduced when also giving quinidine, as digoxin toxicity will likely occur.[144]

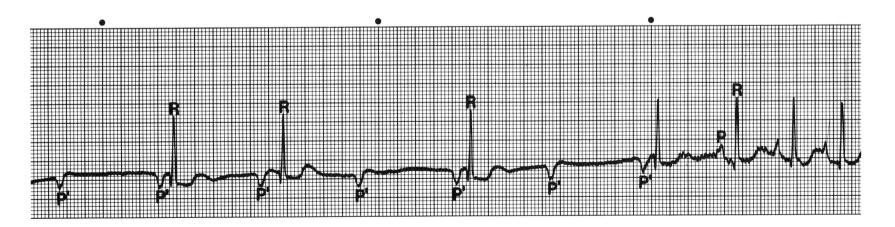

Fig. 6–128. Digitalis toxicity. AV junctional rhythm with second-degree AV block. The abnormal rhythm is only intermittent, with a normal sinus rhythm established at the end of the strip.

Digitalis-induced arrhythmias—cont'd

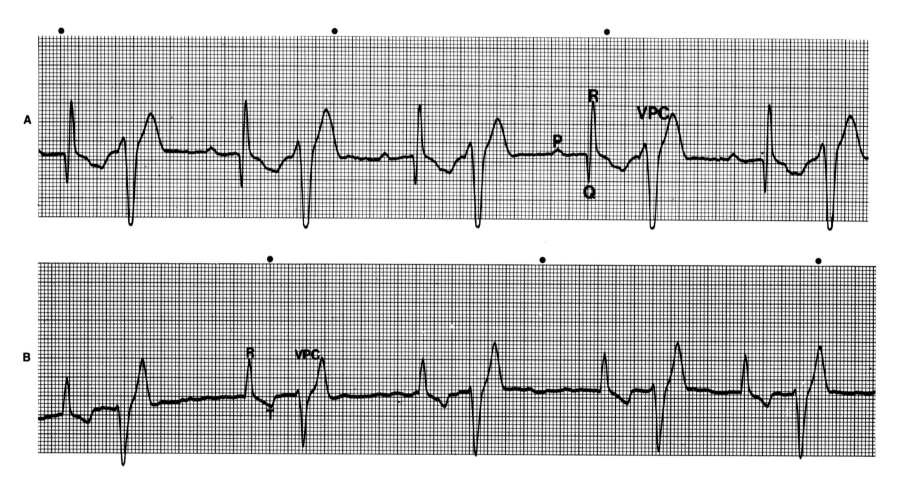

Fig. 6–129. Ventricular bigeminy, not an uncommon manifestation of digitalis toxicity. **A,** With first-degree AV block (P-R interval, 0.18 sec). A regular sinus rhythm alternates with ventricular premature complexes (VPCs). **B,** With atrial fibrillation in another dog with digitalis toxicity. The ventricular rhythm is regular; the rate, excluding the VPCs, averages 65/min. The slow regular ventricular rate also indicates probable block in the AV junction (0.5 cm = 1 mv).

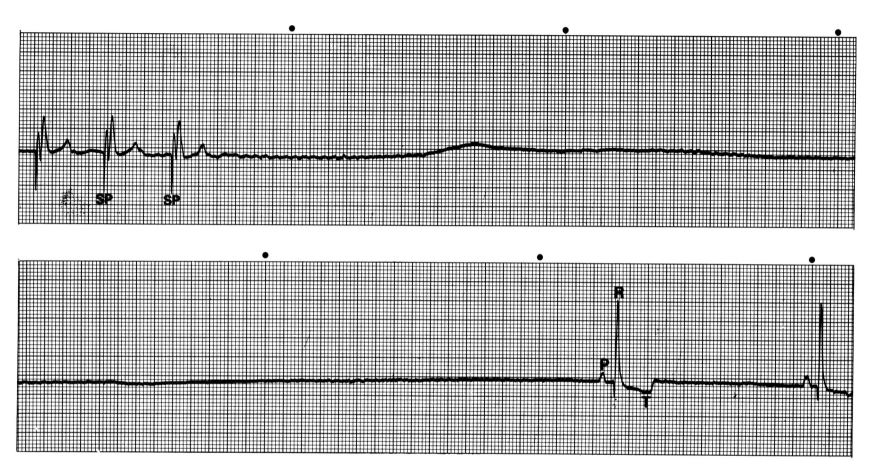

Fig. 6–130.   Toxic effects of a moderate dose of digoxin in a dog with sick sinus syndrome. The dog was first presented with signs of congestive heart failure and a sinus bradycardia. The only demonstrable abnormality at that time was the failure of atropine to increase the heart rate. With diuretics and half the maintenance level of digoxin, episodes of syncope occurred. A temporary artificial pacemaker was used to eliminate the long sinus pauses associated with the syncope. This continuous strip illustrates a long sinus pause (6.5 sec) in the rhythm after the pacemaker was turned off. The SA pacemaker eventually takes over at a slow rate. After the digoxin was stopped, these long pauses in the rhythm stopped. The use of digoxin is probably unwise in cases of severe sinus bradycardia without pacemaker insertion. Digoxin can have an adverse effect on sinus node function.

Artifacts

Since the electrocardiogram is a mechanical recording, a number of technical or mechanical problems can occur while it is being obtained. These technical or mechanical problems superimposed on the normal cardiac complexes cause distortions called artifacts. Artifacts can cause the measurement of the various complexes to be difficult and often simulate disturbances of cardiac rhythm and conduction.[145] Electrocardiographic examples and their causes are presented in this section. Suggestions for obtaining good technical recordings are to be found in Chapter 2.

The causes of artifacts can be placed into two general categories: (1) technical recording problems (fault of the clinician, the machine, or the electrodes and cable) and (2) problems with the animal.

Technical recording problems

1. Lead reversal, incorrect electrode placement, is a frequent mistake. The most common error is reversal of the forelimb electrodes, which simulates the pattern in dextrocardia with negative P waves in leads I and aVL. Other incorrect electrode placements are illustrated in Figure 6–132.
2. If standardizations are improperly labeled, voltages may appear abnormally low or high.
3. Standard paper speed for dogs is 50 mm/sec. If it is slower than this (e.g., 25 mm/sec), false measurements will result.
4. Electrical interference, also called 60-cycle artifact, is due to improper grounding.
5. A poorly defined baseline indicates a dirty stylus or low stylus heat. Reducing the amplitude of large complexes to half is usually helpful.
6. Stylus mounting may be too loose or too tight; overshooting or a slow return to baseline, respectively, can result.
7. Electrodes and cable are often sources of artifacts. Common problems include a broken cable, loose connection of the alligator clip to the cable tip, dirty cable tips, cable wires pulling on the electrodes, or a swinging cable over the table edge.

Animal-related factors

1. Artifacts can result from muscle tremor or from unexpected animal body movements.
2. A wandering baseline, often due to respiratory movements, coughing, or voluntary motion by the animal or handler, can simulate atrial and ventricular arrhythmias.

The electrocardiographic manifestations most helpful in differentiating artifacts from arrhythmias include the rhythm of the artifacts (usually irregular) and the rate of artifacts (usually variable) along with the realization that artifacts do not interrupt atrial or ventricular rhythm.

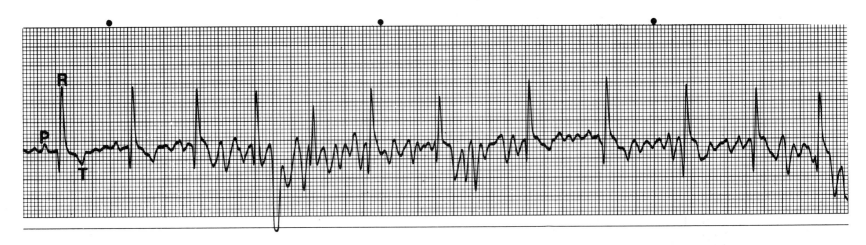

Fig. 6–131. Artifacts simulating atrial and/or ventricular arrhythmias. This strip was recorded from a dog that was trembling.

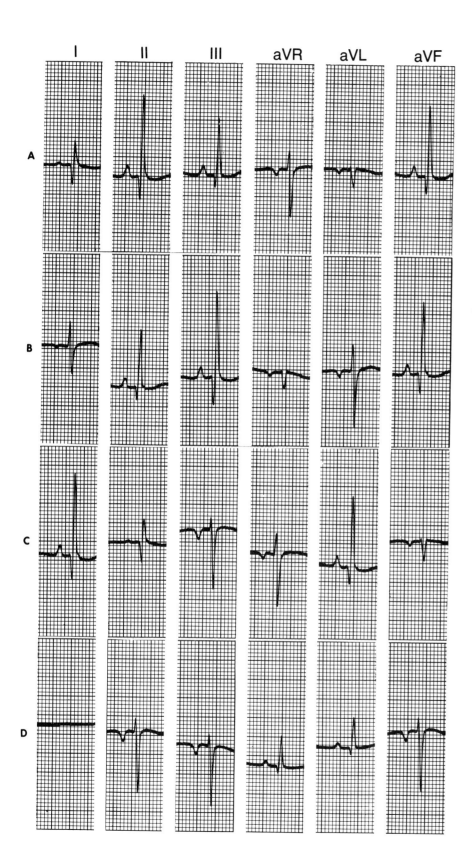

Fig. 6–132. Errors of electrode placement. **A,** Electrodes properly placed. This normal electrocardiogram can be compared with tracings **B, C,** and **D.** **B,** Front limb electrodes reversed. Lead *I* is a mirror image of lead *I* in **A,** *II* is *III* and *III* is *II,* and *aVR* is *aVL* and *aVL* is *aVR.* **C,** Left forelimb and left hindlimb electrodes reversed. Lead *III* is a mirror image of *III* in **A,** *I* is *II* and *II* is *I,* and *aVL* is *aVF* and *aVF* is *aVL.* **D,** Interchange of forelimb and hindlimb electrodes. The tracing is markedly altered compared with leads in **A,** especially in lead *I* (no deflections).

Artifacts—cont'd

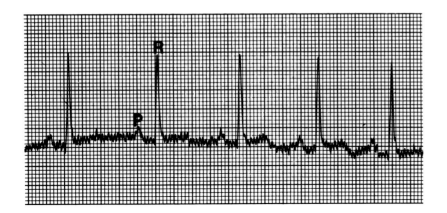

Fig. 6–133. Electrical interference (60-cycle). The electrocardiograph was not properly grounded. The complexes are difficult to measure.

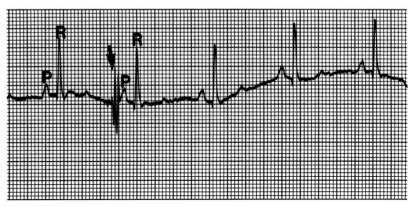

Fig. 6–134. Artifact (arrow) produced when one of the clip electrodes attached to the dog was momentarily touched by the handler.

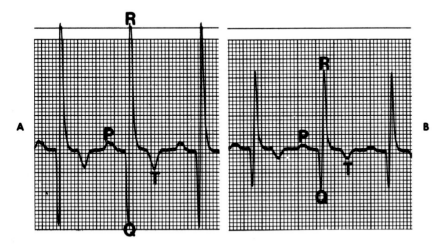

Fig. 6–135. Standardization effect. **A,** Sensitivity switch at position 1 (1 cm = 1 mv), the standard sensitivity setting. **B,** Sensitivity switch at position 1/2 (0.5 cm = 1 mv) for the same tracing as in **A.** A standardization mark should always be made to indicate the change in sensitivity.

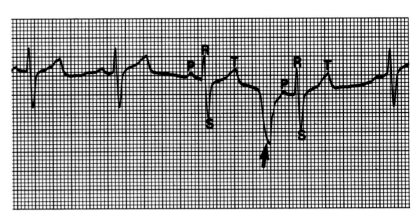

Fig. 6–136. Artifact (arrow) created when the dog jerked its leg. The artifact simulates a VPC but does not interrupt the normal sinus P-QRS-T complexes.

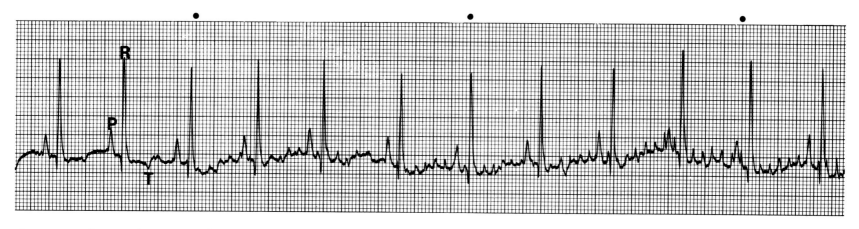

Fig. 6–137. Electrocardiogram recorded from a nervous dog that started to tremble after the second QRS complex. The rapid and irregular vibrations of the baseline resemble atrial ectopic waves.

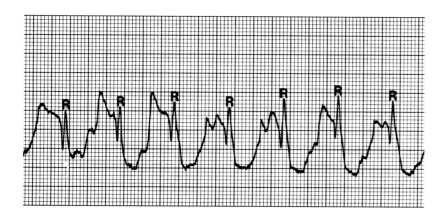

Fig. 6–138. Electrocardiogram recorded from a dog that was panting. The baseline rapidly moves up and down. When the forelimb electrodes were kept from touching the thoracic wall, the tracing improved.

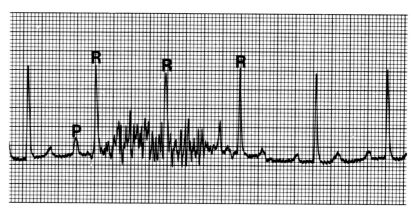

Fig. 6–139. Electrical interference (60-cycle) produced when the clip electrodes attached to this dog were inadvertently touched by the handler.

197

Artifacts—cont'd

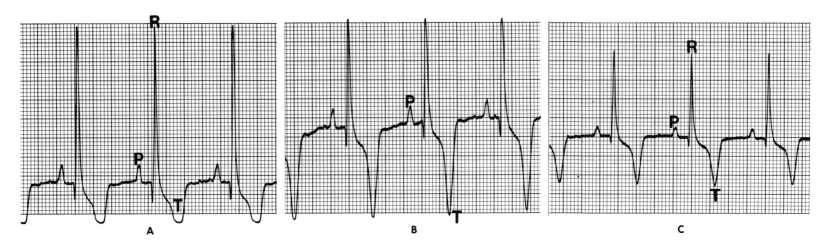

Fig. 6–140. These tracings from a dog with severe hypoxia during anesthesia were obtained at three different sensitivity switch positions. **A,** Sensitivity switch position 2 (2 cm = 1 mv). The QRS complexes are magnified two times. **B,** Normal standard switch position 1 (1 cm = 1 mv). The T wave is of large amplitude, indicating that it was being cut off by the recording in **A. C,** Sensitivity switch at position 1/2 (0.5 cm = 1 mv). The tracing is now half its normal size.

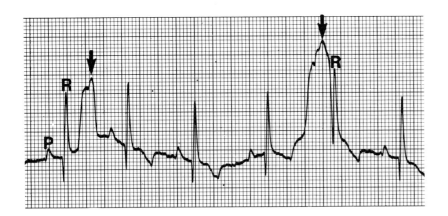

Fig. 6–141. Two large deflections (arrows) mimicking VPCs. Neither artifact interrupts the cardiac rhythm, and both occur too close to the QRS complexes to allow double depolarization of the ventricles.

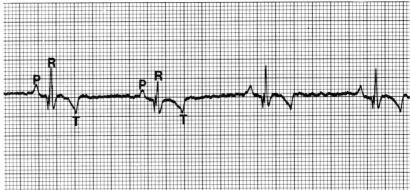

Fig. 6–142. Low-voltage P-QRS-T complexes with a fluctuation in amplitude of complexes in a dog with severe pneumothorax. The air acts like a region of high electrical resistance, a poor conducting medium.

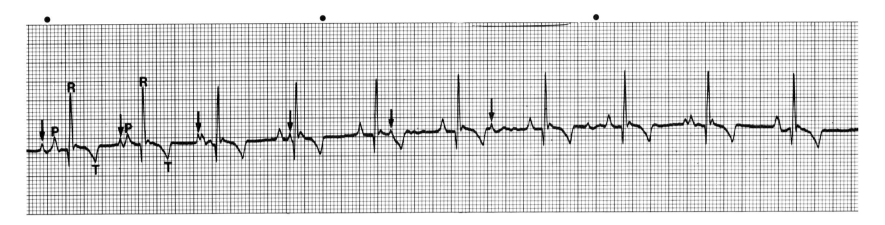

Fig. 6–143. An artifact (arrows) throughout this tracing appears as an extra P wave. The rhythm of the artifact is irregular and does not interrupt the P wave rhythm.

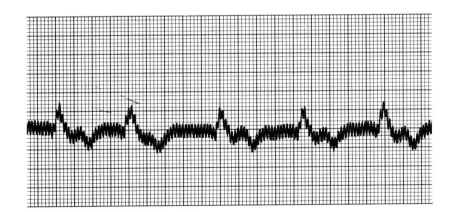

Fig. 6–144. Marked 60-cycle electrical interference caused by an inadequately grounded electrocardiograph.

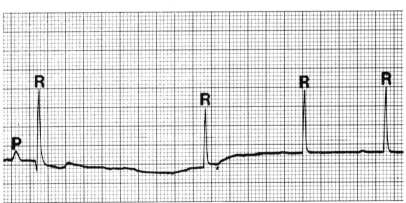

Fig. 6–145. After the first sinus P-QRS-T complex the P wave, Q wave, and T wave have all disappeared. The R wave has decreased in amplitude. This artifact is due to a loose clip electrode connection. The cable tip and alligator clip have only intermittent contact.

REFERENCES

1. Silber, E.N., and Katz, L.N.: *Heart Disease.* New York, Macmillan, 1975.
2. Surawicz, B. (chairman), et al.: Task Force 1: Standardization of terminology and interpretation. Am. J. Cardiol., *41*:130, 1978.
3. WHO/ISC (World Health Organization/International Society for Cardiology) Task Force: Definition of terms related to cardiac rhythm (special report). Am. Heart J., *95*:796, 1978.
4. Patterson, D.F., Detweiler, D.K., Hubben, K., and Botts, R.P.: Spontaneous abnormal cardiac arrhythmias and conduction disturbances in the dog (a clinical and pathological study of 3000 dogs). Am. J. Vet. Res., *22*:355, 1961.
5. Muir, W.W.: Gastric dilatation—volvulus in the dog, with emphasis on cardiac arrhythmias. J. Am. Vet. Med. Assoc., *180*:739, 1982.
6. Calvert, C.A., Chapman, W.L., Toal, R.L.: Congestive cardiomyopathy in Doberman Pinscher dogs. J. Am. Vet. Med. Assoc., *181*:598, 1982.
7. Spaulding, G.L., and Tilley, L.P.: Atrial fibrillation in the dog and cat. Proc. Am. Anim. Hosp. Assoc., *43*:75, 1976.
8. Tilley, L.P.: Transtelephonic analysis of cardiac arrhythmias in the dog—diagnostic accuracy. Vet. Clin. North Am., *13*:395, 1983.
9. Selzer, A.: *Principles of Clinical Cardiology: An Analytical Approach.* Philadelphia, W.B. Saunders, 1975.
10. Tilley, L.P.: *Basic Canine Electrocardiography.* Milton, Wis., The Burdick Corp., 1978.
11. Helfant, R.H.: *Bellet's Essentials of Cardiac Arrhythmias.* 2nd Edition. Philadelphia, W.B. Saunders, 1980.
12. Childers, R.: Classification of cardiac dysrhythmias. Med. Clin. North Am., *60*:3, 1976.
13. Muir, W.W., Werner, L.L., and Hamlin, R.L.: Antiarrhythmic effects of diazepam during coronary artery occlusion in dogs. Am. J. Vet. Res., *36*:1203, 1975.
14. D'Agrosa, L.S.: Cardiac arrhythmias of sympathetic origin in the dog. Am. J. Physiol., *233*:H535, 1977.
15. Hahn, A.W. (chairman), Hamlin, R.L., and Patterson, D.F.: Standards for canine electrocardiography. The Academy of Veterinary Cardiology Committee Report, 1977.
16. Carrig, C.B., Suter, P.F., Ewing, G.O., and Dungworth, D.L.: Primary dextrocardia with situs inversus associated with sinusitis and bronchitis in a dog. J. Am. Vet. Med. Assoc., *164*:1127, 1974.
17. Ettinger, S.J., and Suter, P.F.: *Canine Cardiology.* Philadelphia, W.B. Saunders, 1970.
18. Tilley, L.P., and Weitz, J.: Pharmacologic and other forms of medical therapy in feline cardiac disease. Vet. Clin. North Am., *7*:425, 1977.
19. Moore, E.N., et al.: Studies on ectopic atrial rhythms in dogs. Am. J. Cardiol., *19*:676, 1967.
20. Waldo, A.L., et al.: The P wave and P-R interval. Effects of the site of origin of atrial depolarization. Circulation, *42*:653, 1970.
21. Bolton, G.R.: *Handbook of Canine Electrocardiography.* Philadelphia, W.B. Saunders, 1975.
22. Edwards, N.J., and Tilley, L.P.: Congenital heart defects. In *Pathophysiology of Small Animal Surgery.* Edited by M.J. Bojrab. Philadelphia, Lea & Febiger, 1981.
23. Liu, S.-K., and Tilley, L.P.: Malformation of the canine mitral valve complex. J. Am. Vet. Med. Assoc., *167*:465, 1975.
24. Josephson, M.E., and Kastor, J.A.: Supraventricular tachycardia mechanisms and management. Ann. Intern. Med., *87*:346, 1977.
25. Wit, A.L., Rosen, M.R., and Hoffman, B.F.: Electrophysiology and pharmacology of cardiac arrhythmias. II. Relationship of normal and abnormal electrical activity of cardiac fibers to the genesis of arrhythmias. B. Re-entry. Section 1. Am. Heart J., *88*:664, 1974.
26. Goldman, M.J.: Principles of Clinical Electrocardiography. 11th Edition. Los Altos, Calif., Lange Medical Publications, 1982.
27. Befeler, B.: Mechanical stimulation of the heart, its therapeutic value in tachyarrhythmias. Chest, *73*:832, 1978.
28. Wood, D.S., and Kittleson, M.: ECG of the month. JAMA, *182*:790, 1983.
29. Nakaya, H., Schwartz, A., and Millard, R.W.: Reflex chronotropic and inotropic effects of calcium-blocking agents in conscious dogs. Diltiazem, Verapamil, and Nifedipine compared. Circ. Res., *52*:302, 1983.
30. Robertson, B.T.: Correction of atrial flutter with quinidine and digitalis. J. Small Anim. Pract., *11*:251, 1970.
31. Bilitch, M.: *A Manual of Cardiac Arrhythmias.* Boston, Little, Brown, 1971.
32. Bolton, G.R., and Ettinger, S.J.: Paroxysmal atrial fibrillation in the dog. J. Am. Vet. Med. Assoc., *158*:64, 1971.
33. Mangiola, S., and Ritota, M.C.: *Cardiac Arrhythmias, Practical ECG Interpretation.* Philadelphia, J.B. Lippincott, 1974.
34. Tilley, L.P., and Liu, S.-K.: Cardiomyopathy in the dog. Recent Adv. Stud. Cardiac Struct. Metab., *10*:641, 1975.
35. Bond, B., and Tilley, L.P.: Cardiomyopathy in the dog and cat. In *Current Veterinary Therapy: small animal practice.* Volume 7. Edited by R.W. Kirk. Philadelphia, W.B. Saunders, 1980.
36. Tilley, L.P., Liu, S.-K., Fox, P.R.: Myocardial disease. In *Textbook of Veterinary Internal Medicine.* Edited by S.J. Ettinger. 2nd Edition. Philadelphia, W.B. Saunders, 1983.
37. Bohn, F.K., Patterson, D.F., and Pyle, R.L.: Atrial fibrillation in dogs. Br. Vet. J., *127*:485, 1971.
38. Liu, S.-K., and Tilley, L.P.: Dysplasia of the tricuspid valve in the dog and cat. J. Am. Vet. Med. Assoc., *169*:623, 1976.
39. Alexander, J.W., Bolton, G.R., and Koslow, G.L.: Electrocardiographic changes in nonpenetrating trauma to the chest. J. Am. Anim. Hosp. Assoc., *11*:160, 1975.
40. Ettinger, S.J.: Cardiac arrhythmias. In *Textbook of Veterinary Internal Medicine.* Edited by S.J. Ettinger. 2nd Edition. Philadelphia, W.B. Saunders, 1983.
40a. Harpster, N.: Boxer cardiomyopathy. In *Current Veterinary Therapy: small animal practice.* Edited by R.W. Kirk. Volume 8. Philadelphia, W.B. Saunders, 1983.
41. Hilwig, R.W.: Cardiac arrhythmias in the dog: detection and treatment. J. Am. Vet. Med. Assoc., *169*:789, 1976.
42. Ettinger, S.J.: Conversion of spontaneous atrial fibrillation in dogs, using direct current synchronized shock. J. Am. Vet. Med. Assoc., *152*:41, 1968.
43. Hoffman, B.F., and Cranefield, P.F.: *Electrophysiology of the Heart.* New York, McGraw-Hill, 1960.
43a. Guntheroth, W.G., Selzer, A., and Spodick, D.H.: Atrioventricular nodal rhythm reconsidered. Am. J. Cardiol., *52*:416, 1983.
44. Friedman, H.H.: *Diagnostic Electrocardiography and Vectorcardiography.* 2nd Edition. New York, McGraw-Hill, 1977.
45. Hamlin, R.L., Smetzer, D.L., and Breznock, E.M.: Sinoatrial syncope in miniature Schnauzers. J. Am. Vet. Med. Assoc., *161*:1023, 1972.
46. Muir, W.W.: Effects of atropine on cardiac rate and rhythm in dogs. J. Am. Vet. Med. Assoc., *172*:917, 1978.
47. Carpenter, J.L., et al.: Intestinal and cardiopulmonary forms of parvovirus infection in a litter of pups. J. Am. Vet. Med. Assoc., *176*:1269, 1980.
48. Muir, W.W., and Lipowitz, A.J.: Cardiac dysrhythmias associated with gastric dilatation-volvulus in the dog. J. Am. Vet. Med. Assoc., *172*:683, 1978.
49. Kus, T., and Sasynick, B.I.: Effects of disopyramide phosphate on ventricular arrhythmias in experimental myocardial infarction. J. Pharm. Exp. Ther., *196*:665, 1976.
50. Muir, W.W., and Bonagura, J.D.: Aprindine for treatment of ventricular arrhythmias in the dog. J. Am. Vet. Res., *43*:1815, 1982.
51. Harris, A.S.: Delayed development of ventricular ectopic rhythms following experimental coronary occlusion. Circulation, *1*:1318, 1950.
52. Clark, D.R.: Recognition and treatment of cardiac emergencies. J. Am. Vet. Med. Assoc., *171*:98, 1977.
53. Wiersig, D.O., Davis, R.H., and Szabuniewicz, M.: Prevention of induced ventricular fibrillation in dogs anesthetized with ultrashort acting barbiturate and halothane. J. Am. Vet. Med. Assoc., *165*:341, 1974.
54. DeSilva, R.A., Verrier, R.L., and Lown, B.: The effects of psychological stress and vagal stimulation with morphine on vulnerability to ventricular fibrillation (VF) in the conscious dog. Am. Heart J., *95*:197, 1978.
55. Zenoble, R.D., and Hill, B.L.: Hypothermia and associated cardiac arrhythmias in two dogs. J. Am. Vet. Med. Assoc., *175*:840, 1979.
56. Breznock, E.M., and Kagan, K.G.: Chemical cardioversion of electrically induced ventricular fibrillation in dogs. Am. J. Vet. Res., *39*:971, 1978.
57. Lange, G.: Action of driving stimuli from intrinsic and extrinsic sources on in situ cardiac pacemaker tissues. Circ. Res., *17*:449, 1965.
58. Fox, P.R., and Tilley, L.P.: ECG of the month. J. Am. Vet. Med. Assoc., *176*:978, 1980.
59. Fisher, E.W.: Fainting in Boxers: the possibility of vaso-vagal syncope (Adams-Stokes attacks). J. Small Anim. Pract., *12*:347, 1971.

60. Robertson, B.T.: Bradyarrhythmias. In *Current Veterinary Therapy: small animal practice*. Volume 5. Edited by R.W. Kirk. Philadelphia, W.B. Saunders, 1974.
61. Branch, C.E., Beckett, S.D., and Robertson, B.T.: Spontaneous syncopal attacks in dogs: a method of documentation. J. Am. Anim. Hosp. Assoc., *13*:673, 1977.
62. James, T.N., et al.: De subitaneis mortibus. XV. Hereditary stenosis of the His bundle in Pug dogs. Circulation, *52*:1152, 1975.
63. James, T.N.: The sinus node as a servomechanism. Circ. Res., *32*:307, 1973.
64. James, T.N.: Congenital deafness and cardiac arrhythmias. Am. J. Cardiol., *19*:627, 1967.
65. Brown, K.K.: Bradyarrhythmias and pacemaker therapy. In *Current Veterinary Therapy: small animal practice*. Volume 6. Edited by R.W. Kirk. Philadelphia, W.B. Saunders, 1977.
66. Tanaka, H., et al.: Persistent atrial standstill due to atrial inexcitability. Jap. Heart J., *16*:639, 1975.
67. Woolliscroft, J., and Tuna, N.: Permanent atrial standstill: the clinical spectrum. Am. J. Cardiol., *49*:2037, 1982.
68. Tilley, L.P., and Liu, S.-K.: Persistent atrial standstill in the dog with muscular dystrophy. ACVIM Scientific Proceedings. Seattle, Wash., July 1979 (Abstract).
68a. Tilley, L.P., and Liu, S.-K.: Persistent atrial standstill in the dog and cat. ACVIM, Scientific Proceedings, New York, 1983 (Abstract).
69. Jeraj, K., et al.: Atrial standstill, myocarditis and destruction of cardiac conduction system: Clinicopathologic correlation in a dog. Am. Heart J., *99*:185, 1980.
69a. Bonagura, J.D., and Grady, M.: ECG of the month. J. Am. Vet. Med. Assoc., *183*:658, 1983.
70. Baldwin, B.J., Talley, R.C., Johnson, C., and Nutter, D.O.: Permanent paralysis of the atrium in a patient with fascioscapulohumeral muscular dystrophy. Am. J. Cardiol., *31*:649, 1973.
71. Whitney, J.C.: Progressive muscular dystrophy in the dog. Vet. Rec. *70*:611, 1958.
72. Bharati, S., Rosen, K.M., Miller, R.A., and Lev, M.: Conduction system examination in a case of spontaneous heart block in a dog. Am. Heart J., *88*:596, 1974.
73. Yoneda, S., et al.: Persistent atrial standstill developed in a patient with rheumatic heart disease: electrophysiological and histological study. Clin. Cardiol., *1*:43, 1978.
74. Gross, D.R., Hamlin, R.L., and Pipers, F.S.: Response of P-Q intervals to digitalis glycosides in the dog. J. Am. Vet. Med. Assoc., *162*:888, 1973.
75. Branch, C.E., Robertson, B.T., and Williams, J.C.: Frequency of second-degree atrioventricular heart block in dogs. Am. J. Vet. Res., *36*:925, 1975.
76. Anselmi, A., Giurdiel, O., Saurez, J.A., and Anselmi, G.: Disturbances in the AV conduction system in Chagas' myocarditis in the dog. Circ. Res., *20*:56, 1967.
77. Liu, S.-K., Maron, B.J., and Tilley, L.P.: Canine hypertrophic cardiomyopathy. J. Am. Vet. Med. Assoc., *174*:708, 1979.
78. Watanabe, Y., and Dreifus, L.S.: *Cardiac Arrhythmias, Electrophysiologic Basis for Clinical Interpretation*. New York, Grune & Stratton, 1977.
79. Jenkins, W.L., and Clark, D.R.: A review of drugs affecting the heart. J. Am. Vet. Med. Assoc., *171*:85, 1977.
80. Buchanan, J.W., Dear, M.G., Pyle, R.L., and Berg, P.: Medical and pacemaker therapy of complete heart block and congestive heart failure in a dog. J. Am. Vet. Med. Assoc., *152*:1099, 1968.
81. Dear, M.G.: Complete atrioventricular block in the dog: a possible congenital case. J. Small Anim. Pract., *11*:301, 1970.
82. Dear, M.G.: Spontaneous reversion of complete A-V block to sinus rhythm in the dog. J. Small Anim. Pract., *11*:17, 1970.
83. Ettinger, S.J.: Isoproterenol treatment of atrioventricular block in the dog. J. Am. Vet. Med. Assoc., *154*:398, 1969.
84. Hamlin, R.L.: Heart block. In *Current Veterinary Therapy: small animal practice*. Volume 3. Edited by R.W. Kirk. Philadelphia, W.B. Saunders, 1966.
85. Holmes, J.R., and Wilson, M.R.: Cardiac syncope in a dog associated with a haemangiosarcoma. Vet. Rec., *82*:474, 1968.
86. Jaffe, K.R., and Bolton, G.R.: Myocardial infarction in a dog with complete heart block. Vet. Med. Small Anim. Clin., *69*:197, 1974.
87. James, T.N., and Konde, W.N.: A clinicopathologic study of heart block in a dog, with remarks pertinent to the embryology of the cardiac conduction system. Am. J. Cardiol., *24*:59, 1969.
88. Lev, M., Neuwelt, F., and Necheles, H.: Congenital defect of the interventricular septum, aortic regurgitation, and probable heart block in a dog. Am. J. Vet. Res., *1*:91, 1941.
89. Robertson, B.T., and Giles, H.D.: Complete heart block associated with vegetative endocarditis in a dog, J. Am. Vet. Med. Assoc., *161*:180, 1972.
90. Buchanan, J.W., and Botts, R.P.: Clinical effects of repeated cardiac punctures in dogs. J. Am. Vet. Med. Assoc., *161*:814, 1972.
91. Musselman, E.E., and Hartsfield, S.M.: Complete atrioventricular heart block due to hypokalemia following ovariohysterectomy. Vet. Med. Small Anim. Clin., *71*:155, 1976.
92. James, T.N., and Drake, E.H.: Sudden death in Doberman Pinschers. Ann. Intern. Med., *68*:821, 1968.
93. Meierhenry, E.F., and Liu, S.-K.: Atrioventricular bundle degeneration associated with sudden death in the dog. J. Am. Vet. Med. Assoc., *172*:1418, 1978.
94. Webb, T.J., Clark, D.R., and McCrady, J.D.: Artificial cardiac pacemakers and some clinical indications for pacemaking. Southwest. Vet., *28*:91, 1975.
95. Boineau, J.P., and Moore, E.N.: Evidence for propagation of activation across an accessory atrioventricular connection in types A and B pre-excitation. Circulation, *41*:375, 1970.
96. Boineau, J.P., Moore, E.N., Sealy, W.C., and Kasell, J.H.: Epicardial mapping in Wolff-Parkinson-White syndrome. Arch. Intern. Med., *135*:422, 1975.
97. Burch, G.E.: Of simplifying classification of WPW syndrome (left, right and septal types of WPW syndrome). Am. Heart J., *90*:807, 1975.
98. Lown, B., Ganong, W.F., and Levine, S.A.: The syndrome of short P-R interval, normal QRS complex and paroxysmal rapid heart action. Circulation, *5*:693, 1952.
99. Narula, O.S.: Symposium on cardiac arrhythmias. 4. Wolff-Parkinson-White syndrome. Circulation, *47*:872, 1973.
100. Moore, E.N., Spear, J.F., and Boineau, J.P.: Arrhythmias and conduction disturbances in simulated Wolff-Parkinson-White syndrome in the dog. Am. J. Cardiol., *26*:650, 1971.
101. Lichstein, E., Goyal, S., Chadda, K., and Gupta, P.: Alternating Wolff-Parkinson-White (pre-excitation) pattern. J. Electrocardiol., *11*:81, 1978.
102. Muir, W.W.: Thiobarbiturate-induced dysrhythmias: the role of heart rate and autonomic imbalance. Am. J. Vet. Res., *38*:1377, 1977.
103. Chung, E.K.: Wolff-Parkinson-White syndrome: current views. Am. J. Med., *62*:252, 1977.
103a. Wellens, H.J.J.: Wolff-Parkinson-White syndrome. Part II. Treatment. Mod. Concepts Cardiovasc. Dis., *52*:57, 1983.
103b. Prystowsky, E.N., et al.: Clinical efficacy and electrophysiologic effects of encainide in patients with Wolff-Parkinson-White syndrome. Circulation, *69*:278, 1984.
104. Bashour, T., et al.: Atrioventricular and intraventricular conduction in hyperkalemia. Am. J. Cardiol., *35*:199, 1975.
105. Willard, M.D., Schall, W.D., McCaw, D.E., and Nachreiner, R.F.: Canine hypoadrenocorticism: Report of 37 cases and review of 39 previously reported cases. J. Am. Vet. Med. Assoc., *180*:59, 1982.
106. Coulter, D.B., Duncan, R.J., and Sander, P.D.: Effects of asphyxia and potassium on canine and feline electrocardiograms. Can. J. Comp. Med., *39*:442, 1975.
107. Feldman, E.C., and Ettinger, S.J.: Electrocardiographic changes associated with electrolyte disturbances. Vet. Clin. North Am., *7*:487, 1977.
108. Vander Ark, C.R., Ballantyne, F., and Reynolds, E.W.: Electrolytes and the electrocardiogram. Cardiovasc. Clin., *5*:269, 1973.
109. Morgan, R.V.: Endocrine and metabolic emergencies—Part I. Compend. Contin. Educ. Pract. Vet., *4*:755, 1982.
110. Kaplan, B.M., Langendorf, R., Lev, M., and Pick, A.: Tachycardia-bradycardia syndrome (so-called "sick sinus syndrome"). Am. J. Cardiol., *31*:497, 1973.
111. Clark, D.R., et al.: Artificial pacemaker implantation for control of sinoatrial syncope in a miniature Schnauzer. Southwest. Vet., *28*:101, 1975.
112. Mandel, W.J., Obayoshi, K., and Laks, M.M.: Overview of the sick sinus syndrome. Chest, *66*:223, 1974.
113. Jordan, J.L., Yamaguchi, I., and Mandel, W.J.: Studies on the mechanism of sinus node dysfunction in the sick sinus syndrome. Circulation, *57*:217, 1978.
114. Tilley, L.P.: Feline cardiology. In *Katzen Krankheiten, Klinik und Therapie*. Edited by W.K. Herausgeber and U.M. Durr. Hannover, Germany, Verlag M. & H. Schaper, 1978.
114a. Miller, M.S., and Tilley, L.P.: ECG of the month. J. Am. Vet. Med. Assoc., *184*:423, 1984.
114b. Alpert, M.S., and Flaker, G.C.: Arrhythmias associated with sinus node dysfunction—pathogenesis, recognition, and management. JAMA, *250*:2160, 1983.

115. Fabry-Delaigue, R., et al.: Long-term observation of cardiac rhythm and automaticity in the dog after excision of the sinoatrial node. J. Electrocard., *15*:209, 1982.

116. Beckett, S.D., et al.: Assessment of sinus node overdrive suppression in awake dogs and pups. Fed. Proc., *35*:221, 1976.

117. Bellet, S.: *Clinical Disorders of the Heart Beat.* 3rd Edition. Philadelphia, Lea & Febiger, 1971.

118. Littman, D.: Alternation of the heart. Circulation, *27*:280, 1963.

119. Sbarbaro, J.A., and Brooks, H.L.: Pericardial effusion and electrical alternans, echocardiographic assessment. Postgrad. Med., *63*(3):105, 1978.

120. Cohen, H.C., et al.: Tachycardia and bradycardia-dependent bundle branch block alternans. Circulation, *55*:242, 1977.

121. Scherf, D., and Bornemann, C.: Tachycardias with alternation of the ventricular complexes. Am. Heart J., *74*:667, 1967.

121a.Green, M., et al.: Value of QRS alternation in determining the site of origin of narrow QRS supraventricular tachycardia. Circulation, *68*:368, 1983.

122. Friedman, H.S., et al.: Electrocardiographic features of experimental cardiac tamponade in closed-chest dogs. Eur. J. Cardiol., *6*:311, 1977.

123. Tilley, L.P., and Wilkins, R.J.: Pericardial disease. In *Current Veterinary Therapy: small animal practice.* Volume 5. Edited by R.W. Kirk. Philadelphia, W.B. Saunders, 1974.

124. Bonagura, J.D.: Electrical alternans associated with pericardial effusion in the dog. J. Am. Vet. Med. Assoc., *178*:574, 1981.

125. Navarro-Lopex, F., et al.: Isolated T-wave alternans elicited by hypocalcemia in dogs. J. Electrocardiol., *11*:103, 1978.

126. Muir, W.W.: Electrocardiographic interpretation of thiobarbiturate-induced dysrhythmias in dogs. J. Am. Vet. Med. Assoc., *170*:1419, 1977.

127. Sawyer, D.C.: *The Practice of Small Animal Anesthesia (Major Problems in Veterinary Medicine)* Volume 1. Philadelphia, W.B. Saunders, 1982.

128. Brown, B.R. (Ed.): *Anesthesia and the Patient with Heart Disease.* Philadelphia, F.A. Davis, 1980.

129. Buss, D.D., Hess, R.E., Webb, A.I., and Spencer, K.R.: Incidence of post-anesthetic arrhythmias in the dog. J. Small Anim. Pract., *23*:399, 1982.

130. Klide, A.M., Calderwood, H.W., and Soma, L.R.: Cardiopulmonary effects of xylazine in dogs. Am. J. Vet. Res., *36*:931, 1975.

131. Wright, M.: Pharmacologic effects of ketamine and its use in veterinary medicine. J. Am. Vet. Med. Assoc., *180*:1462, 1982.

132. Mirakhur, R.K.: Premedication with atropine or glycopyrrolate in children. Effects on heart rate and rhythm during induction and maintenance of anesthesia. Anesthesia, *37*:1032, 1982.

133. Rawlings, C.A., and Kolata, R.J.: Cardiopulmonary effects of thiopental/lidocaine combination during anesthetic induction in the dog. Am. J. Vet. Res., *44*:144, 1983.

134. Moore, E.N., Morse, H.T., and Price, H.L.: Cardiac arrhythmias produced by catecholamines in anesthetized dogs. Circ. Res., *15*:77, 1964.

134a.Harvey, R.C., and Short, C.E.: The use of isoflurane for safe anesthesia in animals with traumatic myocarditis or other myocardial sensitivity. Canine Practice *10*:18, 1983.

135. Henderson, B.M., Dougherty, W.J., James, V.C., and Tilley, L.P.: Safety assessment of a new anticancer compound, Mitoxantrone, in Beagle dogs: Comparison with Doxorubicin. I. Clinical observations. Cancer Treat. Rep., *66*:1139, 1982.

136. Kehoe, R., et al.: Adriamycin-induced cardiac dysrhythmias in an experimental dog model. Cancer Treat. Rep., *62*:963, 1978.

137. Hause, W.R., and Bonagura, J.D.: ECG of the month. J. Am. Vet. Med. Assoc., *180*:390, 1982.

138. Susaneck, S.J.: Topics in drug therapy—Doxorubicin therapy in the dog. J. Am. Vet. Med. Assoc., *182*:70, 1983.

139. Bright, J.M.: Controversies in veterinary medicine: Is the long-term use of digitalis for treatment of low output failure unwarranted? J. Am. Anim. Hosp. Assoc., *19*:233, 1983.

140. Ewy, G.A., Marcus, F.I., Fillmore, S.J., and Matthews, N.P.: Digitalis intoxication: diagnosis, management and prevention. Cardiovasc. Clin., *6*:153, 1974.

141. Castellanos, A., Ghafour, A.A., and Soffer, A.: Digitalis-induced arrhythmias: recognition and therapy. Cardiovasc. Clin., *1*:107, 1969.

142. Adams, H.R.: Digitalis and other inotropic agents. In *Veterinary Pharmacology and Therapeutics.* Edited by N.H. Booth and L.E. McDonald. 5th Edition. Ames, Iowa, Iowa State University Press, 1983.

143. Button, C., et al.: Pharmacokinetics, bioavailability and dosage regimens of digoxin in dogs. Am. J. Vet. Res., *41*:1230, 1980.

144. De Rick, A., and Belpaire, F.: Digoxin-quinidine interaction in the dog. J. Vet. Pharm. Therap., *4*:215, 1981.

145. Yurchak, P.M.: Artifacts resembling cardiac arrhythmias. Postgrad. Med., *53*(3):79, 1973.

7 Analysis of common feline cardiac arrhythmias

The general principles of canine arrhythmias are easily applicable to feline arrhythmias. As a supplement to the material in this chapter, the reader is referred to the discussion of canine arrhythmias in Chapter 6.

An arrhythmia can be defined as (1) an abnormality in the rate, regularity, or site of origin of the cardiac impulse and/or (2) a disturbance in conduction of the impulse such that the normal sequence of activation of atria and ventricles is altered.[1]

The anatomic and/or physiologic abnormalities of impulse formation and impulse conduction represent the basic mechanisms that underlie the arrhythmias and give a basis for the following classification. The basic mechanisms underlying arrhythmias are discussed in detail in Chapters 8 and 9.

Sinus rhythm
Normal sinus rhythm
Sinus tachycardia
Sinus bradycardia
Sinus arrhythmia
Wandering sinus pacemaker

Abnormalities of impulse formation
Supraventricular
  Sinus arrest
  Atrial premature complexes (APCs)
  Atrial tachycardia
  Atrial flutter
  Atrial fibrillation
AV junction
  AV junctional escape rhythm (secondary arrhythmia)
Ventricular
  Ventricular premature complexes (VPCs)
  Ventricular tachycardia
  Ventricular flutter, fibrillation
  Ventricular asystole
  Ventricular escape rhythm (secondary arrhythmia)

Abnormalities of impulse conduction
SA block
Atrial standstill (hyperkalemia) (sinoventricular conduction) block
AV block
  First degree
  Second degree
  Third degree (complete heart block)

Abnormalities of both impulse formation and impulse conduction
Pre-excitation (Wolff-Parkinson-White) syndrome, reciprocal rhythm (re-entry)
Parasystole
Other complex rhythms (Chapter 12)

The incidence of the various arrhythmias in the cat has been studied at The Animal Medical Center, and an indication of the frequency of some of these electrocardiographic disturbances has been obtained. Atrial standstill and ventricular arrhythmias are common in cats with hyperkalemia from urethral obstruction. From 1973 to 1975, The Animal Medical Center admitted 1007 cats affected with urethral obstruction. Of these, an average of 50 cats per year, or approximately 1 cat in 10 with urethral obstruction, had severe cardiotoxic signs from associated hyperkalemia.[2,3]

Another study involved the frequency of atrial fibrillation during the 3-year period from 1972 to 1975. Nine cats were diagnosed electrocardiographically at The Animal Medical Center as having atrial fibrillation;[4] all had clinical or postmortem evidence of hypertrophic cardiomyopathy. The inpatient case load for that time period was approximately 7000 cats. A third study from this institution involved a detailed analysis of 34 cats with cardiomyopathy[5] selected from 358 cases diagnosed at necropsy with the requirements of having had at least one physical examination, electrocardiography, radiography, and/or angiocardiographic hemodynamic studies. Cardiac arrhythmias were recorded in 14 of the 34 cats (41.2%).

Table 7–1. Summary of arrhythmias in feline cardiomyopathy

Arrhythmia	AMC*	AMAH†	Total (%)
Supraventricular			
APCs	0	7	7 (13.7)
Atrial tachycardia	2	0	2 (3.9)
Atrial fibrillation	2	1	3 (5.9)
Ventricular			
VPCs	9	15	24 (47.1)
Ventricular tachycardia	1	7	8 (15.7)
Conduction disturbances			
AV block (second and third degree)	2	3	5 (9.8)
Wolff-Parkinson-White syndrome	1	1	2 (3.9)
Total	17	34	51 (100.0)

*Animal Medical Center, New York.[5] Arrhythmias were recorded in 14 (41.2%) of 34 cats studied.

†Angell Memorial Animal Hospital, Boston. Arrhythmias were recorded in 29 (49.2%) of 59 cats studied. Summarized from Harpster, N.K.: Cardiovascular diseases of the domestic cat. Adv. Vet. Sci. Comp. Med., 21:39, 1977.

The types and frequencies of some of the arrhythmias recorded in this study are summarized in Table 7–1.[5] The frequency of each electrocardiographic abnormality in the cat with cardiomyopathy compares closely with the findings of a study reported from Angell Memorial Animal Hospital.[6] The arrhythmias observed in 59 cats with cardiomyopathy in that study are also summarized in Table 7–1. Arrhythmias were recorded in 29 of the 59 cats (49.2%) studied at the Angell Memorial Animal Hospital. In our study at The Animal Medical Center, 14 of the 34 cats (41.2%) had arrhythmias. Nine cats (26.4%) from our study had normal electrocardiograms, whereas 10 (16.9%) cats from Angell were normal.

NORMAL MECHANISM

A knowledge of the anatomic and physiologic properties of the unique impulse-forming and impulse-conducting system of the atria, AV junction, and ventricles is essential for the accurate analysis of cardiac arrhythmias.

Activation of heart muscle results from spontaneous discharge in a pacemaker and conduction of this impulse from cell to cell. The heart's conductive system is composed of the SA node, the internodal tracts, the AV node, the bundle of His, and the bundle branches. This conductive system has many potential pacemaking cells. The SA node exhibits the fastest inherent discharge rate; the cells in the rest of the conduction system exhibit a slower rate. Because the rate and rhythm of the heart are controlled by the SA node, the normal cardiac rhythm is termed *sinoatrial* or sinus rhythm. A pronounced sinus arrhythmia, often normally auscultated in dogs, is rare in cats. An irregular cardiac rhythm auscultated in a cat, then, is generally an abnormal finding. The heart rate is normally accelerated in cats because excitement influences the sympathetic nervous system as part of cardiac regulation. Acceleration often reaches heart rates of up to 240 beats/min and sometimes greater during the period when the electrocardiogram is being recorded. The resting heart rate (telemetrically recorded) for the cat is 128 ± 17 beats/min.[7]

Contrary to what is observed in dogs, atrial and ventricular rates for atrial tachycardia and atrial flutter can be very high in cats. One theory for explaining the mechanism of atrial flutter is the presence of a circus movement in a ring of tissue between the two venae cavae. The faster rates in the cat can possibly be explained by a shorter circuit in the smaller atria, which would require a shorter conduction time.

RECOGNITION OF ARRHYTHMIAS—a systematic approach

With a general knowledge of the normal anatomic and physiologic properties of the impulse-forming and impulse-conducting system of the heart and the use of a systematic approach to analyzing the electrocardiographic strip, the accurate diagnosis of arrhythmias can be greatly simplified. A systematic method for analyzing the electrocardiographic rhythm strip (usually lead II) includes these steps[8–10] (discussed in more detail in Chapter 6).

1. General inspection of the electrocardiogram to show whether the rhythm is a normal sinus rhythm or is characteristic of a type of cardiac arrhythmia
2. Identification of P waves
3. Recognition of QRS complexes
4. Analysis of the relationship between P waves and QRS complexes
5. Summary of findings and final classification of the arrhythmia by answering the following basic questions:
   a. What is the predominant rhythm (e.g., sinus, atrial, AV junction, or ventricular)?
   b. Is the arrhythmia an abnormality of impulse formation or of impulse conduction or both? If either or both, what is the site of the disturbance?

Each of the arrhythmias discussed in this chapter is considered on the basis of the systematic method just described, outlined as follows:

Electrocardiographic features

General inspection: heart rate and rhythm
P waves: present or absent; if present, morphology, uniformity, and regularity
QRS complexes: morphology, uniformity, and regularity
P and QRS relationship: measurement of P-R interval, dominant rhythm

Associated conditions

Treatment

This outline will be used on one page to present and discuss the respective arrhythmia, and representative examples will be arranged on the facing page.

In Section Four, the pathophysiologic basis and effects of cardiac arrhythmias will be discussed. A detailed discussion of the use of antiarrhythmic drugs in the dog and cat can be found in Chapter 10 by Dr. John D. Bonagura and Dr. William W. Muir. *Tables 10–10 and 10–12 list drugs used in the therapy of cardiac arrhythmias.* Special methods for analyzing and treating arrhythmias are discussed in Chapter 11. *Table 11–2 lists drugs used in the management of cardiac resuscitation.*

Specific treatment for many of the arrhythmias present in cats is often not required. In the majority of cases, arrhythmias disappear when the underlying disease is brought under control. For example, the correction of hyperkalemia in urethral obstruction by simply relieving the obstruction and restoring normal acid-base status and intravascular fluid volume may eliminate the associated arrhythmias. A glucose-insulin infusion may also be needed to specifically decrease the serum potassium levels when there are associated life-threatening arrhythmias.[3]

Propranolol and digoxin are the two drugs used commonly in the specific treatment of arrhythmias in the cat. Propranolol is currently the drug of choice in cats because of its broad antiarrhythmic effects. In dogs, propranolol is used primarily when other agents are ineffective, either alone or in combination with other drugs. Propranolol works primarily by blocking the beta-adrenergic receptors. The dosage necessary to obtain this beta-adrenergic effect in cats has been studied.[11] The drug also has a "quinidine-like" effect that provides a further base for its wide antiarrhythmic spectrum, but sometimes only at such high nonphysiologic doses as to create an impractical situation. Propranolol may be beneficial in atrial tachycardia, atrial flutter, Wolff-Parkinson-White syndrome, and ventricular arrhythmias. It also has an additive effect with digitalis in reducing AV conduction, especially atrial fibrillation. Propranolol is contraindicated in allergy, bradycardia, AV block, and some types of cardiac failure. The drug can depress myocardial performance and accentuate cardiac failure.[12–14]

Of the forms of digitalis, only digoxin has been used in cats. The clinical use of digoxin in the cat falls primarily into two categories: (1) control of ventricular rate in atrial fibrillation, atrial tachycardia, and atrial flutter and (2) the inotropic effect in the improvement of cardiac performance in dilated cardiomyopathy. Manifestations of digoxin toxicity include effects on the heart and effects on the gastrointestinal system. The cardiac manifestations can include ventricular arrhythmias, different degrees of AV block, and sinus bradycardia.[12–14]

Normal sinus rhythm

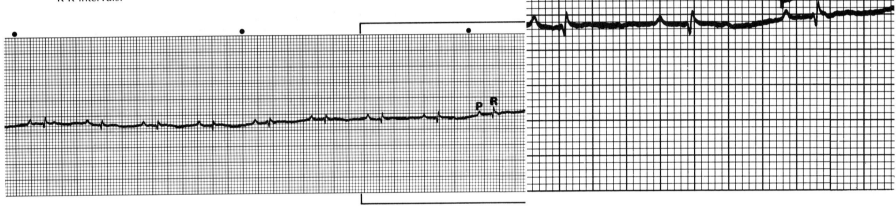

Fig. 7–1. Normal sinus rhythm at a rate of 160 beats/min (8 cycles between two sets of time lines × 20). The rhythm is regular, with no variance in the R-R intervals.

The SA node is the dominant pacemaker and normally depolarizes at a frequency ranging from 160 to 240 per minute in adult cats. The heart rate is normally accelerated in cats because of the influence of excitement on the sympathetic nervous system.

Electrocardiographic features

1. The rhythm is regular at a rate range of 160 to 240 beats/min (mean, 195). The telemetrically recorded resting heart rate for the adult cat is 127 ± 17 beats/min.[7] The difference between the largest and smallest R-R intervals is less than 0.10 second.

2. P waves are positive in lead II with a constant configuration.

3. The QRS complexes are normal or wide and bizarre if an intraventricular conduction defect is present.

4. The P-QRS relationship is normal with a constant P-R interval.

Failure of the rhythm to meet any of these criteria indicates the possible presence of some abnormality of impulse formation and/or impulse conduction, i.e., an *arrhythmia*.

Associated condition

1. Excitement during clinical examination (increase in sinus rate), vagal stimulation (decrease) (The sinus rhythm is the normal rhythm of the heart.)

Treatment

1. There is no treatment.

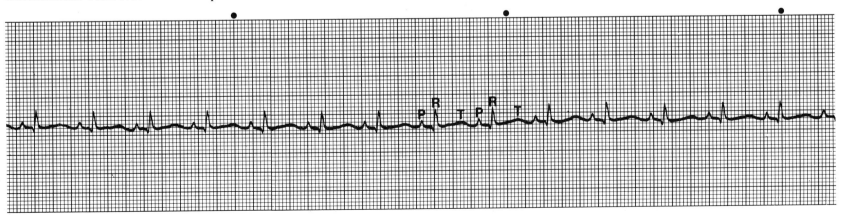

Fig. 7–2. Normal sinus rhythm at an approximate rate of 180 beats/min. The rhythm is regular.

Sinus arrhythmia and wandering pacemaker

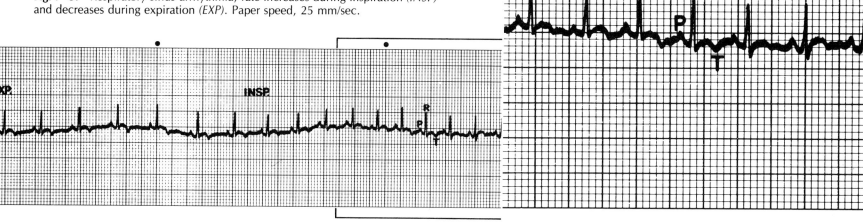

Fig. 7–3. Respiratory sinus arrhythmia; rate increases during inspiration *(INSP)* and decreases during expiration *(EXP)*. Paper speed, 25 mm/sec.

Sinus arrhythmia is an irregular sinus rhythm originating in the SA node. It is represented by alternating periods of slower and more rapid heart rates and is an uncommon and usually abnormal finding in cats (though it is a frequent normal finding in dogs). Contrary to the situation in dogs, sinus arrhythmia in cats usually has no relationship to the phases of respiration. Wandering pacemaker, a variation of sinus arrhythmia, is a shift of the pacemaker within the SA node. A wandering pacemaker is an irregular sinus rhythm with changing P wave morphology.

Electrocardiographic features

1. All criteria of a normal sinus rhythm are met except that a variability of 0.10 second or more exists between successive P waves.

2. A wandering pacemaker within the SA node causes a gradual change in the configuration of the P wave, with the P-R interval being basically constant.

Associated conditions

1. Vagal stimulation from digitalis or from increased intracranial pressure or cerebral dysfunction
2. Digitalis toxicity, severe respiratory disease (atelectasis or pleuritis). Respiratory sinus arrhythmia can be a normal finding.

Treatment

1. Treat the underlying condition.

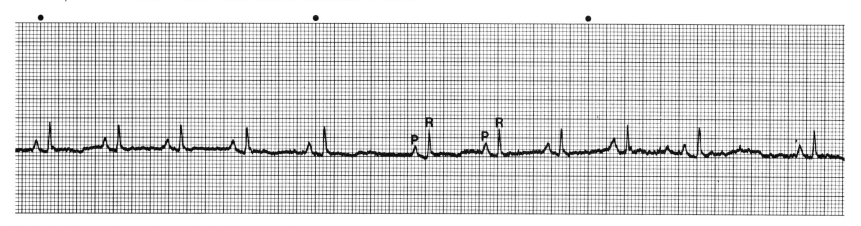

Fig. 7–4. Nonrespiratory sinus arrhythmia in a cat with a severe respiratory infection. Note also the gradual and temporary change in the P waves, a wandering pacemaker.

Sinus tachycardia and sinus bradycardia

Fig. 7–5. Sinus tachycardia at a rate of 250 beats/min in a cat with a fever. The P waves are of a constant configuration, and the rhythm is regular.

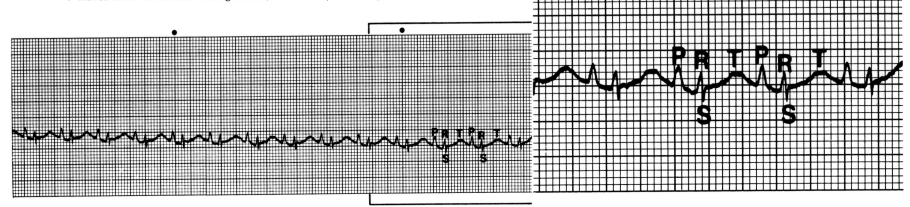

A regular sinus rhythm below the normal heart rate range is a sinus bradycardia; that above the normal heart range is a sinus tachycardia. Sinus tachycardia is the *most common* arrhythmia in cats.

Sinus tachycardia can be associated with the following conditions: as a physiologic mechanism in response to an increase in body metabolism resulting in a greater demand for oxygenation; as a compensatory mechanism to increase cardiac output; resulting from underlying pathology; and in response to pharmacologic agents. The significance of severe sinus bradycardia is its effect upon cardiac output and/or the susceptibility to abnormalities in impulse formation. The arrhythmia can be active (e.g., ventricular tachycardia) or it can be an escape rhythm (e.g., junctional rhythm).

Electrocardiographic features

1. All criteria of a normal sinus rhythm are met except that the heart rate is above 240 beats/min for a sinus tachycardia and below 160 for a sinus bradycardia.

2. The rhythm is regular with a slight variation in R-R intervals; the P-R interval is constant. Ocular pressure usually does not produce a slowing of the heart rate in sinus tachycardia.

Associated conditions

1. Physiologic *(tachycardia):* pain, restraint procedures such as during the clinical examination

2. Pathologic *(tachycardia):* fever, shock, anemia, infection, congestive heart failure, hypoxia, hyperthyroidism; *(bradycardia):* systemic disease with toxicity such as renal failure, dilated cardiomyopathy during end-stage heart failure (Sinus bradycardia can be a warning of an impending cardiac arrest during surgery.)

3. Drugs *(tachycardia):* atropine, epinephrine, ketamine; *(bradycardia):* propranolol, digoxin, anesthetics, lidocaine, propylene glycol in parenteral drugs[12,15]

Treatment

1. The "treatment" of a sinus tachycardia involves merely identifying and controlling the causes. Propranolol in hypertrophic cardiomyopathy counteracts the effects of stress and the accompanying catecholamine effects on the SA node. Propranolol, then, prevents the stress-induced sinus tachycardia that may precipitate heart failure.

2. Sinus bradycardia usually indicates a serious underlying disorder that needs immediate attention. The underlying condition should always be treated. Intravenous atropine or an intravenous infusion of isoproterenol (if atropine is not helpful) is recommended.

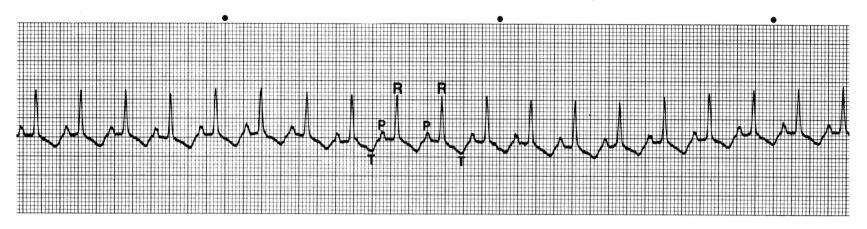

Fig. 7–6. Sinus tachycardia at a rate of 250 beats/min in a cat with congestive heart failure from hypertrophic cardiomyopathy. The P-R interval is constant and the rhythm is regular. The P wave is touching the T wave of the preceding complex. The tall R waves indicate left ventricular enlargement.

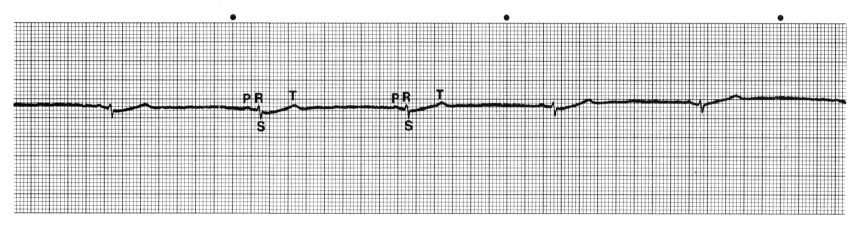

Fig. 7–7. Sinus bradycardia at a rate of 75 beats/min in a cat during anesthetic complications during surgery. Termination of the anesthesia, administration of oxygen and atropine, and close monitoring are immediately indicated.

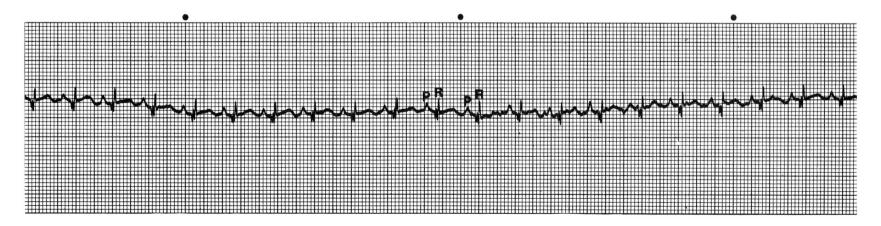

Fig. 7–8. Sinus tachycardia at a rate of 270 beats/min in a cat during an examination. The heart rate dropped to 190 (not shown) after the cat became calm.

Atrial premature complexes

Fig. 7–9. Three APCs occurring in a bigeminal rhythm after the first five sinus complexes. The premature P′ waves are slightly different from the sinus P waves.

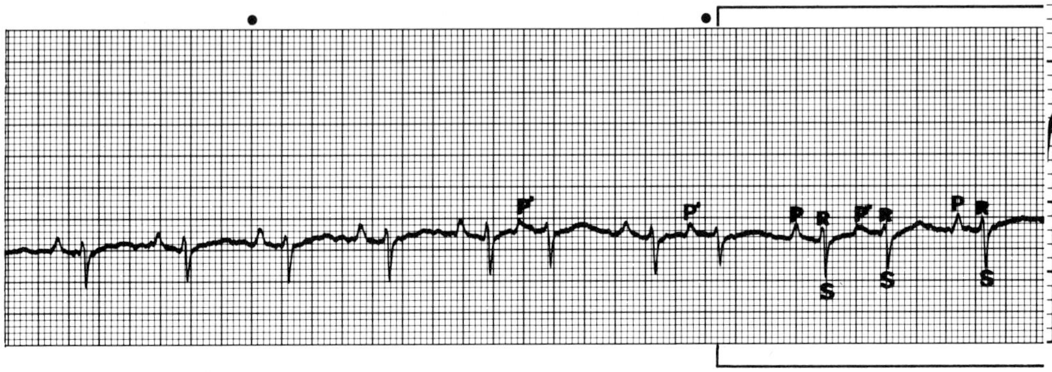

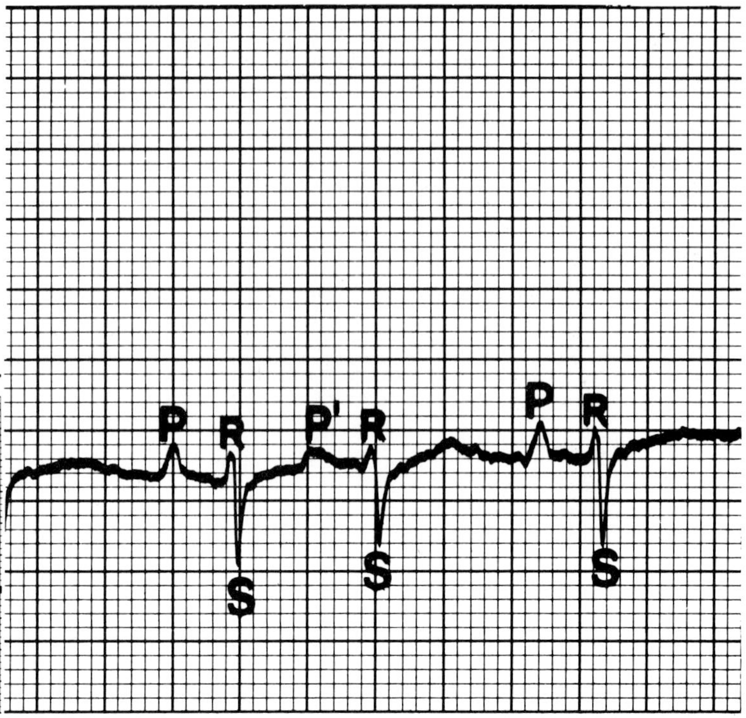

Atrial premature complexes (APCs) (also known as atrial extrasystoles and atrial premature contractions) are impulses that arise from ectopic foci in the atria. They are most often caused by cardiac disease and may lead to atrial tachycardia, atrial flutter, or atrial fibrillation. The impulses spread through the atria to the AV node, and they may or may not reach the ventricle.

Electrocardiographic features

1. The heart rate is usually normal, and the rhythm is irregular owing to the premature P wave (called a P′ wave) that disrupts the normal P wave rhythm.

2. The ectopic P′ wave is premature, and its configuration is different from that of the sinus P waves. It may be negative, positive, biphasic, or superimposed on the previous T wave.

3. The QRS complex is premature, and its configuration is usually normal (same as that of the sinus complexes). It is absent when the P′ wave occurs too early. The AV node is not completely recovered (refractory), so ventricular conduction does not occur (a nonconducted P′ wave). If there is partial recovery in the AV node or the intraventricular conduction systems, the P′ wave is conducted with a long P′-R interval or is conducted with a change in the normal QRS configuration (aberrant conduction). The more premature the complex, the more marked is the aberration.

4. In the P-QRS relationship the P′-R interval is usually as long as or longer than the sinus P-R interval.

5. A noncompensatory pause, i.e., when the R-R interval of the two normal sinus complexes enclosing the atrial premature complex is less than the R-R intervals of three consecutive sinus complexes, usually follows an APC. The ectopic atrial impulse discharges the SA node and resets its cycle.

Associated conditions[13,14]

1. Atrial enlargement secondary to hypertrophic cardiomyopathy[16,17]
2. Any atrial disease: congenital cardiac defects, metastatic tumors, chronic AV valvular insufficiency in older cats
3. Drugs: digitalis toxicity, general anesthesia
4. Hyperthyroidism
5. Atrial premature complexes can be of normal variation in aged cats.

Treatment

1. APCs usually decrease or disappear with rest; specific antiarrhythmic drugs are rarely needed. Propranolol in cats with hypertrophic cardiomyopathy is usually effective.
2. Treat the underlying condition.

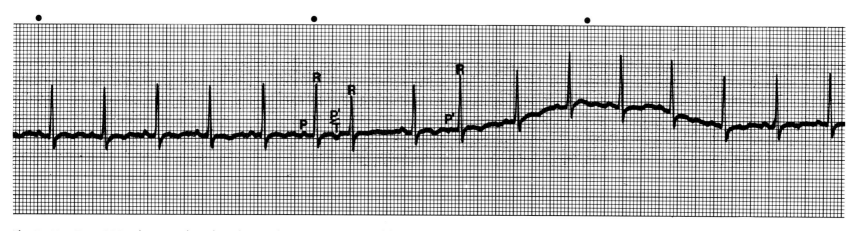

Fig. 7–10. Two APCs, the seventh and ninth complexes, in a 15-year-old cat with chronic mitral insufficiency. The premature P′ waves vary in configuration and are superimposed on the T waves of the preceding QRS complexes. The pause following each APC is noncompensatory.

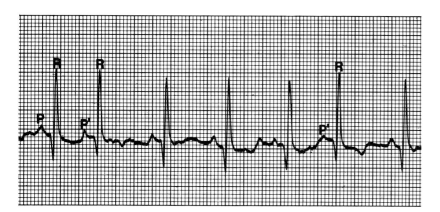

Fig. 7–11. Two APCs, the second and sixth complexes, in a cat with hypertrophic cardiomyopathy. The premature QRS patterns resemble the sinus QRS complexes.

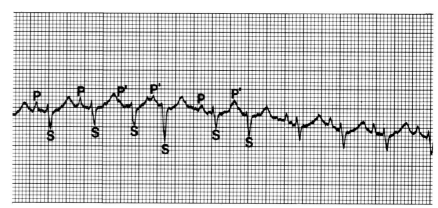

Fig. 7–12. The third, fourth, and sixth complexes are APCs. The fourth impulse is conducted with a change in the normal QRS configuration (aberrant conduction).

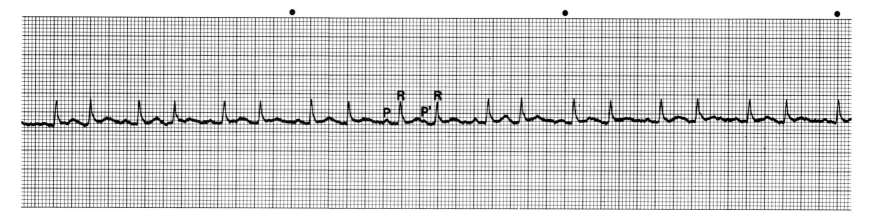

Fig. 7–13. APCs in bigeminy in a cat under general anesthesia. The second complex of each pair is an APC, where the first is a sinus complex. This abnormality in rhythm disappeared after the anesthetic was stopped.

Atrial tachycardia and atrial flutter

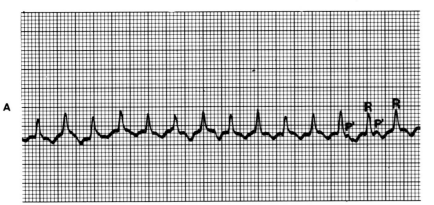
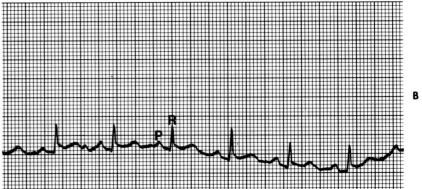

Fig. 7–14. **A,** Supraventricular tachycardia at a ventricular rate of 400 beats/min in a cat with fainting episodes from hypertrophic cardiomyopathy. A 1:1 conduction is suggested; intra-atrial recordings are needed to confirm other atrial waves. (See Fig. 7–18.) **B,** Spontaneous conversion. The rhythm is now sinus with QRS complexes approximately the same as in strip **A.**

Atrial tachycardia is a rapid regular rhythm originating from a focus in the atria away from the SA node. Three or more consecutive APCs are considered atrial tachycardia. There is basically no difference between atrial tachycardia and atrial flutter, except for the atrial rate and the presence of flutter waves in atrial flutter. Atrial flutter usually occurs at atrial rates greater than 300 to 350 beats/min. The term *supraventricular tachycardia* is used when atrial flutter cannot be differentiated from atrial tachycardia.

Electrocardiographic features

1. Atrial rhythm is usually regular with a rate above 240 beats/min in atrial tachycardia and usually above 350 in atrial flutter. The rapid atrial rhythm can be either intermittent (paroxysmal) or continuous. The ventricular rhythm and rate depend on the atrial rate and the state of AV conduction (same as the atrial rate, 1:1 conduction; half the atrial rate, 2:1; 3:1; 4:1; etc.).

2. In atrial tachycardia the P′ waves are usually positive in lead II, with the P′-P′ intervals regular. They may not be easily seen because of the fast ventricular rate. The configuration of the P′ waves is generally somewhat different from that of the sinus P waves. In the typical form of atrial flutter, the normal P waves are replaced by sawtooth flutter waves (F waves).

3. The configuration of the QRS complex is usually normal (same as for the sinus complexes) or wide and bizarre owing to bundle branch block, aberrant ventricular conduction, or ventricular pre-excitation.

4. When the atrial rate is high enough, the normal AV junction may not have enough time to repolarize sufficiently to conduct all atrial impulses to the ventricles. Varying degrees of atrioventricular block usually occur. The most common AV conduction ratio in atrial flutter is 2:1. If 1:1 conduction occurs in spite of a rapid atrial rate, the presence of Wolff-Parkinson-White syndrome should be suspected.

Associated conditions[13,14]

1. Same conditions that caused APCs, those diseases causing atrial enlargement (most often hypertrophic cardiomyopathy[5,16,17])
2. Others: ventricular pre-excitation (Wolff-Parkinson-White syndrome), cardiac neoplasia

Treatment[12] *(See Chapter 10 and Fig. 10–9)*

1. Both atrial tachycardia and atrial flutter usually represent transient arrhythmias. Digoxin is often the drug of choice in dogs. Digoxin is frequently contraindicated in hypertrophic cardiomyopathy unless the arrhythmia is absolutely uncontrollable and no outflow obstruction is present.

2. Intravenous propranolol, along with carotid sinus or ocular pressure, is usually effective. Propranolol is relatively contraindicated in the presence of heart failure and should always be used with great caution. It is useful in preventing atrial arrhythmias in hypertrophic cardiomyopathy.

3. Electrical cardioversion (small doses of electrical energy) or intracardiac pacing may be attempted if the animal is critical and the arrhythmia uncontrollable.

4. A thump delivered to the precordium with a clenched fist can often be used to correct an atrial tachycardia or atrial flutter, especially in emergency when resuscitative drugs and equipment are not available.[18]

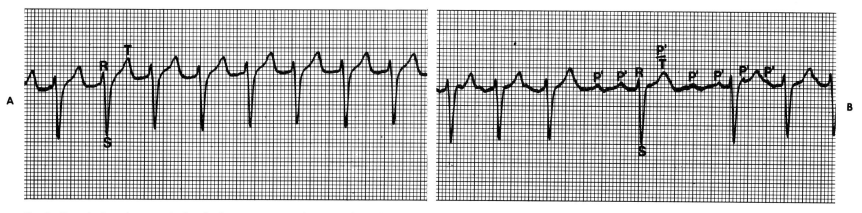

Fig. 7–15. **A,** Regular ventricular rhythm at a ventricular rate of 230 beats/min. P waves cannot be seen. **B,** Ocular pressure with accompanying increase in vagal tone affects AV conduction so the P'-like waves (F waves) are now clearly seen. The atrial rate is 460 beats/min with varying conduction into the ventricles (atrial flutter). Strip **A** then represents 2:1 AV conduction with P waves hidden in the QRS-T complexes. This cat had anterior fascicular block and hypertrophic cardiomyopathy.

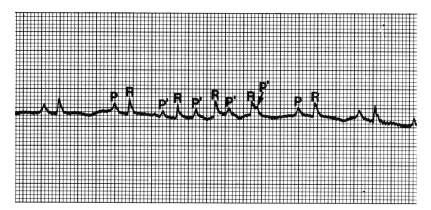

Fig. 7–16. A short period of atrial tachycardia with Wenckebach type (Mobitz I) of AV block induced by an APC (after the first two sinus complexes). The final P' wave is blocked.

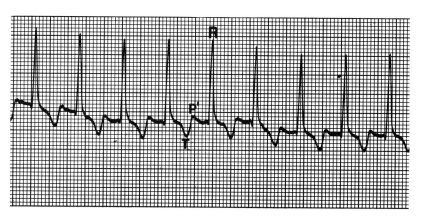

Fig. 7–17. Atrial tachycardia at rate of 250 beats/min in a cat with a pulmonary carcinoma and secondary cardiac involvement. Note the tall and wide QRS complexes, which indicate left ventricular enlargement.

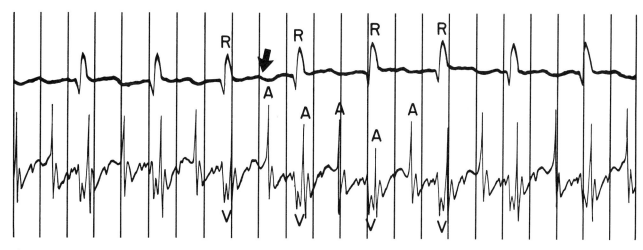

Fig. 7–18. Supraventricular tachycardia in a cat with hypertrophic cardiomyopathy. P waves could not be identified on a lead II electrocardiogram (top strip). Intra-atrial electrocardiography (bottom strip) made identification of the atrial P waves *(A)* easier. Note the ventricular complexes *(V)* that are simultaneous with the QRS complexes *(R)*. With the atrial rate 450 beats/min (2:1 conduction) and at a regular frequency, atrial flutter is the likely diagnosis. The flutter waves *(arrow)* are flat because of the fast paper speed of 100 mm/sec. (From Tilley, L.P.: Vet. Clin. North Am., 7:273, 1977; reprinted with permission.)

Atrial fibrillation

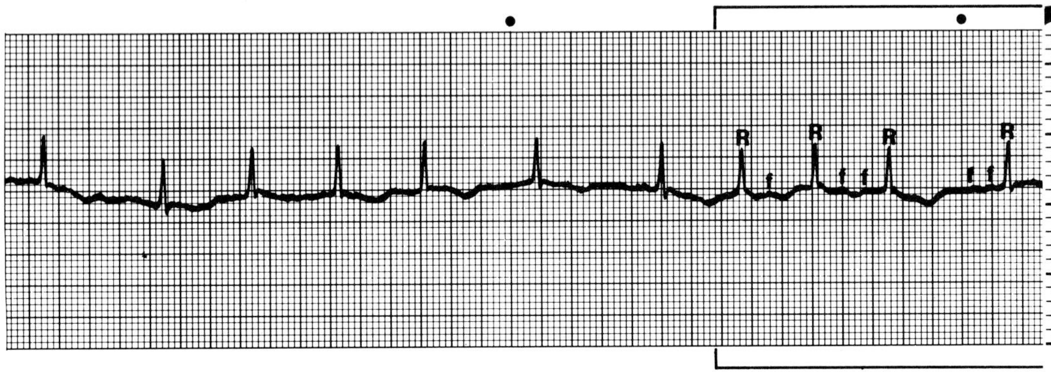

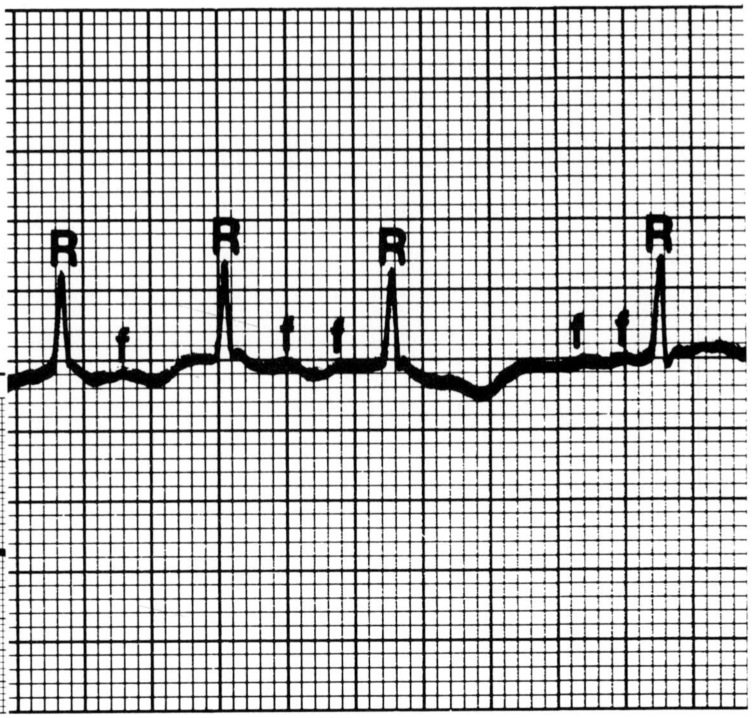

Fig. 7–19. Atrial fibrillation with an average ventricular rate of 200 beats/min in a cat with hypertrophic cardiomyopathy. Note the total irregularity of the R waves and the absence of P waves. The P waves are replaced by f waves.

Four possible mechanisms for atrial fibrillation include: (1) a circus movement of electrical impulses in a ring of tissue between the two vena cavae, (2) unifocal atrial impulse formation, (3) multiple re-entry, and (4) multifocal atrial impulse formation. One or a combination of these may be responsible.[10,19,20]

A reduction in blood flow to the coronary arteries (as much as 40%) and to the cerebral circulation (as much as 20%) can occur with atrial fibrillation.[21] The loss of the "atrial kick" combined with the rapid heart rate, may substantially reduce cardiac output and cause congestive heart failure. A rapid ventricular response in atrial fibrillation may also cause a 20% reduction in renal blood flow, producing oliguria and azotemia.[22]

Atrial fibrillation is rare in cats and is primarily associated with hypertrophic cardiomyopathy.[4,5,23] Hypertrophic cardiomyopathy causes a chronic increasing resistance to left ventricular filling, eventually resulting in severe left atrial enlargement and atrial fibrillation.

Electrocardiographic features

1. Atrial and ventricular rates are rapid and totally irregular.
2. The normal sinus P waves are replaced by fibrillating f waves.
3. The QRS configuration is normal (same as for the sinus com-

plexes) or wide and bizarre owing to an intraventricular conduction defect (especially anterior fascicular block) or ventricular pre-excitation.

4. In the P-QRS the ventricular rate is totally irregular because the AV junction allows only a limited number of fibrillatory waves to be conducted to the ventricles.

Associated conditions[13,14]

1. Same conditions that cause the other atrial arrhythmias, those causing marked atrial enlargement the most common
2. Hypertrophic cardiomyopathy
3. Restrictive cardiomyopathy

Treatment (See Chapter 10)

1. As previously discussed, digoxin should be administered with caution in cats with hypertrophic cardiomyopathy. It is not contraindicated in cats with hypertrophic cardiomyopathy and atrial fibrillation. Digoxin and propranolol should be given together to slow the ventricular rate.[24] Digoxin should be given first and then propranolol because of the negative inotropic effects of the latter.

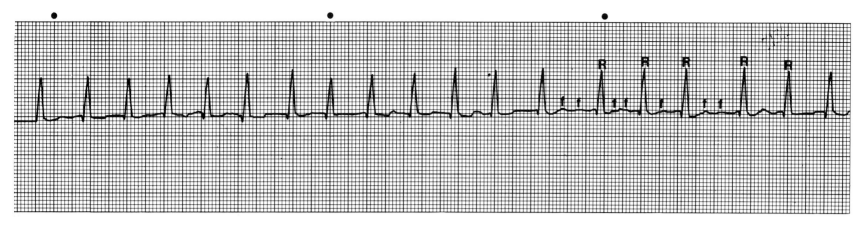

Fig. 7–20. Atrial fibrillation with an average ventricular rate of 240 to 260 beats/min. The ventricular rhythm is markedly irregular. The QRS complexes vary in amplitude, since numerous supraventricular impulses arrive so early that parts of the ventricle are not yet completely recovered.

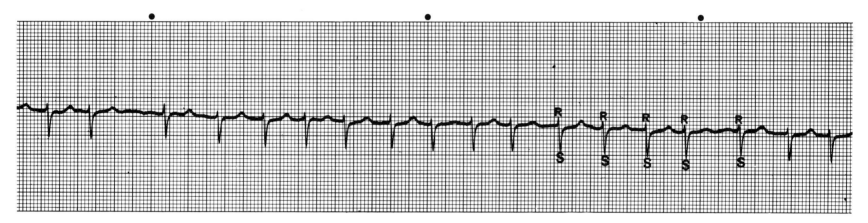

Fig. 7–21. Atrial fibrillation with a rapid ventricular rate averaging 250 beats/min. The other leads (not shown) were compatible with anterior fascicular block and/or left ventricular hypertrophy, the reason for the large S waves in this lead II strip.

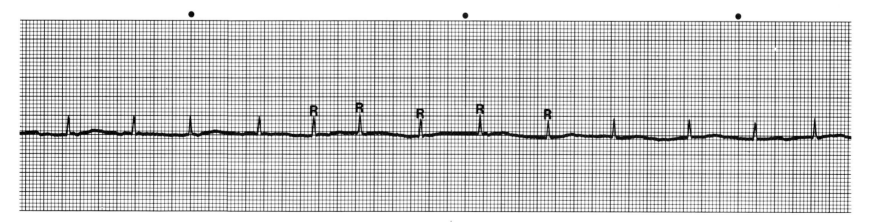

Fig. 7–22. Atrial fibrillation. The ventricular rate has been reduced to an average of 180 beats/min with digoxin and propranolol. Digoxin and propranolol prolong the refractory period in the AV junction, allowing fewer fibrillatory waves to reach the ventricles.

Escape rhythms

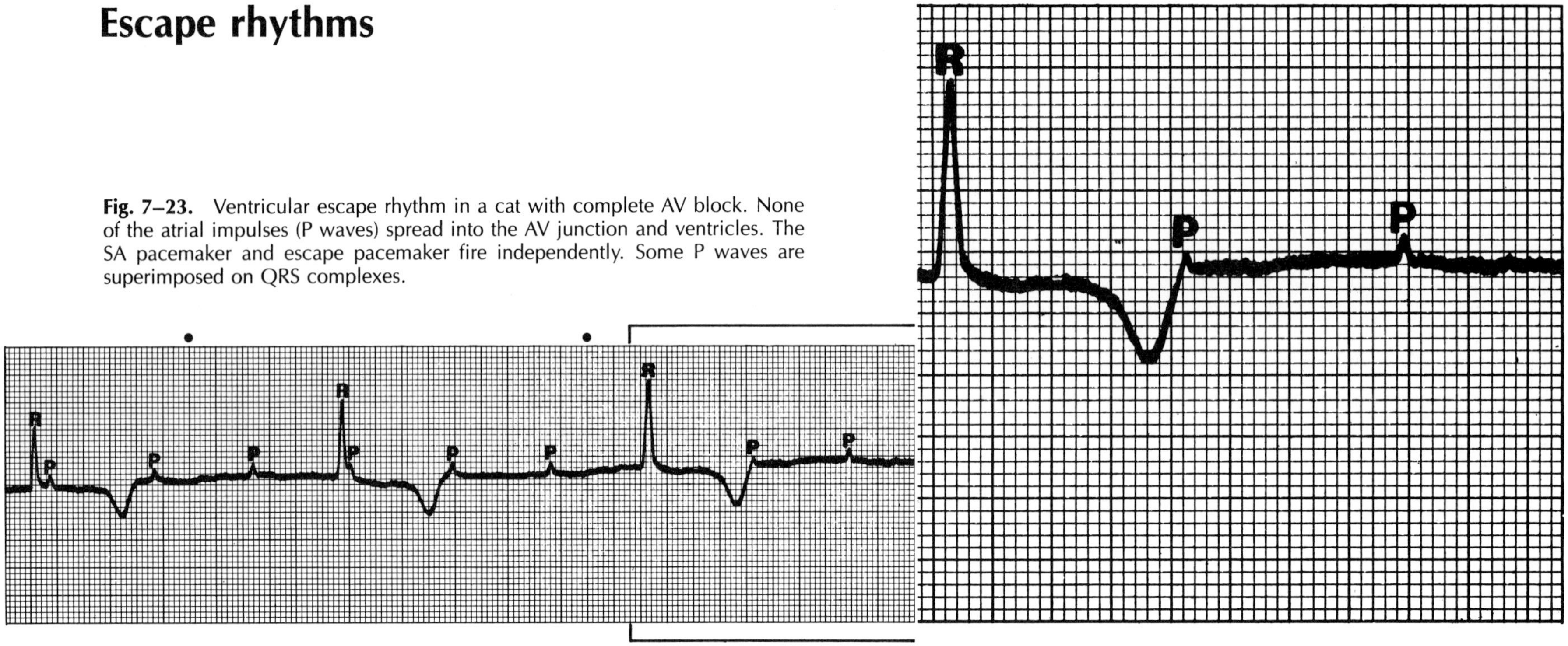

Fig. 7–23. Ventricular escape rhythm in a cat with complete AV block. None of the atrial impulses (P waves) spread into the AV junction and ventricles. The SA pacemaker and escape pacemaker fire independently. Some P waves are superimposed on QRS complexes.

Escape rhythms occur when the pacemaker with the highest automaticity (usually the SA node) either slows down or stops. The intrinsic pacemaker activity of the lower regions of the heart rescues the heart rhythm after a pause in the dominant rhythm. A single spontaneous impulse from a slower subsidiary pacemaker appearing after a pause is called an escape complex. If the subsidiary pacemaker temporarily takes over the role of the cardiac pacemaker, the rhythm is known as an escape rhythm.[25] Escape complexes are most often of AV junctional or ventricular origin. When ventricular escape impulses control the rhythm, the term *idioventricular rhythm* or *idionodal rhythm* is used instead of ventricular escape rhythm.

Electrocardiographic features

Junctional escape rhythms

1. The heart rate is slow. Escape complexes follow a pause longer than the normal cycle length (R-R interval). Rhythm is regular when the AV junction persists as the dominant pacemaker.
2. The P wave is usually negative.
3. The QRS configuration is usually normal.
4. The P wave may precede, be superimposed on, or follow the QRS.

Ventricular escape rhythm (idioventricular rhythm)

1. The heart rate is usually slow. Escape complexes follow a pause longer than the normal sinus cycle length. An idioventricular rhythm is generally regular, with the rate often less than 100 beats/min. The

subsidiary pacemakers in cats seem to discharge more rapidly than in dogs.
2. P waves are usually not present, unless complete AV block or high-grade second-degree AV block exists. The P waves will then be unrelated and precede, be hidden within, or follow the ectopic QRS complexes.
3. The QRS configuration is wide and bizarre, similar to that of VPCs.
4. No relationship exists between the P wave and the QRS complex.

Associated conditions

1. All the causes of sinus bradycardia and AV block (An idioventricular escape rhythm is seen in complete AV block since impulses usually cannot originate from the junctional region.)

Treatment (See Chapter 10)

1. Treat the underlying cause of the arrhythmia, since the escape rhythm is a secondary phenomenon. The actual escape complex or rhythm should *not* be treated. It is a safety mechanism for maintaining cardiac output.
2. Atropine or glycopyrrolate is often indicated. Artificial pacing is used if the arrhythmia is resistant to drug treatment. Causative drugs (e.g., digoxin, propranolol, or anesthetics) should be discontinued.

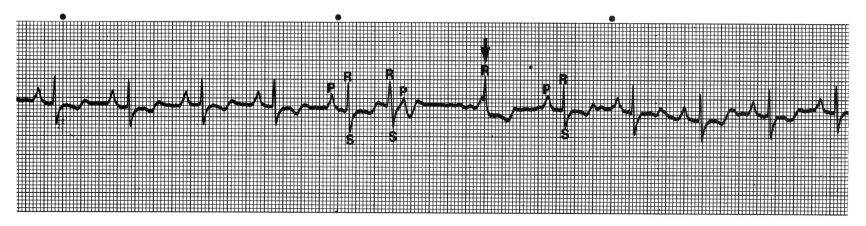

Fig. 7–24. Blocked sinus P waves due to imcomplete recovery of the AV junction after a premature impulse (sixth complex). A long pause is created, causing one escape complex (arrow) to occur. A sinus P wave is superimposed on the escape complex, and its impulse is blocked.

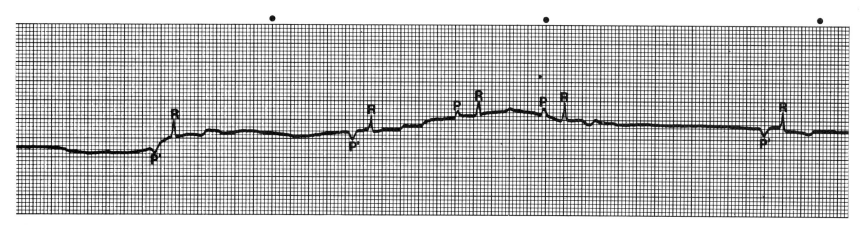

Fig. 7–25. AV junctional escape complexes in a cat with a severe sinus bradycardia and sinus arrest. The inverted P' waves precede the QRS complexes. Atropine later increased the heart rate as well as eliminated the secondary AV junctional escape complexes.

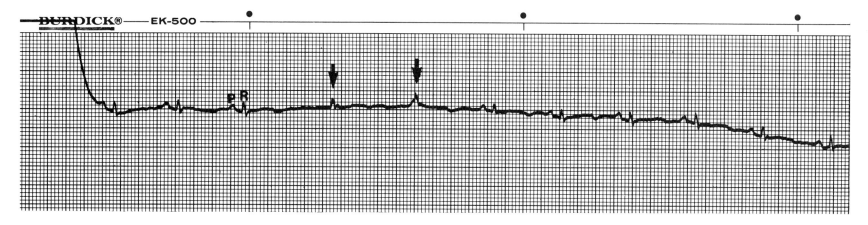

Fig. 7–26. Two escape complexes (arrows) with origin close to the AV junction during a pause in the dominant sinus rhythm in a cat under anesthesia. The sinus rate increased after the anesthesia was stopped, and the escape complexes also were eliminated. Baseline movement is present at first part of tracing.

Ventricular premature complexes

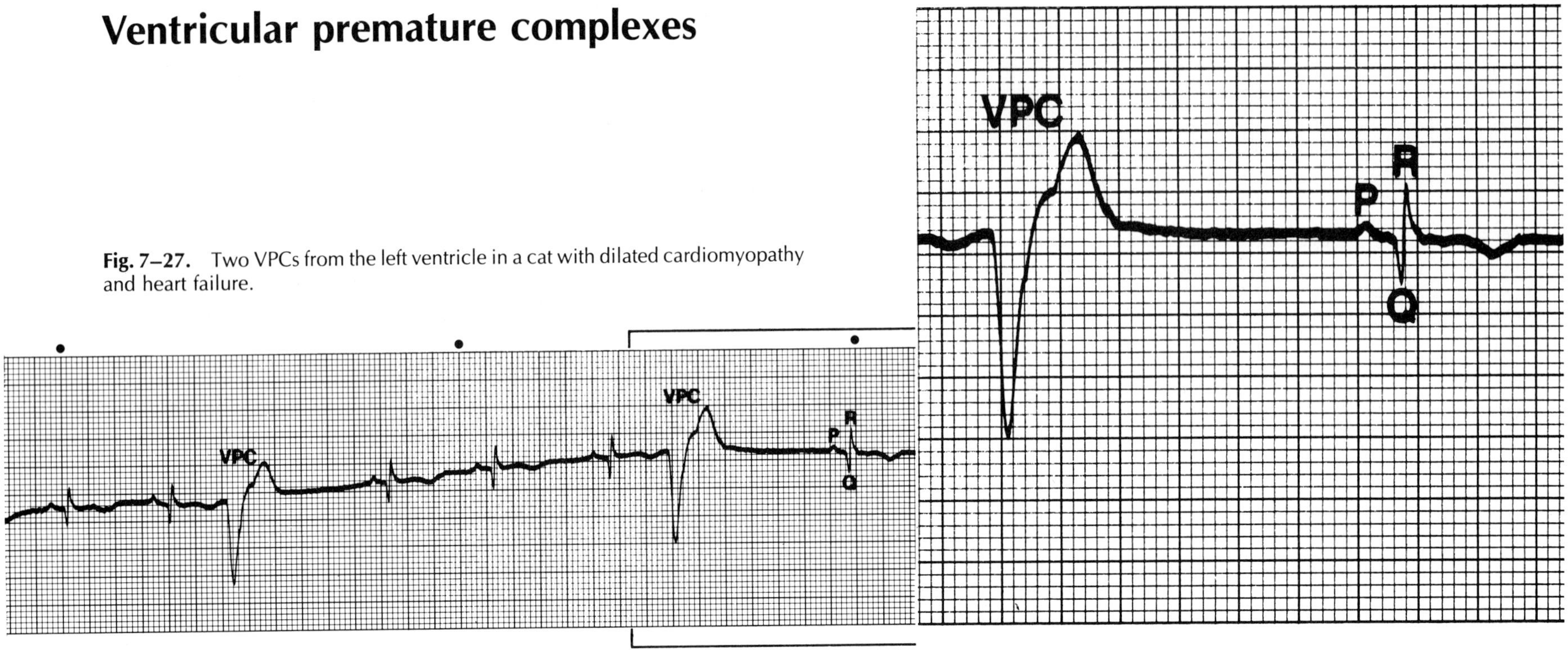

Fig. 7–27. Two VPCs from the left ventricle in a cat with dilated cardiomyopathy and heart failure.

Ventricular premature complexes (VPCs or ventricular premature contractions) are impulses that arise from an ectopic focus in the ventricles. They spread through both ventricles with delay, causing a bizarre widened QRS complex. As in the dog, VPCs in the cat are the most frequent type of abnormal rhythm.[16]

Two possible mechanisms for VPCs are: (1) theory of re-entry (see Chapters 9 and 12) and (2) increased automaticity. Occasional VPCs seldom produce clinical signs. Physical examination usually reveals a pulse deficit during a VPC, as the cardiac output is temporarily increased. A reduction in cardiac output is of greater significance when the cat has pre-existing heart disease.

Electrocardiographic features

1. The heart rate is usually normal and the rhythm irregular owing to the premature QRS complex that disrupts the normal ventricular rhythm.

2. P waves that can be seen are of normal configuration.

3. The QRS complex is premature, bizarre, and often of large amplitude. The T wave is directed opposite the main deflection in the QRS.

4. In the P-QRS complex the VPCs are not associated with the P wave. The independent normal P wave may precede, be within, or follow the VPC.

5. A compensatory pause usually follows a VPC. The R-R interval between two sinus complexes enclosing the VPC is slightly greater than the R-R interval between three sinus complexes.

Associated conditions[13,14]

There are numerous causes of VPCs: primary cardiac diseases, secondary cardiac diseases, and drugs.

1. Cardiac: congestive heart failure (especially in dilated cardiomyopathy[5]), myocardial infarction,[26,27] neoplasia,[28] traumatic myocarditis, bacterial endomyocarditis[6]

2. Secondary: increased sympathetic tone from excitement,[29] hypoxia,[30] anemia, uremia, pyometra, faulty placement of the venous catheter tip in the right ventricle

3. Drugs: digitalis, anesthetic agents, propylene glycol in intravenous diazepam and phenytoin[15]

Treatment (See Chapter 10)

1. Treat the underlying condition. VPCs rarely require aggressive treatment in the cat since they tend to decrease and often disappear spontaneously. Propranolol administered intravenously in small increments may have a possible quinidine-like effect for decreasing ventricular ectopic activity. The drug should be used with caution, especially in cardiac failure.[12]

2. Supportive measures are important; acid-base and electrolyte abnormalities should be corrected.

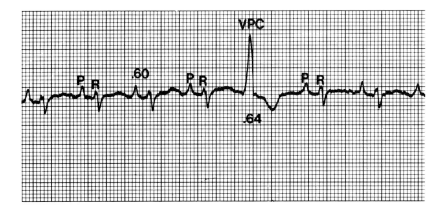

Fig. 7–28. VPC that probably originates in the right ventricle. A compensatory pause is present. The R-R interval (0.64 sec) between the two sinus complexes enclosing the VPC is greater than the R-R interval (0.6 sec) between three adjacent sinus complexes.

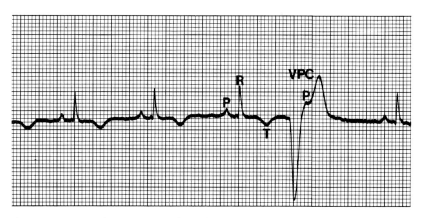

Fig. 7–29. VPC that originates from the left ventricle. Note the superimposed P wave. The atrial impulse is not conducted since the ventricles are in a refractory period.

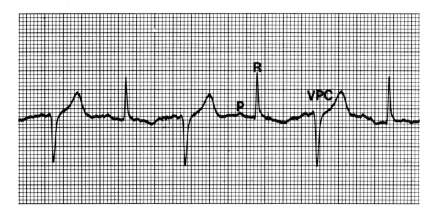

Fig. 7–30. Ventricular bigeminy. Every other complex is a VPC from the same focus. Each is coupled (interval the same between it and the adjacent sinus complex) to the preceding normal complex.

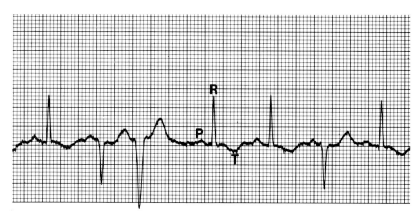

Fig. 7–31. Multiform ventricular ectopic complexes (second, third, and sixth complexes). The second and sixth complexes are of different shape from the third and follow the simultaneous activation of the ventricles from the SA node and the ventricular ectopic foci. The second and sixth complexes both have preceding P waves. These two fusion complexes are late diastolic extrasystoles.

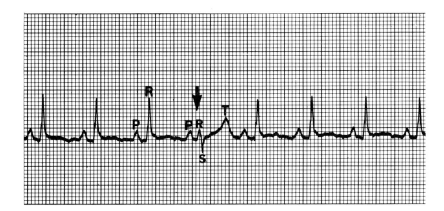

Fig. 7–32. Ventricular fusion complex (arrow). These occur when the ventricles are activated simultaneously by impulses from both the SA node and the ventricular ectopic foci. The result is a complex that has a normal P-R interval and a QRS complex intermediate in configuration. (From Tilley, L.P.: Vet. Clin. North Am., 7:273, 1977; reprinted with permission.)

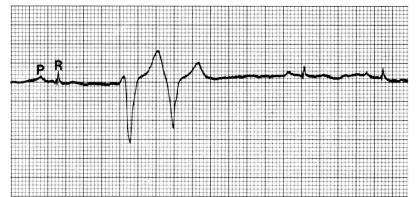

Fig. 7–33. Paired ventricular ectopic complexes occurring late in diastole. The first complex is followed by a second early ectopic complex also from the ventricle. This can represent a serious condition since the second ectopic impulse could easily progress to ventricular tachycardia or ventricular fibrillation.

Ventricular tachycardia

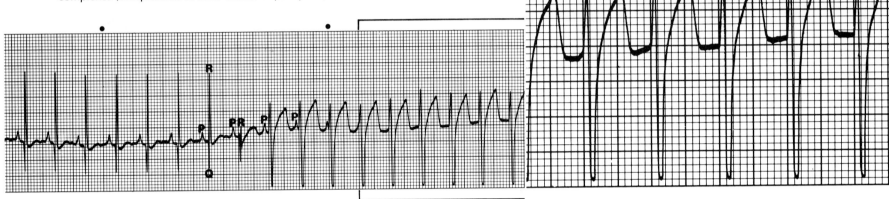

Fig. 7–34. Ventricular tachycardia at a rate of 150 beats/min initiated by a ventricular fusion complex. The first seven complexes are all normal sinus complexes. This cat had dilated cardiomyopathy and heart failure. During the ventricular tachycardia, the P waves have no constant relationship to the ventricular complexes (independent of each other). Paper speed, 25 mm/sec.

Ventricular tachycardia implies a series of repetitive VPCs that are usually of sudden onset. It may be intermittent (three or more VPCs in a row) or persistent (all complexes originating in the ventricles).

The absolute distinction between ventricular tachycardia (at various ventricular ectopic rates) and idioventricular rhythm has not been established in the cat. Ventricular tachycardia is usually above 150 beats/min; an idioventricular escape rhythm, below 100. A slow ventricular tachycardia (sometimes termed *enhanced ventricular rhythm*) probably results from an increased automaticity of certain specialized conducting fibers; by contrast, ventricular tachycardia is caused by re-entry or other mechanisms.[31] The upper rate limits for the various ventricular ectopic rhythms are obviously arbitrary.

Electrocardiographic features

1. The ventricular rate is usually rapid (above 150 beats/min), and the rhythm regular.
2. P waves that are seen are of normal configuration.
3. The QRS complexes are wide and bizarre. Ventricular fusion and capture complexes occur commonly.
4. The QRS complexes are independent of the P waves. P waves may precede, be hidden within, or follow QRS complexes.

Associated conditions[14]

1. VPCs (Ventricular tachycardia is usually a manifestation of significant organic heart disease.)

2. Severe ventricular arrhythmias occurring 2 to 12 hours after acute myocardial infarction,[27] ventricular tachycardia observed after asphyxia in cats under halothane anesthesia,[30] ventricular tachycardia reported with feline cardiomyopathy,[5,16,32] ventricular tachycardia with digitalis[33]

Treatment *(See Chapter 10 and Fig. 10–16)*

1. Treatment should begin as soon as possible. The underlying condition should always be treated.
2. Supportive measures are important; acid-base and electrolyte abnormalities should be corrected.
3. Lidocaine must be used with extreme caution in cats since they are particularly susceptible to its neurotoxic effects.[12] Lidocaine can cause severe sinus bradycardia and sinus arrest. Propranolol can be an effective antiarrhythmic agent and is preferred by some clinicians over lidocaine. The other drugs used for ventricular tachycardia in dogs, quinidine and procainamide, are not recommended in cats.
4. A thump delivered to the precordium with a clenched fist may be successful, especially in an emergency when propranolol is not available or would be contraindicated.[18] This is a commonly used resuscitative maneuver during cardiac arrest.[34] *(See Chapter 11.)*

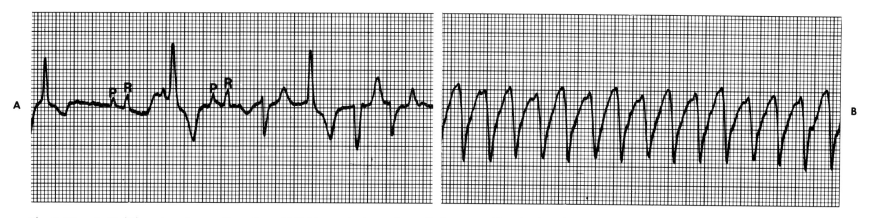

Fig. 7–35. **A,** Multiform (varying configuration of VPCs) ventricular tachycardia in a cat with episodes of fainting. The second and fourth complexes are capture complexes. **B,** The ventricular tachycardia is now an "active" rhythm resulting from the repetitive firing of one ectopic ventricular focus at a rapid rate. A supraventricular tachycardia with abnormal QRS complexes should be considered, but the contour of the capture complexes in **A** is different from that of the ectopic complexes in **B.**

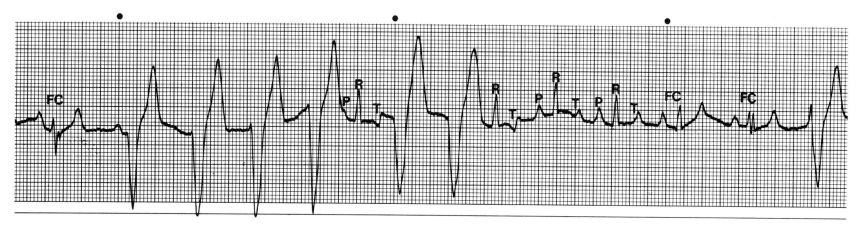

Fig. 7–36. Intermittent ventricular tachycardia in a cat with traumatic myocarditis from an eight-story fall. The ventricular fusion complexes *(FC)* and ventricular capture complexes *(P-R-T)* are the two most reliable criteria for the diagnosis of ventricular tachycardia.

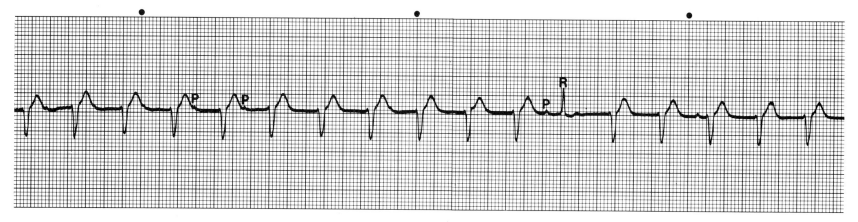

Fig. 7–37. Ventricular tachycardia at a rate of 225 beats/min in a cat with endomyocarditis. The sixth complex from the end of the strip is a capture complex. A normal sinus impulse has reached the AV junction in a recovered state, capturing the ventricles for one complex. No constant relationship exists between the sinus P waves and ventricular complexes; 0.5 cm = 1 mv.

Ventricular fibrillation and ventricular asystole

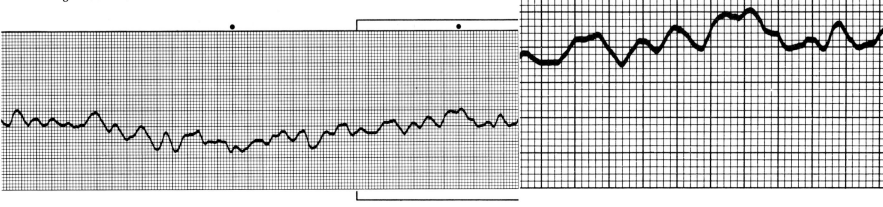

Fig. 7–38. "Coarse" ventricular fibrillation.

Ventricular fibrillation and ventricular asystole both represent *cardiac arrest*. If the ventricular rhythm is not restored in 3 to 4 minutes, irreversible brain damage can occur. Cardiac arrest can also be detected by the dissociation between a recordable electrocardiogram (P-QRS-T complexes) and no palpable femoral pulse, termed *electrical-mechanical dissociation*.

Electrocardiographic features

Ventricular fibrillation

1. The heart rate is rapid with irregular, chaotic, and bizarre waves. Ventricular flutter, by contrast, is a rhythmic series of bizarre and uniform undulating waves which eventually progress to ventricular fibrillation.
2. P waves cannot be recognized.
3. The QRS and T deflections cannot be recognized.
4. There are two types of fibrillation: one with large *(coarse)* oscillations and the other with oscillations that are small and *fine*.

Ventricular asystole

1. This condition may be caused by severe sinus arrest or SA block or by severe third-degree AV block (without an escape rhythm).
2. There is no ventricular rhythm. P waves are present if complete AV block exists.
3. P waves are of normal configuration with complete AV block.
4. No QRS complexes are seen.

Associated conditions[34]

1. Ventricular fibrillation: shock, anoxia, myocardial damage (trauma or infarction), acid-base imbalances, hyperkalemia (serum potassium above 12 mEq/L[30]), anesthetic agents, myocarditis with VPC during the apex of the T wave of the preceding complex
2. Ventricular asystole: ventricular fibrillation and complete AV block (Ventricular asystole and especially electrical-mechanical dissociation often result when a severe underlying electrolyte and acid-base imbalance, particularly hyperkalemia in urethral obstruction, is not treated.)

Treatment[34] *(See Chapter 11, Fig. 11–50, and Table 11–2)*

1. Initiate the "A-B-C-D-E" of cardiac resuscitation.
2. The basic cause of cardiac arrest should be treated, e.g., regular insulin with dextrose, intravenous fluids and bicarbonate for severe hyperkalemia. It has been shown that cats with ventricular fibrillation can recover spontaneously[30] since their small heart size decreases the possibility of maintaining the fibrillation.
3. For ventricular fibrillation, defibrillate with direct-current shock (10 to 50 watt-seconds); repeat if ineffective. Epinephrine and calcium chloride can be used to "coarsen" the fibrillation.
4. For ventricular asystole, specific drugs include epinephrine, sodium bicarbonate and calcium chloride, atropine sulfate (for severe sinus arrest), and intravenous or intracardiac isoproterenol (for severe AV block).
5. For electrical-mechanical dissociation, use dopamine hydrochloride, epinephrine, or calcium chloride.

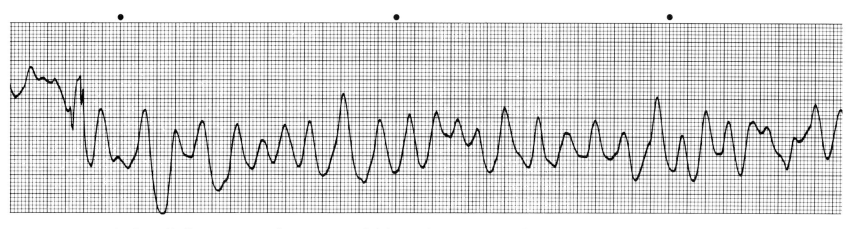

Fig. 7–39. Ventricular flutter-fibrillation in a cat with severe myocardial damage from an 11-story fall. The complexes are very wide, bizarre, tall, and rapid.

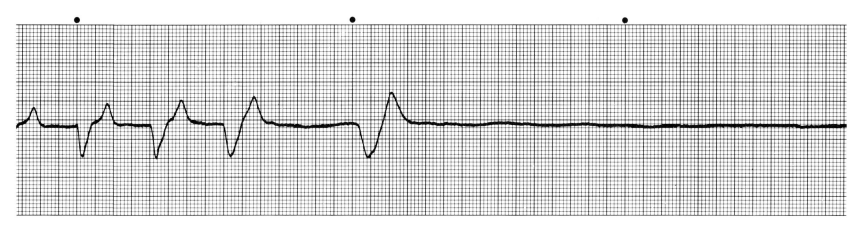

Fig. 7–40. Ventricular asystole in a cat with severe hyperkalemia (11 mEq/L) from urethral obstruction. No P waves or QRS complexes are seen after four wide and bizarre QRS complexes (atrial standstill with delayed ventricular conduction).

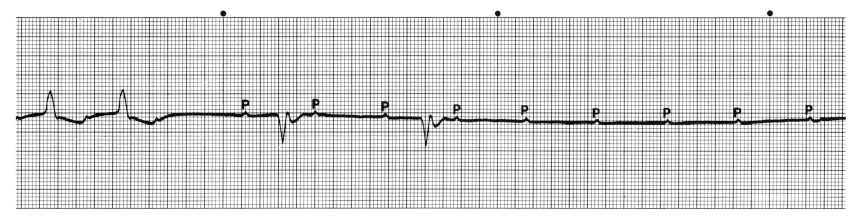

Fig. 7–41. Ventricular asystole in a cat with complete heart block from hypertrophic cardiomyopathy. Only P waves are seen for 2 seconds after the fourth ventricular escape complex.

223

Sinoatrial block (sinus arrest)

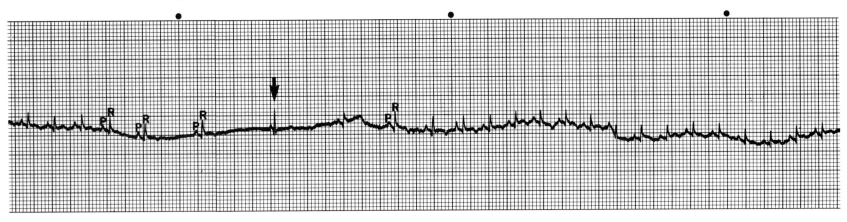

Fig. 7–42. Intermittent sinus arrest in a cat with an upper respiratory infection. After the first five sinus complexes, pauses occur with an escape complex (arrow). A sinus P wave just happens to precede the complex at a short P-R interval. Paper speed, 25 mm/sec.

Sinus arrest is the failure of impulses to be formed within the SA node because the automaticity in the node has been depressed. SA block, the same electrocardiographic pattern, represents a disturbance of conduction from a regularly firing SA node. The two are difficult to differentiate.

Electrocardiographic features

1. The heart rate can be variable. The rhythm is regular with pauses demonstrating a lack of P-QRS-T complexes. The pauses are twice or greater than twice the normal R-R interval; escape complexes are possible.
2. The P wave and QRS complex are usually of normal configuration.
3. The P-R interval is essentially constant.

Associated conditions

SA block (sinus arrest) is rare in the cat. Causes include the following:

1. Irritation of the vagus nerve, e.g., surgical manipulation, thoracic neoplasm, severe respiratory disorders, and vomiting (increased vagal tone)
2. Pathologic conditions of the atria: dilatation, fibrosis of the SA node, cardiomyopathy, drug toxicity (propranolol, anesthetics, and especially digitalis), and electrolyte imbalances

Treatment *(See Chapter 10)*

1. The underlying cause should be treated, the causative drug removed, and atropine or glycopyrrolate given if the animal is symptomatic.

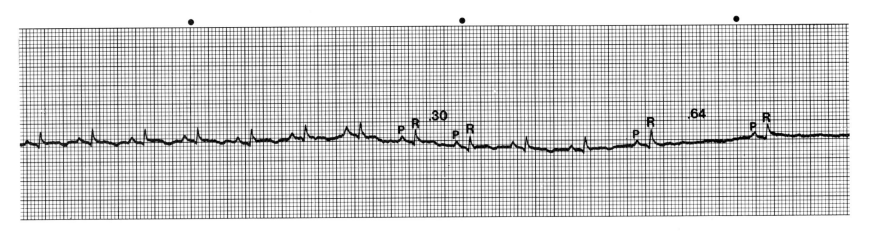

Fig. 7–43. Sinus arrest or block in a cat during anesthesia. The one long pause (0.64 sec) is greater than twice the normal R-R interval (0.30 sec).

First-degree atrioventricular block

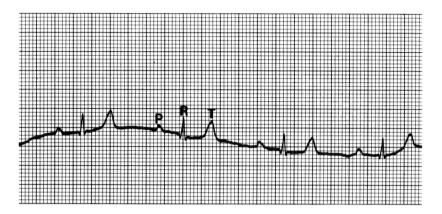

Fig. 7–44. First-degree AV block in a cat with hyperkalemia (serum potassium, 7.5 mEq/L). The P-R interval is 0.12 second (6 boxes). Note the large T waves.

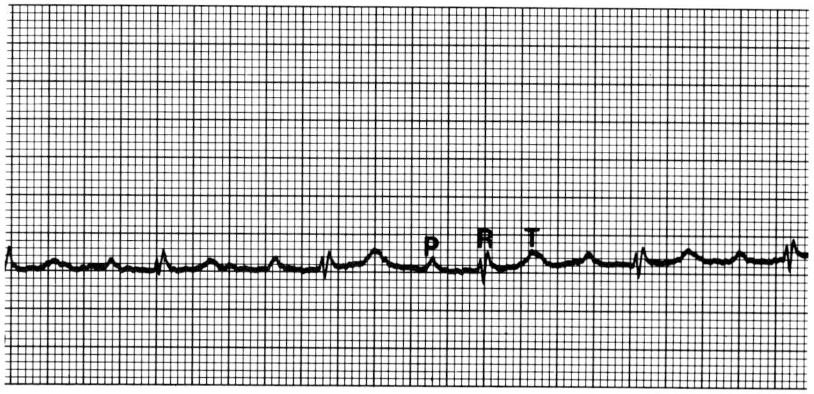

Fig. 7–45. First-degree AV block in a cat with the effects of propranolol. Note the slow heart rate of 140 beats/min and the long P-R interval of 0.14 second (7 boxes).

A delay or interruption in conduction of a supraventricular impulse through the AV junction and bundle of His is called AV block. There are three types or degrees: (1) first degree, a delay in conduction, (2) second degree, intermittent interruptions of conduction, and (3) third degree, complete or permanent interruption of conduction.

Since the P-R interval represents the total time of impulse conduction from the atria to the ventricles, the exact site of the delay is not found on the electrocardiogram. Bundle of His recordings can be done to delineate the exact site of delay or block. A prolonged P-R interval with a normal QRS complex often indicates a delay in conduction within the AV node or His bundle. With a widened QRS complex, the delay is often beyond the His bundle.[35]

Electrocardiographic features

1. The rate and rhythm depend on the presence of other arrhythmias.

2. The P wave and QRS are usually of normal configuration.

3. In the P-QRS the P-R interval is longer than 0.09 second. This applies only to a sinus rhythm and not to an APC (which often has a long P-R interval, a physiologic first-degree AV block).

Associated conditions[14]

First degree AV block may occur in cats that are clinically normal and healthy. The P-R interval tends to lengthen with age and shorten with rapid heart rates.

1. Digitalis intoxication[36,37]
2. Propranolol

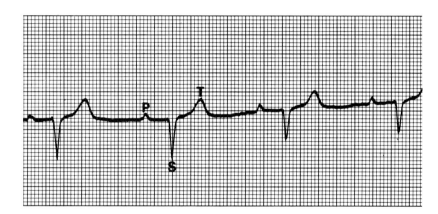

Fig. 7–46. First-degree heart block (P-R interval, 0.14 sec) in combination with an intraventricular conduction defect. The block may be caused by the presence of conduction delay in the other branches or fascicles.

3. All the causes of hyperkalemia and hypokalemia
4. Cardiomyopathy (AV fibrosis); especially dilated form

Treatment

1. Treat the underlying condition. Observe for signs of progression to higher degrees of AV block if an intraventricular conduction defect also exists.

Second-degree AV block

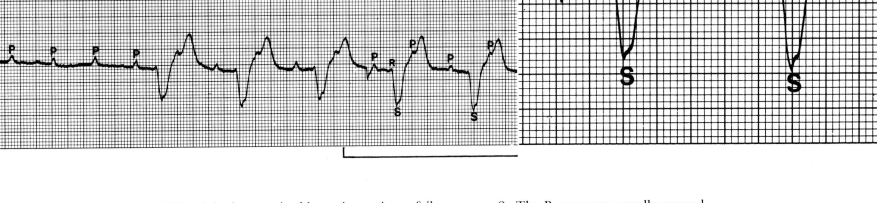

Fig. 7–47. Advanced AV block (type B) with right bundle branch block secondary to metastatic lymphosarcoma. Every other P wave is conducted (2:1 block) after the first three P waves.

Second-degree AV block is characterized by an intermittent failure or disturbance of AV conduction. One or more P waves are not followed by QRS-T complexes. Second-degree AV block can be classified into two types: Mobitz type I and Mobitz type II. As in the dog, the classification can also be based on the QRS duration: type A (lesion above the His bundle), with a normal QRS duration, and type B (lesion below the His bundle) with a wide QRS.[31] Experience at this time indicates that the clinical course and prognosis can be roughly estimated by studying the QRS duration. The conduction lesions in the cat are often quite variable and may be located in the AV node or His-Purkinje system or below the His bundle bifurcation.[38]

Electrocardiographic features

Mobitz type I, usually type A

1. The ventricular rate is slower than the atrial rate because of blocked P waves. The rhythm is usually irregular in the typical form. The R-R interval becomes progressively shorter as the P-R interval becomes longer until a P wave is blocked.

2. The P wave and QRS complex are usually of normal configuration. Bundle branches have no conduction disturbances.

3. In the typical Mobitz type I (also called Wenckebach phenomenon), there is a progressive prolongation of the P-R interval with successive complexes until a P wave is blocked.

Mobitz type II, usually type B

1. The ventricular rate is slower than the atrial rate because of blocked P waves.

2. The P waves are usually normal.

3. The QRS complexes are often of abnormal configuration, having features of bundle branch block.

4. The P-R interval is always constant.

In the majority of our cases, Mobitz type II AV block (type B) has progressed to higher degrees of atrioventricular block: either advanced or complete block (Figs. 7–47 and 7–49). Two or more consecutive blocked P waves are called advanced AV block. The occurrence of ventricular capture complexes proves that the AV block is not complete.

Associated conditions[14]

1. Supraventricular tachycardia, e.g., atrial tachycardia or atrial flutter (The block is physiologic.)
2. Increased vagal tone
3. Hypertrophic cardiomyopathy[17] (Infiltrative cardiomyopathy secondary to tumor metastasis is possible.[28])

Treatment (See Chapter 10 and Fig. 10–18)

1. The majority of cases usually develop an advanced or complete AV block, with accompanying clinical signs (e.g., fainting and weakness). These cases are usually resistant to medical management, and artificial pacing is the only treatment.

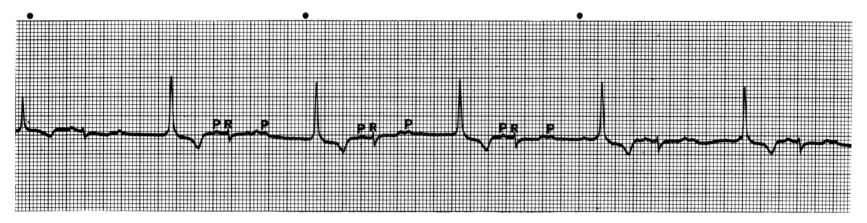

Fig. 7—48. Second-degree AV block. The P-R interval is constant in all conducted beats. A blocked P wave and a ventricular escape complex (large positive configuration) follow each conducted beat. Blocked P waves are also superimposed on the escape rhythm.

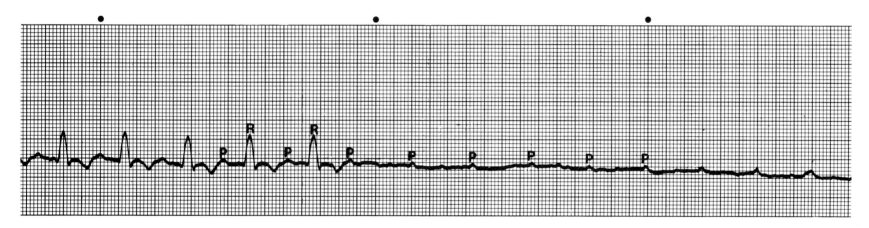

Fig. 7—49. Type B advanced AV block produced by carotid sinus massage (vagal stimulation). The first five complexes are conducted P-QRS complexes. The QRS complexes are wide (0.07 sec), with a prolonged P-R interval (0.12 sec). Normal automaticity of the AV junction and ventricles may also be lacking since no escape complexes occur. Hypertrophic cardiomyopathy was found at necropsy.

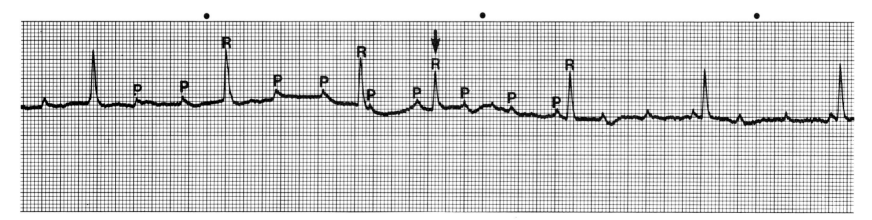

Fig. 7—50. Advanced AV block in a cat with hypertrophic cardiomyopathy and episodes of fainting. Numerous P waves are blocked, producing an escape rhythm that resembles complete heart block. The escape rhythm (AV junctional region) is interrupted by a ventricular capture complex (arrow).

Third-degree AV block (complete block)

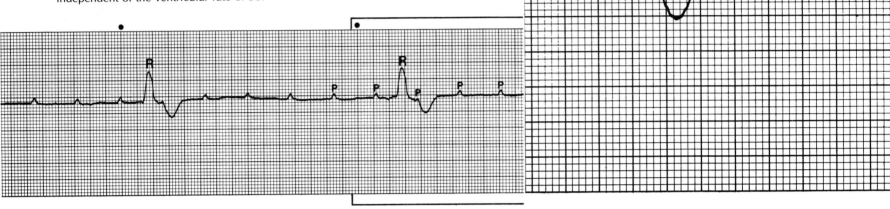

Fig. 7–51. Complete heart block. The P waves occur at a rate of 210/min, independent of the ventricular rate of 30.

Complete AV block occurs when AV conduction is absent and the ventricles are under the control of pacemakers below the area of the block. The atria are thus activated by one pacemaker, usually the SA node, and the ventricles by another. No relationship exists between the P waves and the QRS complexes.

The clinical signs associated with complete heart block are syncope and sometimes congestive heart failure. The fainting episodes are caused by either sudden asystole or the development of ventricular tachyarrhythmias, which lead to circulatory arrest. The location of the pacemaking site to which the ventricles respond will have an effect on heart rate and finally on cardiac output. The heart rate is usually very slow which can be dangerous when the pacemaker site is located in the lower portions of the ventricles.

Electrocardiographic features

1. The ventricular rate is slower than the atrial rate (more P waves than QRS complexes).
2. P waves are usually of normal configuration.
3. The QRS is wide and bizarre when the rescuing pacemaker is located in either the ventricle or the lower AV junction with bundle branch block. It is normal when the escape pacemaker is located in the lower AV junction (above the His bundle bifurcation).
4. The P waves bear no constant relationship to the QRS complexes. The P-P and R-R intervals are relatively constant.

Associated conditions[14]

A review of eight cases with complete AV block from The Animal Medical Center included the following causes:

1. Hypertrophic cardiomyopathy (six cats) (Complete heart block from hypertrophic cardiomyopathy has been reported in man.[39])
2. Infiltrative cardiomyopathy (one cat with metastatic lymphosarcoma)
3. Dilated cardiomyopathy (one cat)

Three cats with complete AV block have been reported in the literature: one with dilated cardiomyopathy,[16] one with coronary arteriosclerosis and myocardial fibrosis,[40] and one with no necropsy diagnosis.[41]

Syncope and sudden death have been associated with AV conduction defects.[16] Degeneration or fibrosis of the AV node and its bundle branches associated with endocardial and myocardial fibrosis was consistently observed in the hearts of 63 cats with cardiomyopathy.[38]

Treatment (See Chapter 10 and Fig. 10–18)

1. Treatment with drugs is usually futile. Artificial pacing is necessary, especially in symptomatic animals.[12] The smaller size of cats makes pacemaker implantation difficult. Ventricular antiarrhythmic drugs are contraindicated because they tend to suppress lower escape foci.

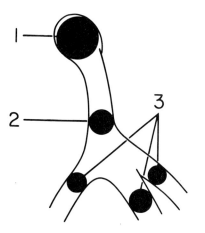

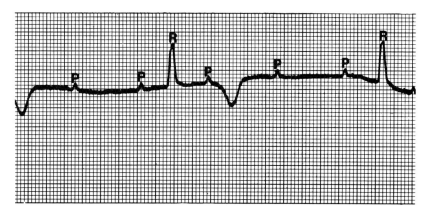

Fig. 7–52. The three possible sites of lesions in complete heart block: *1*, AV node; *2*, bundle of His; *3*, right bundle branch and left bundle branch (anterior and posterior fascicles).

Fig. 7–53. Complete heart block in a cat with fainting episodes due to hypertrophic cardiomyopathy. The P waves are totally independent of the R waves.

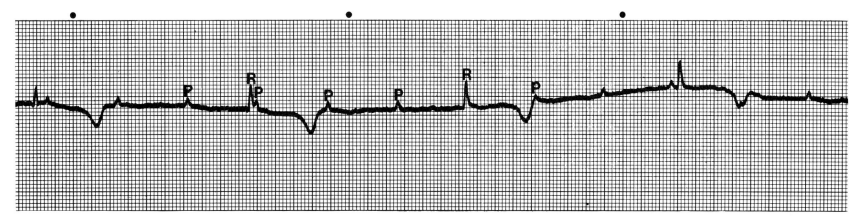

Fig. 7–54. Complete heart block. The P waves occur at a rate of 160/min, independent of the ventricular rate of 50. Because the QRS complex is of normal duration and configuration, the ventricular pacemaker must be above the His bundle bifurcation.

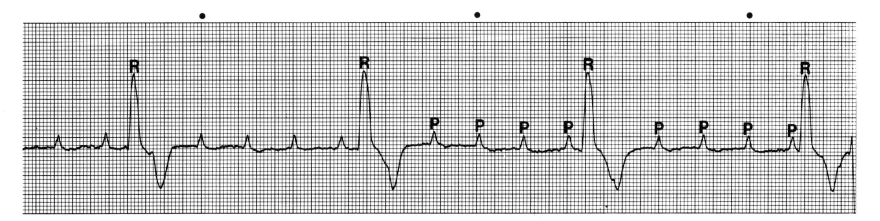

Fig. 7–55. Complete heart block. The P waves occur at a rate of 240/min, independent of the ventricular rate of 48. The QRS configuration is a left bundle branch block pattern.

Ventricular pre-excitation and the Wolff-Parkinson-White syndrome

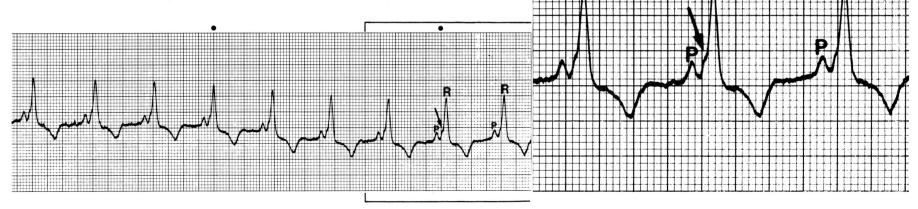

Fig. 7–56. Ventricular pre-excitation in a cat with episodes of fainting. The P waves are normal, the P-R interval is short, and the QRS complex is wide; delta waves (arrow) are present.

Ventricular *pre-excitation* occurs when impulses originating in the SA node or atrium activate a portion of the ventricles prematurely through an accessory pathway without going through the AV node. The Wolff-Parkinson-White syndrome (WPW) consists of ventricular pre-excitation with episodes of paroxysmal supraventricular tachycardia[25] (Chapter 12).

The sinus or atrial impulses conducted via the accessory pathway activate a portion of the ventricle without passing through the bundle of His; the rest of the ventricle is activated via the normal AV pathway. The pre-excitation shortens the P-R interval and widens the QRS complex with a slurred upstroke. If the atrial impulse is conducted over the James bypass fibers, a short P-R interval with a QRS complex of normal duration will result (Lown-Ganong-Levine syndrome).[12] A heightened adrenergic state secondary to fever, hyperthyroidism, and anemia, can cause a short P-R interval, but is usually considered a normal variant.[43]

The paroxysmal tachycardias associated with ventricular pre-excitation (WPW) can be explained by the mechanism *re-entry*. An impulse traveling to the ventricles through the AV junction may turn around and re-enter the atria through the accessory pathway. A reciprocal rhythm or "electrical circuit" is thus established.[44]

Electrocardiographic features[25,45]

1. Heart rate and rhythm are normal in ventricular pre-excitation. In the WPW syndrome the heart rate is extremely rapid, often approaching 400 to 500 beats/min.

2. Sinus P waves are normal in ventricular pre-excitation but difficult to recognize in the WPW syndrome.

3. The QRS in ventricular pre-excitation is widened with slurring or notching of the upstroke of the R wave (delta wave). In the WPW syndrome the configuration of the QRS complexes can be normal, wide with a delta wave, or very wide and bizarre.

4. The P-R interval of the P-QRS in ventricular pre-excitation is short. In the WPW syndrome there is usually a 1:1 conduction (P wave for every QRS complex).

Associated conditions

1. Hypertrophic cardiomyopathy[9,5] At necropsy, five of our nine cats with pre-excitation had hypertrophic cardiomyopathy. Episodes of fainting in two cats were probably due to supraventricular tachycardia (WPW syndrome). In man, the association also exists between hypertrophic cardiomyopathy and the WPW syndrome.[46]

2. Congenital disorders, e.g., atrial septal defect or Ebstein's anomaly

Treatment[46a] *(See Chapters 10 and 12)*

1. Ventricular pre-excitation without tachycardia does not require therapy.

2. The WPW syndrome (supraventricular tachycardia) requires for conversion (a) ocular or carotid sinus pressure, (b) propranolol, the drug of choice, or (c) direct-current shock, the most effective treatment. Calcium-blocking agents may be effective. Digitalis should be used with care since anterograde conduction can be accelerated.

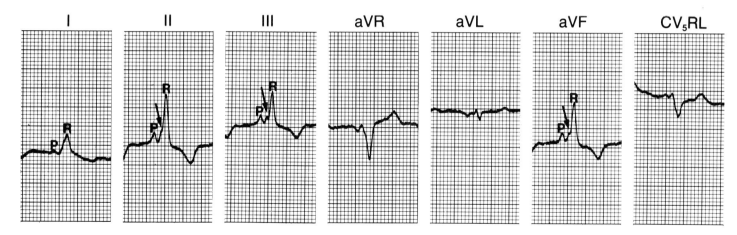

Fig. 7–57. Ventricular pre-excitation from the same cat as in Fig. 7–56. Note the short P-R interval in all leads, the easily recognized slur or notch (arrows) in the upstroke of the wide R wave.

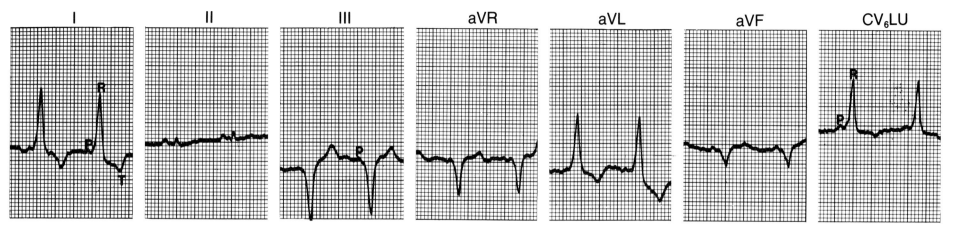

Fig. 7–58. Ventricular pre-excitation. The P-R interval is short in all leads and the QRS complexes are wide. Note the negative QRS complexes in leads *III* and *aVF*, indicating a different accessory pathway from that in Fig. 7–57.

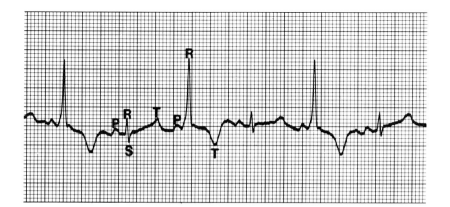

Fig. 7–59. Ventricular pre-excitation alternating with sinus complexes. The regular sinus complexes *(RS)* have a normal P-R interval. This strip can easily be confused with ventricular bigeminy (VPCs), but other strips did show a regular pre-excitation rhythm.

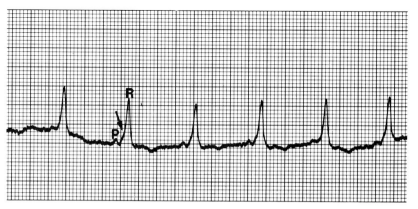

Fig. 7–60. Ventricular pre-excitation delta waves (arrow) broaden the QRS complexes to a width of 0.07 second.

Hyperkalemia (atrial standstill)

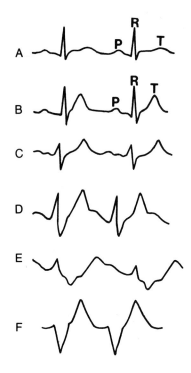

Fig. 7–61. Progressive effects of hyperkalemia on the P-QRS-T complex. **A** is a normal electrocardiogram. **B** through **F** represent serial changes (From Schaer, M.: Vet. Clin. North Am., 7:407, 1977; reprinted with permission.)

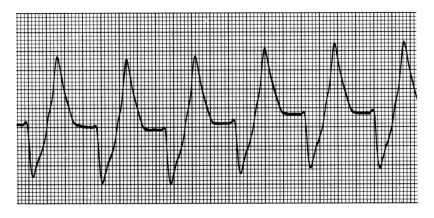

Fig. 7–62. Atrial standstill (sinoventricular rhythm). Hyperkalemia (serum potassium, 9.5 mEq/L) in a cat with urethral obstruction. Immediate treatment is necessary.

Hyperkalemia, an increase in the serum potassium level, is a common clinical problem in cats primarily because of the feline urethral obstruction syndrome. The effects of hyperkalemia on cardiac rhythm are severe and often lethal. Intraventricular conduction defects are common in hyperkalemia.[9] The wide and bizarre QRS complexes simulate an idioventricular rhythm. Experimental studies indicate, however, that the SA node continues to fire and its impulse is transmitted via the internodal pathways to the AV junction and ventricles. The rhythm should be termed *sinoventricular*. No P wave is recorded because the atrial myocardium is not activated.[47]

Electrocardiographic features[3,30,48,49]

The following sequential electrocardiographic changes are observed (Fig. 7–61), *with no sharp* distinctions between the levels of serum potassium:

1. Serum potassium greater than 5.5 mEq/L (T waves larger and peaked)
2. Serum potassium greater than 6.5 mEq/L (decreased amplitude of the R wave, prolonged QRS and P-R intervals, S-T segment depression)
3. Serum potassium greater than 7 mEq/L (decreased amplitude of the P wave with increased duration, longer QRS and P-R intervals, Q-T interval prolonged)
4. Serum potassium greater than 8.5 mEq/L (disappearance of the P wave with *atrial standstill;* a sinoventricular rhythm is the result)
5. Serum potassium greater than 10.0 mEq/L (increased widening of the QRS complex, with eventual replacement by a smooth biphasic curve; final stage is ventricular flutter, ventricular fibrillation, or ventricular asystole)

Associated conditions[3]

1. Feline urethral obstruction syndrome, especially after a 24-hour period of complete obstruction
2. Other conditions: renal insufficiency (oliguric renal failure), untreated diabetic ketoacidosis, excessive potassium infusion, metabolic acidosis, adrenocortical insufficiency (rare)

Treatment

1. Treat the underlying cause, i.e., relieve the urethral obstruction and maintain patency with an indwelling urinary catheter.

2. Lowering the serum potassium includes fluid therapy, sodium bicarbonate (1 to 2 mEq/kg body weight), regular insulin for emergency treatment (0.5 to 1 unit/kg body weight with 2 g dextrose/unit insulin), and calcium gluconate (10% solution, 0.5 to 1 ml/kg body weight) (antagonizes the cardiotoxic effects of potassium).

3. The electrocardiogram should be monitored throughout treatment.

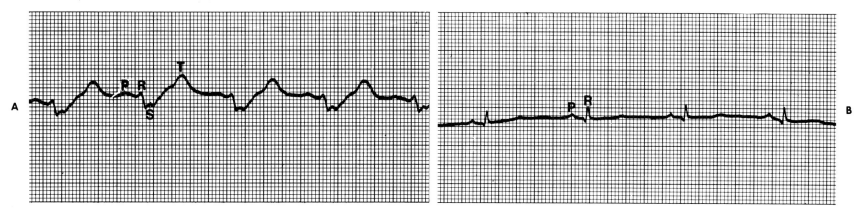

Fig. 7–63. **A,** Hyperkalemia in a cat with urethral obstruction (serum potassium, 8.4 mEq/L). The P waves are of small amplitude and increased duration. The markedly widened QRS complexes represent an intraventricular conduction abnormality. **B,** After therapy. The life-threatening effects of hyperkalemia have been eliminated.

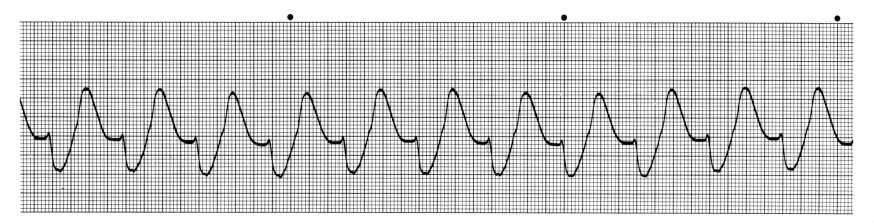

Fig. 7–64. Severe hyperkalemia (serum potassium, 10.5 mEq/L). No P waves are visible. The QRS complexes are wide and bizarre. The rhythm is sinoventricular. Ventricular fibrillation will eventually occur.

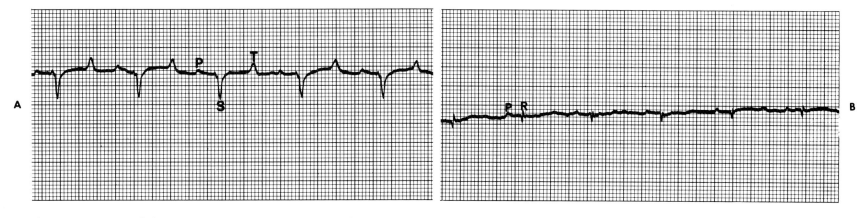

Fig. 7–65. **A,** Hyperkalemia (serum potassium, 7.5 mEq/L). Changes include a prolonged P-R interval, negative QRS complexes (anterior fascicular block pattern based on other leads), and a tall peaked T wave. **B,** 30 minutes after therapy. The QRS-T complexes are now normal.

Drug-induced arrhythmias

The secondary effects of drugs on the heart may or may not be of clinical significance. Some of the more commonly used drugs with their undesirable arrhythmias are summarized in this section. The effects of these drugs on the electrocardiogram have been reviewed in the literature.[25,50–52] The antiarrhythmic agents commonly used in the dog, quinidine, procainamide, and phenytoin, have not been used extensively in cats. The toxic signs of the various antiarrhythmic drugs are discussed in detail in Chapter 10.

Because of the increased frequency of surgical procedures performed on older cats, the importance of arrhythmias in the anesthetized animal should be emphasized even more. Alterations in vagal and sympathetic tone as well as electrolyte and acid-base disturbances that occur during anesthesia and surgery are a major factor. The anesthetic agents themselves, intubation, and surgical manipulation can also promote arrhythmias. Pre-existing cardiac and respiratory diseases can also affect the frequency of arrhythmias during surgery. Intraoperative arrhythmias can be frequent, but the majority are usually clinically insignificant.[10]

For successful nonarrhythmogenic anesthesia, the following principles should be applied: minimal stress of induction, proper ventilation of the patient, light plane of anesthesia, gentle surgical manipulation, proper fluid and electrolyte balance during surgery, and maintenance of a normal body temperature. If arrhythmias occur during anesthesia, the anesthetic concentration should first be lowered and the patient ventilated with higher oxygen concentration. Most arrhythmias can be eliminated by implementing these simple steps. The common preanesthesia medication, intravenous anesthetics, and inhalation anesthetics will first be reviewed[51,52] before discussing the other drug-induced arrhythmias.

Acetylpromazine. The phenothiazine derivatives all possess alpha-adrenergic blocking activity; sinus bradycardia is often seen. The drug also can depress myocardial contractility and excitability and slow impulse conduction.[53]

Xylazine (Rompun). Xylazine causes an increase in vagal tone and interferes with cardiac conductivity. It can cause sinus bradycardia, SA block, and varying degrees of AV block.[54] An anticholinergic such as atropine or glycopyrrolate should be used. Xylazine also may induce a variety of ventricular arrhythmias in the presence of epinephrine and halothane. Both blood pressure and sympathetic tone can be altered.

Ketamine. Ketamine, an analogue of phencyclidine, causes an increase in the heart rate (Fig. 7–66), cardiac output, and arterial blood pressure.[54] The drug also appears to have an antiarrhythmic quality. Ketamine has been shown to abolish epinephrine-induced ventricular arrhythmias in dogs anesthetized with halothane. In cats with primary cardiac disease, ketamine can decrease the contractility of the myocardium.[55]

Glycopyrrolate (Robinul-V). This anticholinergic has some advantages over atropine. It has a longer vagal blocking effect, and ventricular premature complexes occur less frequently following its use.

Barbiturates and Thiobarbiturates. These include thiopental, thiamylal, methohexital, and pentobarbital. A tachycardia may occur because of a transient rise in arterial pressure and a decrease in stroke volume. Especially in cats, laryngospasm is greater with thiobarbiturates than with inhalation anesthetics.[51] An increase in vagal tone may take place. Ventricular arrhythmias may persist into the anesthetic period with thiobarbiturates.

Inhalation Anesthetics. These include halothane, methoxyflurane, isoflurane, and nitrous oxide. Halothane and methoxyflurane cause a dose-related depression of sinus node automaticity.[52] Halothane sensitizes the myocardium to catecholamines, causing severe ventricular arrhythmias. This is usually of no significance unless a cardiac emergency develops in which epinephrine is used. Great care should be used to minimize palpation of the adrenal glands and in the use of epinephrine as a hemostatic agent.[51]

Cardiac arrhythmias are rare with methoxyflurane, and sensitivity to catecholamine-induced changes is less than the sensitivity caused by halothane. Halothane anesthesia in the cat sometimes causes AV dissociation secondary to an accelerated junctional rhythm and/or AV block (Fig. 7–68). Arrhythmias associated with inhalation anesthesia are dose related; most can be controlled by decreasing the concentration of anesthetic delivered to the animal. Nitrous oxide rarely produces arrhythmias. Isoflurane should be considered when there is a need for reducing anticipated arrhythmias during anesthesia.[55a]

Norepinephrine and Isoproterenol. These sympathomimetic drugs are able to stimulate the beta receptors, causing an increased ventricular excitability and an increase in pacemaker automaticity (e.g., sinus tachycardia or atrial tachycardia).

Propranolol (Inderal). The drugs work primarily by blocking the beta-adrenergic receptors. Toxic effects of this drug are bradycardia (Fig. 7–69) and myocardial contractile depression. Heart block may be induced in the presence of diseased conduction system.

Lidocaine. This antiarrhythmic drug should be used with care in cats with severe cardiac disease. Heart failure can cause a significant reduction in both the volume of distribution and the plasma clearance of lidocaine.[56] Severe sinus bradycardia and sinus arrest can result (Fig. 7–67).

Digitalis. The arrhythmias seen in digitalis toxicity are the result primarily of two effects of the drug (occurring either alone or in combination):[36,37] (1) acceleration of pacemaker cells throughout the heart and (2) depression of the pacemaker cells in the SA node and AV junction. Digitalis can cause any cardiac arrhythmias.

Propylene Glycol. This diluent, used in intravenous diazepam and phenytoin sodium, can cause ventricular arrhythmias.[15]

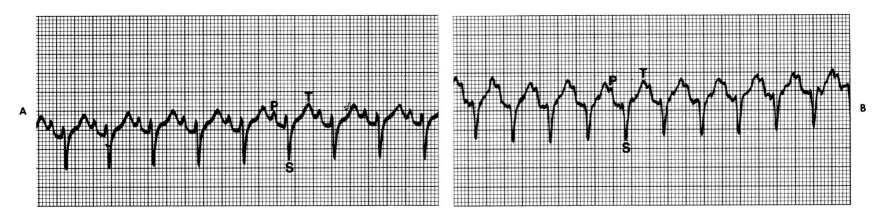

Fig. 7–66. **A,** A heart rate of 250 beats/min. The large S waves in this lead were due to an intraventricular conduction defect. **B,** After intravenous ketamine. The heart rate has now increased to 300. This increase in heart rate could represent serious hemodynamic consequences in a cat with an underlying heart condition.

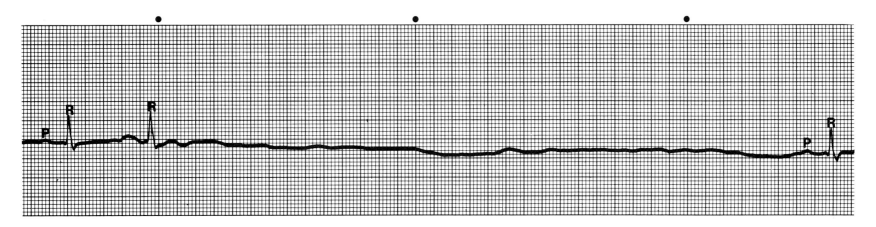

Fig. 7–67. Severe sinus bradycardia with over a 3-second sinus pause (sinus arrest) after the intravenous use of lidocaine. Subsidiary pacemakers were probably also suppressed since the long pause failed to evoke escape complexes. Atropine reversed the bradycardia.

Drug-induced arrhythmias—cont'd

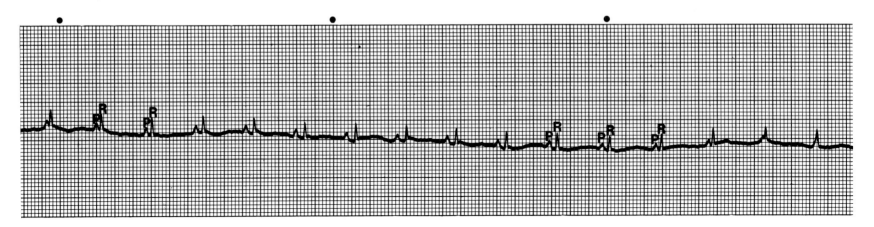

Fig. 7–68. Complete AV dissociation between the SA node and the AV junction due to an accelerated AV junctional focus and/or AV block. The P waves travel toward, inside, and away from the QRS complexes. The arrhythmia stopped when the halothane anesthesia was switched to methoxyflurane.

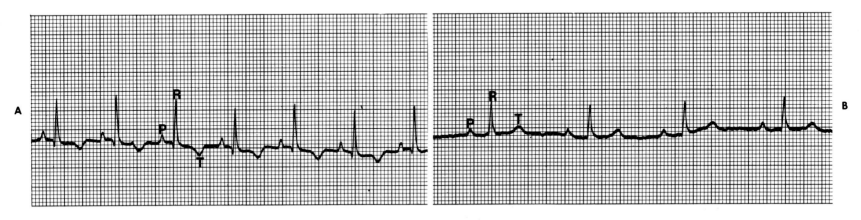

Fig. 7–69. Effect of 2 weeks' administration of propranolol to a cat with hypertrophic cardiomyopathy. **A,** Before and, **B,** after propranolol. The heart rate is much slower with the P-R interval now prolonged. Propranolol prevents a stress-induced tachycardia, subsequently preventing any decreased filling of the left ventricle. The dosage should be reduced in this case, for the heart rate is only 120 beats/min. Note the change in the polarity of the T wave, an indication of probable myocardial changes.

Electrical alternans

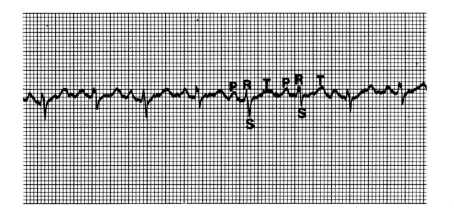

Fig. 7–70. Electrical alternans in a cat with pericardial effusion. The QRS-T complexes alternate in amplitude.

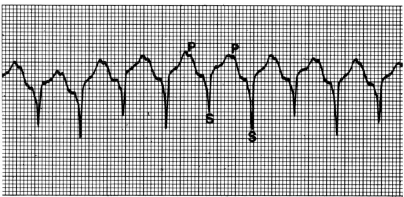

Fig. 7–71. Supraventricular tachycardia with alternation in amplitude of these QS complexes. A P wave is superimposed on each T wave in this cat with tetralogy of Fallot. After ocular pressure (not shown), the tachycardia and electrical alternans were eliminated.

Electrical alternans is diagnosed when the P, QRS, or T complexes (or any combination) alter their configuration on every other complex, every third complex, every fourth complex, etc.; each complex, however, must originate from the same focus.[57] The most common alternating ratio is every other complex (2:1 electrical alternans). Electrical alternans usually involves the QRS complex alone.

Two theories have been proposed to explain the mechanism of electrical alternans: the actual anatomic motion of the whole heart or the alternating conduction within the myocardium.[58] Cardiac motion is accepted as essentially the source of electrical alternans in pericardial effusion.[59] At very fast heart rates or in certain types of bundle branch block, electrical alternans results from the differences in recovery rate of the individual fibers; the refractory phase of the heart can also become prolonged on an alternating basis. In man, the presence of QRS alternation during sustained narrow QRS supraventricular tachycardia is highly indicative of a retrograde accessory AV pathway in the tachycardia circuit.[59a]

Electrocardiographic features

The three causes of electrical alternans that I have recognized are pericardial effusion, alternating bundle branch block, and supraventricular tachycardia. True electrical alternans should not be confused with ventricular bigeminy (the second complex, a VPC) or the effects of respiration.

1. The heart rate is usually normal in pericardial effusion.
2. The P wave may be of alternating amplitude and hidden in supraventricular tachycardia.
3. The QRS may show alternating amplitudes and configurations.
4. The P waves are always related to the QRS complexes; all complexes must be from the same pacemaker.

Associated conditions

My own experience includes only four cats with true electrical alternans.

1. Pericardial effusion: septic pericarditis, right-sided heart failure (two cats)
2. Supraventricular tachycardia, a cat with tetralogy of Fallot
3. Alternating conduction in the ventricular specialized conduction system, a cat with cardiomyopathy

Treatment

1. Pericardiocentesis is usually indicated if pericardial effusion is the cause.
2. Electrical alternans in bundle branch block and in supraventricular tachycardia is usually of no added significance.

Persistent atrial standstill ("silent atrium")

Atrial standstill is characterized by an absence of P waves and by a regular escape rhythm with a supraventricular-type QRS. It may be temporary, terminal, or persistent.[60] Temporary atrial standstill occurs with digitalis toxicity and hyperkalemia. Terminal atrial standstill is associated with a dying heart or with severe hyperkalemia.

Persistent atrial standstill has not been previously reported in the cat and is rare in man.[60] The disorder occurs in man along with various types of muscular dystrophy, amyloidosis, familial heart disease, coronary heart disease, and longstanding cardiac disease.[61]

I have recognized 11 cats, including 8 Siamese, 1 Burmese, and 2 Domestic Shorthair. The clinical signs included weakness, fainting, and congestive heart failure. The dilated forms of cardiomyopathy were found at necropsy in 7 cats.[61a]

Electrocardiographic features[60,61]

1. The heart rate is slow, usually 160 beats/min or less, and the rhythm is often regular.

2. No P waves are observed in any lead, including intracardiac electrograms. Low-voltage atrial activity may be found.

3. The QRS is of nearly normal configuration with supraventricular-type escape QRS complexes, or of increased duration in bundle branch block and/or ventricular enlargement.

4. There is no increase in heart rate, nor are P waves evident after injection of atropine sulfate or exercise.

5. The atria are immobile at fluoroscopy, and they cannot be stimulated electrically or mechanically. With echocardiography, there is no evidence of "atrial kick" on recordings of the mitral valve indicating absence of left atrial mechanical activity.

6. Serum electrolytes are normal.

Associated conditions

Persistent atrial standstill (Fig. 7–72) can be divided into three clinical groups.[61]

1. Longstanding cardiac disease. Diffuse involvement of the atria from the increased load due to hemodynamic dysfunction in mitral valvular fibrosis, congenital heart disease, or cardiomyopathy can result in fibrous replacement of normal atrial muscle cells.[20,62] The dilated form of cardiomyopathy was found most often in the cat with persistent atrial standstill. At necropsy, greatly enlarged and paper-thin atria were observed. At microscopic examination, little atrial myocardium was present.

2. Neuromuscular disease associated with cardiomyopathy; in man, the common diseases include Duchenne muscular dystrophy and myasthenia gravis.

3. Without known cardiac disease or neuromuscular disease; a familial occurrence in the Siamese should be suspected for dilated cardiomyopathy and/or persistent atrial standstill.

Treatment

1. The complications of heart failure should be treated. Implantation of a permanent pacemaker is difficult in the cat, and also the prognosis for the dilated form of cardiomyopathy is guarded.

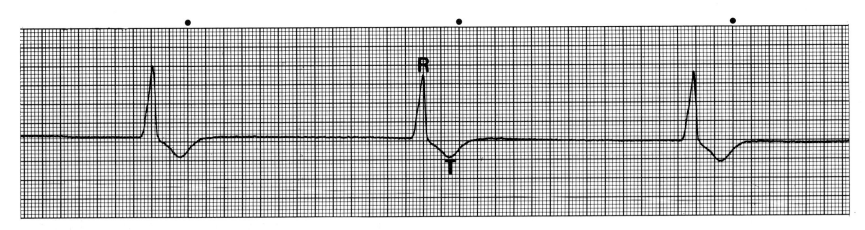

Fig. 7–72. Persistent atrial standstill in a 4-year-old Siamese cat with clinical signs of dyspnea. Pleural effusion and cardiomegaly were found on thoracic radiographs. No P waves are present with the QRS complexes increased in voltage and duration, indicating left bundle branch block and/or left heart enlargement. The heart rate is only 40 beats/min. An idioventricular rhythm should also be considered.

Hyperthyroidism

Hyperthyroidism (thyrotoxicosis) is a common disease in the cat, although just recently documented.[63,64,64a] In the cat, the excessive production of the thyroid hormones, thyroxine (T_4) and tri-iodothyronine (T_3), usually results from one or more functional adenomas that involve one or both thyroid lobes. Hyperthyroidism affects predominantly older cats. Clinical signs include weight loss despite an increased appetite, hyperexcitability, polydipsia/polyuria, diarrhea, frequent defecation, increased heart rate and size, sometimes with arrhythmias, and palpable enlargement of one or both thyroid lobes. The diagnosis of hyperthyroidism can be confirmed on the basis of high serum concentrations of T_4 (usually >6.0 µg/dl) and T_3 (usually >300 µg/dl).

Cardiac abnormalities are a common feature of feline hyperthyroidism. Radiographic evidence of mild to severe cardiomegaly is frequently observed; pleural effusion or pulmonary edema may occur if congestive heart failure is present.

Electrocardiographic abnormalities (Fig. 7–73)

In one study,[64,64a] tachycardia (≥ 240 beats/min) and increased R wave amplitude in lead II (≥ 0.9 mv) were the most frequent abnormalities. Electrocardiographic changes were recorded in 131 cats with hyperthyroidism, with 66% of the cats having tachycardia and 29% an increase in R wave amplitude. Atrial and ventricular arrhythmias were recorded in 14% of the cats. Atrial and ventricular arrhythmias included atrial premature complexes, atrial tachycardia, ventricular premature complexes, and ventricular tachycardia. Sinus tachycardia, increased R wave amplitude, and the arrhythmias usually resolved in all cats following successful therapy. The abnormal electrocardiographic changes resemble the electrocardiographic findings of hyperthyroidism in man.[65]

The majority of the cardiovascular manifestations of hyperthyroidism are due to sympathoadrenal activity.[66] Recent studies explain the hyperadrenergic cardiovascular manifestations in thyrotoxicosis.[66] The possibilities include an increase in the number of myocardial beta-adrenergic receptors; an increase in the sensitivity of cardiac beta-adrenergic receptors to the effects of catecholamines; and an increase in myocardial tissue levels of free catecholamines. Thyroid hormone itself also has potent positive chronotropic and inotropic effects on the heart. The beta-adrenergic blocking agent, propranolol, has been shown to improve cardiac functions in cats with experimentally induced hyperthyroidism.[67]

Treatment[64,65a,66a]

Because of the direct tissue actions of thyroid hormone, propranolol is not the only therapy for hyperthyroidism. Definitive therapy requires the use of antithyroid drugs or surgical removal of the affected thyroid lobe, or radioactive iodine therapy. Bilateral thyroidectomy should be performed if both glands are abnormal in appearance at surgery. At least one parathyroid gland should be left. Careful monitoring of the serum Ca level is indicated to detect hypocalcemia. Replacement therapy with thyroxine is sometimes required to maintain a euthyroid state.[14]

Because hyperthyroidism is a systemic illness, the cats should be prepared for surgery by administration of either propranolol or propylthiouracil (PTU), or methimazole. Propranolol should be given for 7 to 14 days before surgery at the dosage of 2.5 to 5.0 mg three times a day, as required to decrease resting heart rate within normal range. In some cats, the hyperthyroidism can be controlled with antithyroid drugs. The possible toxic effects of PTU have just been recently reported.

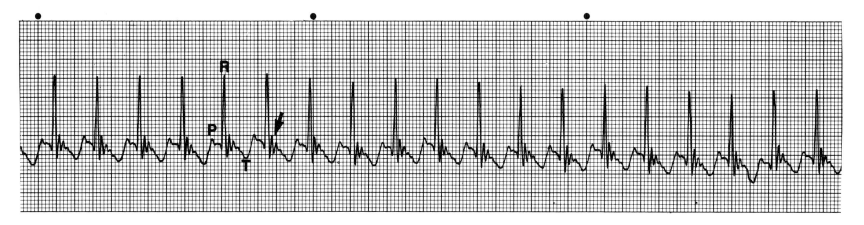

Fig. 7–73. Sinus tachycardia at a rate of 260 beats/min from a 14-year-old cat with hyperthyroidism. The R wave voltage is 1.8 mv (or 18 boxes), indicating left ventricular enlargement. The S-T segment artifact (arrow) is due to inadequate low-frequency response during the transtelephonic transmission.

Artifacts

The electrocardiogram is a mechanical recording; therefore a number of technical or mechanical problems can occur while it is being obtained. These technical or mechanical problems superimposed on the normal cardiac complexes produce distortions called artifacts which can not only cause the measurement of the various complexes to be difficult but also simulate disturbances of cardiac rhythm and conduction.[68] Electrocardiographic examples and their causes are presented in this section. The reader can find suggestions for obtaining good technical recordings in Chapter 2.

The causes of artifacts can be placed into two general categories: (1) technical recording problems (fault of the clinician, the machine, or the electrodes and cable), and (2) problems with the animal.

Technical recording problems

1. Lead reversal, incorrect electrode placement, is a frequent mistake. The most common error is reversal of the forelimb electrodes, which simulates the pattern in dextrocardia with negative P waves in leads I and aVL. Other incorrect electrode placements are illustrated in Figure 7–87.
2. If standardizations are improperly labeled, voltages may appear abnormally low or high.
3. Standard paper speed for cats is 50 mm/sec. A paper speed of 25 mm/sec will create false measurements.

4. Electrical interference, also called 60-cycle artifact, is due to improper grounding.
5. A poorly defined baseline indicates a dirty stylus or a low stylus heat. Reducing the amplitude of large complexes to half is usually helpful.
6. Stylus mounting should not be too loose or too tight, for it can cause overshooting or a slow return to baseline, respectively.
7. Electrodes and cable are often sources of artifacts, e.g., broken cable, loose connection of the alligator clip to the cable tip, dirty cable tips, cable wires pulling on the electrodes, or a swinging cable over the table edge.

Animal-related factors

1. Artifacts can be produced by muscle tremor, as when a cat is purring, or by unexpected animal body movements.
2. Wandering baseline, often due to respiratory movements, coughing, or voluntary motion by the animal or handler, can simulate atrial and ventricular arrhythmias.

The electrocardiographic manifestations most helpful in differentiating artifacts from arrhythmias include (1) the rhythm of the artifacts (usually irregular) (rate of artifacts is variable) and (2) the realization that artifacts do not interrupt atrial or ventricular rhythm.

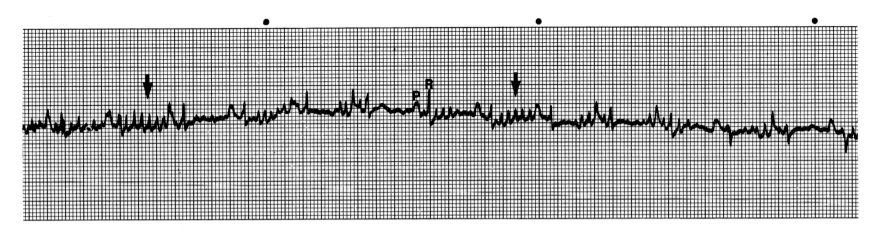

Fig. 7–74.   Effect of intermittent purring on the electrocardiogram. The P-QRS-T complexes are difficult to identify. The artifacts (arrows) mimic a rapid atrial mechanism. Patience, changing the cat's position, and gentle manipulation of the larynx may be helpful.

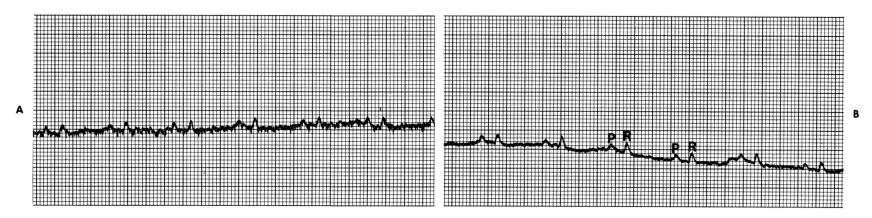

Fig. 7–75. **A,** Electrical interference. The electrocardiograph was not properly grounded. **B,** Most of the artifact has been eliminated; the P waves and R waves are now well defined. Some machines have a frequency response switch to reduce the effects of interference.

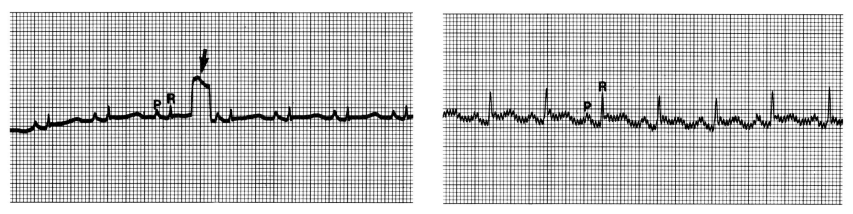

Fig. 7–76. Standardization deflection (arrow) that happens to fall between two sinus complexes. A T wave is superimposed on the standard. The standardization of the machine should be checked frequently so voltages will not be abnormally low or high.

Fig. 7–77. Electrical interference (60-cycle). The artifact was corrected by reapplying the electrode clips to the fleshy part of the limbs, not the large skin folds often seen in cats.

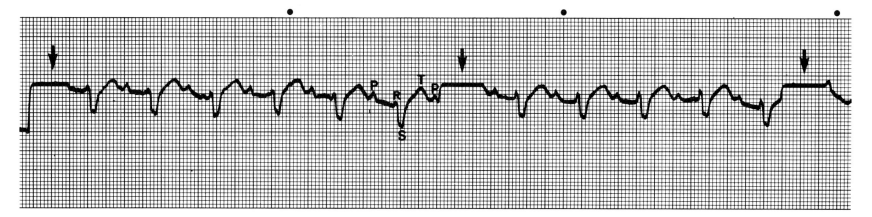

Fig. 7–78. Pauses (arrows) apparently due to sinus arrest or blocked P waves (AV block). This was created by moving the lead selector switch from lead 2 to lead 3 without turning the record switch off. Such a procedure is correct, but realize that pauses will occur between the lead recordings, with P waves and QRS complexes sometimes being separated.

Artifacts—cont'd

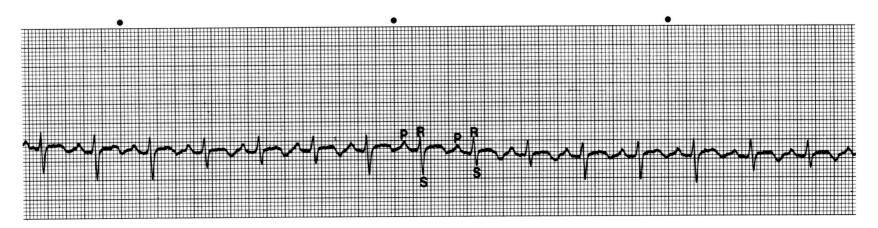

Fig. 7–79. Fluctuation in amplitude of complexes in a cat due to inspiration and expiration. The air acts as a region of high electrical resistance, a poor conducting medium. This artifact can be especially pronounced in pneumothorax.

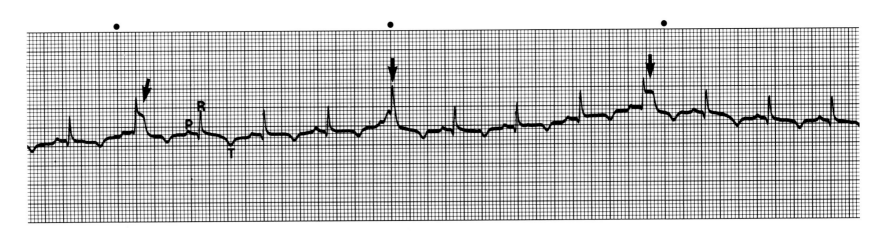

Fig. 7–80. Artifacts (arrows) that happen to fall on the QRS complexes, due to movements of the cat. The artifacts simulate ventricular ectopic complexes but do not interrupt the normal sinus rhythm.

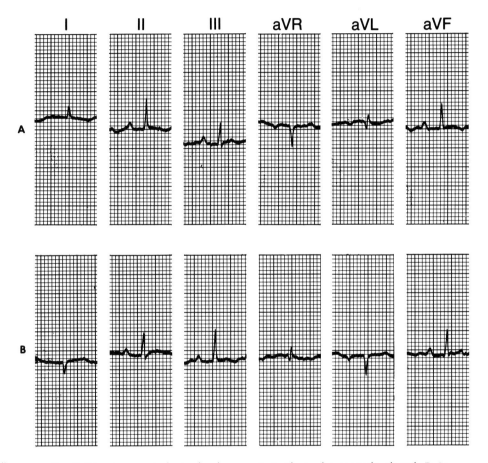

Fig. 7–81. Incorrect electrode placement. **A,** Electrodes properly placed. **B,** In this tracing the front limb electrodes have been reversed. Lead *I* is a mirror image of lead *I* in **A,** *II* is *III* and *III* is *II, aVR* is *aVL* and *aVL* is *aVR,* and *aVF* is *aVF*.

Artifacts—cont'd

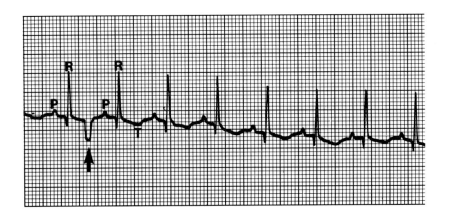

Fig. 7–82. Normal sinus rhythm. A sudden shift of the baseline (arrow) causes an artifact resembling an ectopic complex that is interpolated. The artifact does not interrupt the sinus rhythm.

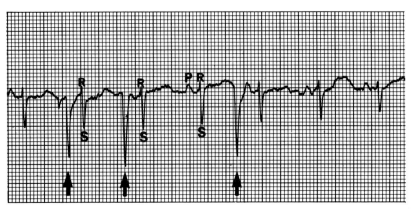

Fig. 7–83. Normal sinus rhythm. Artifacts (arrows) created when the cat intermittently jerked its leg easily resemble ventricular ectopic complexes. The intervals of the artifact to sinus complexes are too short to allow double depolarization of the ventricles.

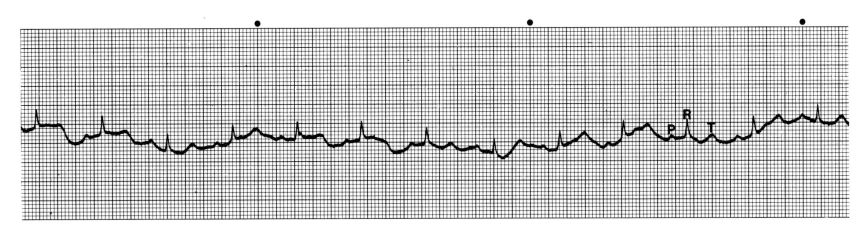

Fig. 7–84. Effect of respirations and movement of the cat on the electrocardiogram. The baseline moves up and down, causing the T wave to change size and shape. The position of sternal recumbency could be used instead, since cats tolerate this position well and values are not significantly different.

REFERENCES

1. Silber, E.N., and Katz, L.N.: *Heart Disease.* New York, Macmillan, 1975.
2. Schaer, M.: Polemical forum on the article Induced feline urethral obstruction: response of hyperkalemia to relief of obstruction and administration of parenteral electrolyte solution. J. Am. Anim. Hosp. Assoc., *12*:673, 1976.
3. Schaer, M.: Hyperkalemia in cats with urethral obstruction: electrocardiographic abnormalities and treatment. Vet. Clin. North Am., *7*:407, 1977.
4. Spaulding, G.L., and Tilley, L.P.: Atrial fibrillation in the dog and cat. Proc. Am. Anim. Hosp. Assoc., *43*:75, 1976.
5. Tilley, L.P., et al.: Primary myocardial disease in the cat. Am. J. Pathol., *86*:493, 1977.
6. Harpster, N.K.: Cardiovascular diseases of the cat. Adv. Vet. Sci. Comp. Med., *21*:39, 1977.
7. Beglinger, R., Heller, A., and Lakotos, L.: Elektrokardiogramme, Herzschlagfrequenz and Blutdruck der Hauskatze (Felis catus). Zentralbl. Veterinaermed., (A) *24*:252, 1977.
8. Selzer, A.: *Principles of Clinical Cardiology: An Analytical Approach.* Philadelphia, W.B. Saunders, 1975.
9. Tilley, L.P., and Gompf, R.E.: Feline electrocardiography. Vet. Clin. North Am., *7*:257, 1977.
10. Helfant, R.H.: *Bellet's Essentials of Cardiac Arrhythmias.* 2nd Edition. Philadelphia, W.B. Saunders, 1980.
11. Hoffman, A., and Meier, M.: Importance of cardiac and vascular beta-receptors in the action of phentolamine. Agents Actions, *7*:399, 1977.
12. Tilley, L.P., and Weitz, J.: Pharmacologic and other forms of medical therapy in feline cardiac disease. Vet. Clin. North Am., *7*:425, 1977.
13. Tilley, L.P., Liu, S.-K., and Fox, P.R.: Myocardial disease. In *Textbook of Veterinary Internal Medicine.* Edited by S.J. Ettinger. 2nd Edition. Philadelphia, W.B. Saunders, 1983.
14. Fox, P.R., Tilley, L.P., Liu, S.-K.: The cardiovascular system. In *Feline Medicine.* Edited by P.W. Pratt. Santa Barbara, Calif., Am. Vet. Publ., Inc., 1983.
15. Louis, S., Kutt, H., and McDowell, F.: The cardiocirculatory changes caused by intravenous Dilantin and its solvent. Am. Heart J., *74*:523, 1968.
16. Harpster, N.K.: Feline cardiomyopathy. Vet. Clin. North Am., *7*:355, 1977.
17. Tilley, L.P.: Feline cardiac arrhythmias. Vet. Clin. North Am., *7*:273, 1977.
18. Befeler, B.: Mechanical stimulation of the heart, its therapeutic value in tachyarrhythmias. Chest, *73*:832, 1978.
19. Blok, J., and Boeles, J.T.F.: The electrocardiogram of the normal cat. Acta Physiol. Pharmacol., *6*:95, 1957.
20. Boyden, P., Tilley, L.P., Liu, S.-K., and Wit, A.L.: Effects of atrial dilation on atrial cellular electrophysiology: studies on cats with spontaneous cardiomyopathy, Circulation, *56*(Suppl. 3):48, 1977 (Abstract.)
21. Chung, E.K.: *Principles of Cardiac Arrhythmias.* 2nd Edition. Baltimore, Williams & Wilkins, 1977.
22. Irving, D.W., and Corday, E.: Effect of the cardiac arrhythmias on the renal and mesenteric circulation. Am. J. Cardiol., *8*:32, 1961.
23. Ettinger, S.J.: Cardiac arrhythmias. In *Textbook of Veterinary Internal Medicine.* Edited by S.J. Ettinger. 2nd Edition. Philadelphia, W.B. Saunders, 1983.
24. Tilley, L.P.: Feline cardiomyopathy. In *Current Veterinary Therapy: Small Animal Practice.* Volume 6. Edited by R.W. Kirk. Philadelphia, W.B. Saunders, 1977.
25. Friedman, H.H.: *Diagnostic Electrocardiography and Vectorcardiography.* 2nd Edition. New York, McGraw-Hill, 1977.
26. Harris, A.S.: Delayed development of ventricular ectopic rhythms following experimental coronary occlusion. Circulation, *1*:1318, 1950.
27. Colcolough, H.L.: A comparative study of acute myocardial infarction in the rabbit, cat and man. Comp. Biochem. Physiol., *49A*:121, 1974.
28. Tilley, L.P., Bond, B., Patnaik, A.K., and Liu, S.-K.: Cardiovascular tumors in the cat. J. Am. Anim. Hosp. Assoc., *17*:1009, 1981.
29. Lown, B., Verrier, R.L., and Rabinowitz, S.H.: Neural and psychologic mechanisms and the problem of sudden cardiac death. Am. J. Cardiol., *39*:890, 1977.
30. Coulter, D.B., Duncan, R.J., and Sander, P.D.: Effects of asphyxia and potassium on canine and feline electrocardiograms. Can. J. Comp. Med., *39*:442, 1975.
31. Watanabe, Y., and Dreifus, L.S.: *Cardiac Arrhythmias, Electrophysiologic Basis for Clinical Interpretation.* New York, Grune & Stratton, 1977.
32. Harris, S.G., and Ogburn, P.N.: The cardiovascular system. In *Feline Medicine and Surgery.* Edited by E.J. Catcott. 2nd Edition. Santa Barbara, Calif., American Veterinary Publications, 1975.
33. Lathers, C.M., Kelliher, G.J., Roberts, J., and Besley, A.B.: Nonuniform cardiac sympathetic nerve discharge, mechanism for coronary occlusion and digitalis-induced arrhythmias. Circulation, *57*:1058, 1978.
34. Bonagura, J.D.: Feline cardiovascular emergencies. Vet. Clin. North Am., *7*:385, 1977.
35. Goldschlager, N., and Scheinman, M.M.: Diagnosis and clinical significance of atrioventricular conduction disturbances. Practical Cardiol., *4*:43, 1978.
36. Bolton, G.R., and Powell, A.A.: Plasma kinetics of digoxin in the cat. Am. J. Vet. Res., *43*:1994, 1982.
37. Erichsen, D.F., Harris, S.G., and Upson, D.W.: Therapeutic and toxic plasma concentrations of digoxin in the cat. Am. J. Vet. Res., *41*:2049, 1980.
38. Liu, S.-K., Tilley, L.P., and Tashjian, R.J.: Lesions of the conduction system in the cat with cardiomyopathy. Recent Adv. Stud. Cardiac Struct. Metab., *10*:681, 1975.
39. Chmielewski, C.A., Riley, R.S., Mahendran, A., and Most, A.S.: Complete heart block as a cause of syncope in asymmetric septal hypertrophy. Am. Heart J., *93*:91, 1977.
40. Buss, D.D., Pyle, R.L., and Chacko, S.K.: Clinico-pathologic conference. J. Am. Vet. Med. Assoc., *161*:402, 1972.
41. Orsini, D., and Buss, D.D.: Complete atrioventricular block in a cat (clinical report). J. Am. Vet. Med. Assoc., *172*:158, 1978.
42. Lown, B., Ganong, W.F., and Levine, S.A.: The syndrome of short P-R interval, normal QRS complex and paroxysmal rapid heart action. Circulation, *5*:693, 1952.
43. Chung, E.K.: Wolff-Parkinson-White syndrome: current views. Am. J. Med., *62*:252, 1977.
44. Narula, O.S.: Symposium on cardiac arrhythmias. 4. Wolff-Parkinson-White syndrome. Circulation, *47*:972, 1973.
45. Ogburn, P.N.: Ventricular pre-excitation (Wolff-Parkinson-White syndrome) in a cat. J. Am. Anim. Hosp. Assoc., *13*:131, 1977.
46. Perosio, A.M., and Suarez, L.O.: Pre-excitation syndrome and hypertrophic cardiomyopathy. J. Electrocardiol., *16*:29, 1983.
46a.Wellens, H.J.J.: Wolff-Parkinson-White syndrome. Part II. Treatment. Mod. Concepts Cardiovasc. Dis., *52*:57, 1983.
47. Goldman, M.J.: *Principles of Clinical Electrocardiography.* 11th Edition. Los Altos, Calif., Lange Medical Publications, 1982.
48. Parks, J.: Electrocardiographic abnormalities from serum electrolyte imbalance due to feline urethral obstruction. J. Am. Anim. Hosp. Assoc., *11*:102, 1975.
49. Vander Ark, C.R., Ballantyne, F., and Reynolds, E.W.: Electrolytes and the electrocardiogram. Cardiovasc. Clin., *5*:269, 1973.
50. Jenkins, W.L., and Clark, D.R.: A review of drugs affecting the heart. J. Am. Vet. Med. Assoc., *171*:85, 1977.
51. Sawyer, D.C.: *The Practice of Small Animal Anesthesia (Major Problems in Veterinary Medicine).* Volume 1. Philadelphia, W.B. Saunders, 1982.
52. Brown, B.R. (Ed.): *Anesthesia and the Patient with Heart Disease.* Philadelphia, F.A. Davis, 1980.
53. Booth, N.H.: Intravenous and other parenteral anesthetics. In *Veterinary Pharmacology and Therapeutics.* Edited by L.M. Jones, N.H. Booth, and L.M. McDonald. 4th Edition. Ames, Iowa, Iowa State University Press, 1977.
54. Haskins, S.C., Peifter, R.L., and Stowe, C.M.: A clinical comparison of CT1341, ketamine, and xylazine in cats. Am. J. Vet. Res., *36*:1537, 1975.
55. Wright, M.: Pharmacologic effects of ketamine and its use in veterinary medicine. J. Am. Vet. Med. Assoc., *180*:1462, 1982.
55a.Harvey, R.C., and Short, C.E.: The use of isoflurane for safe anesthesia in animals with traumatic myocarditis or other myocardial sensitivity. Canine Practice, *10*:18, 1983.
56. Pfeifer, M.J., Greenblatt, D.J., and Weser, J.K.: Clinical use and toxicity of intravenous lidocaine. Am. Heart J., *92*:168, 1976.
57. Bellet, S.: *Clinical Disorders of the Heart Beat.* 3rd Edition. Philadelphia, Lea & Febiger, 1971.
58. Littman, D.: Alternation of the heart. Circulation, *27*:280, 1963.
59. Sbarbaro, J.A., and Brooks, H.L.: Pericardial effusion and electrical alternans, echocardiographic assessment. Postgrad. Med., *63*(3):105, 1978.
59a.Green, M., et al.: Value of QRS alternation in determining the site of origin of narrow QRS supraventricular tachycardia. Circulation, *68*:368, 1983.
60. Tanaka, H., et al.: Persistent atrial standstill due to atrial inexcitability. Jpn. Heart J., *16*:639, 1975.
61. Wooliscroft, J., and Tuna, N.: Permanent atrial standstill: the clinical spectrum. Am. J. Cardiol., *49*:2037, 1982.

61a.Tilley, L.P., and Liu, S.-K.: Persistent atrial standstill in the dog and cat. ACVIM Scientific Proceedings, New York, NY, 1983 (Abstract).

62. Yoneda, S., et al.: Persistent atrial standstill developed in a patient with rheumatic heart disease: electrophysiological and histological study. Clin. Cardiol., *1*:43, 1978.

63. Holzworth, J., et al.: Hyperthyroidism in the cat: ten cases. J. Am. Vet. Med. Assoc., *176*:345, 1980.

64. Peterson, M.E., Keene, B., Ferguson, D.C., and Pipers, F.S.: Electrocardiographic findings in 45 cats with hyperthyroidism. J. Am. Vet. Med. Assoc., *180*:934, 1982.

64a.Peterson, M.E., et al.: Feline hyperthyroidism: pretreatment clinical and laboratory evaluation of 131 cases. J. Am. Vet. Med. Assoc., *183*:103, 1983.

65. Surawicz, B., and Mangiardi, M.L.: Electrocardiogram in endocrine and metabolic disorders. Cardiovasc. Clin., *8*:243, 1977.

65a.Turrel, J.M., Feldman, E.C., Hayes, M., and Hornof, W.: Radioactive iodine therapy in cats with hyperthyroidism. J. Am. Vet. Med. Assoc., *184*:554, 1984.

66. Skeleton, C.L.: The heart and hyperthyroidism. N. Engl. J. Med., *19*:1206, 1982.

66a.Klein, I., and Levey, G.S.: New perspectives on thyroid hormone, catecholamines, and the heart. Am. J. Med., *76*:167, 1984.

67. Strauer, B.E., and Scherpe, A.: Experimental hyperthyroidism III: Contractile responses to propranolol of the intact heart and of the isolated ventricular myocardium. Basic Res. Cardiol., *70*:237, 1975.

68. Yurchak, P.M.: Artifacts resembling cardiac arrhythmias. Postgrad. Med., *53*(5):79, 1973.

Section Four

Pathophysiologic Basis and Effects of Cardiac Arrhythmias

8 Pathophysiologic basis and hemodynamic effects of cardiac arrhythmias

long slow pulse beats mark its good regulation
short empty beats prove its disorderly condition
quick pulse with more than six heart beats per one
   respiratory cycle proves a sickness of the heart
a broadly slow pulse signifies a deterioration of the disease.

From the Yellow Emperor's Book of Medicine
(Twenty-sixth century BC)[1]

As early as the twenty-sixth century BC, there was already some understanding of the pathophysiologic basis and hemodynamic effects of cardiac arrhythmias. Today, it is vitally important that the clinician understand the basis and effects, as well as the normal and abnormal electrocardiographic patterns, of cardiac arrhythmias. Such knowledge helps the clinician to better understand the rationale for treatment and the possible outcome of therapy.

For this reason, throughout the chapters on cardiac arrhythmias and the self-assessment section, I have inserted comments on the hemodynamic effects and clinical features of arrhythmias. The purpose of this chapter is to discuss the pathophysiologic basis and effects of cardiac arrhythmias, the extracardiac causes of arrhythmias (especially originating in the central nervous system), and the pathology of the conduction system (by Dr. Si-Kwang Liu).

Hopefully, the clinician, after reading this chapter, will ask the following questions[2] when an abnormality in rhythm is diagnosed:

1. What caused the abnormality in rhythm and conduction?
2. What clinical features will the animal show based on the hemodynamic effects of the arrhythmia?
3. How can any complications be anticipated and prevented?
4. At what level of cardiac physiology is therapy directed?

In review, the electrocardiogram has the following characteristics,[3] some of which are unique: (1) it may aid in the diagnosis of myocardial disease; (2) it often reflects anatomic, metabolic, and hemodynamic changes, knowledge of which has resulted from studies correlating the electrocardiogram with clinical, necropsy, and experimental findings; (3) it is a unique model for illustrating a variety of complex electrophysiologic concepts through deductive reasoning (see Chapter 12); (4) it serves as a stimulus for the laboratory confirmation of various mechanisms; (5) it is crucial for the proper diagnosis and treatment of many diseases in dogs and cats; and (6) it is without question necessary in the diagnosis of arrhythmias.

CAUSES OF ARRHYTHMIAS

It is important to establish the causes of arrhythmias, since such information may affect prognosis and therapy. The possible sources of arrhythmias in dogs and cats can be divided into three basic categories: (1) autonomic nervous system; (2) cardiac sources; and (3) extracardiac sources involving pathophysiologic factors. Some of the more common causes of arrhythmias in the dog and in the cat are listed in Tables 8–1[4–7] and 8–2,[6–12] respectively (See also Table 10–3).

EXTRACARDIAC CAUSES OF ARRHYTHMIAS

From the viewpoint of the electrophysiologist, arrhythmias arise from alterations in either automaticity or conductivity or both. Alterations in automaticity include enhancement or depression of automaticity, abnormal automaticity, and triggered activity. Alterations in conductivity include slowing of conduction, conduction block, and reentrant arrhythmias. The fundamental mechanisms for the electrophysiologic basis of arrhythmias are discussed in detail in Chapter 9. The classification of these mechanisms implies that the heart itself is

Table 8–1. Causes of arrhythmias in the dog

I. Autonomic nervous system
  A. Respiratory influences on vagal tone (called sinus arrhythmia)—a normal variation
  B. Severe respiratory disorders or gastrointestinal disease (parasympathetic influence)—bradycardia, SA arrest
  C. Excitement, exercise, pain, or fever (sympathetic influence on the SA node)—sinus tachycardia, AV junctional and ventricular tachycardia
  D. Organic brain disease causing sympathetic or vagal stimulation[13]

II. Cardiac sources
  A. Heredity (believed to be genetic)[14]—AV block, Wolff-Parkinson-White syndrome, His bundle degeneration (sudden death syndrome in Dobermans),[15] persistent atrial standstill, sick sinus syndrome,[16] SA arrest (congenital deafness in Dalmatians),[17] stenosis of the His bundle (AV block and SA arrest in Pugs)[18]
  B. Acquired damage to the conduction system—hypertrophic cardiomyopathy,[19] degenerative myocardial disease (microscopic intramural myocardial infarction, MIMI), AV bundle degeneration (sudden death, personality changes),[20] neoplasia, surgical interruption
  C. Diseases of the atria—atrial arrhythmias occurring in mitral valvular disease (congenital or acquired) (mitral valve leaflet as site of ectopic impulses),[21] neoplasia, dilated cardiomyopathy with secondary atrial dilatation
  D. Diseases of the ventricles—myocarditis (many causes, often not proved conclusively), cardiomyopathy,[22] neoplasia, trauma,[23,24] myocardial ischemia secondary to heart failure

III. Extracardiac sources
  A. Hypoxia[25]
  B. Disturbances of the acid-base balance
  C. Electrolyte imbalance (especially hyperkalemia associated with uremia and adrenocortical insufficiency)
  D. Hypothermia[26]
  E. Drugs, e.g., digoxin, thiamylal sodium, and atropine
  F. Endocrine diseases—hyperthyroidism, hypothyroidism, pheochromocytoma, diabetes mellitus, Addison's disease
  G. Mechanical stimulation—faulty placement of the intravenous fluid catheter in either the right atrium or the right ventricle, cardiac catheterization procedures

Table 8–2. Causes of arrhythmias in the cat

I. Autonomic nervous system
  A. Excitement, exercise, pain, or fever (sympathetic influence)—sinus tachycardia, junctional and ventricular arrhythmias
  B. Respiratory influences on vagal tone (not as pronounced in the cat as in the dog; thus, marked sinus arrhythmias rare)
  C. Organic brain disease causing sympathetic or vagal stimulation[13,27]
  D. Cardiac sympathetic neural discharge as a possible mechanism for digitalis-induced arrhythmias[28]

II. Cardiac sources
  A. Heredity (rare)[14]
  B. Acquired damage to the conduction system—hypertrophic cardiomyopathy (high predilection for the conduction system),[29] neoplasia[30]
  C. Diseases of the atria—atrial arrhythmias occurring in neoplasia, hypertrophic cardiomyopathy, and in various congenital heart defects with secondary left atrial enlargement
  D. Diseases of the ventricles—myocarditis (many causes); neoplasia, myocardial ischemia secondary to heart failure in cardiomyopathy

III. Extracardiac sources
  A. Hypoxia
  B. Disturbances of the acid-base balance
  C. Electrolyte imbalance (particularly hyperkalemia associated with urethral obstruction)
  D. Drugs, e.g., digoxin, halothane (accelerated junctional rhythm and AV block), propylene glycol diluent (used in both intravenous diazepam and phenytoin sodium),[31,32] ketamine hydrochloride (increased heart rate), propranolol (AV block, SA arrest, and severe bradycardia), lidocaine (severe bradycardia)
  E. Endocrine diseases—hyperthyroidism, diabetes mellitus
  F. Mechanical stimulation—faulty placement of the venous catheter tip in either the right atrium or the right ventricle, cardiac catheterization procedures

the primary source of arrhythmias, but there are multiple extracardiac causes, as outlined in Tables 8–1 and 8–2.

The hypotheses derived from the study of the electrical activity of single cardiac cells, utilizing intracellular microelectrodes, have been tested by experiments on the in situ canine heart.[33] Important factors that can affect the action potential and influence automaticity and/or conductivity are as follows:[34]

1. Autonomic nervous system
2. Temperature
3. Hypoxemia
4. Potassium concentration
5. Calcium concentration
6. Endocrine diseases
7. Drugs and therapeutic agents

It is important to determine the extracardiac causes of arrhythmias, since correcting the underlying disorder may terminate the arrhythmia.[35] Also, antiarrhythmic drugs are often ineffective when an extracardiac condition, such as an electrolyte abnormality, persists.

The clinician not only must treat the electrocardiogram as a source of highly specific and sensitive diagnostic information, but must also consider it a source of clues as to what is happening in the patient. These clues are an important part of the clinician's data base and his approach to the diagnosis and management of the patient. Atrial

tachycardia with AV block may accompany digitalis toxicity. Atrioventricular block may indicate an irreversible anatomic lesion in the conduction system or may represent reversible changes produced by drugs or electrolytes. Ventricular arrhythmias may be compatible with cardiac irritability produced by myocardial hypoxia, neurogenic factors, electrolyte imbalances, or other metabolic disorders. One possible explanation for the frequent ventricular arrhythmias associated with gastric dilatation is the reduced venous return caused by mechanical obstruction of the caudal vena cava. A subsequent decrease in cardiac output results in reduced coronary blood flow and myocardial ischemia.[36] Repolarization changes such as large T wave inversion may represent myocardial injury, e.g., in central nervous system disorders (to be discussed in this section). The extracardiac causes of arrhythmias are discussed in various chapters of this textbook, except for the central nervous system, which plays a significant role in cardiovascular regulation.[13] The central nervous system as a causative factor of arrhythmias has not been discussed extensively in the veterinary field. In the following section, the relationship between functional and organic disturbances in the brain and the accompanying disorders of cardiac rhythm will be discussed.

THE NERVOUS SYSTEM AND CARDIAC ARRHYTHMIAS

Various central nervous system disorders may be associated with electrocardiographic abnormalities and cardiac arrhythmias. A cause-and-effect relationship between disturbances in the brain and cardiac abnormalities has been established.[13,35,37–39] This association of neurogenic factors with cardiac disturbances and abnormalities is important to the clinician who may administer cardiac drugs while the diagnosis and treatment of central nervous system disease is delayed.

The neurogenic causes of cardiac arrhythmias include neural reflexes from cerebrovascular accidents (e.g., embolism, thrombosis, hemorrhage, tumor in the brain), and from central nervous disorders secondary to other primary diseases such as hepatic coma, advanced renal failure, and diabetic coma.[40] Psychologic stress can also be a

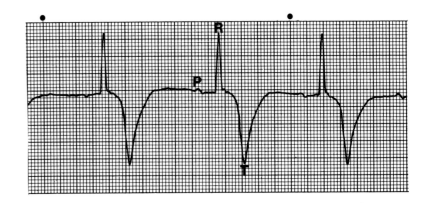

Fig. 8–1. Deep, broad, and negative T waves with a prolonged Q-T interval in a dog with cerebral disease secondary to trauma.

factor. Stimulation of the autonomic nervous system and of the various parts of the brain can produce major electrocardiographic changes. For example, sinoatrial arrest with junctional and/or ventricular escape complexes is often seen in cases of cervical neoplasia, severe respiratory disease, and increased vagal tone in brachycephalic breeds of dog. It should also be known that certain arrhythmias may produce a decrease in cerebral blood flow, resulting in cerebral ischemia. After recovery from cardiopulmonary arrest, the electrocardiogram may show findings characteristic of a neurologic disorder.

The most common electrocardiographic findings associated with central nervous system disease are prolongation of the Q-T interval, S-T segment elevation or depression, and deeply inverted or abnormally tall and broad T waves (Fig. 8–1).[13,40] Also associated with central nervous system stimulation and disease are various arrhythmias, including sinus tachycardia, paroxysmal atrial tachycardia, ventricular premature complexes, and ventricular tachycardia. Stimulation of portions of the hypothalamus (Fig. 8–2) and of the reticular formation in cats produces QRS-T abnormalities and serious arrhythmias via sympathetic and parasympathetic effects.[41] Propranolol has been shown to prevent the appearance of arrhythmias as well as to abolish them.[13] In dogs, electrical stimulation of the diencephalon and mesencephalon results in ventricular arrhythmias, including ventricular tachycardia and fibrillation.[42]

Because of direct actions of the autonomic nervous system on cardiac rate, regularity, and sequence of cardiac activation, an imbalance in this system may play an important role in the genesis of cardiac arrhythmias.[43,44,44a] It has been demonstrated in the dog (Fig. 8–3) that, if all cardiac nerves are severed except for the left ventrolateral cervical cardiac nerve, the heart is vulnerable to arrhythmia. There was no arrhythmia with an intact nerve supply or after complete denervation. Propranolol, by blocking the sympathetic nervous system, controls the arrhythmia.[45] Abnormalities of the cardiac nerves and ganglia (termed cardioneuropathies) have a destabilizing influence on cardiac electrical activity, as well as altering an animal's response to pharmacologic treatment.[45a,b]

In man, an unbalanced sympathetic outflow from the right and left sympathetic system has been suspected as a factor in the etiology of sudden death associated with a prolonged Q-T interval.[35] Arrhythmias provoked during psychophysiologic stress may involve similar mechanisms. Ventricular arrhythmias and a lowering of the threshold for ventricular fibrillation in association with a psychologically stressful environment has been demonstrated in the dog.[46] A similar mechanism may explain sudden death and/or syncope in dogs taken to the dog groomer or to an unusual environment. Beta-adrenergic blockade with propranolol may be indicated when anti-arrhythmic drugs like procainamide fail to control ventricular arrhythmias associated with neurologic disease.[43]

A new disease entity of cats has appeared in the British veterinary literature called autonomic polyganglionopathy, or "Key-Gaskell syndrome."[47] One of the major clinical signs reported is a marked sinus bradycardia from 90 to 120 beats/min. Autonomic imbalance has been reported as one of the explanations for the initiation of cardiac ar-

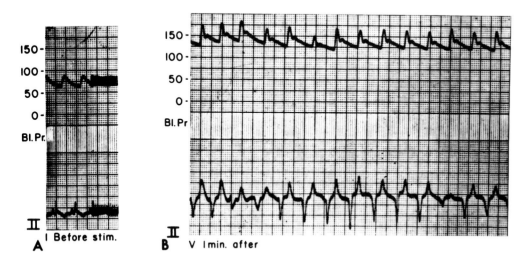

Fig. 8–2. Effect of hypothalamic stimulation on the production of arrhythmias (experiment in the cat). **A,** Control before stimulation. Blood pressure is 85/60, and the electrocardiogram shows normal sinus rhythm. **B,** 1 minute after stimulation. Note rise in blood pressure to 175/135. An idioventricular pacemaker now controls the heart rhythm. Note the widened QRS complexes and the irregularity in rhythm. Normal rhythm returned after cessation of the stimulation. (From Attar, H.J., et al.: Circ. Res., *12*:14, 1963.)

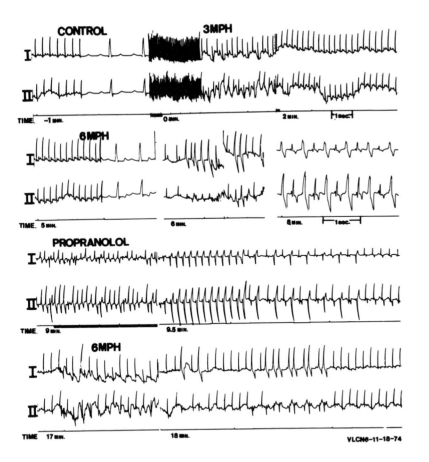

Fig. 8–3. 157 days after partial cardiac denervation eliminating all nervous connection except for the (left) ventrolateral cervical cardiac nerve. At rest (control), regular sinus rhythm is present. Running on 10% grade at 3 min/hour accelerates the heart rate promptly, as expected, from 160 to 240 beats/min. While running at 6 mph, the P waves disappear, the rate slows, and the rhythm becomes irregular. Runs of irregular beats with aberrant ventricular conduction are followed by bigeminy, coupling a supraventricular beat with its follower, manifesting aberrant conduction. Propranolol was administered while supraventricular tachycardia with aberrant conduction was present, and within 30 seconds, the rate slowed with gradual recovery, returning to a regular sinus rhythm and normal conduction, which was maintained. Return to the treadmill, again at 6 mph produced only several ectopic beats, which then disappeared in spite of continuing exercise. Atropine did not prevent this dysrhythmia. (From Wehrmacher, W.H., et al.: The unbalanced heart. Animal models of cardiac dysrhythmias. Cardiology, 64:65, 1979, with permission.)

rhythmias in dogs with gastric dilatation.[36] Myocardial lesions secondary to neural lesions have been reported in the dog[48,48a] and cat.[49] The neural lesions found resulted from trauma, infection, and space-occupying lesions. Increased sympathetic activity is the most popular hypothesis for explaining these myocardial lesions. Similar myocardial lesions have been seen with catecholamine excess in the dog.[49]

It is important to understand that certain arrhythmias may produce a decrease in cerebral blood flow, resulting in cerebral ischemia and

neurologic signs. Aged dogs with atrial arrhythmias such as atrial fibrillation often develop syncopal attacks or seizures. Many times the electrocardiogram is normal, and in such cases, long-term ambulatory electrocardiography is indicated.

Pressure changes within the heart may initiate an arrhythmia. Unbalancing the pressure relationship between the ventricles, either by giving vasopressor drugs or by obstructing the ventricular outflow into the aorta or pulmonary artery, can cause ventricular premature complexes (Fig. 8–4).[45] This arrhythmia is similar to those produced by stimulation of the central nervous system; however, it has been shown that pressure changes within the heart may initiate an arrhythmia independent of neural influence. It has been suggested that stretch-enhancing phase 4 depolarization of Purkinje fibers may be responsible for creating ectopic complexes utilizing adrenaline and a sensitized heart.[50]

HEMODYNAMIC EFFECTS OF CARDIAC ARRHYTHMIAS

The various rhythm disturbances affect the normal hemodynamics of dogs and cats[51,52] by: (1) changing the heart rate (tachycardia, bradycardia); (2) altering the regularity of the heartbeats; (3) changing the time relationship of atrial and ventricular contractions; (4) losing the atrial assistance and regularity of the ventricles in atrial fibrillation; (5) creating a loss of synchrony in ventricular contractions; and (6) causing an increase in cardiac contractility independent of ventricular filling (potentiation). All these hemodynamic effects are more prominent if myocardial function is impaired by heart disease. For example, ventricular tachycardia in a normal heart may cause no major hemodynamic problems, whereas its occurrence in an animal with a diseased heart will usually cause congestive heart failure. The hemodynamic effects of antiarrhythmic drugs should also be considered (Table 10–6).

Clinical signs in dogs with a cardiac arrhythmia can include weakness, lethargy, lack of tolerance to exercise, ataxia, dyspnea, fainting, personality changes, seizures, and even sudden death.[53] Animals showing any of these signs should be carefully evaluated. Sudden death, sudden episodes of viciousness, and seizure disorders in 12 dogs with degeneration of the AV bundle were recently reported by veterinarians at The Animal Medical Center in New York.[20] Hypoxic-type degeneration changes were found in the brains of these dogs, leading to the speculation that occult or transient arrhythmias probably produced the hypoxia. Psychologic abnormalities have been reported in man with chronic cerebral hypoxia and occult arrhythmias.[54] A marked pulse deficit is almost always correlated with clinical signs—weakness, fainting, dyspnea, or even sudden death. Hypertrophic cardiomyopathy and accompanying cardiac arrhythmias are probably the most common cause of sudden death in cats.[29]

In a given animal, some techniques performed during the physical examination may be helpful in diagnosing an arrhythmia even before an electrocardiogram is obtained. These include examination for the presence of a jugular pulse and auscultation of the heart simultaneously with palpation of the femoral pulse. Jugular pulsations occur

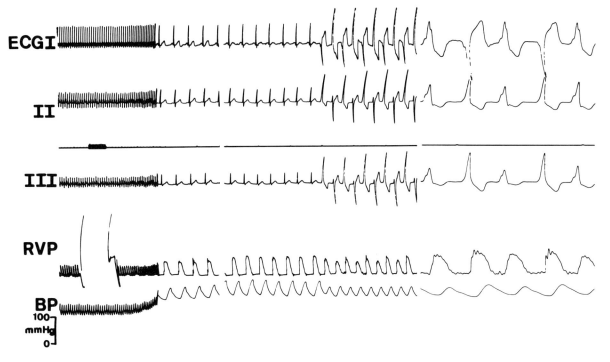

Fig. 8–4. Bidirectional tachycardia induced in dog with totally denervated heart by intravenous injection of phenylephrine. During the recording, the paper speed was accelerated to 100 mm/sec to show details more clearly after the bidirectional tachycardia appeared. Bidirectional tachycardia is a rapid regular rhythm, in which there are alternating rightward and leftward axis shifts. One possible mechanism is the result of alternating routes of ventricular depolarization by a single ectopic left ventricular focus or of alternating discharge of two separate left ventricular foci.[34] RVP is the right ventricular pressure curve, and BP is the aortic pressure curve. (From Wehrmacher, W.H., et al.: The unbalanced heart. Animal models of cardiac dysrhythmias. Cardiology, 64:65, 1979, with permission.)

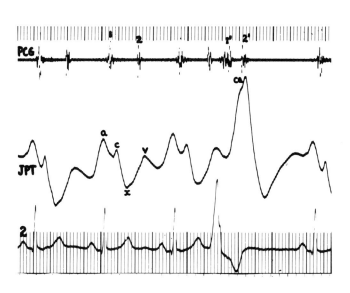

Fig. 8–5. PCG, phonocardiogram; JPT, jugular pulse tracing. Lower panel shows sinus rhythm interrupted by a ventricular premature beat (fourth beat). This closes the atrioventricular valves so that the next atrial contraction forces the blood retrogradely into the neck veins to produce a "cannon wave" (ca). Note also wide splitting of the first sound of the ventricular premature beat (1'). (From Marriott, H.J.L.: *Ventricular Ectopic Beats—I. Contemporary Electrocardiography.* Baltimore, Williams & Wilkins, 1979, with permission.)

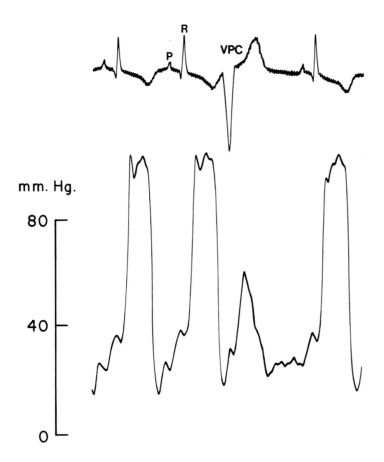

Fig. 8–6. Effect of a ventricular premature complex (VPC) on the left ventricular pressure of a cat with dilated cardiomyopathy. Note the marked drop in blood pressure after the VPC. A very early VPC is usually unable to open the aortic valve and generate a stroke output. A pulse deficit results; heart rate on auscultation is higher than that simultaneously palpated in the femoral artery. Paper speed, 100 mm/sec; amplitude 1 cm = 1 mv.

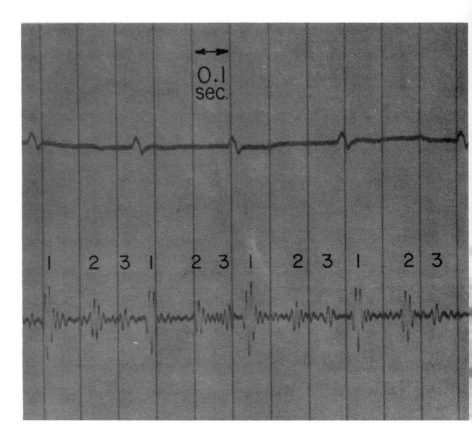

Fig. 8–7. Lead II electrocardiogram from a cat recorded simultaneously with a medium-frequency band phonocardiogram. Hypertrophic cardiomyopathy was found at necropsy. Atrial fibrillation is present. Note the varying intensity of the second sound (2) and the gallop rhythm (third heart sound); often associated with atrial fibrillation. A fixed time relation of the gallop (3) to the second sound (2) is present. Paper speed = 100 mm/sec. (From Tilley, L.P., et al.: Primary myocardial disease in the cat. Am. J. Pathol., 86:493, 1977, with permission.)

when an arrhythmia causes the right atrium to contract on a closed AV valve, thus forcing the blood backward into the jugular vein (Fig. 8–5). The heart rate on auscultation should be routinely correlated with the femoral pulse. There should be a pulse occurring for every heartbeat. Pulse deficits occur when the heart beats without generating a significant flow of blood and usually indicate incomplete ventricular filling often seen with atrial fibrillation, ventricular premature complexes (Fig. 8–6), and atrial premature complexes. In pulse irregularities, the irregularity will be cyclic in sinus arrhythmia, while with other arrhythmias, such as atrial fibrillation, it will be noncyclic. The intensity of the pulse may also vary because of premature complexes or atrial fibrillation.

The heart sounds heard on auscultation are caused by the abrupt acceleration or deceleration of the blood; the first sound is due to closure of the mitral and tricuspid valves, the second to closure of the

aortic and pulmonic valves. These heart sounds may vary in intensity or have extra sounds in the presence of various arrhythmias. For example, atrial fibrillation has a rapid irregular rhythm with variable intensity of the heart sounds (Fig. 8–7). A third heart sound is not uncommon and is usually the result of rapid ventricular filling associated with severe heart failure.

Effects of heart rate and irregularity

In normal large-breed dogs, tachycardia of approximately 140 to 160 beats/min results in an increased cardiac output. Above 160 to 180 beats/min, the rapid heart rate does not have a physiologically useful effect.[51] The phase of rapid ventricular filling is affected, so that stroke filling and stroke output decline. As the heart rate increases, stroke output declines more and more. Also, cardiac oxygen consumption is increased so that more energy is required than is needed by the slow heart to deliver the same output per minute.[55] Tachycardia may also alter blood flow to other organs and produce signs of vascular insufficiency in the central nervous system, the gastrointestinal tract, and the kidneys. In experimental mitral regurgitation in dogs at rates greater than 150 beats/min, the atrial contraction occurs early and increases the amplitude of the left atrial v wave which may contribute to the severity of pulmonary congestion.[55a]

Bradycardia with a heart rate below 40 beats/min results in lowered cardiac output in normal dogs. In dogs with severe ventricular damage, the low heart rate can be a serious condition. For example, the hemodynamics of animals with complete heart block are often similar to those of animals with severe congestive heart failure. Heart failure often results when the animal is excited or exercised, since the demand for greater cardiac output is not satisfied. As the heart fails, heart failure signs increase even with mild activity.[51] Obviously, heart rate is a valuable compensatory mechanism.

In animals with rapid, irregular cardiac rhythm, the average heart rate is an important determinant of performance. The heart's performance can be markedly modified by the irregularity of the beating,[51,56] such as in atrial fibrillation with a rapid ventricular rate.[56a] Many of the beats occur in rapid succession, even though the irregular portion of the rate is not that high. The effects of heart rate and irregular beating on the cardiac hemodynamics can also be demon-strated in animals with slower heart rates, such as in cases of AV block (Fig. 8–8).[2,57]

Significance of atrial contraction

The atrium normally accounts for approximately 10 to 15% of the ventricular filling volume in normal animals.[51] Atrial contraction also contributes to normal closure of the atrioventricular valves. Atrial contraction and its effect on valve closure increases ventricular filling and the force of ventricular contraction, depending on the interval between atrial and ventricular systole. Therefore, any arrhythmia that reduces the contribution of atrial systole reduces ventricular filling. In animals with hypertrophic cardiomyopathy or aortic stenosis, the noncompliant ventricles are more dependent on the extent of atrial contractions for ventricular filling. Atrial fibrillation in these animals markedly diminishes the contribution of atrial systole to ventricular filling.

Echocardiography can provide an excellent opportunity to study cardiac motion in conjunction with various cardiac arrhythmias.[58,58a,59] In 11 dogs with atrial fibrillation examined echocardiographically, there was no evidence of atrial contraction in the left ventricle or aorta, or on the mitral valve leaflets (Fig. 8–9).[58] Not every QRS resulted in systolic or diastolic motion in the mitral and aortic valve leaflets, and this helps to explain the pulse deficits seen during atrial fibrillation.

Atrial fibrillation and atrial tachycardia usually result in reduced

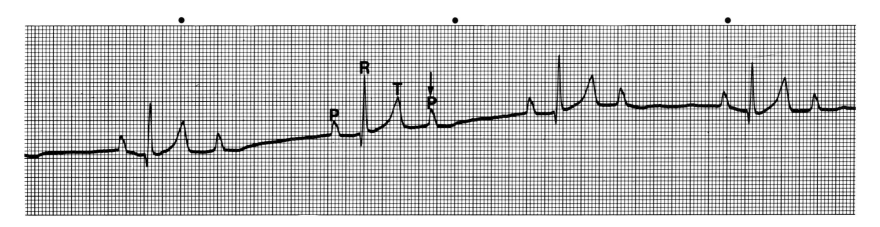

Fig. 8–8. Second-degree 2:1 AV block (arrow) as well as first-degree AV block (P-R interval 0.15 sec). In most cases of advanced second-degree AV block with a 2:1 ratio, a distinctive pattern of the P-P interval often exists. The P-P interval, which includes a QRS complex, is shorter in duration than the P-P interval not containing a QRS complex. One explanation is that the shorter P-P cycle is associated with improved coronary perfusion subsequent to ventricular systole. Another explanation is a baroreceptor response in association with a reduction of vagal tone in response to ventricular systole. Blood supply to the SA node may also be increased following systole. The sinus node responds to the increased perfusion by a more rapid discharge.[2,57]

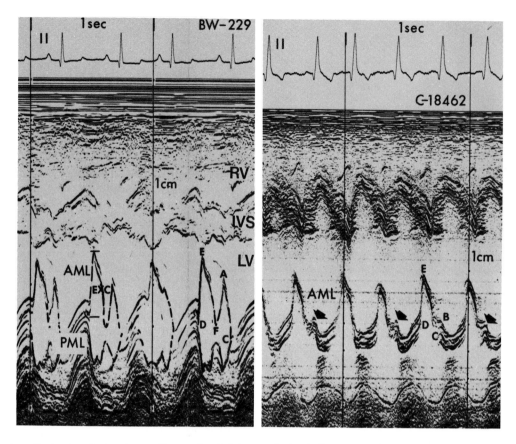

Fig. 8–9. **Left,** Normal motion of a mitral valve during the cardiac cycle. Atrial systole occurs at peak A on the anterior mitral leaflet (AML), the mitral valve closes at point C, diastole occurs at point D, and the valve opens fully at point E, point F occurs just prior to atrial systole. RV = right ventricle; IVS = interventricular septum; LV = left ventricle; PML = posterior mitral leaflet. **Right,** During atrial fibrillation in the dog, there is an absence of an A-point, suggesting lack of effective atrial contractions. Instead of the normal M-shaped excursion of the mitral leaflet, there is only one opening (E-point) of the valve. The descent is delayed by a B-shoulder (arrows). The B-bump can be related to contractions of the fibrillating atrium. (From Lombard, C.W.: Echocardiographic and clinical signs of canine dilated cardiomyopathy. J. Small Anim. Pract., *25*:59, 1984.)

cardiac output, since the rapid atrial contractions reduce venous inflow. In atrial fibrillation, the ventricular rate is rapid and irregular with the sequence of ventricular filling from the atrium lost.[56] The use of digoxin or verapamil in atrial fibrillation often dramatically improves circulatory function since the ventricular rate is slowed and often made more regular.

Ventricular arrhythmias

In ventricular fibrillation, the circulatory effects are obviously major. Arterial pressure is usually absent, and the animal will not survive long without defibrillation. Asynchronous contractions can have a major effect on cardiac output. In ventricular fibrillation, the asynchrony of ventricular contractions is severe, even though mechanical and electrical activity is present. When the cardiac impulse spreads abnormally, the tension energy created in the muscle fibers is dissipated. The fibers that contract early pull upon the fibers not yet contracting, causing internal movements that are ineffective.[51] This asynchronous effect on cardiac efficiency can also be found, for example, in intraventricular block, aberrant ventricular conduction, and in idioventricular rhythms.

Ventricular tachycardia can also be a serious arrhythmia.[59a] The circulatory effects are more serious as the ventricular rate increases.[60,61] In Figure 8–10, circulatory function in a dog deteriorates as the rate of the ventricular tachycardia increases from 100 to 120 to 140 beats/min. Ventricular tachycardia with no major heart disease, such as often seen in dogs with gastric dilatation-volvulus, is not life threatening. It is thus quite important to follow the common statement, "Look at the patient, not just the ECG."[60]

Pulsus alternans and pulsus bigeminus

By palpation of the femoral arterial pulse, beat-to-beat variations in systolic pressure can usually be appreciated. Beat-to-beat alteration of the pulse may occur: (1) during inspiration in animals with pulmonary disease in which the respiratory rate is half the heart rate (called pulsus paradoxus); (2) in animals with bigeminal rhythm; and (3) in animals with severe heart failure (called pulsus alternans).[51]

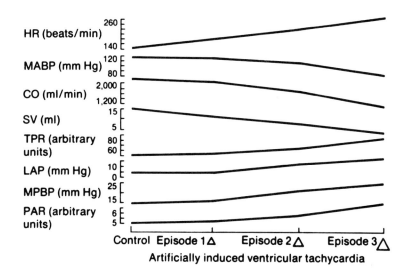

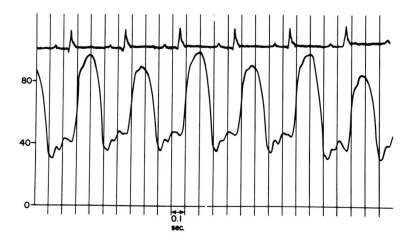

Fig. 8–10. Hemodynamic changes in dog during control and three induced episodes of ventricular tachycardia at progressively faster rates. Note that the third episode resulted in marked deterioration of ventricular function. HR = heart rate; MABP = mean arterial blood pressure; CO = cardiac output; SV = stroke volume; TPR = total peripheral resistance; LAP = left atrial pressure; MPBP = mean pulmonary blood pressure; PAR = pulmonary artery pressure. (From Harrison, D.C.: The circulatory effects of cardiac arrhythmias. In *Cornell Postgraduate Course on Cardiac Arrhythmias.* New York, Cornell University Press, 1979, with permission.)

Fig. 8–11. A tracing from an 8-year-old domestic shorthaired cat with a 1-week history of listlessness and anorexia. There is elevation of the end diastolic pressure together with elevation of both the peak systolic and diastolic pressure tracing. Pulsus alternans is also present, often found with severe heart failure. The cardiac rhythm is regular. Congestive cardiomyopathy was found at necropsy. (From Tilley, L.P., et al.: Primary myocardial disease in the cat. Am. J. Pathol., 86:493, 1977, with permission.)

Pulsus alternans (Fig. 8–11), which is frequently precipitated by a ventricular premature complex, occurs at a regular rhythm. The post-ventricular premature contraction pulsus alternans is probably related to the increased duration of left ventricular filling after the premature beat, resulting in a greater-end-diastolic volume and resultant increased contractile force due to the Frank-Starling mechanism.[62] In animals with severe heart disease, pulsus alternans is often present during a tachycardia.

Pulsus bigeminus (Figs. 8–12 and 8–13) is a bigeminal rhythm caused by the occurrence of premature contractions, usually ventricular. The premature complexes occur after every other beat and result in alternation of the strength of the pulse. The premature beat causes the ventricle to contract too soon, before the chamber has had time to adequately fill with blood. The blood pressure drops when the premature beat occurs.

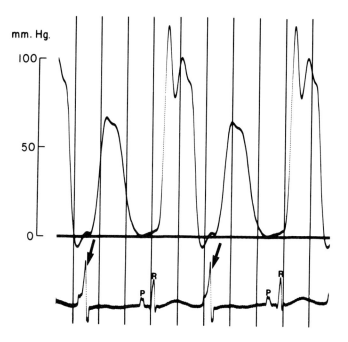

Fig. 8–12. Pulsus bigeminus. Effects of ventricular premature complexes (VPCs) (arrows) on the left ventricular pressure of a dog. Note the drop in blood pressure after each of the premature impulses. Time lines, 0.1 second.

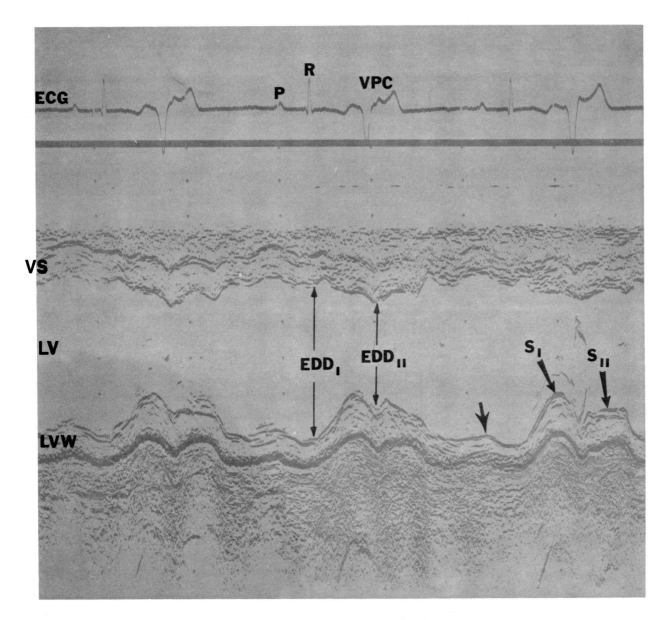

Fig. 8–13. Echocardiogram recorded at a position just below the mitral valve from a 6-month-old male Airedale. The simultaneously recorded electrocardiogram (ECG) shows ventricular bigeminy. The normal contribution of atrial contraction to ventricular filling is illustrated by left ventricular free wall motion (following the large arrow). VS = ventricular septum; LV = left ventricle; LVW = left ventricular wall. It is obvious that the end diastolic dimension of the sinus beat (EDD$_I$) compared to the ventricular premature beat (EDD$_{II}$) is much greater, reflecting a marked difference in ventricular filling and resultant cardiac output. Note that left ventricular wall (LVW) motion during systole is increased during the sinus beat (S$_I$) in contrast to the ventricular premature beat (S$_{II}$). On the right as the transducer is angled dorsally, a portion of the mitral valve appears. Paper speed = 50 mm sec; 1-cm depth markers are recorded every 0.5 sec. (Courtesy of Dr. Gilbert Jacobs, University of Pennsylvania, Philadelphia.)

Histopathologic study of the conduction system

Si-Kwang Liu, D.V.M., Ph.D.

To achieve a better understanding of the pathophysiologic basis and effects of cardiac arrhythmias, it is important to be aware of methods that permit detailed examination of various anatomic lesions involving the conduction system. An anatomic lesion involving the conduction system can explain many clinical signs as well as sudden death. Recent studies in man have emphasized hemodynamic anomalies and the changes that result in both atrial fiber structure and electrical function.[63]

The purpose of this section is to describe the technique for examining the conduction system in the dog and cat.

NECROPSY DISSECTION OF THE HEART

The heart may be removed from the lungs by dissecting between the left atrium and pulmonary veins, and the right atrium and vena cava, ascending aorta, and pulmonary trunk. After the heart has been removed from the lungs and thoracic cavity, the inflow-outflow method of dissection should be employed for examination of the conduction system.[64] The right ventricle is opened by extending an incision from the pulmonary trunk through the pulmonary valve, ventricular free wall, apex, dorsal wall of the ventricle, and dorsal atrial wall to the posterior vena cava without severing the papillary muscles, chordae tendineae, or tricuspid valve.[65,66] The left ventricle is opened by making an incision on the apex extending anteriorly to the aorta, and posteriorly to the left atrium without damaging the papillary muscles, chordae tendineae, or mitral leaflets.[65,66]

GROSS EXAMINATION OF THE CONDUCTION SYSTEM

The conduction system consists of the sinoatrial node, the internodal atrial pathways, the atrioventricular node, the bundle of His, the right and left bundle branches, and the Purkinje fibers (Fig. 8–14). The conduction fiber has a high glycogen content and can be stained easily by applying Lugol's (iodine) solution to the endocardial surface. The bundle branch and its fascicles in the left ventricle of the dog can be identified with this technique (Fig. 8–15). The entire heart should be fixed in 10% cold buffered formalin.

PREPARATION OF TISSUE FOR HISTOLOGIC STUDY

For histologic study of the sinoatrial node, the junction of the anterior vena cava and free wall of the right atrium (Fig. 8–16) are cut into sections 2 and 3 mm thick.[29,67] For study of the atrioventricular node, the entire junction of the interatrial and interventricular septa, from the anterior margin of the coronary sinus of the aorta to the posterior margin of the noncoronary sinus (Fig. 8–17), is sliced into sections 2 to 3 mm thick, perpendicular to the line of junction of the septa.[29,68] One adjacent centimeter of each septum is retained. The slices are embedded in paraffin, and the blocks are serially sectioned

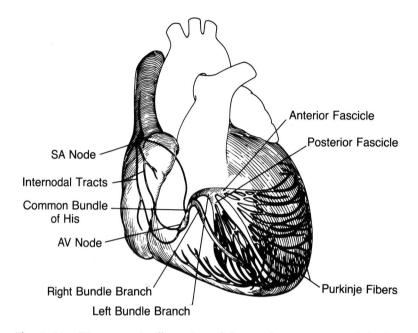

Fig. 8–14. Diagrammatic illustration of the conduction system of the heart. (From De Sanctis, R.W.: Disturbances of cardiac rhythm and conduction. In *SCIENTIFIC AMERICAN MEDICINE*. Edited by R. Rubenstein. New York, Scientific American, 1982, with permission.)

Labels: SA Node, Internodal Tracts, Common Bundle of His, AV Node, Right Bundle Branch, Left Bundle Branch, Anterior Fascicle, Posterior Fascicle, Purkinje Fibers

6 μm in thickness and stained with hematoxylin and eosin, Masson's trichrome, or periodic acid Schiff stains.

LESIONS OF THE CONDUCTION SYSTEM

The conduction system of the hearts of 85 adult cats, ranging in age from 6 months to 16 years (mean age, 7.2 years), has been studied.[69] Clinical findings included dyspnea, anorexia, aortic thromboembolism, abnormal electrocardiograms (various degrees of heart block), syncope, and unexpected death in 30% of the affected cats. Histologic examination of cardiac tissue showed degeneration, vacuolization, and fibrosis of the atrioventricular nodal tissue, and degeneration and infiltration of the fibrous granulation tissue in the left and right bundle branches. Islands of cartilage and bone with marrow in the central fibrous body were often found compressing the adjacent node (Fig. 8–18).[68,69]

Sudden and unexpected death associated with atrioventricular degeneration has been studied in 23 young dogs ranging in age from 7 months to 10½ years (mean age 4.2 years).[69] Doberman Pinschers had a higher occurrence of the syndrome than other breeds. Clinical findings included cardiac arrhythmias, sudden and unexpected death,

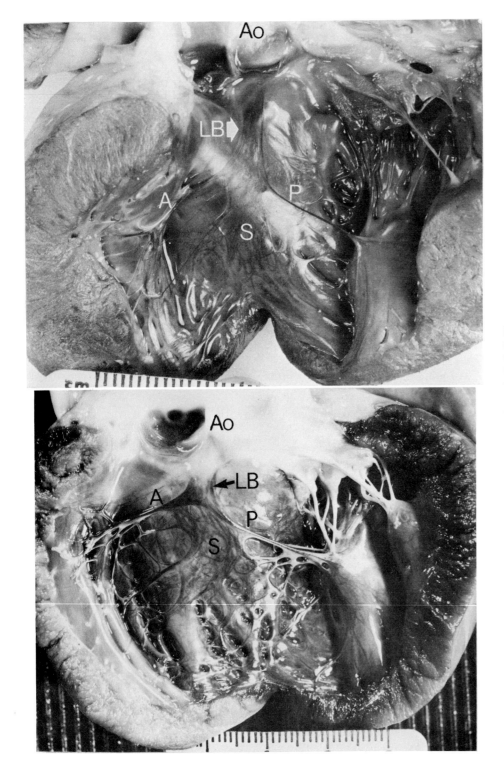

Fig. 8–15. Left ventricular conduction system in two canine hearts. These photographs were taken of the left ventricular septal surface after iodine staining of the endocardium. The left bundle branch (LB) emerges as a bandlike structure below the aortic valve (Ao) in both cases. The left bundle branch bifurcates into the anterior (A) and posterior (P) fascicles, which are attached to the apical portions of the papillary muscles. A network of midseptal Purkinje fibers (S) is distributed throughout the septal surface bordered by the two major fascicles. In the lower photo, the septal fibers are extensive, and the contribution of the posterior fascicle is predominant. Many of the strands on the unstained heart are, in effect, portions of the peripheral and terminal branches of the conduction system.

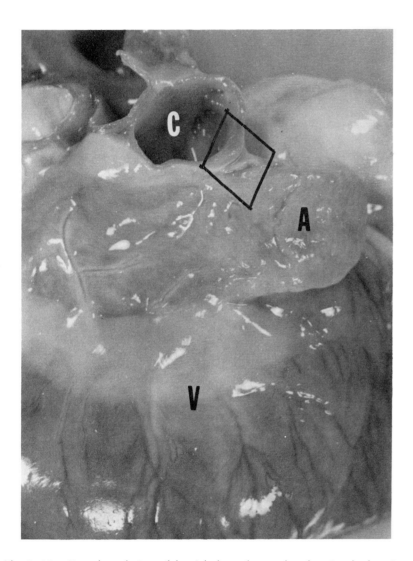

Fig. 8–16. Dorsolateral view of the right heart from a dog showing the location of the sinoatrial node in the square box; note Ventricular free wall (V); Auricle (A); and Anterior vena cava (C).

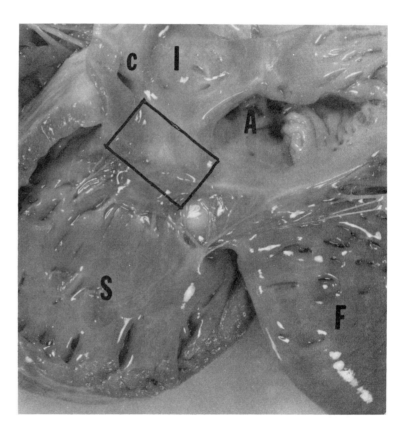

Fig. 8–17. Opened right heart from a dog showing the location of the atrioventricular node in the square box; Ventricular septum (S); Ventricular free wall (F); Atrium (A); Atrial septum (I); and Coronary sinus (C).

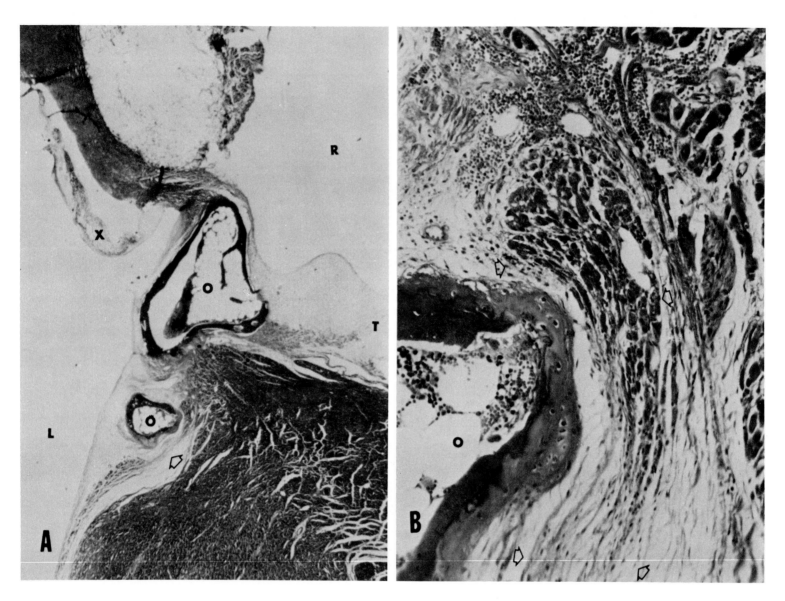

Fig. 8–18. Microphotographs of the atrioventricular septa from a 6-year-old male Siamese cat with a left bundle branch block resulting in sudden death. Note ossifications (O) in the central fibrous body and left ventricular septum; left ventricle (L), aortic valve (X), right atrium (R), and tricuspid valve (T). The bone cysts are compressed and have caused degeneration, fibrosis, and vacuolization of the left bundle fibers (arrows). H & E stain, **A** × 40, **B** × 160.

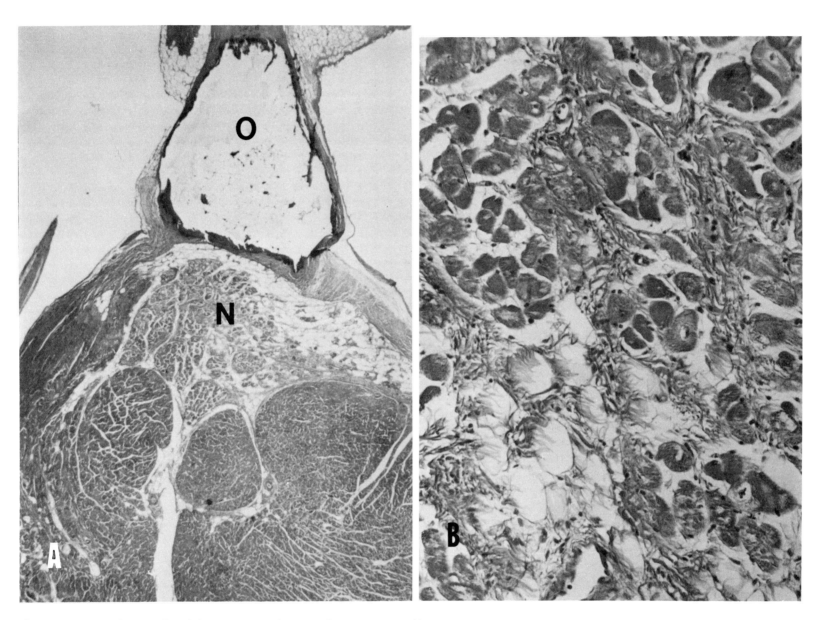

Fig. 8–19. Microphotographs of the atrioventricular septa from an 8-year-old female Doberman Pinscher with multifocal ventricular premature complexes for 1 year prior to sudden death. **A,** Note bone cyst (O) in the central fibrous body, and degeneration, fibrosis, and vacuolization of the AV nodal tissue (N). H & E stain; × 28. **B,** Note fibrosis, degeneration, and vacuolization of the conduction fibers. H & E stain, × 160. (From Liu, S.-K.: Cardiac disease in the dog and cat. *Pig Model for Biomedical Research.* Pig Research Institute, Taiwan, pp. 110–133, 1982, with permission.)

sudden episodes of viciousness, and seizures. Histologic changes in the conduction system included degeneration and fibrosis of the atrioventricular node (Fig. 8–19), or His bundle, cartilage and bone formation in the central fibrous body, and narrowing of the local small coronary arteries.[15,18,20]

Luminal narrowing of small arteries in the region of the His bundle is probably the cause of degenerative changes in the conduction system of dogs that die suddenly.[15,18] The pathogenesis of conduction system lesions is uncertain at present, but hereditary factors may be involved.[18] On the basis of the lesions of the conduction system, and clinical and electrocardiographic findings, it has been postulated that the conduction disturbance, syncope, and sudden death may be caused by atrioventricular nodal lesions and labile left ventricular end diastolic pressure, as described in man.[15] Bone is found in the central fibrous body of the heart in human patients with severe syncope attacks.[70] The presence of cartilage in the central fibrous body may initiate fatal conduction disturbances.[71] In dogs, abnormal presence of bone with lesions in the atrioventricular node of the heart reportedly relate to sudden death, sudden episodes of viciousness, or seizure disorder.[15,18,20]

REFERENCES

1. Veith, I., and Huang, Ti Nei Ching Su Weu: *The Yellow Emperor's Classic of Internal Medicine*. Baltimore, Williams & Wilkins, 1949.
2. Kernicki, J., and Weiler, K.M.: *Electrocardiography for Nurses, Physiological Correlates.* New York, Wiley, 1981.
3. Fisch, C.: The clinical electrocardiogram: a classic (Lewis A. Connor Memorial lecture—American Heart Association). Circulation, 62:III-1, 1980.
4. Bolton, G.R.: *Handbook of Canine Electrocardiography*, Philadelphia, W.B. Saunders, 1975.
5. Tilley, L.P., Liu, S.-K., and Fox, P.R.: Myocardial disease. In *Textbook of Veterinary Internal Medicine*. Edited by S.J. Ettinger. 2nd Edition. Philadelphia, W.B. Saunders, 1983.
6. Rios, J.C. (Ed.): *Clinical Electrocardiographic Correlations. Cardiovascular Clinics* (A.N. Brest; Editor-in-Chief). Philadelphia, F.A. Davis, 1977.
7. Helfant, R.H.: *Bellet's Essentials of Cardiac Arrhythmias.* 2nd Edition. Philadelphia, W.B. Saunders, 1980.
8. Harpster, N.K.: Cardiovascular diseases of the cat. Adv. Vet. Sci. Comp. Med., 21:39, 1977.
9. Tilley, L.P.: Feline cardiac arrhythmias. Vet. Clin. North Am., 7:273, 1977.
10. Tilley, L.P., et al.: Primary myocardial disease in the cat. Am. J. Pathol., 86:493, 1977.
11. Fox, P.R., Tilley, L.P., and Liu, S.-K.: The cardiovascular system. In *Feline Medicine*. Edited by P.W. Pratt. Santa Barbara, Calif., Am. Vet. Publ. Inc., 1983.
12. Tilley, L.P., Bond, B., Patnaik, A.K., and Liu, S.-K.: Cardiovascular tumors in the cat. J. Am. Anim. Hosp. Assoc., 17:1009, 1981.
13. Bodenheimer, M.M.: Brain and heart relationship. In *Bellet's Essentials of Cardiac Arrhythmias*. Edited by R.H. Helfant. 2nd Edition. Philadelphia, W.B. Saunders, 1979.
14. Guntheroth, W.G., and Motulsky, A.G.: Inherited primary disorders of cardiac rhythm and conduction. In *Progress of Medical Genetics—Genetics of Cardiovascular Disease*. Volume 5, Philadelphia, W.B. Saunders, 1983.
15. James, T.N., and Drake, E.H.: Sudden death in Doberman Pinschers. Ann. Intern. Med., 68:821, 1968.
16. Hamlin, R.L., Smetzer, D.L., and Breznock, E.M.: Sinoatrial syncope in miniature Schnauzers. J. Am. Vet. Med. Assoc., 161:1023, 1972.
17. James, T.N.: Congenital deafness and cardiac arrhythmias. Am. J. Cardiol., 19:627, 1967.
18. James, T.N., et al.: De subitaneis mortibus. XV. Hereditary stenosis of the His bundle in Pug dogs. Circulation, 52:1152, 1975.
19. Liu, S.-K., Maron, B.J., and Tilley, L.P.: Canine hypertrophic cardiomyopathy. J. Am. Vet. Med. Assoc., 174:708, 1979.
20. Meierhenry, E.F., and Liu, S.-K.: Atrioventricular bundle degeneration associated with sudden death in the dog. J. Am. Vet. Med. Assoc., 172:1418, 1978.
21. Wit, A.L., et al.: Electrophysiological properties of cardiac muscle in the anterior mitral valve leaflet and the adjacent atrium in the dog, possible implications for the genesis of atrial dysrhythmias. Circ. Res., 32:731, 1973.
22. Calvert, C.A., Chapman, W.L., and Toal, R.L.: Congestive cardiomyopathy in Doberman Pinscher dogs. J. Am. Vet. Assoc., 181:598, 1982.
23. Alexander, J.W., Bolton, G.R., and Koslow, G.L.: Electrocardiographic changes in nonpenetrating trauma to the chest. J. Am. Anim. Hosp. Assoc., 11:160, 1975.
24. Harpster, N.K., Van Zwieten, M.J., and Bernstein, M.: Traumatic papillary muscle rupture in a dog. J. Am. Vet. Med. Assoc., 165:1074, 1974.
25. Muir, W.W., and Lipowitz, A.J.: Cardiac dysrhythmias associated with gastric dilatation-volvulus in the dog. J. Am. Vet. Med. Assoc., 172:683, 1978.
26. Zenoble, R.D., and Hill, B.L.: Hypothermia and associated cardiac arrhythmias in two dogs. J. Am. Vet. Med. Assoc., 175:840, 1979.
27. Corr, P.B., Witkowski, F.X., and Sobel, B.E.: Mechanisms contributing to malignant dysrhythmias induced by ischemia in the cat. J. Clin. Invest., 61:109, 1978.
28. Lathers, C.M., Kelliher, G.J., Roberts, J., and Besley, A.B.: Nonuniform cardiac sympathetic nerve discharge, mechanism for coronary occlusion and digitalis-induced arrhythmias. Circulation, 57:1058, 1978.
29. Liu, S.-K., Tilley, L.P., and Tashjian, R.J.: Lesions of the conduction system in the cat with cardiomyopathy. Recent Adv. Stud. Cardiac Struct. Metab., 10:681, 1975.
30. Tilley, L.P., Bond, B., Patnaik, A.K., and Liu, S.-K.: Cardiovascular tumors in the cat. J. Am. Anim. Hosp. Assoc., 17:1009, 1981.
31. Louis, S., Kutt, H., and McDowell, F.: The cardiocirculatory changes caused by intravenous Dilantin and its solvent. Am. Heart J., 74:523, 1968.
32. Muir, W.E., Werner, L.L., and Hamlin, R.L.: Antiarrhythmic effects of diazepam during coronary artery occlusion in dogs. Am. J. Vet. Res., 36:1203, 1975.
33. Hoffman, B.F., and Rosen, M.R.: Cellular mechanisms for cardiac arrhythmias. Circ. Res., 49:1, 1981.
34. Gallagher, J.J.: Mechanisms of arrhythmias and conduction abnormalities. In *The Heart*. Edited by J.W. Hurst. 5th Edition. New York, McGraw-Hill, 1982.
35. Naylor, R.E., and O'Rourke, R.A.: Extracardiac causes of dysrhythmias. Hosp. Med., 18:91, 1982.
36. Muir, W.W.: Gastric dilatation-volvulus in the dog, with emphasis on cardiac arrhythmias. J. Am. Vet. Med. Assoc., 180:739, 1982.
37. Malliani, A., Schwartz, P.J., and Zanchetti, A.: Neural mechanisms in life-threatening arrhythmias. Am. Heart J., 100:705, 1980.
38. Levitt, B., et al.: Role of the nervous system in the genesis of cardiac rhythm disorders. Am. J. Cardiol., 37:1111, 1976.
39. Abildskov, J.A.: The nervous system and cardiac arrhythmias. Circulation, 51, 52:III-116, 1975.
40. Chung, E.K.: Central nervous system disorders (ECG of the Month). Primary Cardiology, 6:69, 1980.
41. Attar, H.J., Gutierrez, M.T., Bellet, S., and Ravens, J.R.: Effect and stimulation of hypothalamus and reticular activating system on production of cardiac arrhythmias. Circ. Res., 12:14, 1963.
42. Hockman, C.H., Mauck, H.P., and Hoff, E.C.: ECG changes resulting from cerebral stimulation. Am. Heart J., 71:695, 1966.
43. D'Agrosa, L.S.: Cardiac arrhythmias of sympathetic origin in the dog. Am. J. Physiol., 233:H535, 1977.
44. Randall, W.C., et al.: Autonomic neural control of cardiac rhythm: the role of autonomic imbalance in the genesis of cardiac dysrhythmia. Cardiology, 61:20, 1976.
44a. Waxman, M.B., Wald, R.W., and Cameron, D.: Interactions between the autonomic nervous system and tachycardias in man. Cardiology Clin., 1(2):143, 1983.
45. Wehrmacher, W.H., Talano, J.V., Kaye, M.P., and Randall, W.C.: The unbalanced heart. Animal models of cardiac dysrhythmias. Cardiology, 64:65, 1979.
45a. James, T.N.: Primary and secondary cardioneuropathies and their functional significance. J. Am. College Cardiol., 2:983, 1983.
45b. Rardon, D.P., and Bailey, J.C.: Parasympathetic effects on electrophysiologic properties of cardiac ventricular tissue. J. Am. College Cardiol., 2:1200, 1983.
46. Corbalan, R., Verrier, R.L., and Lown, B.: Psychological stress and ventricular arrhythmias during myocardial infarction in the conscious dog. Am. J. Cardiol., 34:692, 1974.

47. Griffiths, I.R., Nash, A.S., and Sharp, N.J.H.: The Key-Gaskell syndrome: the current situation. Vet. Rec., *111*:532, 1982.
48. King, J.M., Roth, L., and Haschek, M.: Myocardial necrosis secondary to neural lesions in domestic animals. J. Am. Vet. Med. Assoc., *180*:144, 1982.
48a.Macintire, D.K., and Snyder, III, T.G.: Cardiac arrhythmias associated with multiple trauma in dogs. J. Am. Vet. Med. Assoc., *184*:541, 1984.
49. Greenhoot, J.H., and Reichenbach, D.D.: Cardiac injury and subarachnoid hemorrhage. A clinical, pathological, and physiological correlation. J. Neurosurg., *30*:521, 1969.
50. Reynolds, A.K., Chiz, J.F., and Tanikella, T.K.: On the mechanism of coupling in adrenal induced bigeminy in sensitized hearts. Can. J. Physiol. Pharmacol., *53*:1158, 1975.
51. Silber, E.N., and Katz, L.N.: *Heart Disease.* New York, Macmillan, 1975.
52. Sinno, M.Z., and Gunner, R.M.: Hemodynamic consequences of dysrhythmias. Med. Clin. North Am., *60*:69, 1976.
53. Beckett, S.D., Branch, C.E., and Robertson, B.T.: Syncopal attacks and sudden death in dogs: mechanisms and etiologies. J. Am. Anim. Hosp. Assoc., *14*:378, 1978.
54. Bellet, S.: *Clinical Disorders of the Heart Beat.* 3rd Edition. Philadelphia, Lea & Febiger, 1971.
55. Wegria, R., et al.: The effect of atrial and ventricular tachycardia on cardiac output, coronary blood flow, and arterial blood pressure. Circ. Res., *6*:624, 1958.
55a.Yoran, C., et al.: Effects of heart rate on experimentally produced mitral regurgitation in dogs. Am. J. Cardiol., *52*:1345, 1983.
56. Morris, J.J., et al.: Experience with cardioversion of atrial fibrillation and flutter. Am. J. Cardiol., *14*:94, 1964.
56a.Wichman, J., Ertl, G., Rudolph, G., and Kochsiek, H.: Effect of experimentally induced atrial fibrillation on coronary circulation in dogs. Basic Res. Cardiol., *78*:473, 1983.
57. Stock, J.P., and Williams, M.B.: *Diagnosis and Treatment of Cardiac Arrhythmias.* 3rd Edition. Boston, Butterworth, 1974.
58. Wingfield, W.E., Boon, J., and Miller, C.W.: Echocardiographic assessment of mitral valve motion, cardiac structures, and ventricular function in dogs with atrial fibrillation. J. Am. Vet. Med. Assoc., *181*:46, 1982.
58a.Lombard, C.W.: Echocardiographic and clinical signs of canine dilated cardiomyopathy. J. Small Anim. Practice, *25*:59, 1984.
59. Feigenbaum, H.: *Echocardiography.* 3rd Edition. Philadelphia, Lea & Febiger, 1981.
59a.Lima, J.A., et al.: Incomplete filling and incoordinate contraction as mechanisms of hypotension during ventricular tachycardia in man. Circulation, *68*:928, 1983.
60. Harrison, D.C.: The circulatory effects of cardiac arrhythmias. In *Cornell Postgraduate Course on Cardiac Arrhythmias.* New York, Cornell University Press, 1979.
61. Lown, B., Temte, J.V., and Arter, W.J.: Ventricular tachyarrhythmias: clinical aspects. Circulation, *47*:1364, 1973.
62. Mitchell, J.H., Sarnoff, S.J., and Sonnenblik, E.H.: Alternating end-diastolic fiber length as a causative factor. J. Clin. Invest., *42*:55, 1963.
63. Mary-Rabine, L., et al.: The relationship of human atrial cellular electrophysiology to clinical function and ultrastructure. Circ. Res., *52*:188, 1983.
64. Liu, S.-K.: Postmortem examination of the heart. Vet. Clin. North Am., *13*:379, 1983.
65. Liu, S.-K., Tashjian, R.J., and Patnaik, A.K.: Congestive heart failure in the cat. Am. J. Vet. Med. Assoc., *156*:1319, 1970.
66. Liu, S.-K.: Acquired cardiac lesions leading to congestive heart failure in the cat. Am. J. Vet. Res., *31*:2071, 1970.
67. James, T.N.: Anatomy of the Sinus Node of the Dog. Anat. Rec., *143*:251, 1962.
68. James, T.B.: Anatomy of the A-V node of the dog. Anat. Rec., *148*:15, 1964.
69. Liu, S.-K.: Cardiac disease in the dog and cat. In *Pig Model for Biomedical Research.* Edited by H.R. Roberts and W.J. Dodds. Pig Research Institute, Taiwan, 1982, p. 110.
70. Tapham, J.A.: Bone formations in the heart. Br. Med. J., *2*:953, 1906.
71. Ferris, J.S., and Aherne, W.A.: Cartilage in relation to the conductive tissue of the heart in sudden death. Lancet, *i*:64, 1971.

9 Cellular electrophysiologic basis of cardiac arrhythmias

PENELOPE A. BOYDEN, Ph.D.

ANDREW L. WIT, Ph.D.

In physiology, as in all other sciences, no discovery is useless, no curiosity misplaced or too ambitious, and we may be certain that every advance achieved in the quest of pure knowledge will sooner or later play its part. . . .*

ERNEST H. STARLING, M.D., 1915

During normal sinus rhythm, the cardiac impulse originates in the sinus node at a rate appropriate to the age and state of activity of the animal and spreads in an orderly fashion throughout the atria, through the AV node and His-Purkinje system, and throughout the ventricles. An arrhythmia is an abnormality in the rate, regularity, or site of origin of the cardiac impulse or a disturbance in conduction of the impulse such that the normal sequence of activation of atria and ventricles is altered.

As discussed throughout this textbook, cardiac arrhythmias and conduction disturbances occur in every region of the heart and are caused by numerous diseases. In the final analysis, however, all arrhythmias and conduction disturbances, regardless of their pathologic cause, result from critical alterations in the electrical activity of the myocardial cell. This chapter will provide basic information on how the normal cardiac electrophysiology can be changed by cardiac disease and how these changes can lead to conduction disturbances and cardiac arrhythmias.

Arrhythmias may be said to result from abnormalities of impulse generation and/or impulse conduction. Table 9–1 shows a current classification of the cellular mechanisms for cardiac arrhythmias.[1] The electrical activity causing these abnormalities of impulse formation and conduction may result from some change in the ionic mechanism responsible for generation of the normal transmembrane action potential (Fig. 9–1). Abnormalities of impulse formation and conduction may also result from a different type of electrical activity with an ionic basis and electrophysiologic characteristics quite unlike those that are normal for cardiac fibers.

EFFECT OF CARDIAC DISEASE ON THE RESTING AND ACTION POTENTIAL

Resting potential

It appears that most diseases affecting the heart cause the resting potential to decrease (become less negative). At the present time,

transmembrane potentials have been recorded from atrial fibers in man and in cats with cardiomyopathy and from ventricular muscle and ventricular specialized conducting fibers in failed and ischemic hearts. In all instances, resting potential has been less negative than in normal regions of the heart.[2]

The reasons for the decline in resting potential are not completely understood, but several factors may be important. In some instances of disease, the extracellular environment can be changed. For example, ischemia causes a decrease in intracellular ATP, which in turn causes a decrease in sodium-potassium ion pumping. Normally the Na^+-K^+ pump removes Na^+ from the cell and returns K^+ into the cell after each action potential. When pumping decreases, K^+ accumulates in the restricted extracellular spaces. This elevation in external K^+ concentration ($[K^+]_o$) can lead to a decrease in resting potential of the cell, because when $[K^+]_o$ is increased, the diffusion gradient for K^+ decreases across the semipermeable membrane. In fact, the resting membrane potential is a linear function of the logarithm of $[K^+]_o$[3] (Fig. 9–2).

In other diseases, intracellular ion concentrations may be altered, as from a decrease in active Na^+-K^+ pumping or from changes in the permeability of the cell membrane to K^+ or Na^+ caused by the cardiac disease. If cardiac disease has caused either decreased pumping or increased permeability of the membrane to K^+, the result may be a decrease in intracellular K^+ concentration ($[K^+]_i$) and/or an increase in intracellular Na^+ concentration ($[Na^+]_i$). Both alterations in internal ion concentration could lead to a decrease in resting potential. Current research has shown that resting potentials are decreased in atrial fibers in hearts of cats with cardiomyopathy.[2] Whether these fibers have a decrease in $[K^+]_i$ or an increase in $[Na^+]_i$, however, is not yet known.

Another possible cause for the decline in membrane potential is a decrease in membrane permeability to K^+. Such a change in permeability characteristics of the cardiac cell membrane might result from alterations in protein or lipid metabolism. In this way, partial depolarization of the cell (a decline in resting potential) might happen even without marked changes in extra- or intracellular electrolytes. As discussed, the high resting potential of normal cardiac fibers results not only from the marked difference in intra- and extracellular K^+ concentrations but also from the fact that the membrane at rest is highly permeable to K^+. If this permeability to K^+ is decreased, fewer K^+ ions will be able to diffuse across the membrane to cause the high resting potential.

Although we have stressed that the resting potential is decreased in many cardiac diseases, in some diseases it does remain normal. Transmembrane potentials have been recorded with microelectrodes

---

*From Starling, E.H.: "The Linacre Lecture on the Law of the Heart" (Cambridge, 1915). London, Longmans, Green and Company, Ltd., 1918.

Table 9–1. Mechanisms for arrhythmias*

I Abnormal impulse generation	II Abnormal impulse conduction	III Simultaneous abnormalities of impulse generation and conduction

A. Normal automatic mechanism
  1. Abnormal rate
    a. Tachycardia
    b. Bradycardia
  2. Abnormal rhythm
    a. Premature impulses
    b. Delayed impulses
    c. Absent impulses
B. Abnormal automatic mechanism
  1. Phase 4 depolarization at low
    membrane potential
  2. Oscillatory depolarizations at low
    membrane potential preceding
    upstroke
C. Triggered activity
  1. Early afterdepolarizations
  2. Delayed afterdepolarizations
  3. Oscillatory depolarizations at low
    membrane potentials following
    action potential upstroke
	A. Slowing and block
	  1. Sinoatrial block
	  2. Atrioventricular block
	  3. His bundle block
	  4. Bundle branch block
	B. Unidirectional block and re-entry
	  1. Random-re-entry
	    a. Atrial muscle
	    b. Ventricular muscle
	  2. Ordered re-entry
	    a. Sinoatrial node and junction
	    b. AV node and junction
	    c. His-Purkinje system
	    d. Purkinje fiber-muscle
	    e. Abnormal AV connection
	      (pre-excitation)
		A. Phase 4 depolarization and
		   impaired conduction
		  1. Specialized cardiac fibers
		B. Parasystole

*Adapted from Hoffman, B.F., and Rosen, M.R.: Cellular mechanisms for cardiac arrhythmias. Circ. Res., *49*:1, 1981, with permission of the American Heart Assoc. Inc.

Fig. 9–1. Normal action potential of a nonpacemaking cell (on the left) with the relationship of the electrocardiogram (on the bottom). The QRS is produced by the upstrokes (phase 0) of all the action potentials in the cells throughout the ventricles during depolarization; the S-T segment corresponds to the plateaus (phase 2); the T wave occurs during repolarization (phase 3) of the ventricular cells; the isoelectric line after the T wave corresponds to ventricular diastole (phase 4). The normal action potential of a pacemaking cell is illustrated on the right. Pacemaker cells (e.g., those in the SA node) are capable of initiating their own impulses without an extrinsic stimulus. They can depolarize spontaneously during phase 4 until threshold potential is reached and an action potential occurs.

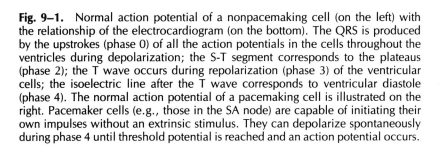

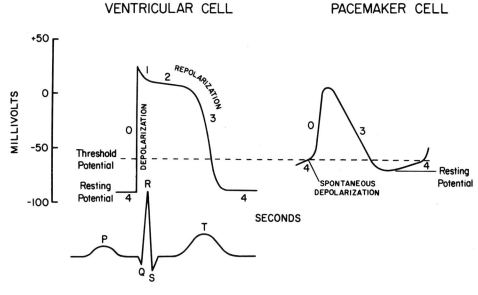

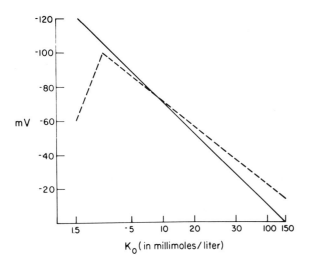

Fig. 9–2. The solid line shows the diffusion potential of a K-concentration cell; the concentration on one side of the cell remains at 150 millimoles, whereas that on the other side varies. When the concentrations on both sides equal 150 millimoles, the measured potential difference is zero; when $[K^+]_o$ decreases to 1.5 millimoles, the potential difference increases up to 123 mv. The broken line shows experimentally determined values of membrane potential of a Purkinje fiber. As $[K^+]_o$ is increased, the potential difference decreases or the resting potential becomes less negative. (From Cranefield, P.F.: *The Conduction of the Cardiac Impulse*. New York, Futura Publishing Co., 1975, reprinted with permission.)

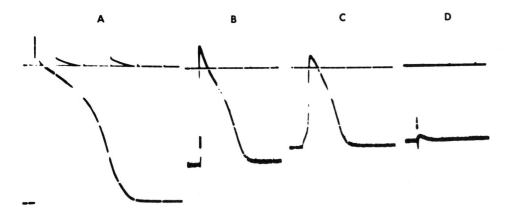

Fig. 9–3. The actual behavior of a Purkinje fiber action potential as resting potential depolarization is caused by an increase in the external potassium concentration ($[K^+]_o$). **A,** Resting potential, -90 mv; $\dot{V}_{max} = 500$ V/sec; $[K^+]_o = 4$ millimoles. **B,** Resting potential, -80 mv; $\dot{V}_{max} = 200$ mv; $[K^+]_o = 8$ millimoles. **C,** Resting potential, -70 mv; $\dot{V}_{max} = 100$ V/sec; $[K^+]_o = 11$ millimoles. **D,** Resting potential, -60 mv; no action potential can be generated (the cell is inexcitable). (From Cranefield, P.F.: *The Conduction of the Cardiac Impulse*. New York, Futura Publishing Co., 1975, reprinted with permission.)

from dogs with mitral valve disease, enlarged atria and atrial fibrillation.[4] The resting potential of most atrial cells was in the normal range of -70 to -85 mv. Therefore, in this example, atrial fibrillation is not caused by low resting potentials but, rather, by other electrophysiologic abnormalities.

Phase 0 depolarization

In most cardiac diseases, the characteristics of the upstroke of the action potential (phase 0) are significantly altered. This may occur because of several reasons. First, a reduction in resting membrane potential may alter the upstroke of the action potential. Second, cardiac disease may directly alter the fast Na^+ and slow Ca^{++} channels through which depolarizing current flows.

A decrease in resting potential of atrial, ventricular, or Purkinje fibers causes decreases in the rate of phase 0 depolarization (V_{max}) and in the amplitude of the action potential. This is due to the effect of membrane potential on the fast inward Na^+ current. When cells with high resting potentials (-90 mv) are excited, most of the Na^+ channels in the membrane open widely, and the fast inward Na^+ current flows through these fast channels to cause depolarization (Fig. 9–3A). When cells with lower resting potentials (-70 mv) are stimulated, fewer Na^+ channels open and the amount of inward Na^+ current decreases, causing a decrease in upstroke velocity and action potential amplitude. When cells with resting potentials of -65 mv are excited, most of the fast Na^+ channels do not open. Since the amount of Na^+ current that can flow through these partially inactivated channels is severely reduced, the upstrokes and amplitudes of action potentials elicited at such resting potentials is reduced even further. Finally, when cells with resting potentials of -55 to -60 mv are stimulated, the fast Na^+ channels do not open at all and, hence, the cells cannot develop an action potential with an upstroke caused by the inward movement of sodium through fast Na^+ channels (Fig. 9–3D).

Action potentials elicited in fibers with low resting potentials and reduced upstrokes dependent on reduced inward Na^+ current flowing through partially inactivated fast channels are called *depressed fast responses*. This term underlines the fact that the depolarization phase is still caused by Na^+ current flowing through the fast channel even though upstroke velocity is slow.

One of the factors that govern the speed of conduction of an impulse is the rate and amplitude of depolarization of the action potential. As the maximum rate of depolarization and amplitude decreases, conduction velocity decreases. Therefore, action potentials arising from reduced resting membrane potentials propagate more slowly than normal and may be more susceptible to block. How this slowed conduction and block may cause arrhythmias is discussed later.

In Chapter 1, the second phase of the action potential (phase 2, slow repolarization) is described as being partially caused by a slow inward current flowing through a slow channel (which is distinct from the fast Na^+ channel). This slow inward current begins to flow during the latter part of phase 0 and is responsible for the plateau of the action potential (Fig. 9–1). The slow current channel still operates normally at the low resting membrane potentials that reduce the function of the fast inward channel. Therefore, under appropriate conditions, cells with very low resting potentials may generate action potentials with a depolarization phase caused entirely by a slow current flowing through the slow channel. Phase 0 is very slow, and the action potential amplitude is reduced owing to the weakness of this slow inward current (Fig. 9–4). Such an action potential is called a *slow response;* this terminology emphasizes the difference between the membrane channels responsible for the upstroke of the slow reponse (slow channel) action potential and those responsible for the upstroke of the depressed fast response (fast channel) action potential. The slow response propagates much more slowly than the normal fast response, and conduction is more likely to be blocked.[5] The blockage may cause arrhythmias, as will be discussed later.

Not all cardiac cells with very low resting potentials caused by disease develop slow response action potentials. One requirement is that the membrane K^+ conductance must be relatively low. Since the slow inward current is a weak current, any significant outward current would prevent it from depolarizing the cell. A significant outward current exists when K^+ conductance is high. If an outward current prevents the slow inward current from depolarizing the cell and causing a slow response action potential, then any influence that increases the magnitude of the slow inward current may result in slow responses. As shown in Figure 9–4, catecholamines can induce slow response action potentials in cells with low resting potentials because they increase the slow inward current. Thus, some arrhythmias caused by sympathetic stimulation may result from slow conduction and block in fibers with slow responses.

We should also mention here that naturally occurring slow response action potentials occur in the normal sinus and AV nodes. In these regions, resting potential is normally low, and the inward current causing depolarization of the action potential flows through slow channels.

At present, it is uncertain which cardiac diseases cause slow responses and which cause depressed fast responses. Most probably both

types of action potentials can be found in diseased areas of the heart. The reduction in resting potential is rarely uniform in diseased areas. There may be regions with very low membrane potentials of less than -60 mv where Na^+ channels are completely inactivated and where slow responses occur, and other regions with membrane potentials of -60 to -70 mv where Na^+ channels are only partly inactivated and depressed fast responses occur. In still other areas of the diseased heart, cells with low resting potentials may not be able to generate either a slow response or a depressed fast response and thus may remain inexcitable.

So far we have considered only changes in phase 0 which are caused by a decrease in the resting potential. Cardiac disease can also directly alter the properties of the fast and slow channels independent of any changes in resting potential. For example, a direct action of disease on the fast Na^+ channel may cause a decrease in the rate of depolarization and amplitude of the action potential even when resting potential remains high.

Repolarization (phases 1 through 3) and refractoriness

Another prominent effect of cardiac disease is on the refractoriness of cardiac fibers. Changes in refractoriness can occur for either of two reasons: (1) A reduction in the resting potential changes the relationship existing between repolarization and recovery of excitability of the fast inward current. Alternatively, (2) the disease can either prolong or shorten action potential duration; and since recovery of excitability depends on the duration of the action potential, refractoriness is altered concomitantly.

Cells with decreased resting membrane potentials may generate depressed fast response action potentials or slow response action potentials. In a fiber with depressed fast response action potentials, recovery of excitability and refractoriness lags far behind the end of repolarization (phase 3); by contrast, in fibers with normal action potentials, recovery of excitability is complete upon complete repolarization. Therefore, fibers with depressed fast response action potentials may not respond to a second stimulus immediately after complete repolarization. After more time elapses from the end of repolarization, a stimulus during phase 4 will elicit an action potential, but this action potential will have a much slower rate of depolarization and decreased amplitude than the original response. A normal response may not be elicited for up to several hundred milliseconds after the end of repolarization. In fibers with slow response action potentials, complete recovery of excitability also requires a longer time than is required for complete repolarization (end of phase 3) (Fig. 9–5).

Not only does complete recovery of excitability occur long after repolarization when membrane potential is decreased, but the effects of the varying heart rate on recovery of excitability are different from the effects seen in fibers with normal action potentials. In normal atrial, ventricular, and Purkinje fibers, the time for repolarization decreases as the rate at which the fiber is driven increases.[6] As the action potential duration becomes shorter, recovery of excitability

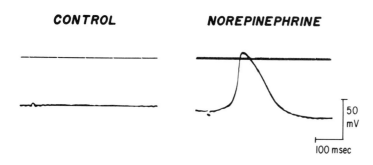

CONTROL　　　**NOREPINEPHRINE**

50 mV

100 msec

Fig. 9–4. A slow upstroke action potential induced with catecholamine was recorded from a left atrial fiber of a cat with severe hypertrophic cardiomyopathy and atrial fibrillation. Resting potential, -57 mv; $\dot{V}_{max} = 1$ V/sec.

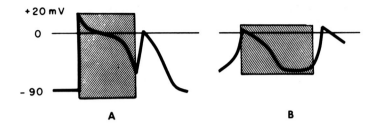

Fig. 9–5. Recovery of excitability in fibers with fast and slow response action potentials. **A,** Fast response action potential. The shaded area indicates the time in the cycle during which the cell is excitable. At approximately −55 mv, an action potential can be elicited by another stimulus. **B,** Slow response action potential. A second action potential cannot be elicited until long after maximum diastolic potential has been reached. (From Wit, A.L., Rosen, M.R., and Hoffman, B.F.: Am. Heart J., 88:517, 1974; reprinted with permission.)

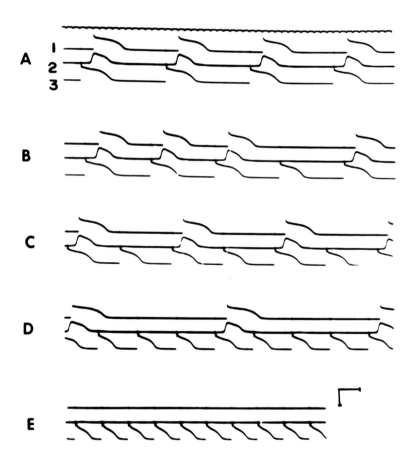

Fig. 9–6. Effects of increasing rate on conduction through a depressed segment in an unbranched bundle of a canine Purkinje fiber. Electrodes *1* and *3* are at either normal end of the fiber whereas electrode *2* is recording from the depressed segment in the middle of the fiber. **A,** At a drive rate of 50 beats/min, every impulse is conducted. **B,** At 60/min, 4:3 conduction block appears. **C** to **E,** At 75/min, 100/min, and 140/min, there is a progressive increase in conduction block. (From Cranefield, P.F., Wit, A.L., and Hoffman, B.F.: Circulation, 47:192, 1973; reprinted by permission of the American Heart Assoc., Inc.)

occurs sooner, and the refractory period is shortened. In fibers with low resting potential, recovery of excitability does not depend on the duration of the repolarization (phase 3). At increased heart rates, action potential duration of these fibers decreases (though not as much as in normal fibers), but the time for recovery of excitability either remains the same or increases (Fig. 9–6). Thus, at increasing rates, recovery of excitability can lag even further behind complete repolarization of the action potential, and conduction block can occur.[7]

Phase 4 depolarization and automaticity

As described in Chapter 1, most specialized cardiac cells—sinus node, AV valves, some parts of the atrium, the distal region of the AV node, and the His-Purkinje system—can develop action potentials without external stimuli (Fig. 9–1). This is normal *automaticity,* and it arises because of slow spontaneous depolarization during diastole (Fig. 9–7). This slow spontaneous depolarization during diastole results from a shift in the specific membrane inward (Na^+) and outward (K^+) currents to net in an inward depolarizing current. When this net depolarization causes the potential to reach threshold potential, an action potential is elicited without an external stimulus. Under disease conditions, atrial and ventricular muscle fibers as well as specialized atrial and ventricular fibers can develop an abnormal type of automatic firing[2] owing to slow phase 4 depolarization at a membrane

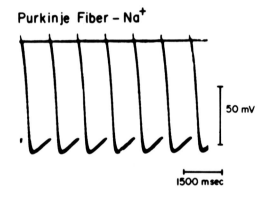

Fig. 9–7. Spontaneous diastolic depolarization in a fast response action potential of a canine Purkinje fiber.

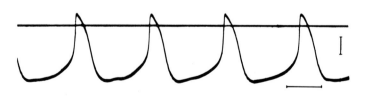

Fig. 9–8. Slow response action potential recorded from a left atrial fiber of a dog with chronic mitral insufficiency and severe left atrial dilatation. Maximum diastolic potential is −57 mv. Note the prominent phase 4 depolarization and automatic activity.

potential much lower than normal (Fig. 9–8). The mechanism responsible for this type of abnormal automaticity appears not to be the same as the type of spontaneous phase 4 depolarization seen at high levels of membrane potentials.

AFTERDEPOLARIZATION AND TRIGGERED ACTIVITY

Automatic rhythms, by definition, occur independently of a prior action potential. Impulses may also originate in cardiac fibers by a mechanism other than automaticity. These impulses are a direct result of prior activity and are called *triggered* impulses. Nondriven triggered action potentials can occur during the plateau phase of an action potential that initially arose at a high resting potential (Fig. 9–9A). Then the repolarization phase does not progress smoothly; rather, low-amplitude action potentials caused by *early afterdepolarizations* arise during repolarization. These action potentials occurring during the repolarization phase are an example of triggered activity since they are nondriven action potentials triggered by the upstroke of the previous action potentials. It is not certain why these early afterdepolarizations sometimes occur in cardiac fibers.

Triggered activity can also arise from low-amplitude depolarizations occurring after the fiber has repolarized completely (Fig. 9–9B). These are called *delayed afterdepolarizations*. Under certain conditions (e.g., increased drive rate), delayed afterdepolarizations increase their amplitude and reach threshold potential. When this occurs, nondriven repetitive action potentials arise from the peak of the delayed afterdepolarizations. Delayed afterdepolarizations can be caused by digitalis toxicity[7a] and have been recorded from diseased atrial[2] and ventricular fibers.

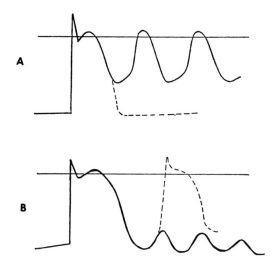

Fig. 9–9. **A,** When a fiber fails to repolarize completely, repetitive depolarizations can originate at a low level of membrane potential. These are called early afterdepolarizations. **B,** A fiber can completely repolarize and then develop one or more small depolarizations. These are called delayed afterdepolarizations.

EFFECTS OF ALTERED TRANSMEMBRANE POTENTIAL ON CONDUCTION OF THE CARDIAC IMPULSE

Alterations in the resting potential (phase 0 depolarization) repolarization and refractoriness affect the conduction of the cardiac impulse, causing atrial and ventricular conduction disturbances and cardiac arrhythmias.

Conduction in depressed cardiac fibers

We have previously stressed that the rate of phase 0 depolarization ($\dot{V}_{max}$) and the amplitude of depolarization are important determinants of conduction velocity. The reduced velocity of phase 0 depolarization and reduced amplitude of the overshoot occurring when membrane potential is decreased or when the inward current channels are directly affected by disease cause conduction to slow. For example, depression of $\dot{V}_{max}$ in a bundle of Purkinje fibers can reduce conduction velocity from 1 to 5 m/sec down to 0.05 to 0.1 m/sec. Both the depressed fast response and the slow response action potentials can conduct slowly. Such depression in a segment of the bundle of His would produce first-degree heart block, and a similar delay in a bundle branch could give rise to ventricular aberration or bundle branch block.

In atrial, ventricular, or Purkinje fibers with low resting potentials, recovery of excitability occurs after repolarization is complete, and the effect of increasing drive rate on recovery of excitability is different from what occurs in fibers with normal resting and action potentials.[8] In the depressed fibers, an increased drive rate causes a longer time for recovery of excitability and can markedly slow conduction velocity since the recovery of excitability lags far behind the end of repolarization (phase 3). In fact, at a critical drive rate, conduction block develops when the next stimulus occurs during the refractory period of the depressed fiber. These conduction properties of depressed fibers provide an explanation for many electrocardiographic observations. A moderate increase in heart rate can cause a transition from normal intraventricular conduction to bundle branch block. An increase in heart rate can lead to a Mobitz type II block in the bundle of His.

Depression of phase 0 depolarization may also cause unidirectional conduction block.[9] In bundles of normal cardiac fibers, an impulse can be conducted equally well in either direction along the bundle. In bundles of diseased cardiac fibers with decreased upstroke velocities and decreased action potential amplitudes, conduction can be slowed in one direction and blocked completely in the other. This type of conduction defect, called *unidirectional block*, may occur in fibers with either depressed fast response or slow response action potentials.

Conduction in fibers with altered repolarization

The duration of the action potential of fibers with high resting potential determines the duration of the refractory period. Therefore, the duration of the action potential can also influence conduction. For conduction of the impulse to be slowed, the action potential must arise prior to completion of phase 3 of the preceding action potential. In fibers with prolonged action potential duration, slowing of conduction occurs when the drive rate is so increased that each action potential arises prior to the end of phase 3 of the preceding action potential. The drive rate at which this occurs is slower than the drive rate needed to cause slowed conduction in fibers with a normal duration of repolarization.

An increase in action potential duration also affects conduction of premature impulses. Premature impulses are conducted slowly through normal atrial, ventricular, or Purkinje tissue when they excite that tissue prior to the end of phase 3 of the preceding action potential. When action potential duration is increased, premature impulses are conducted even more slowly or are blocked owing to the longer refractory period of the cell.[10]

Alterations in conduction caused by changes in passive membrane properties

The action potential upstroke is not the only determinant of conduction velocity. The resistance to the current flow that occurs from one cell to the next and that is responsible for propagation of the impulse also influences conduction velocity. An important determinant of conduction velocity is the degree of coupling of one cell to the next through the intercalated discs. These discs are formed where the membranes of two cells are in apposition (see Fig. 1–6). They represent a fusing of the membranes. Normally the discs provide a low-resistance pathway through which current from one cell flows into and excites the neighboring cell. Sometimes cardiac pathology may cause cellular "uncoupling," e.g., the cells are pulled apart at the location of the intercalated discs and the membranes are separated. This might result from fibrosis in enlarged atria or in the ischemic region of the ventricle. No longer are there the numerous low-resistance pathways for current to flow from one cell to the next. In this case, it is conceivable that although transmembrane current flow, e.g., the resting and action potentials, is normal, patterns of conduction from cell to cell are altered and may result in areas of block, slowed conduction, and, possibly, re-entry.

RELATIONSHIP OF NORMAL AND ABNORMAL ELECTRICAL ACTIVITY OF CARDIAC FIBERS TO THE GENESIS OF ARRHYTHMIAS

The changes in electrophysiologic properties of cardiac fibers caused by cardiac disease can produce arrhythmias. The basic principles underlying abnormal impulse initiation and conduction that cause ectopic beats and tachycardias will be described.

Arrhythmias caused by automaticity

In the normal heart, there are many regions having the capability of impulse formation by normal automaticity: sinus node, atrial specialized fibers, atrial fibers in the coronary sinus and AV valves, atrioventricular nodal fibers, and Purkinje fibers in the ventricular specialized conducting system.

The rate of impulse initiation due to automaticity of cells in the sinus node during sinus rhythm is sufficiently rapid such that potentially automatic cells (latent pacemakers) elsewhere in the heart, are excited by propagated impulses before they can depolarize spontaneously to threshold potential. Not only are these ectopic pacemakers prevented from initiating an impulse because they are depolarized before they have a chance to fire, but also, the diastolic depolarization of the latent pacemaker cells is actually inhibited by the impulses from the sinus node. This inhibition is called overdrive suppression.[11]

Overdrive suppression has been best characterized in microelectrode studies on isolated Purkinje fiber bundles exhibiting pacemaker activity; it results from driving a pacemaker cell faster than its intrinsic spontaneous rate and is mediated by enhanced activity of the Na^+/K^+ exchange pump. Since sodium ions enter the cell during each action potential, the higher the rate of stimulation, the greater will be the amount of Na^+ entering the cell over a given period of time. The rate of activity of the sodium pump is largely determined by the level of intracellular sodium concentration, so that pump activity is enhanced during high rates of stimulation. The sodium pump usually moves more Na^+ outward than K^+ inward, thereby generating a net outward (hyperpolarizing) current across the cell membrane.[12] When subsidiary pacemaker cells are driven faster than their intrinsic rate, the enhanced pump current suppresses spontaneous impulse initiation in these cells. When the dominant (overdrive) pacemaker is stopped, this suppression is responsible for the period of quiescence that lasts until the intracellular Na^+ concentration, and hence the pump current, becomes small enough to allow subsidiary pacemaker cells to depolarize spontaneously to threshold. Intracellular Na^+ and pump current continue to decline after the first spontaneous impulse, causing a gradual increase in the discharge rate of the subsidiary pacemaker. Inhibition can easily be demonstrated by suddenly stopping the sinus node such as by vagal stimulation. Impulses then usually arise from a subsidiary pacemaker, but the impulse initiation is usually preceded by a long period of quiescence.

In normal hearts, the sinus node is the site of the most rapid impulse formation (dominant pacemaker). Shifts in the site of impulse formation can cause many types of cardiac arrhythmias and may result when the rate of impulse generation in the sinus node is too slow or too fast, when impulses generated by the node fail to excite the heart, or when subsidiary pacemaker automaticity is enhanced.

The rate of sinus node impulse formation may be slowed through the influences of the autonomic nervous system or by sinus node disease. Impulse conduction from the sinus node to the atria may also be impaired. Any of these phenomena would remove the dominance of the sinus node as a pacemaker, causing a subsidiary pacemaker to control the rhythm of the heart, and could lead to single or multiple ectopic impulses or to a sustained ectopic rhythm.

Many factors enhance subsidiary pacemaker activity and cause impulse formation to shift to these regions, even when sinus node function is normal. For example, norepinephrine released from sympathetic nerves increases the slope of normal phase 4 depolarization of most ectopic pacemaker cells, enabling the cells to reach threshold potential and fire before normal activation occurs via the sinus node impulse.

Working atrial and ventricular myocardial cells do not normally show spontaneous diastolic depolarization. When the resting potentials of these cells are experimentally reduced to less than -60 mv, however, spontaneous diastolic depolarization may occur and cause repetitive impulse initiation. This is called abnormal automaticity.[13,14] Likewise, cells such as Purkinje fibers, which have the property of normal automaticity at normal levels of membrane potential, also show abnormal automaticity when membrane potential is reduced.

At the low level of membrane potential at which abnormal automaticity occurs, it is likely that at least some of the ionic currents causing the automatic activity are not the same as those causing normal automatic activity. Since the ionic currents causing the abnormal automaticity may not be the same as those causing normal automaticity, the two kinds of automaticity may not respond to antiarrhythmic drugs in the same way. In addition, because of the low level of membrane potential, the spontaneously occurring action potentials may be slow responses (action potentials with upstrokes dependent on the slow inward current). The decrease in membrane potential of cardiac cells required for abnormal automaticity to occur may be caused by a variety of factors related to cardiac disease.

Myocardial fibers with low resting potentials will not fire automatically if the sinus node drives them faster than their intrinsic abnormal, automatic rate. An abnormal automatic focus should manifest itself and cause an arrhythmia when the sinus rate decreases below the intrinsic rate of the focus, as was discussed for latent pacemakers with normal automaticity. There may be an important distinction between the effects of the dominant sinus pacemaker on the two kinds of foci, however. Unlike normal automaticity, abnormal automaticity may not be overdrive suppressed.[15] Therefore, even transient sinus pauses or occasional long sinus cycle lengths may permit the ectopic focus to capture the heart for one or more impulses. On the other hand, an ectopic pacemaker with normal automaticity would probably be quiescent during relatively short, transient sinus pauses because they are overdrive suppressed.

It is also possible that the depolarized level of membrane potential at which abnormal automaticity occurs might cause entrance block into the focus and prevent it from being overdriven by the sinus node. This would lead to parasystole (Fig. 12–8), an example of an arrhythmia caused by a combination of an abnormality of impulse conduction and initiation as outlined in Table 9–1. Entrance block may also occur into regions of normal automaticity if they are surrounded by depolarized or inexcitable fibers.

Arrhythmias caused by triggered activity

Increased sympathetic activity via released norepinephrine may increase the amplitude of delayed afterdepolarizations in the normal mitral valve and coronary sinus atrial fibers. The delayed afterdepolarizations may then reach threshold and initiate triggered activity.

If this rate of activity is faster than the sinus rate, pacemaker function will shift from the sinus node to these regions.

Toxic doses of digitalis can also cause delayed afterdepolarizations in atrial or ventricular fibers, but especially in Purkinje fibers in the ventricular specialized conducting system.[16] These delayed afterdepolarizations cause rapid triggered activity. This is an important mechanism for atrial or ventricular tachycardia associated with digitalis intoxication.

Early afterdepolarizations leading to triggered activity may be caused by hypoxia, high P_{CO_2}, and high concentrations of catecholamines. Since catecholamines, hypoxia, and elevated P_{CO_2} may be present in diseased regions of the ventricles, it is possible that early afterdepolarizations may cause some of the arrhythmias that occur in diseased hearts. Early afterdepolarizations also can be seen occasionally in Purkinje fibers superfused with a normal Tyrode's solution soon after they have been excised from the heart. These early afterdepolarizations might be caused by relatively nonspecific inward current flowing via incompletely healed cuts made at the ends of the fibers or through other regions injured by stretching or crushing during the dissection. This suggests the interesting possibility that mechanical injury or stretch of Purkinje fibers in situ might cause triggering. Stretch of the cardiac fibers in the ventricles might occur in heart failure or in ventricular aneurysms. Mechanical injury might occur also in the area of an infarct or aneurysm. Some drugs that are used clinically and that markedly prolong the time course for repolarization, such as the β-receptor-blocking drug sotalol, and the antiarrhythmic drug N-acetyl procainamide, cause early afterdepolarizations and triggered activity. These drugs can also cause cardiac arrhythmias, which may be a result of this triggered activity. Since early afterdepolarizations may occur when action potential duration is markedly prolonged, arrhythmias associated with clinical syndromes characterized by action potentials of long duration, such as the prolonged QT syndrome, might also be caused by triggered activity.

RE-ENTRY

Under physiologic conditions, the conducting impulse dies out after sequential activation of the atria and ventricles because it is surrounded by refractory tissue that it has recently excited. The heart must then await a new impulse, normally arising in the sinus node, for subsequent activation. The concept of re-entry means that the propagating impulse does not die out after complete activation of the heart but persists to re-excite the heart after the end of the refractory period. For this to happen, the impulse must remain somewhere in the heart while the cardiac fibers it has excited regain excitability so the impulse can re-enter and reactivate them. The refractory period of normal cardiac fibers is long, ranging from 150 msec in the atrium to approximately 500 msec in the ventricular conducting system. An impulse destined to re-enter or re-excite the heart therefore must survive for this period if it is to outlast the refractory period. It cannot remain stationary while awaiting the end of the refractory period, however, but must continue to conduct over a pathway that is functionally isolated from the rest of the heart. Such a conduction pathway must provide a return route to the regions that previously have been excited and must be sufficiently long to permit propagation of the impulse during the refractory period.

Since the normal cardiac impulse is conducted very quickly in fibers other than the SA or AV node, the pathway through which the impulse must travel while waiting for the heart to regain excitability must be very long and functionally isolated from the rest of the heart. Such a pathway would not likely exist in the normal heart. If conduction of the cardiac impulse is slowed, however, this pathway could be shorter and re-entry would be more likely to occur. Conduction is slow enough to enable re-entry to occur in cardiac fibers with slow response action potentials, either after the normally fast response has been converted to a slow response by disease or in fibers with naturally occurring slow responses in the sinus or AV node. Conduction is also slow enough for re-entry in fibers with depressed fast response action potentials.[9,10]

Alterations in refractory period duration brought about by alterations in time of phase 3 may also facilitate re-entry. Shortening of phase 3 and refractoriness reduce the period of time during which

the impulse must linger in the heart to await the recovery of excitability. Lengthening of the phase 3 and time for recovery may lead to marked slowing of conduction of premature impulses that can also cause re-entry.

Random re-entry vs. ordered re-entry

Random re-entry: In random re-entry, continuous propagation of an impulse is due to re-entrant re-excitation over one or more pathways that may change. Fibrillation is thought to be caused by random re-entry of impulses. In random re-entry, a specific anatomic circuit is not required. For example, repetitive activity can be induced in the atria by appropriately timed single premature stimuli. Such activity is caused by re-entrant excitation occurring in the absence of an anatomic obstacle. This kind of re-entry may occur by the leading circle mechanism described by Allessie et al.[17,18] The initiation of re-entry is made possible by the different refractory periods of atrial fibers in close proximity to each other. The premature impulse that initiates repetitive activity blocks in fibers with long refractory periods and conducts in fibers with shorter refractory periods, eventually returning to the initial point of block after excitability recovers there. The

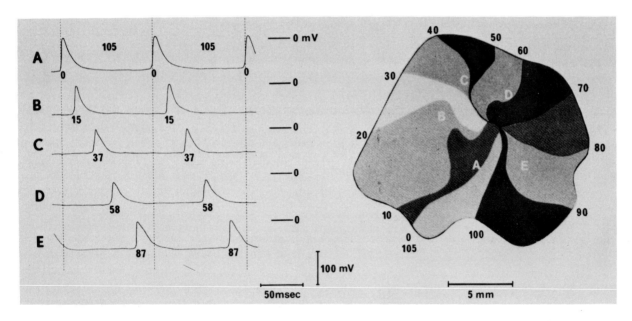

Fig. 9–10. Re-entry in isolated left atrial myocardium of a rabbit heart. On the right is a map of the activation pattern of the atrium during circus movement of the leading circle type and is constructed from time measurements of action potentials of 94 different fibers. The different shadings and numbers indicate the time in milliseconds during which each portion of the tissue is activated. Activation during one complete cycle (0 to 105 msec) is clockwise. At the left are transmembrane potentials (*A* thru *E*) of five of the fibers recorded simultaneously during this single beat of the tachycardia. The location from which these potentials were recorded are shown by the letters on the activation map at the right. (From Allessie, M.A., Bonke, F.I.M., and Schopman, F.J.G.: Circus movement in rabbit atrial muscle as a mechanism of tachycardia. Circ. Res., *41*:9, 1977, with permission.)

impulse may then continue to circulate. Conduction through the re-entrant circuit is slowed because impulses are propagating in partially refractory tissue. The circumference of the pathway may be as small as 6 to 8 mm. Impulses spread centripetally from the circumference of the circulating wave towards the center, maintaining a functionally inactive center. The rates of rise and amplitudes of these action potentials gradually decrease as the center is approached (Fig. 9–10). Cells at the center of the circulating wave show only local responses, since they are kept in a refractory state by the circulating impulse. The length of the circuit is completely defined by the conduction velocity and refractory period of the fibers composing it rather than by some well-defined anatomic pathway around an obstacle.

Ordered re-entry: In ordered re-entry, the occurrence of slowed conduction and unidirectional block set up conditions for re-entrant excitation over a circumscribed pathway that has finite anatomic boundaries. For example, this anatomically determined circuit may be within the AV node and its junction (see Fig. 12–4) or may involve the abnormal AV connection that occurs in hearts with pre-excitation (see Fig. 12–5).

Re-entry caused by slow conduction and unidirectional block in tissue with depressed action potentials

Re-entry of this type is dependent on the presence of slow conduction and unidirectional conduction block and can occur in loops composed of bundles of cardiac fibers—whether atrial, ventricular, or Purkinje.

For example, the anatomy of the ventricular specialized conducting system provides conduction pathways that are functionally suitable for re-entry. Bundles of interconnecting Purkinje fibers are surrounded by connective tissue, which separates them from ventricular myocardium. In peripheral regions of the conducting system, such Purkinje fiber bundles often arborize into many branches. At sites where these Purkinje fiber branches make contact with ventricular muscle, anatomic loops composed of the Purkinje fiber bundles and the muscle are often found. Under normal circumstances, the rapidly conducted impulses of sinus origin invade all the Purkinje fiber bundles of a distal loop and pass into ventricular muscle, where they collide and die out because they are surrounded by refractory tissue (Fig. 9–11*I*). For re-entry to occur in the distal ventricular specialized conducting system, conduction must be slowed and a strategically located region of unidirectional block must be present (Fig. 9–11*II*). The slowed conduction occurs when the loop is in a diseased region of the heart, which decreases the rate of phase 0 depolarization and the overshoot of the action potential. The unidirectional block is also caused by depression of phase 0 depolarization of the action potential. Depression of the resting potential and action potential upstroke is rarely uniform, and therefore, in the loop, some small areas may be more depressed than others. Unidirectional block may occur only in the area of greatest depression.

The mechanism whereby slowed conduction and unidirectional block can produce re-entry is illustrated in Figure 9–12. In the distal

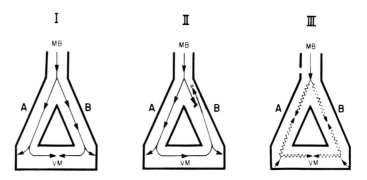

Fig. 9–11. Purkinje fiber bundle *(MB)* in the distal ventricular conducting system. The fiber divides into two branches *(A* and *B)* before making contact with ventricular muscle *(VM)*. **I,** Pathway of the impulse under normal conditions. **II,** Pathway of the impulse if unidirectional block exists (in *B*) but conduction velocity is normal. The impulse is conducted around the loop too rapidly and returns to the Purkinje fiber bundle before the bundle has recovered excitability. Therefore conduction is blocked due to the presence of refractory tissue. **III,** Pathway of impulse excitation if conduction is slowed but no segment of loop exhibits unidirectional conduction block. The impulse is conducted slowly through the Purkinje fiber bundle and both branches to finally collide in ventricular muscle. (From Wit, A.L., Rosen, M.R., and Hoffman, B.F.: Am. Heart J., *88*:664, 1974; reprinted with permission.)

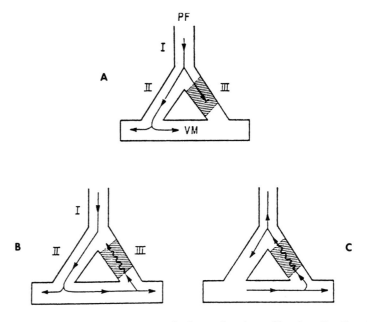

Fig. 9–12. Sequence of activation of a loop of Purkinje fiber bundles (*I* and *II*) and ventricular muscle *(VM)* during re-entry. Unidirectional conduction block is indicated by the darkly shaded area in *III*. Conduction can occur only in the retrograde direction (*VM* to *PF*). Slowed conduction is present throughout the loop. **A,** The impulse travels down the Purkinje fiber bundles, is blocked at *III*, and therefore travels down *II*. **B,** Retrograde conduction through *III* back to *I*. **C,** The impulse meets nonrefractory tissue and can re-excite *I* and *II*. The sequence then repeats itself. This mechanism might cause either premature depolarizations or ectopic rhythms.

loop, composed of Purkinje fiber bundles and ventricular muscle, an area of unidirectional conduction block is located near the origin of branch *III*; impulses can be conducted retrograde but not anterograde through this area. As a result an impulse of sinus origin conducted into the loop through the main Purkinje fiber bundle is obstructed near the origin of branch *III* and can only enter branch *II*, through which it is conducted slowly into ventricular muscle. It then invades branch *III* in a retrograde direction; but branch *III* has not been excited previously because of the area of unidirectional block, so the impulse is conducted retrograde in branch *I*, through the region of unidirectional block to re-excite the main bundle from which it entered the loop. This happens only if conduction has been slow enough that sufficient time has elapsed to allow the main bundle to recover excitability.

When the re-entrant impulse has returned to the main bundle, it is conducted throughout the conducting system to reactivate the ventricles. It also may reinvade the bundle of Purkinje fibers through which it was originally conducted to the ventricular muscle (branch *II* in Fig. 9–12) and again may be conducted back through the re-entrant pathway. The process may result in a continuous circling of the impulse around the loop or "circus movement." The continuous circling would cause repetitive excitation of the ventricles.

If conduction in the loop of Purkinje fibers and ventricular muscle is slowed insufficiently to permit re-entry or if a strategically located site of unidirectional block is absent, re-entry can still be induced by *premature activation*. The basic impulse may spread through the Purkinje bundles and ventricular muscle in any of the ways indicated in Figure 9–12. If these Purkinje fibers are then reactivated prematurely before they have completely recovered excitability, the premature impulse will be conducted even more slowly. Premature activation can also produce unidirectional block because of the lower safety margin for conduction of premature impulses in partially refractory tissue. Therefore, both slowed conduction and unidirectional block induced by premature activation can produce re-entry.

Although we have described the mechanism for re-entry in a loop using the peripheral Purkinje system as an example, re-entry may occur by the same mechanism in other regions of the heart. For example, the two bundle branches and the intervening ventricular muscle may form an anatomically gross loop. An anterograde-conducted impulse from the His bundle might be blocked at the origin of the right bundle branch at a region of unidirectional block, might be conducted slowly through the left bundle branch into ventricular muscle and through the muscle to the right ventricle, and then might invade the distal right bundle branch to be conducted retrograde back to the His bundle. From here, the impulse could pass retrograde to re-excite the atrium or again anterograde through the left bundle to re-excite the heart. Loops of tissue may also be formed in atrial or ventricular muscle as the consequence of disease. Cardiomyopathy in the atrium can produce areas of inexcitable tissue.[2] Conduction around these areas may be circular as described for the Purkinje system and cause re-entrant arrhythmias.

Anatomically discrete loops are not absolutely necessary for slow conduction and unidirectional block to cause re-entry. Re-entry caused by slow conduction and unidirectional block can also occur in unbranched bundles or "sheets" of muscle fibers. These same principles apply for re-entry in loops of tissue.

Re-entry caused by dispersion of refractoriness

Re-entry can also occur without disease-induced reduction in resting membrane potential and depression of phase 0 depolarization. The same basic mechanisms discussed for re-entry in depressed fibers still apply, however: slow conduction and unidirectional block. Both

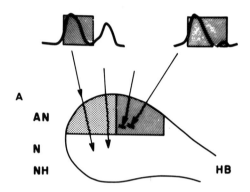

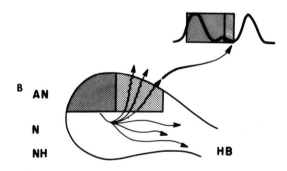

Fig. 9–13. Re-entry of an atrial impulse in the AV node. *AN*, Upper; *N*, middle; *NH*, lower; *HB*, His bundle. **A,** Action potentials recorded from two regions of the upper node are shown at the top. The action potential at the left has a shorter refractory period than does the one at the right (as indicated by the shaded area). Therefore, when an atrial premature complex enters the AV node (arrows), it may be able to excite the part of the upper node with the shorter refractory period but may be blocked in the region with the longer refractory period. This is also indicated in the action potential recordings at the top. **B,** Continuation of these events. The impulse can return to excite the area of the node in which anterograde conduction block occurred and then re-enter the atrium. Action potentials recorded from the return nodal pathway are shown; the first results from conduction of the sinus impulse, followed by low-amplitude depolarization resulting from conduction block of the APC, followed by an action potential resulting from the return impulse. (From Wit, A.L., Rosen, M.R., and Hoffman, B.F.: Am. Heart J., *88*:798, 1974; reprinted with permission.)

may come about as a result of conduction of premature impulses in relatively refractory cardiac fibers.

For example, loss of membrane potential produced by disease is not necessary for re-entry to occur in the AV node. Re-entry can occur because functional differences exist between the different groups of cells that make up the AV node.[10] Generally the time needed for recovery of excitability of AV nodal cells is significantly longer than the time to the end of phase 3 of the cell. This time for recovery of excitability is significantly different for two populations of AV nodal cells; thus, if refractory periods of adjacent groups of cardiac fibers are markedly different, re-entry can result (Fig. 9–13).

A premature impulse can easily initiate re-entry through the AV node. Differences in refractory periods of the two populations of cells functionally divide the AV node into two pathways for the conduction of early premature impulses. (1) If conduction of the premature impulse through the excitable regions of the AV node is slow enough, the impulse may enter the region where conduction block occurred in a retrograde direction once its fibers have recovered excitability and may return to re-excite the atrium as a re-entrant impulse or return extrasystole (Fig. 9–13). (2) If a re-entrant impulse returns to the atrium at a time when the nodal fibers that it previously excited in the anterograde pathway have recovered excitability, it can again enter the AV node and conduct around the circuit. This can become a continuous process, activating the atrium each time the impulse is conducted around the re-entrant loop, and may lead to atrial tachycardia with some degree of AV block.

Differences in refractoriness can also cause re-entry in atrial, ventricular, or Purkinje fibers, which have rapid rates of phase 0 depolarization. Pathologic events accentuating local differences in refractoriness predispose to re-entry, but like the example of re-entry in the AV node, a premature impulse is necessary for re-entry to occur.

REFERENCES

1. Hoffman, B.F., and Rosen, M.R.: Cellular Mechanisms for Cardiac Arrhythmias. Circ. Res., 49:1, 1981.
2. Boyden, P.A., et al.: Mechanisms for atrial arrhythmias associated with cardiomyopathy: A study on the feline heart with primary myocardial disease. Circulation, 69:1036, 1984.
3. Weidmann, S.: Elektrophysiologie der Herzmuskelfaser. Bern, Hans Huber Medical Publisher, 1956.
4. Boyden, P.A., et al.: Effects of left atrial enlargement on atrial transmembrane potentials and structure in dogs with mitral valve fibrosis. Am. J. Cardiol., 49:1896, 1982.
5. Cranefield, P.F.: The Conduction of the Cardiac Impulse. Mt. Kisco, NY, Futura Publishing Co., 1975.
6. Hoffman, B.F., and Cranefield, P.F.: Electrophysiology of the Heart. New York, McGraw-Hill, 1960.
7. Cranefield, P.F., Wit, A.L., and Hoffman, B.F.: Genesis of cardiac arrhythmias. Circulation, 47:190, 1973.
7a. Rosen, M.R., Gelband, H., and Hoffman, B.F.: Correlation between effects of ouabain on the canine electrocardiogram and transmembrane potentials of isolated Purkinje fibers, Circulation 47:65, 1973.
8. Wit, A.L., Rosen, M.R., and Hoffman, B.F.: Electrophysiology and pharmacology of cardiac arrhythmias. II. Relationship of normal and abnormal electrical activity of cardiac fibers to the genesis of arrhythmias. A. Automaticity. Am. Heart J., 88:515, 1974.
9. Wit, A.L., Rosen, M.R., and Hoffman, B.F.: Electrophysiology and pharmacology of cardiac arrhythmias. II. Relationship of normal and abnormal electrical activity of cardiac fibers to the genesis of arrhythmias. B. Re-entry. Section 1. Am. Heart J., 88:664, 1974.
10. Wit, A.L., Rosen, M.R., and Hoffman, B.F.: Electrophysiology and pharmacology of cardiac arrhythmias. II. Relationship of normal and abnormal electrical activity of cardiac fibers to the genesis of arrhythmias. B. Re-entry. Section 2. Am. Heart J., 88:798, 1974.
11. Vassalle, M.: Electrogenic suppression of automaticity in sheep and dog Purkinje fibers. Circ. Res., 27:361, 1970.
12. Glitsch, H.G.: Characteristics of active Na transport in intact cardiac cells. Am. J. Physiol., 236(2):H189, 1979.
13. Katzung, B.O., and Morgenstern, J.A.: Effects of extracellular potassium on ventricular automaticity and evidence for a pacemaker current in mammalian ventricular myocardium. Circ. Res., 40:105, 1977.
14. Surawicz, B., and Imanishi, S.: Automatic activity in depolarized guinea pig ventricular myocardium. Circ. Res., 39:751, 1976.
15. Dangman, K.H., and Hoffman, B.F.: Effects of overdrive and premature stimuli on abnormal automaticity in canine cardiac Purkinje fibers. Circulation (Suppl. III), 62:III–55, 1980.
16. Cranefield, P.F.: Action potentials, after potentials and arrhythmias. Circ. Res., 41:415, 1977.
17. Allessie, M.A., Bonke, F.I.M., and Schopman, F.J.G.: Circus movement in rabbit atrial muscle as a mechanism of tachycardia. Circ. Res., 32:54, 1973.
18. Allessie, M.A., Bonke, F.I.M., and Schopman, F.J.G.: Circus movement in rabbit atrial muscle as a mechanism of tachycardia. III. The "leading circle" concept. A new model of circus movement in cardiac tissue without the involvement of an anatomical obstacle. Circ. Res., 41:9, 1977.

Section Five

Management of Cardiac Arrhythmias

10 Antiarrhythmic therapy

JOHN D. BONAGURA and WILLIAM W. MUIR

*. . . . . Even therapeutics, I am convinced, will take a definite step forward when an attempt is made in a systematic way to modify the disease processes produced in animals by the well known drugs.**

LUDWIG TRAUBE, 1871

Disorders of heart rate, rhythm, and conduction are commonly encountered in clinical practice. Although some rhythm disturbances are clinically benign, a significant number of animals develop arrhythmias that are serious enough to be life threatening or to lead to physical impairment. Since the ability of the heart to pump blood effectively is linked closely to the electrical activity of cardiac muscle, it follows that arrhythmias may dramatically impair hemodynamics. Studies in animals and man have documented the deleterious effects of bradycardias, premature beats, tachyarrhythmias, accessory atrioventricular (AV) pathways, and myocardial fibrillation on cardiac output, arterial blood pressure, coronary circulation, electrical properties of the heart, and extracardiac organ perfusion (see Chapter 8).[1-5] Such circulatory alterations are recognized in affected animals by the clinical signs that occur, including: depression, weakness, hypotension, syncope, congestive heart failure, renal failure, further deterioration of the cardiac rhythm, and sudden death.[6,7]

Prompt intervention with antiarrhythmic therapy may allow the reestablishment of normal hemodynamics. Before initiating therapy, however, the clinician must accurately describe the arrhythmia,[8] ascertain its probable cause and its effect on the patient,[7] and appreciate the properties of the therapeutics available for treatment of that specific rhythm disorder (Tables 10–1 and 10–2).[9] The purpose of this chapter is to acquaint the student and veterinary practitioner with the types of therapeutic agents available for the management of cardiac arrhythmias and to provide a framework for the clinical management of these disturbances in the dog and the cat.

Before embarking on a description of antiarrhythmic therapy, some general comments about arrhythmias are required. Accurate rhythm diagnosis is essential if arrhythmias are to be treated successfully. Detailed information pertaining to cardiac rhythm diagnosis can be found elsewhere in this volume. Etiologic considerations are relevant (Table 10–3), since arrhythmias can occur secondary to essentially noncardiac conditions and may abate when the primary disorder is corrected. Examples of noncardiac disturbances that can lead to arrhythmias include acid-base and electrolyte disorders, hypoxemia, hypothermia, toxemia, sepsis, trauma, hypovolemia leading to myo-

---

*From Ludwig Traube: Gesammelte Beiträge zur Pathologie und Physiologie. Berlin, A. Hirschwald, 1871–1878 (Introduction).

Table 10–1. Methods available for the termination of arrhythmias

PHYSIOLOGIC MANEUVERS
  Ocular pressure
  Carotid sinus pressure (massage)
  Diving reflex
ALTERATION OF RECEPTORS
  Alpha and Beta adrenergic
  Dopaminergic
  Histaminic (H1, H2)
  Purinergic
CORRECTION OF ACID-BASE, ELECTROLYTE, AND FLUID DISORDERS
OXYGEN THERAPY
DC CARDIOVERSION
ATRIAL AND VENTRICULAR PACING
DRUG THERAPY
  Vagomimetics
  Anticholinergics
  Sympathomimetics
  Alpha and Beta-adrenergic blocking agents
  Antiarrhythmic drugs
  Calcium channel blocking agents
  Inotropic agents
OTHER THERAPY
  Blood transfusion
  Rest
  Surgery
  Corticosteroids
  Antibiotics
  Analgesics

Table 10–2. Classification of antiarrhythmic agents

Electrophysiologic group	Agent	Presumed antiarrhythmic mechanism
I	Quinidine Procainamide Disopyramide Lidocaine Phenytoin Aprindine* Encainide* Flecainide* Mexiletine* Tocainide*	Primary action is to decrease the membrane conductance to Na^+
II	Propranolol Nadolol Timolol Metoprolol Atenolol Pindolol	Reduce sympathetic excitation of the heart
III	Bretylium Amiodarone*	Primary effect is to lengthen action potential duration and refractoriness. Antiadrenergic effects
IV	Verapamil Diltiazem Nifedipine	Primary action is to decrease the slow inward current, particularly the Ca^{++} component

*Investigational drug

Table 10–3. Causes of cardiac arrhythmias*

Cardiac rhythm	Clinical disorder	Cardiac rhythm	Clinical disorder
SINUS RHYTHMS		Atrial flutter/fibrillation	CARDIAC: Atrial enlargement from any cause, cardiomyopathy, atrioventricular valvular regurgitation, untreated congenital heart defect, cardiac catheterization
Normal sinus rhythm	Normal rhythm but can be associated with intermittent rhythm disturbances and conduction defects		NONCARDIAC: Trauma, drugs, dysautonomia (vagotonia)
Sinus arrhythmia	Normal rhythm, less common in the cat; may be pronounced in conditions of high vagal tone or after vagotonic drugs	Junctional escape rhythm	A protective rhythm associated with sinus bradycardia, sinus arrest, and atrioventricular blocks
Sinus bradycardia	CARDIAC: Sick sinus syndrome, dilated cardiomyopathy	VENTRICULAR ARRHYTHMIAS	
	DRUGS: Propranolol, digitalis, anesthetic agents	Premature ventricular complexes/ ventricular tachycardia	CARDIAC: Congenital heart disease, cardiomyopathy (particularly Boxer dogs and Doberman Pinschers), chronic valvular heart disease, pericarditis, cardiac tumor, congestive heart failure, myocardial ischemia, endomyocarditis, parvovirus infection, heartworm disease, ventricular pacemaker wire, cardiac catheterization, ventricular dilatation from any cause
	NONCARDIAC: Vagotonia, elevated cerebrospinal fluid pressure, brainstem lesions, head trauma, hypoxia, hypothermia, hypothyroidism, hyperkalemia, systemic hypertension		
Sinus tachycardia	CARDIAC: Sick sinus syndrome, heart failure, cardiac trauma		DRUGS: Digitalis, sympathomimetic agents, anesthetic agents, phenothiazine tranquilizers, atropine, antiarrhythmic drugs
	DRUGS: Sympathomimetic drugs, atropine, glycopyrrolate, vasodilators, drugs with vagolytic properties		NONCARDIAC: Hypoxia, acidosis, alkalosis, electrolyte disorder (particularly potassium), dysautonomia, high sympathetic tone, pheochromocytoma, CNS disease, thyrotoxicosis, sepsis and toxemia, thoracic and abdominal trauma, gastric dilatation-volvulus, pulmonary disease, renal failure, fever, hypothermia
	NONCARDIAC: Increased sympathetic tone, pain, fear, excitement, exercise, hypovolemia, hypotension, anemia, hypoxemia, hypokalemia, hyperthyroidism, CNS hemorrhage		
Sinoatrial arrest	Vagotonia, surgical manipulation, digitalis glycosides	Ventricular escape rhythm	As per AV junctional escape rhythm
	Atrial myocarditis, fibrosis, or muscular dystrophy	CONDUCTION DISTURBANCES	
Sick sinus syndrome	Common in Miniature Schnauzer, Pug, Dachshund, Cocker Spaniel; can alternate with sinus or supraventricular tachycardias	Atrial standstill	CARDIAC: Muscular dystrophy (Springer Spaniels), chronic atrial myocarditis, dilated cardiomyopathy
SUPRAVENTRICULAR ARRHYTHMIAS			DRUGS: Anesthetics (barbiturates), antiarrhythmics
Atrial/junctional premature complexes	CARDIAC: Atrial distension, atrioventricular valvular regurgitation, cardiomyopathy, congenital heart disease, atrial tumors (hemangiosarcoma), pericarditis, heartworm disease, endocarditis		NONCARDIAC: Hyperkalemia, Addison's disease, urinary obstruction
		Incomplete AV block (first/second degree)	CARDIAC: AV nodal or bundle branch disease, cardiomyopathy, bacterial endocarditis
	DRUGS: Digitalis glycosides, sympathomimetics, anesthetic agents		DRUGS: Digitalis, xylazine, doxorubicin
	NONCARDIAC: Increased sympathetic tone, dysautonomia, chronic obstructive lung disease, hypokalemia, hypoxia, toxemia, anemia, thyrotoxicosis		OTHER: Normal variation, vagotonia
Supraventricular tachycardia: Atrial, AV junctional and re-entrant	Causes of atrial/junctional premature complexes	Complete AV block	Cardiac and drug causes of incomplete AV block CARDIAC: Degeneration, infarction, inflammation, or neoplastic invasion of AV conduction system or bundle branches, cardiomyopathy
	CARDIAC: Atrial septal defect, tricuspid valve dysplasia, accessory atrioventricular pathway, cardiac catheterization	Intraventricular conduction defect (fascicular/bundle branch block)	Congenital or acquired heart disease, acute ventricular dilatation, ischemia, acute cor pulmonale, heart rate-dependent bundle branch block, doxorubicin toxicity, digitalis toxicity
	NONCARDIAC: Electrocution, thyrotoxicosis		

*Modified from Bonagura, J.D.: Therapy of cardiac arrhythmias. In *Current Veterinary Therapy*. Volume 8. Edited by R.W. Kirk. Philadelphia, W.B. Saunders, 1983.

cardial ischemia, thyrotoxicosis, dysautonomia caused by central nervous system, pulmonary, or gastrointestinal disease, and drug therapy. The integrity of myocardial structure and contractile function greatly influences the severity of a cardiac rhythm disturbance.[1] Accordingly, arrhythmias that complicate congenital heart disease, cardiomyopathy, valvular heart disease, pericardial effusion, and endomyocarditis often precipitate or aggravate heart failure. Arrhythmias that occur in the setting of myocardial ischemia potentiate hypoperfusion and may lead to even more serious arrhythmias. Some arrhythmias appear to be spontaneous, with no obvious cause.

Such disturbances may represent primary degeneration or malfunction of the impulse-forming and conduction systems. Others are likely the result of previously occult heart disease or the influence of the autonomic nervous system. Finally, the clinician must recognize that an arrhythmia may change: modified by drug therapy, autonomic responses to changing blood pressure, intraluminal cardiac pressures, and heart rate.[10]

When approaching the patient with a cardiac arrhythmia, the veterinarian must assess the severity of the disturbance and examine the risk-benefit ratio and the practicality of therapy. There is little reason

Table 10–4. Evaluation of the patient with a cardiac arrhythmia

HISTORY
    Clinical signs of disease, including impaired hemodynamics (e.g., syncope)
    General medical history
    Drug and medication history
PHYSICAL EXAMINATION
    Cardiovascular examination—evidence for organic heart disease or failure
    General physical examination
ASSESSMENT OF HEMODYNAMIC STATE
    Level of consciousness, muscle strength
    Arterial blood pressure, arterial pulse pressure, capillary refill time
    Urine output
    Central venous pressure/adequate plasma volume
    Thoracic radiographs: cardiac size, evidence for congestive heart failure
    Cardiac output determination
METABOLIC STATE
    Blood pH, PO_2, PCO_2, packed cell volume
    Serum potassium, sodium, chloride, bicarbonate, calcium, magnesium
    Renal function—capacity for drug elimination
    Hepatic function—capacity for drug metabolism and elimination
    Plasma proteins, albumin (protein binding)
IDENTIFICATION OF INTERCURRENT EXTRACARDIAC DISEASE
ACCURATE ASSESSMENT OF THE ELECTROCARDIOGRAM
EVALUATION OF PREVIOUS AND CURRENT DRUG THERAPY
    Response to previous medication/adverse reactions
    Current medication—dose, route, and frequency of administration/adverse drug
        reactions
    Potential for reduced hepatic or renal drug clearance
    Potential for drug interactions

to administer anticholinergic drugs to a Miniature Schnauzer with periods of sinus arrest, if the pauses do not result in clinical signs. Similarly, overaggressiveness in the suppression of isolated premature ventricular complexes only increases the probability of a drug-related adverse effect and provides little benefit to the patient. Some forms of antiarrhythmic therapy are not feasible for certain practice situations. For example, it is hazardous to administer constant-rate infusions if the drip rate cannot be carefully controlled or monitored. This must be considered in primary care practices. The practitioner must be familiar with the myriad of drugs and nonpharmacologic methods currently used for the treatment of arrhythmias (Tables 10–1 and 10–2). The safe and effective use of these potent agents can be guided only through a knowledge of pharmacology and pharmacokinetics. These topics are addressed in the next two sections of this chapter. Eventually, the clinical use of any antiarrhythmic treatment must be guided by an overall assessment of the patient (Table 10–4), and experience with the arrhythmia and antiarrhythmic drugs in that animal and in other similar patients.

PHARMACOKINETICS OF ANTIARRHYTHMIC DRUGS

The successful treatment of cardiac arrhythmias is based upon a thorough knowledge of the arrhythmia to be treated and the pharmacology and pharmacokinetics of the drugs available for treatment. Previous discussions in this text have described the factors believed to be responsible for cardiac arrhythmias. Ischemia, hypoxia, acidosis, electrolyte abnormalities, acute inflammatory lesions, fibrosing lesions, drugs, humoral factors, and alterations in autonomic nervous system activity are experimentally used, either individually or in combination, to produce cardiac arrhythmias.[11] Ultimately, these abnormalities result in profound derangements in the movement of ionic-induced currents across the cell membrane, causing abnormal impulse formation in normally automatic tissues, the development of automaticity in tissues not normally possessing the ability to initiate an impulse, and functional disturbances in conduction leading to re-entry and increased temporal dispersion of refractoriness.[12,13] Antiarrhythmic drugs are a unique group of diverse chemical compounds that, based upon their ability to further modify membrane ionic conductances, possess the ability to normalize heart rate and rhythm. Fundamental experimental electrophysiologic studies of antiarrhythmic drugs in isolated tissues, intact animals, and humans have resulted in their classification based upon hypothesized primary mechanisms of action (Table 10–2).[14,15] Although controversial, this classification serves as a basis for categorizing and comparing the various drugs developed for the treatment of cardiac arrhythmias.

The successful treatment of disease with chemical compounds is predicated upon a working knowledge of drug behavior within the body. Pharmacokinetics is the science that describes drug absorption, distribution, biotransformation, and elimination. Nowhere in medicine is the knowledge of pharmacokinetics more crucial than in the successful treatment of cardiac arrhythmias. This assertion derives from the experimental and clinical observations that antiarrhythmic drugs have a relatively narrow therapeutic ratio and exert both beneficial and deleterious effects that are predictably related to the unbound or free drug plasma concentration.[16] The unbound drug concentration at the receptor site determines the magnitude and time course of the drug's pharmacologic effects. In practice, total drug concentration, both unbound drug and drug bound to protein, is measured, emphasizing the importance of plasma protein binding in determining drug activity. The ability to determine drug plasma concentration serves as an important guide for establishing drug dosage requirements, confirming therapeutic failures or toxicity, determining patient compliance, and investigating drug interactions. Once a drug is absorbed or injected into the body, knowledge of the drug's plasma concentration (Cp) is used to calculate the drug's volume of distribution (Vd), total body clearance (Cl_T), and half-life ($t_{1/2}$). These pharmacokinetic indices in turn are used to establish initial dosage guidelines, which are then modified by the patient's response and by determinations of drug concentration. Additional determinants of activity that must be considered when establishing dosage guidelines include the potential for the production of pharmacologically active drug metabolites, changes in the ratio of unbound to bound drug, and alterations in drug metabolism and excretion.[17]

Once a drug has entered the blood stream, it is subjected to two basic processes, distribution and elimination. Most antiarrhythmic drugs are eliminated by a first-order process, that is, their rate of

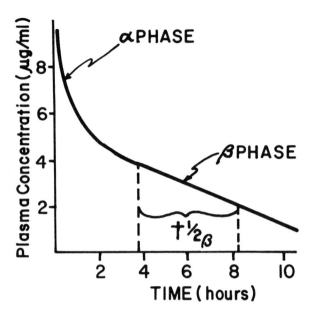

Fig. 10–1. Drug concentration time curve after intravenous administration. The rapid decrease in drug concentration (alpha phase) represents drug distribution. The slow decrease in drug concentration (beta phase) represents drug elimination. The drug half-life ($t_{1/2_\beta}$) is determined by noting the time taken for plasma concentration to decrease by 50% during the beta phase.

disappearance is dependent upon the plasma concentration.[18,19] Initial rapid declines in drug concentration occur because of distribution throughout the blood volume and to tissues receiving relatively large blood flows. This is termed the rapid (alpha) phase of disposition. Further decreases in plasma drug concentration are more gradual and include renal and hepatic phases of elimination of the drug from the body. The later phase of drug elimination is called the slow (beta) phase (Fig. 10–1). Extrapolation of the slow phase of elimination to zero time allows the determination of a theoretical plasma concentration (Cp_0), which is used to calculate a drug's Vd. The Vd is the hypothetical volume of plasma into which a drug would have to be distributed in order to give a value equal to Cp_0. Vd is calculated by using the formula

$$Vd \ (L/kg) = \frac{Drug\ dose\ (mg/kg)}{Cp_0\ (mg/L)}$$

Calculation of Vd is used clinically to determine the loading dose. A drug with a large Vd requires larger initial dosages to attain a given plasma concentration than the same drug with a small Vd. The Vd of a drug can be changed by those factors that affect Cp_0. Factors that can change Cp_0 include alterations in plasma volume or blood volume, binding of the drug to plasma proteins, and uptake of drug by tissues. Diseases that decrease plasma volume (dehydration), decrease plasma albumin (renal or liver disease), or decrease peripheral tissue binding

(circulatory failure) result in an increased amount of drug in the plasma, a smaller Vd, and a decrease in the loading dose.[17]

Total body clearance (Cl_T) is an important determinant of drug elimination from the body and is the sum of all organ clearances. Since renal excretion and hepatic metabolism are the predominant routes for drug elimination, total body clearance is usually approximated by $Cl_T = Cl_R + Cl_H$, where $Cl_R + Cl_H$ are renal and hepatic clearances, respectively. Drug clearance values are used clinically to determine drug dosages necessary to maintain a relatively constant or steady state drug concentration (Cp_{ss}). Obviously, in order to maintain Cp_{ss} a dose of drug equal to the amount of drug being eliminated must be added. The Cp_{ss} of drugs that are administered by infusion is dependent solely upon drug clearance and infusion rate (I), according to the formula

$$Cp_{ss} = \frac{I}{Cl_T}$$

The Cp of drugs administered intermittently (oral or intramuscular) increases and decreases based upon the dose (D), Cl_T, and T, the time interval between doses. The average plasma drug concentration (Cp_{av}) can be calculated by the formula

$$Cp_{av} = \frac{D}{Cl_T \times T}$$

and is identical to Cp_{ss} if the drug were to be given by infusion. Ideally, the peaks and troughs in C_p are maintained within the therapeutic range (see Fig. 10–3). Clinically it is assumed that drug concentrations are maintained in the therapeutic range if the drug is administered every half-life. The elimination half-life ($t_{1/2_\beta}$) of a drug is the amount of time required for half of the drug in the body to be eliminated. This value can be determined by plotting Cp versus time on semilogarithmic paper; it is determined during the slow elimination phase and is expressed as a function of the drug elimination slope. A common expression for $t_{1/2_\beta}$ is

$$t_{1/2_\beta} = Vd \times \frac{0.693}{Cl_T}$$

which illustrates the fact that drug half-life is ultimately dependent upon both the volume of distribution and total body clearance.[17] In addition to defining the rate of drug elimination and drug dosage interval, $t_{1/2_\beta}$ is also used to determine the time required to reach Cp_{ss} during constant infusion. The time course for drug accumulation during infusion is the mirror image of drug elimination. After one $T_{1/2}$, 50% of a drug is eliminated and 50% retained. Because drug elimination for most antiarrhythmic drugs follows first-order kinetics, both the Cp and drug elimination will have increased during the second $t_{1/2}$, 75% being eliminated and an additional 25% of the dose retained. This process continues until the drug infusion rate equals the elimination rate. Clinically, it is assumed that Cp_{ss} is reached within three to four drug half-lives, which actually represents about 90% of

Cp_{ss} (Fig. 10–2A). Because the $t\frac{1}{2}\beta$ and, therefore, the time to attain Cp_{ss} is too long for patients requiring immediate antiarrhythmic therapy, single or multiple intravenous bolus injections or "loading" doses are often recommended (Figs. 10–2B and 10–3). These therapeutic techniques possess the advantage of immediately establishing the therapeutic Cp of the drug, but they often produce signs of toxicity. If

loading doses are reduced in order to avoid toxicity, therapeutic effects may be relatively short lived. One method of avoiding this predicament is to administer several small loading doses combined with a constant infusion of the same drug (Fig. 10–4). This technique is commonly used clinically in dogs for the management of ventricular arrhythmias with lidocaine.[20] An alternative approach that is equally as acceptable for all intravenous antiarrhythmic drugs, although not quite as rapid in establishing Cp_{ss}, is the double-infusion technique. This technique is performed by administering a rapid infusion followed by a maintenance infusion (Fig. 10–2C). During life-threatening situations, a single bolus injection followed by the double-infusion technique can be used.

The only practical method of administering antiarrhythmic drugs for long periods of time is by adjusting dosages of drugs that can be administered orally. Oral administration of drugs, however, assumes that a significant percentage of the active drug will be absorbed (F) and that metabolism in the intestine or liver prior to reaching the systemic circulation is small. Inactivation of drugs by the liver during the absorption process is called presystemic or "first-pass" elimination and is important during disopyramide, propranolol, and verapamil administration.[19,21] Oral lidocaine therapy, for example, is totally ineffective because of first-pass metabolism. Poor mucosal blood flow from heart failure, gut hypermotility, and malabsorption syndromes may further decrease the amount of drug reaching the systemic cir-

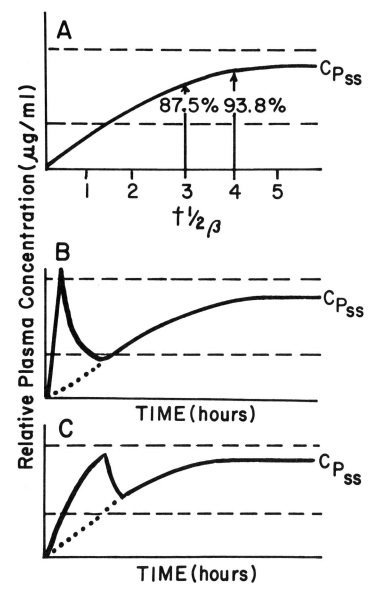

Fig. 10–2. Examples of various methods of drug administration. The therapeutic range is enclosed by the dashed lines. **A,** The constant infusion of drug. The percent of the final Cp_{ss} at three and four half-lives is noted. **B,** A single intravenous loading dose followed by a constant infusion. Plasma drug concentration may dip below the minimum effective concentration during drug distribution. **C,** The change in Cp when the double infusion technique is used to administer drug. This technique avoids the initial dip that occurs with bolus doses **(B)**.

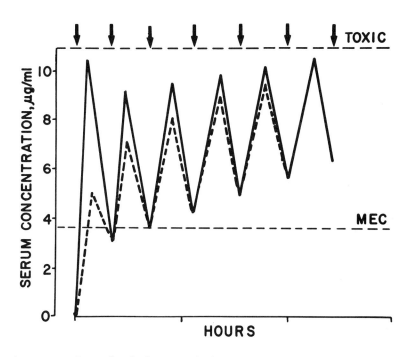

Fig. 10–3. Plasma levels during oral administration of drug at intervals equal to one half-life (dotted line). Note that the peak drug level at steady state is twice the first dose peak level. Therapeutic drug concentrations can be reached immediately by doubling the first oral dose (solid line).

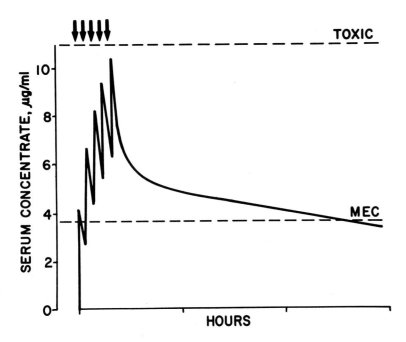

Fig. 10–4. The administration of multiple intravenous boluses at reduced dosages causes therapeutic drug concentrations to be reached rapidly without toxicity (arrows indicate drug administration).

culation. Alternatively, alkalinization of the stomach by antacids increases gastric absorption of antiarrhythmic drugs that are weak bases. This knowledge has been used in developing sustained-release preparations of quinidine, procainamide, and disopyramide that exhibit slow absorption and decreased F but long elimination times, thus permitting less frequent dosing. Alterations in client compliance must also be considered when administering oral antiarrhythmic drugs to patients. Most antiarrhythmic drugs that are administered intermittently are given every $t_{1/2_\beta}$. When this is done, the peaks and troughs in Cp generally do not differ by a factor of more than two (Fig. 10–3). When patients begin to demonstrate signs of drug toxicity followed by periods of drug ineffectiveness, one approach to therapy is to maintain the same daily dosage but to divide the drug dosage into smaller portions and administer the drug at more frequent intervals. The daily dosage of digoxin, a drug with a relatively long $t_{1/2_\beta}$, for example, is frequently divided and administered up to four times daily in patients demonstrating poor compliance.[22] Since this technique more closely approximates constant infusion, the peaks and troughs in Cp are reduced, providing a therapeutic effect.

Other biologic determinants known to affect drug distribution and elimination during health and disease are the activity of basic removal processes (collectively referred to as the "intrinsic clearance"), alterations in organ blood flow, and changes in drug binding in blood and tissues.[17] These factors can effect $t_{1/2_\beta}$, Vd, and Cl_T of antiarrhythmic drugs, and need to be considered when designing or adjusting drug

dosages. For example, most antiarrhythmic drugs are weak bases and bind reversibly to macromolecules such as albumin and alpha$_1$-acid glycoprotein. Concentrations of alpha$_1$-acid glycoprotein increase during heart failure and inflammatory disease, thereby decreasing the unbound or free drug fraction in the plasma. Since decreases in unbound drug concentration result in a reduction in pharmacologic activity, the quantity of drug necessary for loading doses must be adjusted. Similarly, propranolol, lidocaine, disopyramide, and verapamil are extremely dependent upon hepatic metabolism and are all cleared from the plasma at rates that approach liver blood flow rates.[19] Reductions in liver blood flow secondary to decreases in cardiac output or drugs like cimetidine will reduce the clearance of these drugs, necessitating reductions in dosing rates and increases in dosing intervals. Similar arguments are used during renal disease for drugs that are highly dependent upon renal elimination, such as bretylium and digoxin.[16,22]

In summary, knowledge of Vd, Cl_T, and $t_{1/2_\beta}$ are useful guides when initially designing drug dose regimens. Dosage recommendations for many of the standard antiarrhythmic drugs used to treat cardiac arrhythmias are developed using these indices. Thereafter, drug dosages are titrated to produce therapeutic effects without producing toxicity. Determination of plasma drug concentrations, when possible, can be valuable for determining if therapeutic or toxic drug concentrations have been attained. When this is not possible, 30% to 50% reductions in drug dosages are prudent in patients with obvious cardiac disease.

PHARMACOLOGY OF ANTIARRHYTHMIC DRUGS

Quinidine

Quinidine is a class I antiarrhythmic drug capable of producing profound electrophysiologic and hemodynamic effects in dogs and cats. The pharmacologic activity of quinidine on the heart and circulation is the result of both direct effects and reflexly mediated alterations in autonomic tone.[16] Isolated tissue experiments using a variety of different types of cardiac tissues indicate that quinidine has little effect upon isolated sinus node preparations but substantially depresses automaticity in atrial and ventricular specialized fibers.[23,24] Quinidine shifts threshold in all cardiac tissues toward zero potential, making it more difficult for the heart to be excited. In addition to its depressive effects upon automaticity and excitability, quinidine also depresses impulse conduction throughout the heart.[25] These effects are concentration dependent, becoming particularly pronounced in diseased tissues or when toxic concentrations are administered. Quinidine produces significant prolongation of the effective refractory period (ERP) in atrial and ventricular muscle and in Purkinje fibers. Prolongation of ERP is considered the most likely method by which quinidine exerts its antiarrhythmic effect (Table 10–5).[16,18] Another possible mechanism for antiarrhythmic activity is a decrease in dispersion of repolarization in working myocardium and Purkinje fibers.[18] Dispersion of repolarization was recently demonstrated to fa-

Table 10–5. Electrophysiologic properties of antiarrhythmic drugs

Drug*	Isolated tissues			Intact hearts				
	Automaticity	Conduction velocity	Effective refractory period	PR	QRS	QT	Ventricular rate during atrial fibrillation	Conduction in accessory pathway
Approved								
Quinidine	↓	↓	↑	—	↑	↑	↑	↓
Procainamide	↓	↓	↑	—	↑	↑	↑	↓
Disopyramide	↓	↓	↑	—	↑	↑	↑	↓
Lidocaine	↓	↓	↓	—	—	↓	↓ – ↑	↓
Phenytoin	↓	↓	↓	—	—	↓	↓ – ↑	↓
Propranolol†	↓	—	— ↑	↑	—	—	↓	↓
Bretylium	—	—	↑	— ↑	—	↑	↑ ↓	—
Verapamil	—	—	— ↑	↑	—	—	—	—
Digoxin†	↓ ↑	— ↓	↓	— ↑	—	↓	↓	↑ ↓
Investigational								
Amiodarone	↓	— ↓	↑	↑	— ↑	↑	↓	↓
Aprindine	↓	↓	— ↓	↑	↑	—	↓	↓
Encainide	↓	↓	↑	↑	↑	↑	↓	↓
Flecainide	↓	↓	↑	—	↑	↑	—	↓
Mexiletine	↓	↓	↓	—	—	— ↓	↓ – ↑	↓
Tocainide	↓	↓	↓	—	—	— ↓	↓ – ↑	↓

*Assumes therapeutic drug concentrations
†Includes all other drugs with similar activity
↓ = decrease or shorten; ↑ = increases or lengthen; — = no change

cilitate the development of conduction delay necessary for the induction and maintenance of sustained re-entrant arrhythmias.[13]

All of quinidine's direct effects upon isolated cardiac tissues are due to interaction with receptors in individual membrane channels that alter ionic permeabilities. Although a plethora of basic experimental studies originally suggested that quinidine produces its electrophysiologic effects by depressing transmembrane fluxes of sodium, potassium, and calcium ions, recent experimental evidence suggests that most, if not all, of quinidine's activities are due to inhibition of sodium currents alone.[24] This inhibition is exquisitely sensitive to extracellular potassium concentration.[16,18] These facts are particularly important when considering quinidine as therapy in hypokalemic patients suffering from cardiac arrhythmias from multiple causes.

Therapeutic direct actions of quinidine in intact animals are modified by a purported "atropine-like" action and alpha adrenergic blocking properties.[26] Quinidine's "atropine-like" activity, however, was recently suggested to be inappropriate and misleading based upon evidence that cardioacceleration is caused by an adrenergic mechanism involving beta receptors.[27] Regardless of mechanism—cholinergic blockade, beta-adrenergic stimulation or alpha-adrenergic blockade—the net result is an increase in sinus rate and enhancement of atrioventricular conduction. Quinidine's depressant effect upon conduction in isolated tissues is evidenced electrocardiographically by prolongation of the P-R, QRS, and Q-T intervals (Table 10–5). Increases in the QRS duration to values 25% greater than baseline values, the development of conduction abnormalities (right bundle

branch block) and marked prolongation of the Q-T interval are clinically useful as indications of quinidine toxicity (Fig. 10–5).

Quinidine's hemodynamic effects are well described and based upon clinical impression cannot be underestimated (Table 10–6). The intravenous administration of up to 5 mg/kg of quinidine gluconate or quinidine sulfate to normal dogs produces no change in stroke volume, cardiac output, left ventricular end diastolic pressure, or indices of left ventricular contractility.[16,26,27] Peripheral vascular resistance decreases. Intravenous dosages of quinidine in excess of 5 mg/kg produce depression in all of these variables except left ventricular end diastolic pressure, which increases. These effects are extremely important when considering quinidine as antiarrhythmic therapy in patients with known cardiac disease or in patients with a depressed myocardium from other causes and suggest that quinidine be administered intravenously with caution.

Quinidine is most frequently used clinically as an oral preparation, although it is occasionally administered intramuscularly and, in special situations, intravenously. Most oral quinidine preparations are rapidly absorbed from the gastrointestinal tract of the dog, with the drug reaching maximum effect within 1 to 2 hours of administration. The bioavailability (F) of quinidine is excellent (greater than 75%); this less-than-optimal systemic bioavailability is due to quinidine's first-pass hepatic metabolism (Table 10–7). Recently, sulfate, gluconate, and polygalacturonate salts of quinidine have been developed as slow-release preparations. These preparations are absorbed more slowly from the gastrointestinal tract and take longer to reach peak effect;

Table 10–6. Hemodynamic effects of antiarrhythmic drugs

Drug*	Sinus rate	Contractility	Cardiac output	Arterial blood pressure	Peripheral vascular resistance	Comments
Approved						
Quinidine	− ↑	↓	↓	↓	↓	Anticholinergic; adrenergic; alpha-adrenoceptor blockade; sympatholytic
Procainamide	−	↓	− ↓	↓	↓	Anticholinergic; ganglionic blockade
Disopyramide	− ↑	↓	↓	↓	↓	Anticholinergic
Lidocaine	−	−	− ↓	− ↓	↓	Mildly sympatholytic
Phenytoin	−	−	− ↓	− ↓	↓	Central sympatholytic effect
Propranolol†	↓	↓	↓	↓	↑ ↓	Beta-adrenoceptor blockade
Bretylium	− ↓	− ↑	−	− ↑	↑ ↓	Releases norepinephrine then prevents this release
Verapamil	− ↓	↓	↓ ↑	↓	↓	Calcium antagonist; vasodilation
Digoxin†	− ↓	↑	− ↑	↑ ↓	↑ ↓	Positive inotrope; increases vagal tone
Investigational						
Amiodarone	↓	↓	↓	↓	↓	Sympatholytic vasodilator
Aprindine	↓	↓	↓	↓	↓	Not defined
Encainide	−	− ↓	↓	↓	↓	Not defined
Flecainide	−	− ↓	↓	↓	↓	Not defined
Mexiletine	−	−	− ↓	− ↓	↓	Similar to lidocaine
Tocainide	−	−	− ↓	− ↓	↓	Similar to lidocaine

*Assumes therapeutic drug concentrations
†Includes all other drugs with similar activity
↓ = decreases; ↑ = increases; − = no change

Table 10–7. Pharmacokinetics of antiarrhythmic drugs in dogs and cats*

Drug	Common routes of administration	Oral availability (F, %)	Protein binding (5)	Volume of distribution (L/kg)	Clearance (ml/min/kg)	Elimination Half-life: t½ (hrs)	Therapeutic range	Major method of elimination	Comments
Approved									
Quinidine	PO, IM, IV	60–90	80	2.9 [2.2]	6,0 [15.0]	6.0 [1.9]	3–5 µg/ml	Hepatic	Active metabolites accumulate in liver failure
Procainamide	PO, IM, IV	80–90	60–80	2.1	12.5	2.5	3–8 µg/ml	Hepatic	Negligible metabolites
Disopyramide	PO	70	20–40	3.0	8.0	1.5	3–8 µg/ml	Hepatic	
Lidocaine	IM, IV	<25	40–60	5.7	62.0	0.7	2–6 µg/ml	Hepatic	Clearance dependent upon liver blood flow
Phenytoin	PO, IV	40	50–70	1.2	4.0	3.5 [>24]	10–16 µg/ml	Hepatic	Variable protein binding
Propranolol	PO, IV	<20 [low]	90	3–6 [1.6]	30–70 [30]	0.5–1.0 [.5]	50–150 ng/ml	Hepatic	Clearance dependent upon liver blood flow
Bretylium	IV							Renal	Accumulates in renal failure
Verapamil	PO, IV	low	90	4.5	65	0.8		Hepatic	Clearance dependent upon liver blood flow
Digoxin	PO, IV	80–90	10–20	9.5	3.9	15–23 [33]	0.5–2 ng/ml	Hepatic Renal	Accumulates in renal failure and in the presence of quinidine
Investigational									
Amiodarone	PO							Hepatic	
Aprindine	PO, IV	85	—	7	11.6	10	1–3 µg/ml	Hepatic	Unknown
Encainide	PO						2–5 µg/ml	Hepatic	Active metabolites
Flecainide	PO						2–5 µg/ml	Hepatic	Active metabolites
Mexiletine	PO, IV						0.5–2 µg/ml	Hepatic	Unknown Similar to lidocaine
Tocainide	PO	85	50	1.7	4.2	4.7 (8–12 PO)	6–10 µg/ml	Hepatic Renal	Similar to lidocaine

* [ ] Refer to values in cats.

however, they have the advantage of a long duration of action. Quinidine has a $t_{1/2\beta}$ of approximately 6 hours when administered intravenously and from 6 to 10 hours after oral administration.[28,29] These values are probably lower in cats, but definitive pharmacokinetic studies are needed.

Quinidine is metabolized in the liver in dogs and cats, and although metabolites have been identified, their antiarrhythmic effects are uncertain. A small percentage of unchanged quinidine (parent compound) and metabolites is excreted by the kidney.[28,29] Studies in man and dogs suggest that quinidine dosages should be reduced in patients with congestive heart failure and hepatic disease, while the dosage need not be reduced in patients with renal failure.[19,29] Animals with congestive heart failure have a decreased Vd, predisposing to higher peak plasma levels. Patients with liver disease demonstrate reduced hepatic enzyme activity and become hypoalbuminemic. Hypoalbuminemia decreases quinidine binding and promotes toxicity by allowing more free drug to interact with cardiac cellular membranes. Conversely, phenobarbital and phenytoin, known hepatic enzyme inducers, increase quinidine elimination, which may require an increase in drug dosages. Simultaneous administration of cimetidine impairs the absorption and elimination of oral quinidine and can lead to quinidine toxicity. Finally, it must be noted that concurrent quinidine and digoxin therapy can result in signs of digitalis toxicity.[30] The mechanism whereby quinidine increases serum digoxin levels is controversial, although most authors believe that quinidine-induced decreases in digoxin tissue binding sites, decreased renal clearance, and decreases in digoxin Vd are responsible.

Regardless of the development of new antiarrhythmic drugs, quinidine remains one of the most effective drugs in the treatment of both atrial and ventricular arrhythmias, including arrhythmias dependent upon accessory pathways. Quinidine is particularly effective in the management of ventricular arrhythmias and is occasionally used in terminating acute atrial flutter or fibrillation.[16,31] In the latter instance, quinidine therapy may be combined with digitalis or a beta-adreno-ceptor blocking drug in order to avoid quinidine-induced increases in atrioventricular conduction and an accelerated ventricular response. Quinidine is a relatively ineffective therapy for preventing paroxysmal supraventricular tachycardias originating from the atrioventricular node and is contraindicated in patients with sick sinus syndrome, in which it can induce a dramatic depression in sinus discharge rate.[16] Quinidine is of limited value in controlling digitalis-induced cardiac arrhythmias and may potentiate digitalis toxicity owing to the previously described quinidine-digoxin interaction.

Quinidine toxicity is pronounced and can be life threatening. Rapid intravenous administration of quinidine can cause hypotension, ventricular arrhythmias and acute myocardial decompensation.[18,32] Electrocardiographically, quinidine produces first-, second-, and third-degree heart block, conduction disturbances, and ventricular tachycardia, including torsade de pointes (Fig. 10–5) (see Chapter 12). The sudden development of ventricular tachyarrhythmias may be responsible for "quinidine syncope." Gastrointestinal upset, inappetence, nausea, and diarrhea are the most common side effects observed during chronic oral therapy, although urine retention, skin lesions, fever, and thrombocytopenia are occasionally observed (Table 10–8). These toxic effects usually abate within a short period of time following discontinuation of drug therapy and are directly related to chronically elevated quinidine plasma concentrations. One antidote that is worth remembering during an episode of acute intravenous quinidine toxicity is to administer sodium bicarbonate (1.0 mEq/kg) intravenously if ventricular tachyarrhythmias or hypotension develops. Alkalinization of the plasma increases quinidine protein binding, thereby decreasing the amount of unbound or active drug available for interaction with cardiac membranes.

Procainamide

Procainamide, a weak local anesthetic and class I antiarrhythmic, has many electrophysiologic and hemodynamic properties similar to those of quinidine. Following the administration of procainamide to isolated tissue baths, spontaneous electrical activity is unaffected or decreased, conduction velocity in specialized conducting tissues is decreased, particularly in diseased heart tissue, and Purkinje fibers become less excitable.[16,23] Procainamide exerts little or no effect on the pacemaker current in dog Purkinje fibers but depresses spontaneous automaticity in partially depolarized or chemically stimulated specialized tissues.[18] Therapeutic concentrations of procainamide produce little to no effect upon sinus node or atrioventricular node auto-

QUINIDINE / PROCAINAMIDE / LIDOCAINE

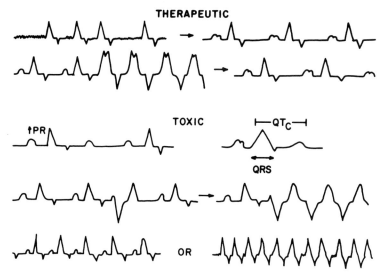

Fig. 10–5. Therapeutic plasma concentrations of quinidine and procainamide can convert acute atrial fibrillation to sinus rhythm. Quinidine, procainamide, and lidocaine can convert ventricular tachycardia to sinus rhythm (top two traces). Toxic concentrations of these drugs can produce prolongation of the P-R interval, ventricular conduction disturbances, ventricular tachycardia, and supraventricular tachyarrhythmias (bottom three traces).

Table 10–8. Toxic effects of antiarrhythmic drugs

Drug	Electrocardiographic	Hemodynamic	Other	
Approved				
Quinidine	Atropine like effects; pacemaker suppression; sinus arrest; asystole; ventricular tachycardia; ventricular fibrillation; first-, second-, and third-degree heart block	Hypotension; negative inotropes; disopyramide may aggravate or induce heart failure	Quinidine: Nausea Vomiting Diarrhea Circhonism Urine retention	Procainamide: Nausea Agranulocytois Lupus syndrome Disopyramide: Nausea Urine retention Constipation
Procainamide				
Disopyramide				
Lidocaine	Pacemaker suppression; sinus arrest; asystole; atrioventricular block; ventricular tachycardia	Hypotension	Lidocaine: Convulsions Respiratory arrest Vomiting	Phenytoin: Depression Convulsions
Phenytoin				
Propranolol	Pacemaker suppression, atrioventricular block	Hypotension; may aggravate or induce heart failure	Lethargy, bronchospasm, hyperglycemia, syncope	
Bretylium	Ventricular tachycardia	Hypotension	Nausea, vomiting, diarrhea	
Verapamil	Pacemaker suppression, atrioventricular block	Hypotension; may aggravate or induce heart failure	Nervousness, pruritus, syncope	
Investigational				
Amiodarone (a)	Exacerbation or induction of arrhythmias; conduction disturbances; bradycardia or asystole	Hypotension; aggravation or induction of heart failure	(a) Nausea, vomiting, bluish skin discoloration in humans; pulmonary fibrosis; hepatitis	
Aprindine (b)				
Encainide (c)			(b) Nausea, convulsions, acute reversible hepatitis, leukopenia	
Flecainide (d)			(c) Nausea, weakness, disorientation (d) Nausea, weakness, disorientation	
Mexiletine	Similar to lidocaine	Hypotension	Similar to lidocaine	
Tocainide	Similar to lidocaine	Hypotension	Similar to lidocaine	

maticity. Atrioventricular nodal conduction velocity is unchanged except at toxic concentrations, when depression may occur. Procainamide, like quinidine, produces significant prolongation of the ERP in atrial and ventricular muscle and Purkinje fibers (Table 10-5).[23] This latter property, combined with depression of conduction, is believed to be responsible for procainamide's ability to turn unidirectional into bidirectional block, thereby abolishing re-entrant arrhythmias. Procainamide's electrophysiologic activities, like those of quinidine, are directly linked to the amount of free or unbound drug available for interaction with cardiac membranes. Procainamide binding with cardiac membranes inhibits transmembrane currents carried by sodium ion. These electrophysiologic effects are exquisitely sensitive to extracellular potassium concentration and pH. Procainamide is relatively ineffective during hypokalemia and produces pronounced myocardial depression during hyperkalemia and acidosis.[33–35]

Studies in intact animals indicate that relatively rapid infusions of procainamide, in dosages of up to 10 mg/kg, produced insignificant changes in cardiac output, cardiac contractility, and left ventricular end diastolic pressure (Table 10–6).[34] Heart rate increases slightly, while arterial blood pressure and total peripheral vascular resistance decrease.[35] These latter effects may be partially attributed to procain-

amide's purported anticholinergic activity and ganglionic blocking action.[36] Vasodilation could be particularly deleterious in patients dependent upon compensatory increases in sympathetic vasomotor tone in order to maintain adequate arterial pressures. Renal function is significantly depressed by procainamide owing to drug-induced decreases in glomerular filtration rate and effective renal plasma flow.[37] Electrocardiographically, therapeutic concentrations of procainamide produce insignificant prolongation of the QRS and Q-T intervals, while toxic concentrations may cause marked prolongation in the QRS, Q-T, and P-R intervals (Table 10–5). These effects are exaggerated by metabolic acidosis and hyperkalemia.

Procainamide is rapidly and completely absorbed after oral administration, although first-pass elimination reduces bioavailability to 80% to 90% in dogs. Plasma $t\frac{1}{2}_\beta$ following intravenous administration is approximately 2.5 hours, with the liver serving as the major elimination pathway (Table 10–7).[38] N-acetylprocainamide (acecainide) is the major metabolite of procainamide metabolism in man and has been demonstrated to possess potent antiarrhythmic properties that may necessitate dosage readjustments.[38] Only negligible quantities of N-acetylprocainamide have been identified in dogs and cats, thereby minimizing this potential effect during therapy.[39] Procainamide's short

$t\frac{1}{2}_\beta$ and relatively minimal hemodynamic effects compared to quinidine are responsible for its clinical popularity as intravenous therapy. Intravenous bolus dosages combined with constant- or double-infusion techniques are used initially to eradicate cardiac arrhythmias in emergency situations. This initial therapy can be followed by either intermittent intramuscular or oral therapy to maintain antiarrhythmic protection. Absorption from intramuscular sites is rapid but may be erratic, leading to variable antiarrhythmic activity. The short $t\frac{1}{2}_\beta$ may require that procainamide be dosed four to six times daily. For this reason, several sustained-release procainamide preparations have been developed. These preparations demonstrate a half-life of from 3 to 6 hours after oral administration, thereby reducing dosing frequency to a minimum of three or four times per day.[39] Procainamide elimination is altered significantly in patients with severely compensated heart failure. The Cl_T is reduced because of depression of liver enzymatic activity. In addition, the Vd for procainamide may be decreased secondary to decreases in the effective circulating blood volume. Decreases in plasma protein binding and renal function apparently demonstrate little effect upon procainamide disposition in the dog and cat. Additional studies are needed to clarify the importance of renal disease on procainamide elimination in the dog and cat.

Procainamide can be used as therapy for the majority of cardiac arrhythmias, although its efficacy in converting supraventricular arrhythmias is poorly documented. Acute atrial flutter or fibrillation can be treated with procainamide, although our clinical impression is that quinidine is better suited for this task. Like quinidine, procainamide can accelerate atrioventricular conduction in dogs with atrial fibrillation resulting in an increase in ventricular rate.[36] It also has the potential to produce marked depression in sinus rate in dogs with sick sinus syndrome. Ventricular arrhythmias are excellently managed by procainamide, particularly since intravenous therapy can be followed by oral medication. Procainamide is compatible with digitalis glycosides in the management of ventricular arrhythmias associated with heart failure in dogs. Procainamide is also extremely effective in prolonging the ERP in an accessory pathway, thereby abolishing or preventing arrhythmias dependent upon this mechanism.

When administered at usual therapeutic concentrations or by slow infusion rates, procainamide produces no significant deleterious effects, but myocardial depression does occur after rapid intravenous dosing. Procainamide-induced hypotension can be treated with fluids and catecholamines (dopamine) if necessary. Toxic concentrations of procainamide can produce anorexia, emesis, fever, depression, and cardiac arrhythmias (Table 10–8).[18,32] Prolongation of the P-R, QRS, and Q-T intervals, atrioventricular block, and ventricular tachyarrhythmias may occur after rapid intravenous procainamide administration (Fig. 10–5). Neither quinidine nor procainamide should be administered in patients with third-degree heart block or idioventricular rhythms without evidence of P waves for fear of eliminating the ventricular pacemaker. Syncopal episodes caused by paroxysmal ventricular tachycardia have not been reported during procainamide therapy in dogs. A form of systemic lupus erythematosus with a positive antinuclear antibody test is possible during chronic procainamide therapy in dogs, but clinical cases of autoimmune disease have been poorly documented in the dog and cat.

Disopyramide

Disopyramide is a class I antiarrhythmic drug whose direct electrophysiologic effects are almost identical to those of quinidine. Disopyramide depresses automaticity, diminishes myocardial conduction velocity, and prolongs the ERP in atria, atrioventricular node, and ventricles in isolated tissues (Table 10–5). These effects are dependent upon extracellular potassium concentration.[40,41] Anticholinergic properties similar to those reported for procainamide nullify or even reverse any direct effects upon the atrioventricular node in intact dogs, resulting in accelerated atrioventricular conduction and an increased ventricular response during atrial fibrillation.[18] Electrocardiographically, disopyramide produces dose-dependent widening of the QRS and Q-T intervals and can exaggerate pre-existing conduction abnormalities (Table 10–5). These effects are linked to disopyramide's suppression of sodium transport across cardiac membranes and resultant changes in ionic currents.[40]

Hemodynamic studies in dogs indicate that disopyramide produces increases in heart rate, mean aortic pressure, and systemic vascular resistance and decreases in stroke volume and cardiac contractility (Table 10–5). These changes are observed after infusion of 1 mg/kg disopyramide over 5 minutes and could have important deleterious effects in patients with myocardial dysfunction.[26] Increases in heart rate and arterial pressure result in increased myocardial oxygen demand and decreases in cardiac output, thereby exacerbating tissue hypoxia and potentially resulting in shock or acute heart failure.

The metabolism and disposition of disopyramide in the dog varies dramatically from that reported for humans. Following oral administration, disopyramide is rapidly absorbed, demonstrating a bioavailability of approximately 70%. The liver is the major organ responsible for disopyramide biotransformation in the dog.[42] Clearance is particularly dependent upon liver blood flow rate. Active metabolites have not been identified in either the dog or the cat. The mean elimination $t\frac{1}{2}_\beta$ after intravenous administration of disopyramide to dogs is less than 2 hours and after oral administration less than 3 hours (Table 10–7). This fact, coupled with concentration-dependent protein binding, makes it difficult to achieve and maintain therapeutic drug concentrations in the dog unless doses are administered at frequent intervals. Clinically, this requires oral dosing of at least six to eight times daily. Disopyramide elimination is reduced in animals with chronic congestive cardiac disease.

Disopyramide is effective as therapy for the same types of arrhythmias that quinidine and procainamide are used to treat. Clinically, however, limited experience in dogs indicates that disopyramide is best suited for the treatment of ventricular tachyarrhythmias. Since atrioventricular conduction is not impaired, supraventricular arrhythmias resulting from atrioventricular re-entry respond poorly to disopyramide therapy, and this drug may produce an acceleration of the ventricular response during atrial flutter or fibrillations.[16] Disopyramide is effective in controlling ventricular response in atrial arrhythmias complicating pre-excitation syndromes because of prolongation of the ERP of the accessory pathway.

The toxic manifestations associated with oral disopyramide administration are not well documented in dogs and cats but are believed to be similar to those of quinidine and include nausea, urine retention, and constipation (Table 10–8). Occasionally, depression is observed. Toxic electrocardiographic effects are similar to those of quinidine (Fig. 10–5). Disopyramide is contraindicated in patients with atrioventricular block or sick sinus syndrome, and ventricular arrhythmias may be produced or exacerbated following administration.[32] These side effects result from the known parasympatholytic and electrophysiologic actions of the drug. Toxic concentrations of disopyramide produce significant depression of cardiac output and left ventricular performance in normal dogs, and this effect could be pronounced in patients with pre-existing ventricular failure. This latter effect, coupled with its rapid clearance, makes disopyramide relatively unsuitable as therapy for arrhythmias in dogs or cats.

Lidocaine

Lidocaine is a class I antiarrhythmic drug that has undergone extensive experimental and clinical evaluation in both the dog and the cat. Despite extensive investigation, it is only within the past several years that the electrophysiologic effects of lidocaine have been elucidated. Lidocaine, like other membrane stabilizers, depresses automaticity in normal Purkinje fibers and in Purkinje fibers and ventricular muscle tissue preparations made automatic by hypoxemia, catecholamines, digitalis, and other pharmacologic manipulations. Lidocaine has no effect on the rate of isolated sinus node preparations.[16,18,43] The threshold for excitation or inducement of ventricular fibrillation is increased by lidocaine (Table 10–5). Lidocaine, however, differs from quinidine, procainamide, and disopyramide. Conduction velocity in isolated tissues is not changed by therapeutic concentrations of lidocaine and was originally thought to be increased. Recently, however, lidocaine was shown to produce minimal depression in conduction velocity in normal cardiac tissue.[25] Lidocaine produces dramatic decreases in conduction velocity in ischemic or hypoxic cardiac tissues. Conversely, lidocaine hyperpolarizes and improves conduction in tissues depolarized by stretch or hypokalemia.[44] The duration of the action potential and ERP are decreased in Purkinje fibers and ventricular muscle (Table 10–5). The ratio between ERP and action potential duration is increased, however, resulting in decreases in the time during which the cell can be re-excited before repolarization occurs (decreases the supernormal period). Lidocaine abolishes disparities in action potential duration in Purkinje fibers and ventricular muscle, thereby making it suitable in the management of re-entrant arrhythmias. Lidocaine is relatively ineffective in prolonging refractoriness or decreasing atrial excitability.[18] The reasons for this are unclear at present. Recent data suggest that most, if not all, of lidocaine's electrophysiologic effects are mediated by inhibition of sodium channels located in the cardiac cell membrane. The disparity in the effects of lidocaine versus quinidine, procainamide, and disopyramide upon action potential duration and ERP are explained by different effects on repolarizing potassium currents.[43] Electrocardiographically, lidocaine may shorten the Q-T interval but does not affect the P-R interval or QRS duration (Table 10–5). The refractory period of the atrioventricular node may decrease, causing a marked increase in ventricular response in patients with atrial flutter or fibrillation (Fig. 10–5).

Hemodynamically, therapeutic concentrations of lidocaine produce negligible effects upon cardiac output, cardiac contractility, or arterial blood pressure (Table 10–6). Lidocaine occasionally produces sinus tachycardia secondary to peripheral vasodilation and reflex increases in sympathetic tone.[18] Peripheral vasodilation is caused by ganglionic blockade. Glomerular filtration rate and effective renal plasma flow are not affected by lidocaine administration.[37]

Lidocaine is metabolized by the liver to such an extent that greater than 70% of an intravenous dose is biotransformed on a single pass. It is this tremendous first-pass elimination that has made lidocaine virtually ineffective when administered orally. Lidocaine clearance is extremely dependent on liver blood flow; thus, alterations in plasma protein binding and renal elimination do not affect its clearance.[45,46] Several metabolites of lidocaine, monoethylglycine xylidide and glycine xylidide, have been identified in dogs but have not been developed for clinical use because of toxic side effects.[47] The $t_{\frac{1}{2}\beta}$ in dogs following intravenous lidocaine administration is approximately 1 to 1.5 hours (Table 10–7). This predicts that Cp_{ss} during constant infusion is reached in between 3 and 4 hours and makes lidocaine the drug of choice for the rapid control of ventricular arrhythmias. Intravenous bolus dosages ("loading doses") are used to establish therapeutic plasma concentrations rapidly. Liver disease and cardiac failure reduce lidocaine clearance and Vd, thereby requiring dosage readjustments if these disorders are present. Furthermore, the simultaneous administration of drugs that reduce liver blood flow (propranolol, cimetidine) or decrease hepatic clearance may increase lidocaine plasma levels.[48,49] If lidocaine therapy is required in these situations, both loading dosages and the infusion rate should be reduced in order to avoid toxicity. Measurement of plasma drug levels has proved useful in verifying therapeutic concentrations in patients with questionable liver function and congestive heart failure.

Lidocaine is the agent of choice for the treatment or prevention of ventricular tachyarrhythmias from any cause. It is effective in treating catecholamine-induced arrhythmias during inhalation anesthesia, and in suppressing digitalis-induced arrhythmias. It also reduces ventricular response in pre-excitation associated with atrial flutter or fibrillation. Lidocaine's effectiveness in converting ventricular arrhythmias to sinus rhythm is extremely dependent upon extracellular potassium concentration.[44] Hypokalemia negates most of lidocaine's beneficial antiarrhythmic effects. Lidocaine is ineffective in the treatment of most supraventricular arrhythmias, although we have observed the occasional conversion of atrial premature contractions and atrial fibrillation to sinus rhythm during lidocaine treatment of ventricular rhythm disturbances. The inability of lidocaine to convert supraventricular arrhythmias to sinus rhythm correlates well with its lack of electrophysiologic effects upon isolated atrial tissues. Lidocaine is contraindicated in patients with sick sinus syndrome, second- or third-degree heart block, idioventricular rhythms with no evidence of P waves, and in patients with sinus bradycardia in which the predominant rhythm is due to ventricular escape.

Toxic signs associated with lidocaine overdosage are relatively common but are comparatively less dramatic than those observed with quinidine and disopyramide. Hypotension, occasional exacerbation of ventricular arrhythmias, and acceleration in ventricular rhythms have been observed (Fig. 10–5). The most common side effects are nausea, disorientation, depression, neuromuscular excitability (twitching), and convulsions (Table 10–3). Lidocaine-induced seizures are self-limiting, abating as plasma concentration decreases, but they may be accompanied by respiratory arrest or airway obstruction. Lidocaine-induced seizures are particularly common in cats and are believed to be due to local anesthetic reduction in the release of gamma-aminobutyric acid from nerve terminals in the central nervous system.[50] The central nervous signs associated with lidocaine toxicity can be managed by intravenous diazepam.

Phenytoin

Phenytoin is an antiepileptic drug that possesses class I antiarrhythmic activity. Therapeutic concentrations of phenytoin produce electrophysiologic and electrocardiographic effects identical to those observed with lidocaine (Table 10–5). In addition, phenytoin is capable of inhibiting slow-response action potentials that may be important in the initiation and maintenance of ventricular arrhythmias caused by myocardial ischemia and digitalis preparations.[51] Phenytoin produces minimal hemodynamic effects when administered intravenously, provided that infusion is slow (Table 10–6). Slight decreases in heart rate and blood pressure are attributed to decreases in central nervous system sympathetic activity. Propylene glycol, a diluent of intravenous preparations of phenytoin, produces decreases in cardiac output, hypotension, bradycardia, and, potentially, cardiac arrest if administration is rapid.[16] Phenytoin is most frequently administered orally, although intravenous administration has been used for treating acute digitalis toxicity. Absorption from the gastrointestinal tract is erratic, giving a systemic bioavailability of only 40% (Table 10–7). Phenytoin is metabolized by the liver, and the parent compound and metabolites are excreted in the urine. Hepatic clearance in the dog is affected by changes in plasma protein binding and not by liver blood flow, making hypoalbuminemia and decreases in Vd secondary to congestive heart failure the most important causes of increases in phenytoin plasma concentrations. The $t_{1/2_\beta}$ for phenytoin in dogs is 3 to 5 hours compared to values in excess of 20 hours in the cat (Table 10–7). The reasons for this large difference are due to differences in hepatic clearance.[52] A variety of drugs may produce increases in phenytoin plasma concentrations, presumably by interfering with hepatic

microsomal enzyme activity. Simultaneous administration of chloramphenicol or cimetidine, for example, will decrease phenytoin clearance to approximately 25% of its original value.

A lack of clinical effectiveness and difficulty in determining dosage rates and techniques have limited phenytoin to the treatment of digitalis-induced arrhythmias. Although potentially beneficial for treating a wide variety of ventricular tachyarrhythmias, phenytoin has not gained popularity in veterinary medicine.

Toxic signs associated with intravenous phenytoin therapy include respiratory arrest, bradycardia, progressive hypotension, atrioventricular heart block, and asystole (Table 10–8). Transient sinoatrial arrest and atrial standstill has been reported after acute intravenous phenytoin therapy in man. Occasionally, phenytoin enhances atrioventricular conduction, an effect that is potentially beneficial in digitalis toxicity, but one that could result in accelerated ventricular response during re-entrant supraventricular arrhythmias.[32] Other signs of phenytoin toxicity include nausea, ataxia, polydipsia, hepatopathy, and depression. Lupus erythematosus and lymphadenopathy reportedly can occur associated with chronic phenytoin therapy but have not been documented in the dog or cat.

Propranolol

Propranolol, a class II antiarrhythmic, is a relatively short-acting, nonselective (blocks both beta$_1$ and beta$_2$ adrenoceptors) beta-adrenoceptor blocking drug. The basis for propranolol's therapeutic benefits in the treatment of cardiac arrhythmias originates from its membrane-stabilizing (quinidine-like) activity and beta-adrenoceptor blocking effects. Membrane-stabilizing drugs are capable of decreasing spontaneous frequency, depressing conduction velocity, and increasing the electrical threshold for excitability (Table 10–5). Although potentially important during drug overdose, it is questionable whether membrane-stabilizing effects are of therapeutic value at currently recommended dosage schedules. Propranolol therefore produces its most important clinical effects by antagonizing the actions of catecholamines released by an increased frequency of sympathetic discharge from the central nervous system or from the release of catecholamines from the adrenal medulla. Propranolol demonstrates its most profound therapeutic effects in the presence of elevated sympathetic tone. Beta-adrenoceptor blockade reduces sinus rate, prolongs the atrioventricular conduction time and therefore the P-R interval, decreases the rate of atrial and ventricular premature depolarizations, and prevents reflex tachycardia due to hypotension.[53] Hemodynamically, propranolol can produce decreases in cardiac output, cardiac contractility, and arterial blood pressure with increases in total peripheral resistance (Table 10–6).

Propranolol is extensively metabolized by oxidation and glucuronidation in the liver, leading to low bioavailability after oral administration. At least one metabolite, 4-hydropropranolol, has beta-adrenoceptor blocking activity, but concentrations in dogs are too low for this compound to be considered significant. Hepatic clearance of propranolol approaches hepatic blood flow; consequently, elimination depends primarily upon changes in hepatic blood flow rate.[54,55] Since propranolol reduces cardiac output, and hence hepatic blood flow rate, it reduces its own clearance. Similarly, propranolol can reduce the clearance of other drugs that are highly extracted by the liver and dependent upon liver blood flow rate (e.g., lidocaine). The $t_{1/2\beta}$ for propranolol is less than 1.5 hours, potentially necessitating large or frequent dosages (Table 10–7). Alterations in cellular metabolism during chronic propranolol administration or during simultaneous administration of cimetidine, however, may permit the use of lower-than-expected doses.[53] Because of wide variability in plasma concentration after oral dosing and the variability in drug response owing to prevailing sympathetic activity, propranolol should be administered with caution and initially at low dosages. Dogs and cats with failing hearts may have a reduced liver blood flow and increased reflex sympathetic activity, thereby potentiating the effects of propranolol. Interestingly, decreases in propranolol protein binding and renal disease do not affect propranolol elimination. Conversely, increases in plasma levels of alpha$_1$-acid glycoprotein secondary to heart failure or inflammatory diseases may increase propranolol protein binding, resulting in a decrease in Vd and a shortened $t_{1/2\beta}$.

Propranolol is particularly effective therapy in reducing heart rate caused by increased sympathetic tone or by thyrotoxicosis.[56] Sinus tachycardia caused by hypokalemia, fever, and abnormal forms of automaticity do not respond favorably to propranolol. Clinically, propranolol is frequently combined with digitalis preparations to decrease ventricular response during atrial fibrillation. Propranolol is useful in treating supraventricular arrhythmias, including atrial premature depolarizations and paroxysmal supraventricular or ventricular tachycardias, particularly when sympathetic tone is high. Propranolol can be combined with class I antiarrhythmic drugs (quinidine, procainamide, lidocaine) in the treatment of refractory cardiac arrhythmias.

Excessive dosages of propranolol or poor clinical judgment can result in bradyarrhythmias, hypotension, heart failure and sudden death, bronchospasm, and hypoglycemia (Table 10–8). Signs of toxicity are frequent in aged animals. Interestingly, the frequency and severity of side effects in humans is independent of the dose administered. Based upon clinical impression, it is presumed that the frequency of side effects in dogs and cats is also independent of dose.

Intravenous dobutamine (3–5 μg/kg/min), furosemide (1.0 mg/kg), and glycopyrrolate (0.05 mg/kg), can be administered if propranolol toxicity is recognized early.

It should be noted that, in the past several years, the Food and Drug Administration has approved five additional beta-adrenoceptor blocking drugs for clinical use in the United States. These compounds include metoprolol, nadolol, timolol, atenolol, and pindolol.[57,57a] Differences in their pharmacologic activity, relative beta$_1$- versus beta$_2$-adrenoceptor blocking activity, and ability to stimulate while blocking beta-adrenoceptors are listed in Table 10–9. Regardless of these differences, all possess equally effective antiarrhythmic activity when proper adjustments in dosage have been made.

Bretylium

Bretylium, a class III antiarrhythmic, is an antihypertensive drug that is promoted as an antifibrillatory agent. The electrical threshold for ventricular fibrillation in dogs is increased by bretylium.[16] Bretylium increases spontaneous rate, action potential duration, and ERP in isolated tissue preparations (Table 10–5). Resting membrane potential becomes more negative in partially depolarized tissues.[58,59] The mechanism for these effects is not known, but the fact that they occur may be responsible for improving conduction and abolishing re-entrant circuits in diseased myocardium. Electrocardiographic effects are unremarkable. Hemodynamically, bretylium administration results in acute increases in cardiac contractility, cardiac output, and arterial blood pressure (Table 10–6). These transient effects are followed by little to no change in most hemodynamic indices except arterial blood pressure, which is mildly decreased.[60] Bretylium's hemodynamic effects parallel an initial increase in catecholamine release, followed by an inhibition of catecholamine release. The pharmacokinetics of bretylium in the dog and cat are unknown.

Bretylium is recommended as therapy for the treatment of refractory ventricular tachyarrhythmias and recurrent ventricular fibrillation in humans.[18] Some experimental studies in dogs and cats do not

Table 10–9. Important properties of beta-adrenergic blocking drugs

Drug	Beta$_1$-blocking potency ratio*	Relative beta$_1$ selectivity	Intrinsic sympatho-mimetic activity	Heart rate	Cardiac output	Arterial blood pressure	Peripheral vascular resistance	AV conduction velocity	Broncho-constriction	Platelet aggregation
Propranolol	1.0	No	No	↓	↓	↓	↑	↓	↑ —	↓
Nadolol	1.0	No	No	↓	↓	↓	↑	↓	↑ —	↓
Timolol	8.0	No	No	↓	↓	↓	↑	↓	↑ — ?	ND
Metoprolol	1.0	Yes	No	↓	↓	↓	↑ —	↓	— ?	ND
Atenolol	1.0	Yes	No	↓	↓	↓ —	↑ —	↓	—	ND
Pindolol	5.0	No	Yes	↓	↓	↓ —	↓ —	↓	—	↓

* = Compared to propranolol = 1.0.
↑ = Increase; ↓ = decrease; — = no change; ND = not determined
† = Bronchoconstriction observed at large dosages

support this recommendation and in fact suggest that bretylium may precipitate the production of ventricular tachycardia, increase the rate of chemically induced ventricular tachycardias, and precipitate ventricular fibrillation.[61,62] The reason for the disparity between human and animal studies is unclear but may be related to the absence in animals of large areas of infarcted myocardium usually being responsible for ventricular fibrillation in man.

Bretylium toxicity has not been reported in dogs or cats but would be expected to include nausea, vomiting, hypotension, and potentially an aggravation of pre-existing rhythm disturbances (Table 10–8). Recently, an orally absorbed analogue of bretylium, bethanidine sulfate, has been shown to exert an antifibrillatory effect in the dog.[63]

Verapamil

Verapamil, a class IV antiarrhythmic drug, is one of a number of compounds that have been termed calcium channel blocking drugs. These drugs inhibit transmembrane calcium transport. In contradistinction to the majority of the class I antiarrhythmic drugs, verapamil produces its most pronounced electrophysiologic effects on both the sinoatrial and atrioventricular nodes. Isolated sinus node discharge rate is depressed, and conduction velocity through the atrioventricular node is decreased following verapamil administration.[64,65] These effects are dependent on dose and not on autonomic tone, and are reversed by calcium addition to the bathing solution, pointing out the importance of calcium currents in the normal function of both of these tissues. In contrast to its effects upon nodal tissues, therapeutic concentrations produce little, if any, measurable effects upon atrial and ventricular myocardium and Purkinje fibers. Normal spontaneous automaticity arising from Purkinje fibers is not affected by verapamil (Table 10–5). Spontaneous and electrically stimulated rhythmic activity originating from depolarized cardiac tissues are depressed. In addition, spontaneous depolarizations resulting from "triggered" repetitive activity are abolished.[18,66] The electrical current required to produce electrical fibrillation in dogs is increased following verapamil administration. These electrophysiologic effects are attributed to verapamil's ability to inhibit both sodium and particularly calcium currents in cardiac tissues. Electrocardiographic and hemodynamic studies indicate that verapamil produces marked prolongation in the P-R interval but has little or no effect on sinus rate or on QRS or Q-T intervals in patients in sinus rhythm (Table 10–5). Peripheral vasodilation, coronary arterial dilation, and negative inotropic effects are the three principal responses to intravenous verapamil therapy (Table 10–6). Vasodilation is due to direct vasodilation and a minor alpha-adrenergic blocking activity.[66–68] Clinically, verapamil's negative inotropic and hypotensive effects could induce congestive symptoms in patients with compensated heart failure.

Verapamil is poorly absorbed from the gastrointestinal tract of dogs and is subject to first-pass metabolism by the liver.[69] Like lidocaine, disopyramide, and propranolol, verapamil clearance in dogs approaches liver blood flow rates. This indicates that diseases, drugs, or manipulations that reduce liver blood flow will prolong verapamil elimination. Although verapamil is highly protein bound, alterations in plasma protein binding and renal elimination do not affect clearance. The intravenous $t_{1/2\beta}$ for verapamil is less than 1 hour in dogs, indicating that frequent dosing may be necessary to maintain a sustained effect (Table 10–7). Pharmacokinetic data from cats are unavailable. Verapamil may cause an increase in serum digoxin levels if therapy is initiated in chronically digitalized animals, thereby necessitating digoxin dosage readjustments.[70]

The major therapeutic use for verapamil is in controlling supraventricular tachyarrhythmias. Although most documented instances of arrhythmia control are from studies conducted in humans, verapamil should be equally effective in animals. Verapamil can slow sinus rate in atrial tachycardia, is extremely effective in terminating reentrant supraventricular tachycardia, and abolishes re-entrant tachycardia owing to an accessory pathway. Ventricular response during atrial flutter or fibrillation is dramatically slowed following verapamil administration in dogs. Verapamil is of limited value as therapy for ectopic atrial tachycardias, in converting atrial fibrillation, and in converting ventricular tachycardias to sinus rhythm.[68] More clinical experience in dogs and cats is required before firm therapeutic indications can be made.

Acute toxic manifestations associated with verapamil therapy are caused by sinus or atrioventricular node suppression and hypotension (Table 10–8). Verapamil therapy may induce first degree, second degree, or complete heart block and is contraindicated in patients with sinus bradycardia or sick sinus syndrome. We have produced marked hypotension and cardiogenic shock when attempting to slow ventricular response during atrial fibrillation in cardiomyopathic dogs. Intravenous fluids, calcium salts, calcium chloride, and catecholamines (dobutamine, dopamine) should be administered if circulatory failure occurs.

Two relatively new calcium entry blocking drugs, nifedipine and diltiazem, have recently become available for use as antianginal agents in humans. These drugs possess many direct electrophysiologic and hemodynamic effects similar to those of verapamil.[71] Diltiazem may be of some value in treating supraventricular tachyarrhythmias, but nifedipine is totally ineffective because it produces intense reflex increases in adrenergic tone. A great deal of clinical experience is needed before either of these drugs can be administered safely to dogs and cats.

Digitalis

The digitalis glycosides, digoxin and digitoxin, are potentially useful for the treatment of cardiac arrhythmias; the majority of their antiarrhythmic effects stemming from indirect actions.[72] Therapeutic concentrations of digitalis produce minimal changes in sinus node rate, conduction velocity, ERP, or excitability in isolated cardiac tissue preparations (Table 10–5). Toxic concentrations of digitalis can depolarize cardiac cells, depress conduction velocity, and shorten ERP. Oscillations in the resting membrane potential can occur during toxicity, leading to spontaneous automaticity in specialized cardiac fibers.[72] These effects are responsible for the development of cardiac arrhythmias from either re-entrant or ectopic automatic mechanisms. Digitalis also lowers the ventricular fibrillation threshold. Digitalis effects upon electrical and mechanical activity in intact dog or cat heart are the result of glycoside-induced alterations in automatic tone and the sensitivity of the heart to parasympathetic and sympathetic neurotransmitters. Therapeutic concentrations of digitalis increase vagal tone, sensitize arterial and ventricular baroreceptors, and increase the activity of the central nervous system vagal nuclei. Toxic concentrations of digitalis may also enhance central nervous system efferent sympathetic activity.[72] The clinical result of these diverse pharmacologic effects is a reduction in sinus rate, prolongation in atrioventricular conduction, and improvement in intra-atrial conduction velocity.[18] These actions are consistent with the effects of acetylcholine upon cardiac cell membranes and reflect its ability to depress automaticity and hyperpolarize cardiac tissues, resulting in improved conduction. Hemodynamically, therapeutic concentrations of digitalis increase cardiac contractility and produce variable effects upon cardiac output and arterial blood pressure (Table 10–6). Increases in inotropic activity are produced by inhibition of the sodium-potassium ATP-dependent membrane pump, resulting in intracellular calcium accumulation and increased actin-myosin interaction.[72] Cardiac output increases and heart rate declines in patients with heart failure due to digitalis-induced increases in cardiac contractility and withdrawal of sympathetic tone.

Digitalis is uncommonly used intravenously to treat cardiac arrhythmias. Oral preparations usually suffice for this purpose but are subject to variable degrees of absorption and biotransformation by the liver (Table 10–7). Problems with absorption of various oral formulas of digitalis have been minimized in recent years. Digoxin plasma concentrations are partially dependent upon renal elimination, plasma protein binding, and intrinsic clearance mechanisms.[72,73] These factors may be responsible for frequent dosage adjustments in patients with renal disease or heart failure and emphasize the value of periodic determinations of plasma digitalis concentration. Furthermore, uremia displaces digitalis from skeletal muscle-binding sites, resulting in an increase in active plasma digoxin concentrations.[74] As previously discussed, both quinidine and verapamil can increase plasma digoxin concentrations by decreasing renal digoxin clearance.[70]

The indirect effect of digitalis upon supraventricular tissues makes it ideally suited for the treatment of a wide variety of supraventricular tachyarrhythmias. Digitalis is effective therapy for sinus tachycardia, ectopic atrial pacemakers, and atrial flutter or fibrillation.[72] Occasionally, atrial fibrillation is converted to sinus rhythm in dogs, although the more frequent response is a decrease in ventricular rate. Digitalis may be effective in the treatment of ventricular arrhythmias owing to its potential to decrease cardiac size, improve hemodynamics, and normalize acid-base status. The use of digitalis as therapy for sinus tachycardia associated with sick sinus syndrome and atrial fibrillation associated with an accessory pathway is controversial and has not been defined in dogs or cats.

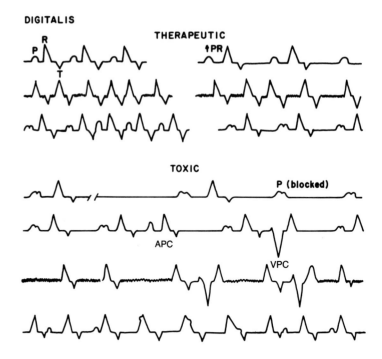

Fig. 10–6. Therapeutic concentrations of digitalis increase the P-R interval, slow ventricular rate during atrial fibrillation, and may prevent atrial tachycardia (top three traces). Toxic concentrations of digitalis produce second-degree atrioventricular block, premature atrial and ventricular complexes, and ventricular bradycardia during atrial fibrillation and induce atrioventricular nodal rhythms with atrioventricular dissociation (bottom four traces).

Toxic manifestations associated with digitalis administration are frequent and usually include lethargy, anorexia, vomiting, and diarrhea.[72,73] Potassium depletion may occur with chronic therapy.[73] Hypokalemia exaggerates the effects of digitalis glycosides on cardiac membranes. Electrocardiographically, toxic concentrations of digitalis produce sinus bradycardia, first- and second-degree atrioventricular block, sinus arrest, sinus block, ST changes, conduction abnormalities, junctional rhythms, and ventricular arrhythmias (Fig. 10–6). Ventricular arrhythmias are attributed to digitalis-induced membrane oscillations and respond favorably to lidocaine or phenytoin therapy. Bradycardia can be treated with atropine or glycopyrrolate.

CLINICAL MANAGEMENT OF CARDIAC ARRHYTHMIAS

General principles

The significance of a cardiac arrhythmia depends on both the type of rhythm disturbance and the underlying or associated clinical disorder. Many arrhythmias do not require therapy or prove to be self-limiting when the underlying disorder is treated. The decision to treat an arrhythmia and the selection of specific therapy are based on consideration of the following:[75]

1. The degree of hemodynamic or functional impairment

2. The natural history of the arrhythmia based on literature and personal experience
3. The history of the arrhythmia in the individual patient
4. The potential for development of further electrical instability such as ventricular tachycardia or fibrillation
5. The potential for development of congestive heart failure as may occur with atrial fibrillation or complete atrioventricular block
6. The availability of methods or drugs that have been proven to correct the rhythm disturbance
7. The assurance that the drug can be administered correctly
8. The potential risk of adverse effects due to the antiarrhythmic therapy
9. The potential for adverse drug interactions with currently administered medications

It is imperative to recognize that, although some arrhythmias cannot be completely controlled, antiarrhythmic therapy may reduce the risk of more serious arrhythmias or may improve the clinical well-being of the patient. Procainamide, for example, may prevent syncope-causing paroxysmal ventricular tachycardia in a Boxer dog with cardiomyopathy, but may not totally abolish isolated ventricular premature complexes (VPCs). Similarly, the Saint Bernard dog in atrial fibrillation may improve clinically if the ventricular rate is reduced via digitalization and beta-adrenergic blockade. Such a patient may benefit even though the digoxin-propranolol combination therapy will not convert atrial fibrillation to normal sinus rhythm.

The *initial evaluation* of the patient with an arrhythmia should encompass the following points: patient history, medication history, physical examination, cardiovascular examination, assessment of hemodynamic and metabolic states, identification of intercurrent extracardiac disease, accurate interpretation of previous and current electrocardiograms, and evaluation of current medication (Table 10–4). Following the completion of this type of evaluation, the clinician can usually determine if the arrhythmia is caused by a noncardiac or cardiac disorder and can assess the risks and benefits of antiarrhythmic therapy.

Table 10–4 provides an outline for the evaluation of a patient with a cardiac arrhythmia. One can offer numerous examples that emphasize the importance of such an evaluation prior to the initiation of therapy. For instance, if the history is suggestive of abrupt reductions in blood pressure, and the ECG shows evidence for sinoatrial arrest or frequent VPCs, it is probable that the arrhythmia has led to the clinical signs, and a course of antiarrhythmic therapy would be reasonable. When physical and radiographic examinations indicate heart failure due to valvular or myocardial heart disease, it may be essential to direct inotropic, diuretic, or vasodilator therapy to control the predisposing problem. Some arrhythmias will spontaneously abate when congestive heart failure is controlled and heart size is reduced. Antiarrhythmic therapy is probably unwarranted in the postoperative patient with isolated VPCs when that animal is otherwise hemodynamically stable. Frequently, the identification and the correction of hy-

povolemia, anemia, acidosis, hypoxemia, hypokalemia, or hyperkalemia will suffice to correct a rhythm disturbance. At other times, prompt drug therapy is imperative to prevent progressive hypotension, congestion, or organ hypoperfusion. This is particularly true in traumatized animals, high-risk surgical patients, and pets in congestive heart failure. As might be expected, there are "grey zones"—cases that defy hard and fast rules for treatment. Clinical judgment is required to successfully manage such cases. A good example of this is found in the dog with an idioventricular tachycardia that is hemodynamically stable, despite the occurrence of frequent ventricular beats.

Of course, no set of guidelines can adapt to every clinical situation, and the experienced clinician will be best served by a thorough knowledge of the patient and of the therapy that can be directed to an arrhythmia. Without accurate interpretation of the ECG rhythm, most types of therapy are futile. An example: it is not uncommon to observe cases in which the patient is treated with lidocaine for ventricular tachycardia when the actual rhythm is sinus tachycardia with right bundle branch block. Current knowledge of pharmacokinetics and drug pharmacology,[21,75,76] as presented in the previous sections, is essential for appropriate use of antiarrhythmic drugs in patients that have altered renal or hepatic clearance mechanisms. In the age of multiple pharmacotherapy, the potential for drug interaction must always be realized. With these concepts and comments in mind, we can proceed to a description of general guidelines for the treatment of specific cardiac arrhythmias.

SINUS RHYTHMS

Regular sinus rhythm and sinus arrhythmia are the normal cardiac rhythms in the dog and in the cat. Sinus arrhythmia is mediated by fluctuations in vagal tone; therefore, conditions that result in enhancement of vagal tone may lead to marked sinus arrhythmia. Pronounced sinus arrhythmia is frequently noted with pulmonary, central nervous system, and gastrointestinal disorders or following the administration of cholinergic drugs such as pilocarpine, pyridostigmine bromide, narcotics, and xylazine. Sinus pauses on occasion can be relatively long and accompanied by escape beats and thus mimic the findings of sinus arrest. Nevertheless, sinus arrhythmia should not be treated unless it is associated with profound bradycardia and signs of hypotension.

Sinus bradycardia. Sinus bradycardia is observed with organic heart disease, endocrinopathies, hypothermia, drug administration, and clinical disorders that reflexively increase vagal tone (Table 10–3). Most cases of sinus bradycardia are self-limiting, resolving with correction of the underlying disorder. In dogs with otherwise normal hearts, ventricular rates as low as 40 to 50 per minute may supply a normal cardiac output at rest. Thus, sinus bradycardia is treated when it results in symptoms of hypotension or when associated with potentially dangerous circumstances such as hypovolemia or anesthesia.

Management of sinus bradycardia must involve the identification and elimination of the underlying disorder since bradycardia asso-

Table 10–10. Drugs used in the therapy of cardiac arrhythmias

Generic name	Commonly used preparations	Indications	Adverse effects	Approximate dosage*
Atropine	Atropine sulfate USP 0.4 mg/ml	Sinus bradycardia Sinoatrial arrest Incomplete AV block	Sinus tachycardia, ectopic complexes, ocular, gastrointestinal, and pulmonary side effects, paradoxic vagomimetic effects	0.01–0.2 mg/kg IV, IM 0.02–0.04 mg/kg SQ (Dog and cat)
Digitoxin	Crystodigin 0.2 mg/ml 0.1, 0.2 mg tablets Foxalin 0.1, 0.25, 0.5 mg	Supraventricular premature complexes, supraventricular tachycardia, atrial flutter/ fibrillation	Anorexia, depression, vomiting, diarrhea, AV block, ectopia, junctional tachycardia	Oral Maintenance: 0.04 to 0.1 mg/kg divided BID to TID. Rapid IV digitalization: 0.01 to 0.03 mg/kg; administer ½ of calculated dose IV, wait 30 to 60 minutes and administer ¼ of dose, wait 30 to 60 minutes and administer remaining dose if necessary.
Digoxin	Lanoxin elixir 0.05 mg/ml, 0.125, 0.25, 0.5 mg tablets; Cardoxin elixirs 0.05, 0.15 mg/ml	Same as digitoxin	Same as digitoxin	Oral Maintenance: 0.01 to 0.02 mg/kg divided BID. Rapid IV digitalization: 0.01–0.02 mg/kg IV as per digitoxin. Rapid Oral Digitalization: 0.02 to 0.06 mg/kg divided BID for one day. Cat: 0.007–0.015 mg/kg divided BID
Glycopyrrolate	Robinul injection 0.2 mg/ml	Sinus bradycardia Sinoatrial arrest	As per atropine	0.005–.01 mg/kg IV, IM 0.01–0.02 mg/kg SQ (Dog and Cat)
Isopropamide	Darbid 5 mg tablets	Incomplete AV block Sinoatrial arrest	As per atropine, keratoconjunctivitis sicca	2.5–5 mg BID-TID
Isoproterenol	Isuprel HCl injection 0.2 mg/ml; 1- and 5-ml ampuls Proternol 20-, 40-mg tablets; Isuprel glossets, 10 mg	Sinoatrial arrest Sinus bradycardia Complete AV block	CNS stimulation, ectopic complexes Tachycardia, emesis	0.4 mg in 250 ml D5W, drip slowly to effect. Proternol—10–20 mg q 4–6 hours, Isuprel glossets—5–10 mg sublingual or per rectum q 4–6 hours
Lidocaine HCl	Xylocaine (without epinephrine) 2% (20 mg/ml)	Ventricular premature complexes, ventricular tachycardia	CNS excitation, seizures, tremors, emesis, (R$_x$ with diazepam), other rhythm disturbances	2–4 mg/kg IV slowly, repeat to maximum of 8 mg/kg. For the *cat:* 0.25–1 mg/kg IV over 5 minutes. Constant-rate infusion† for the dog: 25–75 μg/kg/min.
Procainamide	Pronestyl injection of 100 or 500 mg/ml, 250- and 500-mg tablets; Procan sustained release (SR) 250, 500 mg	Ventricular premature complexes, ventricular tachycardia	Weakness, hypotension, decreased contractility, anorexia, vomiting, diarrhea, widening of QRS and QT interval, AV block	6–8 mg/kg IV over 5 min, CRI: 25–40 μg/kg/min, 6–20 mg/kg IM q 4–6h, (See text) Tablets—8–20 mg/kg q 6h Procan SR—8–20 mg/kg q 6–8h
Propranolol HCl	Inderal 1 mg/ml vials, 10-, 20-, 40-, 80-mg tablets	Supraventricular premature complexes and tachyarrhythmias, atrial fibrillation, ventricular premature complexes	Decreased contractility, bronchoconstriction, loss of compensatory mechanisms	0.04–0.06 mg/kg IV slowly 0.2–1.0 mg/kg orally TID (Dog, Cat)
Quinidine sulfate gluconate polygalacturonate	Quinidine gluconate USP injection 80 mg/ml; Quinidine sulfate tablets USP 200 mg, Quinidex (sustained release) tablets, 300 mg, Quinaglute Dura-tabs (quinidine gluconate) 324 mg; Cardioquin tablets (quinidine polygalacturonate) 275 mg	Ventricular premature complexes, ventricular tachycardia, acute atrial fibrillation, refractory supraventricular tachycardias	As per procainamide, drug interaction with digoxin; urine retention	6–20 mg/kg IM, q 6h (See text) 6–16 mg/kg orally q 6h Quinaglute Dura-tabs (quinidine gluconate) and Cardioquin tablets (quinidine polygalacturonate) 8–20 mg/kg orally q 6–8h

*All dosages are for the *dog* unless otherwise noted.
†Formula for CRI: Body weight (in kg) × dose (in μg/kg/min) × 0.36 = total dose in mg to administer intravenously over 6 hours
   e.g., 20-kg dog, 50-μg/kg/min infusion
   e.g., (20) (50) (.36) = 360 mg over 6 hours
   Modified from Bonagura, J.D.: Therapy of cardiac arrhythmias. In *Current Veterinary Therapy.* Volume 8. Edited by R.W. Kirk. Philadelphia, W.B. Saunders, 1983.

ciated with hypothermia, hypothyroidism, hyperkalemia, hypoglycemia, and inhalation anesthetics may be refractory to treatment with anticholinergic medication. Symptomatic sinus bradycardia is treated with parenteral atropine or glycopyrrolate. Whenever possible, the intramuscular or subcutaneous routes of administration are selected (Table 10–10), since the intravenous administration of atropine frequently results in disparate effects on the SA and AV node[77] and can enhance sinus bradycardia or cause temporary AV block.[78,79] The rapid intravenous injection of atropine can also predispose to ventricular arrhythmias by altering autonomic balance.[78] During cardiovascular emergencies, sympathomimetic agents like epinephrine, isoproterenol, and dopamine HCl can be used to stimulate the SA node. Some cases require placement of a temporary transvenous pacing wire. Expansion of the blood volume is a valuable adjunctive treatment for hypotension caused by sinus bradycardia.

Sinus tachycardia. Sinus tachycardia invariably indicates an increase in sympathetic tone (Table 10–3). Specific antiarrhythmic therapy is seldom necessary provided that the underlying abnormality is corrected. Cage rest, administration of analgesics, antipyretics, oxygen, and fluid therapy are examples of treatments that often reduce the need for sympathetic compensation. Sinus tachycardia associated with congestive heart failure may abate with digitalization. Propranolol is used to control sinus tachycardia associated with thyrotoxicosis and hypertrophic cardiomyopathy in cats. Beta-adrenergic blockers are indicated to protect the heart in animals with persistent sinus tachycardia and other arrhythmias associated with central nervous system lesions ("brain-heart syndrome").[80] When given parenterally, sympathetic blocking drugs like propranolol should first be diluted and then administered with extreme caution over 5 to 10 minutes.

Sick sinus syndrome. The term "sick sinus syndrome" encompasses a complex of cardiac rhythm disturbances that include sinus bradycardia, sinus tachycardia, sinoatrial arrest, supraventricular premature complexes, supraventricular tachycardia, and often accompanying AV nodal and intraventricular conduction disturbances. One or all of these abnormalities may be present in a single patient.[81–83] The condition demonstrates distinctive breed predispositions (Table 10–3). Fortunately, sudden death is uncommon, even in dogs with frequent syncopal episodes. Inasmuch as weakness and syncope are consequences of these arrhythmias, the clinician must be prepared to evaluate and treat this disorder (Fig. 10–7).

Asymptomatic dogs are not treated, while symptomatic patients are grouped as follows: Group I dogs are those that show predominantly sinus bradycardia and sinus arrest; Group II dogs have periods of sinus arrest that are preceded by sinus or supraventricular tachycardias. As a general rule, digitalis glycosides are not given to Group I dogs, whereas a trial course of digitalis, or even propranolol, may be given to Group II dogs in an attempt to limit the atrial tachycardias that predispose the sick sinoatrial node to overdrive suppression. Dogs with sinus arrest are evaluated by an atropine response test. Atropine is administered at a dose of 0.04 mg/kg intramuscularly, and an ECG

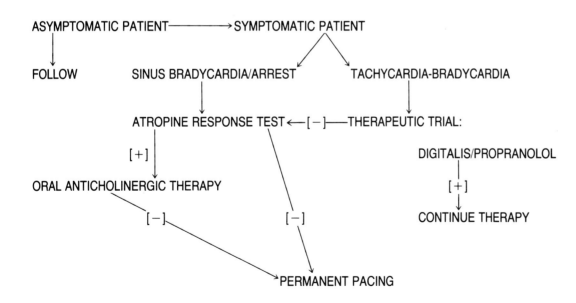

Fig. 10–7. Management of the sick sinus syndrome. [+] = therapeutic response to therapy; [−] = inadequate response to therapy.

is recorded 15 minutes later. Dogs that develop a regular sinus rhythm or sinus tachycardia after atropine may benefit from oral anticholinergic therapy and are given either isopropamide tablets (Darbid—2.5 to 5 mg, BID-TID) or propantheline bromide (Pro-banthine—3.75 to 7.5 mg BID-TID) for 1 week. Dogs that fail to respond to vagolytic therapy, or those that cannot tolerate the anticholinergic side effects (emesis, sicca, diarrhea), are treated with a permanent pacemaker. The prognosis with pacemaker therapy, in the absence of concurrent congestive heart failure (CHF), is quite good.[84] Clinical responses to medical therapy are inconsistent, and therapeutic failures are common when oral anticholinergic therapy is the principal mode of treatment.

SUPRAVENTRICULAR ARRHYTHMIAS

Atrial and junctional premature complexes. Premature complexes arising from the atria and junction are common and are associated with numerous cardiac and noncardiac causes (Table 10–3).[6,8,85] The clinical significance of premature complexes of supraventricular origin relates to their frequency and distributional pattern and to the underlying clinical problems. In animals with cardiomegaly, these arrhythmias can be harbingers of more serious rhythm disturbances, including supraventricular tachycardia, paroxysmal and sustained atrial tachycardia, atrial flutter, and atrial fibrillation.

Detailed clinical studies relating the type of supraventricular arrhythmia to the efficacy of drug therapy have not been published; however, clinical experience has indicated that many of these arrhythmias spontaneously resolve with correction of underlying metabolic disturbances or treatment of congestive heart failure. Infrequent or isolated premature complexes are not treated unless the animal experiences syncope or the veterinarian suspects (undocumented) paroxysmal tachycardia. Antiarrhythmic therapy is initiated under the following circumstances: (1) clinical signs of low cardiac output; (2) repetitive complexes (pairs, paroxysmal tachycardia), or (3) frequent occurrence of premature complexes (usually greater than 20 to 30 per minute). When associated with heart failure, these arrhythmias are managed through maintenance digitalization and by controlling congestive heart failure with diuretics and vasodilators. Frequently, a reduction in heart size is associated with a decrease in the number of

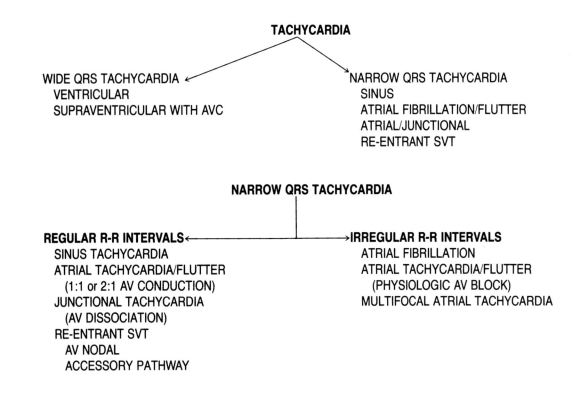

Fig. 10–8. Approach to supraventricular tachyarrhythmias. AVC = aberrant ventricular conduction, e.g., bundle branch or fascicular block; SVT = supraventricular tachycardia.

premature beats. As the effect of digitalis is variable—some patients develop an increase in abnormal complexes—the ECG must be re-evaluated following digitalization. Patients refractory to digitalization may benefit from the addition of propranolol, which is given in graded doses to achieve an antiarrhythmic effect. Dogs respond to oral quinidine, but this agent is less commonly used.

Supraventricular tachycardia. Supraventricular tachycardia (SVT) is a general term used to describe a rapid heart rate caused by abnormal impulse generation in the atrial and AV junctional tissues.

Sinus tachycardia, atrial fibrillation, and atrial flutter are usually not included in this group, although they also constitute types of supraventricular tachyarrhythmias. Supraventricular tachycardias are generated by both automatic and re-entrant mechanisms and can arise in the SA and AV nodes (junction), atria, and accessory atrioventricular pathways (bypass tracts of Kent, James, Mahaim—see Chapter 6). Supraventricular tachycardias can be very brief (paroxysmal), nonsustained, or sustained, and it is the nonparoxysmal forms that cause the particularly serious hemodynamic consequences of hypotension

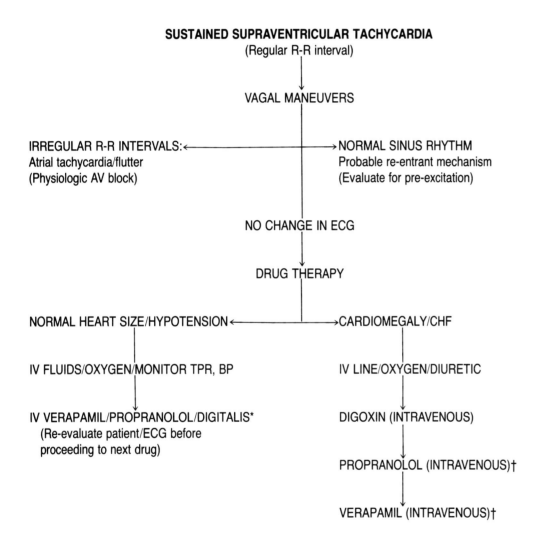

*Selection of drug depends on suspected mechanism of arrhythmia, arterial blood pressure, and experience with individual therapeutic agents.
†If needed.

Fig. 10–9. Treatment of sustained supraventricular tachycardia. TPR = body temperature, pulse and respiration; BP = blood pressure.

and venous congestion.[86] While paroxysmal SVT is relatively simple to diagnose, the ECG interpretation of sustained narrow QRS tachycardias can be uncertain and requires that the clinician perform vagal maneuvers and administer drugs to identify the cardiac rhythm (Figs. 10–8, 10–9, and 10–10). Vagal maneuvers applicable to animals include ocular pressure (application of gradually increasing pressure to each globe for 10 to 30 seconds), carotid sinus massage (application of gradually increasing pressure to one or both carotid arteries for 10 to 30 seconds), and stimulation of the face with cold water (this diving reflex is activated by applying towels soaked in ice water to each side of the face, over the masseter muscle groups). Each of these veterinarian-activated reflexes causes increased vagal efferent traffic to the heart. Unfortunately, the failing heart may respond poorly to autonomic stimulation. Furthermore, the response to these maneuvers varies among individuals. The administration of vagomimetic drugs such as morphine (0.2 mg/kg IM) and edrophonium HCl (Tensilon: 1 to 5 mg IV), or pressor agents such as phenylephrine may serve to enhance responsiveness to a vagal maneuver.[10,87]

Vagal maneuvers can provide information of diagnostic significance and can actually terminate SVT in some patients (Figs. 10–10 and 10–11). The expected response of a properly applied vagal maneuver depends on the underlying rhythm. In sinus tachycardia, a slight temporary slowing of the heart rate usually occurs. With atrial tachycardia or flutter, physiologic AV block generally occurs, and the R-R intervals become irregular, thus proving the atrial origin of the impulses (Fig. 10–10). The atrial rate may actually increase while the ventricular rate declines owing to the disparate effects of vagal traffic on refractoriness in atrial muscle and the AV node. Supraventricular tachycardias that arise from AV junctional tissues or that depend on a circus or re-entrant movement may respond to a vagotonic maneuver by: (1) speeding or slowing of the heart rate, (2) normalization of previously aberrant ventricular conduction, or (3) abrupt termination of the tachycardia (Fig. 10–11). These responses occur because some automatic tachycardias depend on sympathetic tone and because re-entrant (circus movement) tachycardias depend on conduction through the AV node to complete the circus pathway. Abrupt increases

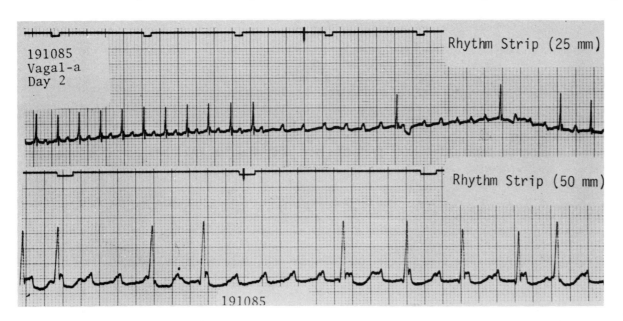

Fig. 10–10. Lead aVF ECG from a dog with chronic valvular heart disease and atrial tachycardia. The top strip demonstrates the effect of vagal tone on an atrial tachyarrhythmia. The left half of the ECG shows a narrow QRS tachycardia with a ventricular rate of about 260/min. One cannot be certain if the small positive deflections between QRS complexes are P waves or T waves. Following the application of ocular pressure, an atrial tachycardia is uncovered. Atrioventricular block occurs owing to impeded conduction through the AV node and indicates that the initial rhythm was atrial tachycardia with 1:1 AV conduction. Following the vagal maneuver, the atrial rate increases slightly to 300/min demonstrating the effect of increased vagal tone on atrial muscle refractoriness and intra-atrial conduction. The bottom panel is a close-up taken at higher paper speed and indicates the effect of declining vagal influence. The ventricular rate is irregular owing to variable conduction through the AV node. Each QRS is related to a P wave, but most P waves are blocked owing to physiologic refractoriness of the node.

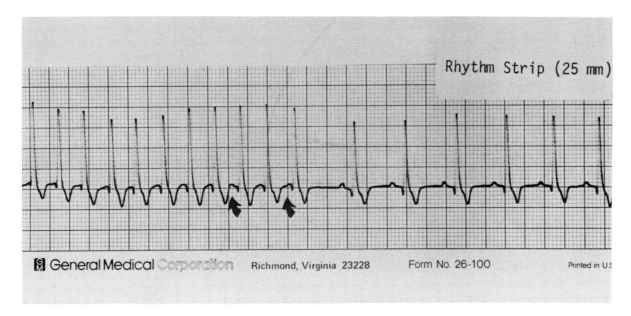

Rhythm Strip (25 mm)

General Medical Corporation   Richmond, Virginia 23228   Form No. 26-100   Printed in U.S

Fig. 10–11. Monitor (lead 2) ECG from a dog with sustained narrow QRS tachycardia. The left portion of the ECG shows a ventricular rate of approximately 230 beats/min. Although P waves are not obvious, one can appreciate deflections that probably represent atrial activity (arrows), but that appear to be slower and unrelated to the ventricular activity. Atrioventricular dissociation is suspected. Since the QRS complexes appear nearly normal, the ventricular rhythm probably originates in the AV junction or His bundle. Following the application of ocular and carotid sinus pressure, the tachyarrhythmia terminates abruptly and normal sinus rhythm with 1:1 AV conduction ensues. There is no conclusive evidence of AV nodal re-entry using the atrium (owing to the lack of retrograde P waves throughout the tachycardia and the fact that the tachycardia does not terminate with a P wave). The P-R interval is normal (0.12 sec) following conversion and is not indicative of an overt pre-excitation pathway. Inasmuch as the vagal maneuver appeared to terminate the arrhythmia, but the underlying electrophysiologic mechanism for the tachyarrhythmia cannot be stated from this record, the potential use of drugs that increase vagal tone (digitalis) or block sympathetic tone (propranolol) might be considered for repeated attacks of this arrhythmia.

in vagal tone impede AV nodal transmission, and the abolition of conduction in any part of a circus pathway usually will extinguish the abnormal rhythm. Although conversion to normal sinus rhythm may be only temporary, the identification of an SVT that terminates with increased vagal tone is significant. Restoration of normal sinus rhythm (NSR) may uncover a pre-excitation syndrome (see Chapter 6) or recommend the use of drugs, like verapamil, that are potent suppressors of AV nodal conduction, or agents like propranolol that block sympathetic activity.

The administration of antiarrhythmic drugs to dogs with SVT may eliminate the arrhythmia or simply slow the ventricular response—particularly when the underlying rhythm is actually atrial tachycardia or flutter. Either response may be of benefit to the patient. The *paroxysmal* type of SVT is seldom an emergency, and the animal can be treated per os with medications, such as digitalis[22,73] and propranolol,[54,88–90] that are effective in the suppression of atrial and junctional

premature complexes. Although propranolol suppresses myocardial contractility, the negative chronotropic effects of the drug appear to outlast the inotropic effects,[89] and the drug can be administered to dogs in heart failure provided it is given cautiously. If analysis of the ECG preceding and following the paroxysmal SVT indicates a pre-excitation syndrome, verapamil may be considered as a potential alternative for chronic oral therapy.

An approach to the patient with *sustained* SVT is outlined in Figures 10–8 and 10–9. The goals of therapy in this group of patients are either conversion of the abnormal rhythm to NSR or slowing of the ventricular rate via AV nodal blockade (see sections on atrial flutter and fibrillation). From a practical standpoint, patients can be divided into two groups: animals with obvious cardiomegaly and congestive heart failure, and animals with SVT but without demonstrable organic heart disease or CHF. The majority of patients have CHF, and many cases of regular SVT are ultimately diagnosed as atrial flutter or sustained atrial tachycardia with 1:1 AV conduction. This can usually be proven with a vagal maneuver or by evaluating the ventricular rate after therapy with digitalis or propranolol. While the occasional animal with atrial tachycardia and 1:1 AV conduction reverts to sinus rhythm, the majority will maintain the rapid atrial rhythm but will experience a decline in the ventricular rate owing to delayed conduction in the AV node. For this reason, digitalis and propranolol are the most commonly used preparations when sustained SVT complicates CHF. Less commonly, a pet is examined for sustained SVT that has led to weakness or syncope but is unassociated with obvious signs of CHF. Such animals may have abnormal atrioventricular connections and are more likely to convert to NSR following a vagal maneuver or administration of verapamil. Inasmuch as clinical experience with calcium channel blockers is limited, it is difficult to advocate verapamil over more conventional drugs like digitalis or propranolol for SVT. As the clinical experience approaches that of the laboratory,[65–69,91] however, greater use of verapamil may be indicated for therapy of SVT. Finally, it should be noted that DC cardioversion or quinidine occasionally has been used to convert sustained SVT to NSR.

Atrial flutter. Atrial flutter is relatively uncommon in dogs and is rare in cats, but this arrhythmia has been observed in association with myocardial disease, atrial enlargement, and cardiac catheterization. Atrial flutter is similar to other supraventricular tachycardias since the rapid and regular atrial activation results in a rapid ventricular response. Consequently, treatment can involve either attempted conversion to NSR using quinidine, or control of the ventricular rate with digitalis and a beta-blocker such as propranolol. While atrial pacing or direct current countershock can also be used to convert this arrhythmia to NSR, special equipment and training are required; thus, these techniques are seldom employed. Atrial flutter does not appear to be a very stable rhythm is small animal patients, and spontaneous conversion to NSR or progression to atrial fibrillation is common. Actual drug therapy of this arrhythmia is similar to that described in the following for atrial fibrillation.

Atrial fibrillation. Atrial fibrillation, one of the most commonly encountered arrhythmias in small animal practice, complicates the clinical course of the cardiomyopathies, chronic valvular disease, and untreated congenital heart disease (Table 10–3).[6,92–94] Although atrial fibrillation is occasionally paroxysmal,[93] the majority of patients have sustained atrial fibrillation with a rapid ventricular rate. As with other atrial tachyarrhythmias, the ventricular rate is principally controlled by the rapidity of AV nodal conduction. This concept is important, as the approach to treatment usually involves administration of drugs that slow AV conduction. Since the degree of ventricular filling is directly related to the previous R-R intervals, a slower ventricular rate allows more time for passive diastolic filling and leads to a longer ventricular ejection time.[95]

Drug and electrical conversion of atrial fibrillation to NSR is frequently employed in man and in the horse, yet this approach has only limited applications in the dog and cat. Most small animals with atrial fibrillation have serious, progressive heart disease, and atrial fibrillation may be either refractory to conversion or may recur within a short period following cardioversion. Nevertheless, we have used

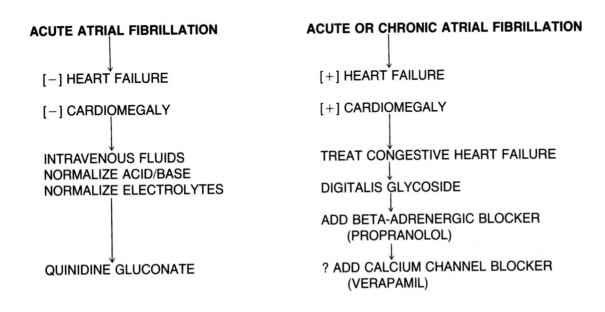

Fig. 10–12. Management of atrial fibrillation. [+] = present; [−] = absent.

quinidine for conversion to NSR in a subset of patients who have atrial fibrillation of recent onset (often postanesthetic or post-traumatic) and do not exhibit other signs of organic heart disease (Fig. 10–12). In such dogs, the intramuscular (or occasionally oral) adminstration of quinidine at a dose of 6 to 10 mg/kg every 6 hours, for three to four doses, has often been successful in causing conversion. Most of these animals have maintained NSR in the hospital, and some for longer than 3 months (Fig. 10–13).

The vast majority of small animal patients with atrial fibrillation are treated for accompanying heart failure and are given digitalis and propranolol to control the heart rate. In a review of 82 hospitalized dogs with atrial fibrillation, it was found that at least two subsets of patients could be identified. The majority of dogs were presented in atrial fibrillation with a rapid ventricular response (greater than 210 beats/min), and these dogs required the combined use of digoxin and propranolol to lower the ventricular rate to an average of less than 150 beats/min. A smaller subset was presented with slightly slower ventricular rates and responded well to digoxin alone (Bonagura and Ware, unpublished observations). Thus it has been our practice to administer digoxin, by maintenance dosing, starting on the first hospital day, and to add a beta-adrenergic blocker on the second or third hospital day using propranolol[96] at an initial dose of 0.2 mg/kg every 8 hours, by the oral route (oral or intravenous loading doses of digoxin are used if the heart rate at admission is greater than 240/min or if circulatory collapse is evident). The *daily* dose of propranolol is then increased by increments of 0.3 mg/kg (in three divided doses) up to a maximum of 1 mg/kg/TID (Fig. 10–14). In clinical practice, most giant-breed dogs require a maintenance dose of between 20 and 50 mg of propranolol every 8 hours to maintain the heart rate between 100 and 140 beats/min. It is imperative that propranolol be given in graded dosages, with frequent monitoring of the ECG, and that the *lowest* effective maintenance dose be chosen. We have used digoxin-propranolol in an attempt to lower the ventricular rate to an arbitrary range of 100 to 140 beats/min, and we will adjust the maintenance dose as dictated by follow-up examinations. The adverse effects of beta-blockers like propranolol must be appreciated (Table 10–10) and the dosage lowered when drug-induced cardiopulmonary complications are suspected.

Since most dogs with atrial fibrillation are in CHF, symptomatic therapy of CHF is usually necessary to control edema. Of particular relevance is the determination of serum digoxin or digitoxin concentrations to ensure that the patient is optimally digitalized. We obtain these after 7 to 10 days of constant maintenance dosing and titrate the dosage to obtain a serum concentration of 1 to 2 ng/ml (measured 8 to 12 hours after the previous drug dose). In the future, longer-acting beta-adrenergic blockers like nadolol or blockers with intrinsic sympathomimetic activity may be substituted for propranolol. Clinical trials are currently progressing to evaluate the effectiveness of verapamil for slowing the ventricular rate in atrial fibrillation. Preliminary experience indicates that IV dosages of 0.1 to 0.3 mg/kg will slow ventricular response but can be very hypotensive in dogs with CHF. Combination therapy of verapamil-digoxin has been employed in man[70] to blunt the tachycardia that occurs in both human and animal patients with atrial fibrillation.

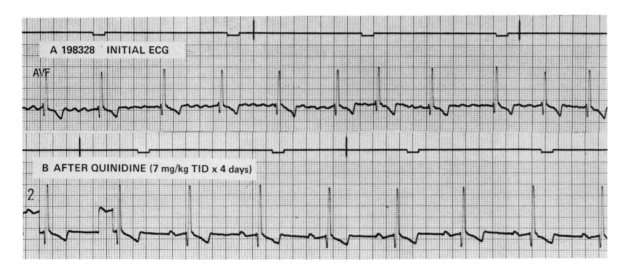

Fig. 10–13. ECG taken from a 5-year-old Doberman Pinscher with atrial fibrillation of 2 weeks' duration. The initial strip was taken at admission. Cardiac auscultation and thoracic radiography were normal; however, an echocardiogram showed a possible decrease in left ventricular systolic function. Following the oral administration of quinidine sulfate, the ECG shows normal sinus rhythm. Follow-up ECGs indicated that NSR was maintained for 7 months after initial conversion with quinidine.

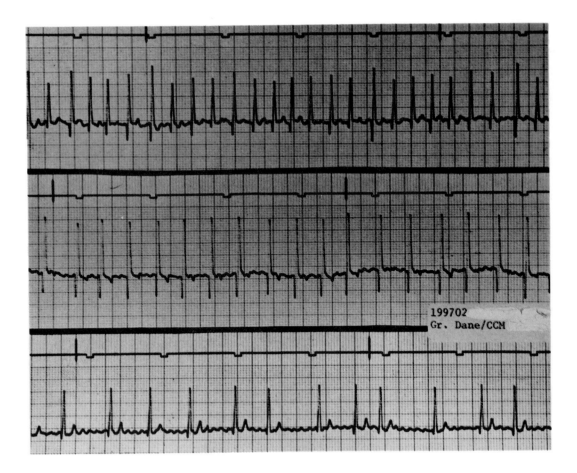

Fig. 10–14. ECG from a Great Dane with atrial fibrillation and congestive heart failure. The ventricular response to combination therapy with digoxin and propranolol is demonstrated in the three traces obtained at admission (top), after 3 days of digoxin (middle), and after 7 days of drug therapy (bottom). The final tracing, obtained while the dog received 0.5 mg digoxin per day and 40 mg propranolol TID shows atrial fibrillation with a ventricular rate of 110 beats/min. This rate is considerably slower than the initial ventricular rate of 225 beats/min and the rate of 180 beats/min noted in the middle tracing, and it illustrates the additive effects of digitalis and propranolol in depressing AV nodal conduction. The serum digoxin concentration (day 7) was 1.7 ng/ml. Monitor leads (2 and aVF) recorded at 25 mm/sec; 1 cm = 1 mV. One-second time markers are evident above each tracing.

VENTRICULAR ARRHYTHMIAS

Premature ventricular complexes or ventricular premature complexes (VPCs) indicate the existence of organic heart disease or of an alteration in cardiac electrical activity brought about by disorders remote to the heart. A list of the causes of VPCs is almost endless (Table 10–3),[97–102] and the clinical interpretation of ventricular arrhythmias must include identification of the probable cause and significance of the rhythm disorder (Table 10–4). Rhythms that originate within the ventricles assume a number of distributional patterns: from isolated single premature complexes to single VPC in bigeminal (paired), tri-geminal, or quadrigeminal distributions to repetitive (linked) VPCs at a variety of rates. The clinician must be careful to accurately identify and classify ventricular complexes. Not all VPCs require therapy and ventricular escape complexes—those that occur as rescue mechanisms for sinus bradycardia and AV block—should not be suppressed with drugs (see Chapter 6).

Ventricular premature complexes. The clinician must recognize that VPCs need not always be treated with antiarrhythmic agents. Major concerns in assessing the significance of VPCs are hemodynamic embarrassment and ventricular instability.[103,104] Although it is impossible to accurately gauge these problems in all patients, we generally administer antiarrhythmic agents when any of the following occur: (1) frequent VPCs (greater than 20 to 30 beats/min), (2) repetitive complexes (pairs, paroxysms) that occur at a rate of greater than 120 to 130 beats/min, (3) multiform (multifocal) QRS configurations, (4) VPCs with a short coupling intervals—R on T phenomena (the VPCs occur at the apex of the previous T wave), and (5) clinical signs of decreased cardiac output such as weakness, depression, or syncope. Drug therapy of isolated VPCs can usually be initiated using oral preparations of quinidine or procainamide in the dog and propranolol in the cat. Specific therapeutic guidelines[105,106] are similar to those for ventricular tachycardia and are described in the following section.

Ventricular tachycardia. Ventricular tachycardia can be a medical emergency and may require prompt antiarrhythmic therapy when it leads to hypotension or myocardial ischemia. From a clinical standpoint, it is useful to identify ventricular tachycardia as paroxysmal or sustained, unifocal or multiform ("multifocal"), and to observe the rate of the ventricular tachycardia. Relatively "slow" ventricular rhythms, often termed *idioventricular tachycardias*, are quite common in the dog[107] and are not as serious as ventricular tachycardias that occur at rates of greater than 130 beats/min. Idioventricular tachycardia is often recognized as a competing ventricular rhythm that alternates with sinus arrhythmia and manifests a rate of between 60 and 120 beats/min. Such rhythms tend to warm up and to be affected by autonomic tone.[108] Most idioventricular tachycardias are clinically benign, associated with a near-normal arterial pulse pressure, and abate spontaneously in 24 to 48 hours. It is doubtful whether such arrhythmias need to be suppressed, although it may prove difficult for a clinician not to intervene when he identifies a ventricular focus that discharges at a regular rate. We have identified idioventricular

tachycardia in many dogs and have usually opted to simply monitor such animals. In the vast majority of patients, the arrhythmia abates without proceeding to a more serious (or rapid) rhythm. However, since rapid ventricular rhythms impair hemodynamics and promote inhomogeneity of myocardial cell refractoriness, idioventricular rhythms should be suppressed when they progress to ventricular tachycardia or aggravate hypotension.

The *initial therapy* of ventricular tachycardia involves correction of the underlying disorder. Drugs useful in the treatment of ventricular arrhythmias in the dog include lidocaine,[20,46–48,109–114] quinidine,[6,28] procainamide,[34,36,39] propranolol,[54,89] phenytoin,[51] and, occasionally, digitalis (Fig. 10–15). Low-dose lidocaine and propranolol have proved most useful for the cat.[6] It is emphasized that patients with frequent VPCs or with ventricular tachycardia should not be given digitalis unless myocardial failure or a supraventricular arrhythmia is also present. The use of digitalis, in the setting of VPCs, must be accompanied by frequent ECG monitoring and possibly by the use of another antiarrhythmic drug. Clinical experience in dogs and in man[115] has indicated that digitalis can be administered safely to many patients with VPCs; however, if the frequency of the VPCs increases following digitalization or if repetitive ventricular complexes are present, other antiarrhythmic drugs are given prior to or with digitalis.

Antiarrhythmic therapy for ventricular tachycardia can be given by the intravenous, intramuscular, and oral routes. The method of administration depends on the clinical circumstances. The intravenous route is obviously preferred in the hemodynamically impaired, anesthetized, or critical patient, whereas the intramuscular or oral routes are appropriate for animals without clinical signs of hemodynamic or electrical instability and with normal gastrointestinal function.

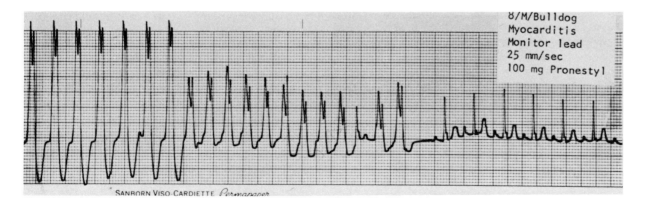

Fig. 10–15. ECG from a Bulldog with nonsuppurative myocarditis. The initial rhythm was ventricular tachycardia at an average rate of 220 beats/min. This arrhythmia was refractory to intravenous boluses of lidocaine but responded to approximately 5 mg/kg of procainamide administered intravenously over 5 minutes. Note that the rate and the configuration of the ventricular tachycardia is altered prior to conversion to normal sinus rhythm. This is probably due to the effect of procainamide on intraventricular conduction.

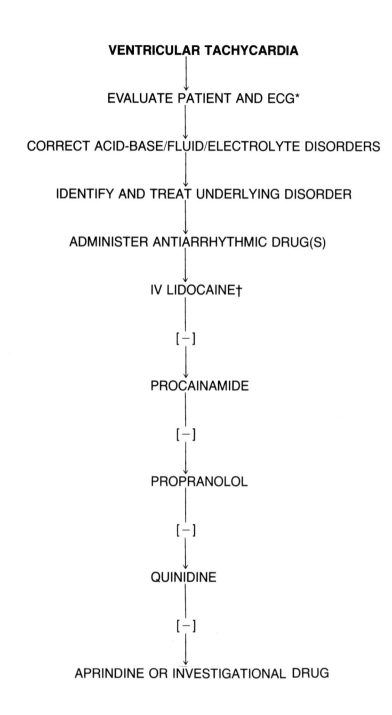

VENTRICULAR TACHYCARDIA

↓

EVALUATE PATIENT AND ECG*

↓

CORRECT ACID-BASE/FLUID/ELECTROLYTE DISORDERS

↓

IDENTIFY AND TREAT UNDERLYING DISORDER

↓

ADMINISTER ANTIARRHYTHMIC DRUG(S)

↓

IV LIDOCAINE†

↓

[−]

↓

PROCAINAMIDE

↓

[−]

↓

PROPRANOLOL

↓

[−]

↓

QUINIDINE

↓

[−]

↓

APRINDINE OR INVESTIGATIONAL DRUG

*See Table 10–4.
†Use low-dose lidocaine or propranolol in the cat.

Fig. 10–16. Management of ventricular tachycardia. [−] = inadequate response to therapy.

In most situations, lidocaine HCl is the intravenous agent of choice for immediate control of VPC or ventricular tachycardia (Fig. 10–16). Lidocaine has minimal adverse hemodynamic effects, and the neurotoxic signs associated with higher doses are readily controlled by intravenous diazepam (2 to 5 mg). Initial doses of 2 to 3 mg/kg IV for dogs (LOWER DOSES for cats; see Table 10–10), are usually effective within 2 to 3 minutes of administration. An initial total dose of 8 mg/kg can be given to dogs with refractory arrhythmias; however, some dogs exhibit toxicity at this dosage level. Lidocaine is injected slowly over 1 to 2 minutes and must be used with extreme caution in cats since this species is particularly susceptible to the neurotoxic effects. An alternative to an intravenous bolus in the dog is a rapid lidocaine infusion (0.8 mg/kg/min) administered over 10 minutes.

When parenteral therapy is indicated and lidocaine is ineffective, procainamide, quinidine, propranolol, phenytoin, or an investigational antiarrhythmic drug (Table 10–11) are administered. Many of these drugs have significant cardiodepressant effects when given intravenously; therefore, they must be injected slowly and carefully, with attention directed to cardiac rhythm and arterial pulse pressure. Procainamide, the first drug chosen for the dog when lidocaine is ineffective, is particularly versatile in clinical situations since it also can be given by intravenous, intramuscular, and oral routes. In dogs requiring long-term antiarrhythmic therapy, procainamide is almost ideal, since the initial intravenous bolus (if effective) can be followed with a constant-rate infusion, intramuscular injections, and eventual oral administration. Propranolol is an effective intravenous antiarrhythmic agent in the cat and is preferred by some clinicians over lidocaine for this species. Propranolol is particularly beneficial in ventricular arrhythmias associated with sympathetic excess and hyperthyroidism, and is also effective in some dogs that do not respond to lidocaine or procainamide. In order to administer this agent safely, it should be diluted to a concentration of 0.1 mg/ml and administered by intravenous injection of 1 ml of the dilution (0.1 mg) every minute until the arrhythmia is controlled or until a maximum acceptable dosage is delivered (Table 10–10). The intravenous use of quinidine

Table 10–11. Investigational antiarrhythmic drugs

Drug classification*	Drug	Potential use
I	Aprindine HCl	Ventricular arrhythmias
		Supraventricular arrhythmias
	Mexiletine	Ventricular arrhythmias
	Tocainide	Ventricular arrhythmias
	Encainide	Ventricular arrhythmias
		Blocking accessory pathway
	Flecainide	Ventricular arrhythmias
III	Amiodarone	Supraventricular arrhythmias
		Atrial fibrillation
		Ventricular arrhythmias
		Blocking accessory pathway

*Additional class I agents, beta-adrenoceptor blockers (class II), and class III (calcium channel blockers) antiarrhythmic drugs have been developed and tested, but are not considered here.

is limited owing to its hypotensive properties; however, this drug is useful as an intramuscular or orally administered preparation. We use phenytoin infrequently, although it is effective in preventing digitalis-induced VPCs. Lidocaine is still preferred over phenytoin when it is effective for digitalis-associated ventricular tachycardia. A final method available for the termination of ventricular tachycardia is DC cardioversion. Lack of availability of ECG-synchronized equipment and the need for anesthesia have limited the use of this technique.

Following the initial conversion of ventricular tachycardia to normal sinus rhythm, the ECG must be re-evaluated since most serious arrhythmias tend to recur within 30 minutes. This is particularly true when drugs that are rapidly redistributed and eliminated, like lidocaine, are administered. In order to maintain effective blood concentrations, repeated administration of an antiarrhythmic drug is nec-

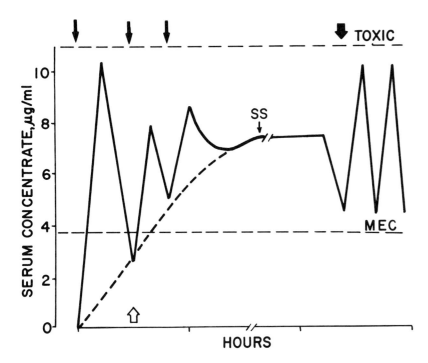

Fig. 10–17. Highly schematic drawing of serum drug concentrations following the use of intravenous bolus, constant-rate infusion, and intramuscular or oral antiarrhythmic drug therapy. If the drug is merely infused (dotted line), a considerable delay occurs between the onset of treatment and the establishment of minimal effective concentrations (MEC). This can be avoided by administering an initial intravenous bolus (top left arrow), starting the constant-rate infusion, and administering small supplemental intravenous injections of the drug as needed (second and third arrows) to prevent a decline in blood levels below the MEC. Supplemental doses generally are 25% to 50% that of the initial bolus. Following the establishment of steady-state concentrations (SS) in 4 to 6 half-lives, the infusion can be continued or replaced with an intramuscularly or orally administered preparation of the same drug (bold arrow). Drugs such as procainamide are well suited for intravenous bolus, constant-rate infusion, and eventual intramuscular or oral administration. Alternately, one can administer lidocaine intravenously to control the arrhythmia and follow this with an intramuscular or orally given preparation of quinidine or procainamide.

essary. This can be done by giving multiple intravenous boluses (which is impractical), by establishing a *constant-rate infusion*,[20,113,114a,116,117] or by administering intramuscular or oral dosages of a drug. We have found that constant rate infusions are an excellent method to control ventricular arrhythmias in critically ill canine patients (see Figs. 10–2 and 10–17). Since it generally takes 4 to 6 hours to obtain steady-state plasma concentrations with lidocaine (much longer with procainamide), supplemental intravenous bolus injections or a double-infusion technique may be needed to control arrhythmias during the initial infusion period. These supplemental low-dose boluses are designed to prevent the dip in plasma concentration that occurs after the initial intravenous boluses. Constant-rate infusions are continued for 2 to 3 days, if necessary. Of particular importance is the maintenance of normal serum potassium levels during this treatment period, as hypokalemia will blunt the effectiveness of these drugs. Once the patient is stabilized, the infusion can be tapered, discontinued, combined with another drug (e.g., lidocaine plus quinidine) or replaced with intramuscularly or orally administered agents (quinidine, procainamide, or propranolol), depending on the clinical circumstances.

Intravenous antiarrhythmic therapy is not feasible in some practice situations or may not be necessary in some dogs. In such cases, the *intramuscular* or oral administration of procainamide or quinidine can be quite effective in controlling ventricular tachycardia. Typically, a single intramuscular or oral loading dose (14 to 20 mg/kg) is given to evaluate the effectiveness of the antiarrhythmic drug, and an ECG is repeated 2 hours later. If effective, the drug is given every 4 to 6 hours at a dosage of 6 to 12 mg/kg IM. Intramuscular therapy can be successfully followed with administration of an oral preparation of the same drug given at the appropriate maintenance dosing interval (Table 10–10).

Certain patients require long-term *maintenance therapy* for ventricular arrhythmias, and these animals are managed with available oral preparations of quinidine, procainamide, or propranolol (see Table 10–10). The choice of an oral drug depends on numerous factors including the species, efficacy of parenteral therapy with a particular agent, dosing frequency, owner compliance, concurrent drug medication, response to oral therapy, and adverse drug effects. Recent evidence suggests that, in the dog, new sustained-released preparations of quinidine and procainamide[39] may be superior to other formulations inasmuch as TID dosing may be adequate to obtain therapeutic blood concentrations. Although quinidine has been used in cats,[6] most clinicians suggest that propranolol is the drug of choice for chronic oral therapy of VPCs in this species.

Antiarrhythmic therapy must be reassessed periodically for need, efficacy, and safety. Many animals develop severe ventricular arrhythmias that require only short-term therapy, generally involving 1 to 2 weeks of treatment. If weekly check-ups indicate that there is no evidence of recurrent ventricular ectopic activity, then it is reasonable to discontinue treatment and re-evaluate the ECG in 1 to 2 days. At that time a decision can be made to reinstitute therapy or to merely reassess the ECG in a week. Other patients continue to demonstrate ventricular ectopic activity even when receiving antiarrhythmic drugs. Since drugs frequently reduce the number of repetitive complexes or VPCs, but may not totally restore sinus rhythm, some clinical judgment is required in directing further treatment. The presence or absence of clinical signs, the current ECG trace, and the daily drug dosage should be considered before the dose is increased. If the animal is showing clinical signs that are related to the arrhythmia, or if the ECG shows repetitive complexes, the total daily dose is increased. If this is not effective, or results in toxicosis, other approaches may be necessary (see section on management of refractory arrhythmias).

CONDUCTION DISTURBANCES

Atrial conduction disturbances. Atrial conduction disturbances occur in the setting of sick sinus syndrome, muscular dystrophy, hyperkalemia, and congestive cardiomyopathy. Toxicosis with antiarrhythmic drugs can also lead to marked depression of intra-atrial conduction. The treatment of atrial conduction disorders must be tailored to the underlying problem. Withdrawal of a drug is prudent if a new conduction disturbance has emerged since the onset of therapy. Treatment of atrial standstill ("silent atrium") caused by muscular dystrophy or myocardial disease involves implantation of a pacemaker to increase the heart rate (see Chapter 6). Sinoatrial exit block is managed as previously described for sinus arrest under the heading of sick sinus syndrome.

Hyperkalemia is the most common cause of temporary atrial standstill. In addition to atrial inexcitability, intraventricular conduction may be prolonged, resulting in widening of the QRS complexes. The ventricular rate is usually slow but can be regular or irregular. Immediate therapy consists of the IV administration of sodium bicarbonate (0.5–1 mEq/kg slowly over 3 to 4 minutes). This is given in order to drive potassium into the cells. Sodium bicarbonate is repeated in 10 minutes, and further doses are guided by measurement of blood pH, bicarbonate, and CO_2. Correction of the primary problem (Table 10–3) and intravenous administration of 0.9% saline solution are important adjunctive treatments. Hyperkalemia can cause cardiac arrest and if bicarbonate therapy is ineffective, a *slow* intravenous infusion of calcium gluconate (1 ml of a 10% solution/10 kg of body weight) is used to antagonize the effects of potassium on the heart.

Atrioventricular block. Treatment of atrioventricular block requires identification of the type and severity of the block (incomplete vs. complete) and an appreciation of the multiple causes of abnormal AV conduction (Table 10–3). Most cases of incomplete AV block do not result in clinical signs and are either physiologic or self-limiting when the cause is eliminated. When incomplete AV block leads to dangerous bradycardia, either atropine or glycopyrrolate is given.

High-grade second-degree AV block (greater than 3:1 P:QRS) and complete AV block generally indicate severe drug toxicity or organic disease of the AV conduction system. Since syncope, sudden death, and congestive heart failure can occur secondary to advanced AV blocks, patients with these arrhythmias are treated with implantation of a pacemaker (Fig. 10–18).[84,118] Catecholamines can be given in an emergency in an attempt to stimulate ventricular escape rhythms.

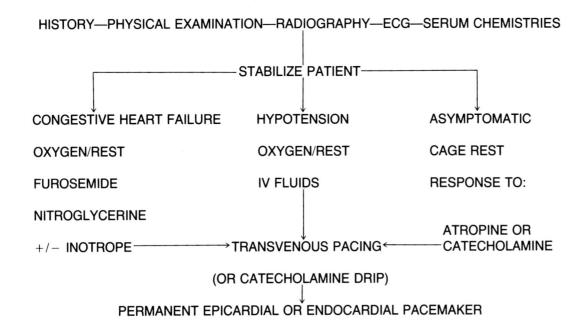

HISTORY—PHYSICAL EXAMINATION—RADIOGRAPHY—ECG—SERUM CHEMISTRIES

STABILIZE PATIENT

CONGESTIVE HEART FAILURE	HYPOTENSION	ASYMPTOMATIC
OXYGEN/REST	OXYGEN/REST	CAGE REST
FUROSEMIDE	IV FLUIDS	RESPONSE TO:
NITROGLYCERINE		ATROPINE OR
+/− INOTROPE ——→ TRANSVENOUS PACING ←—— CATECHOLAMINE

(OR CATECHOLAMINE DRIP)

PERMANENT EPICARDIAL OR ENDOCARDIAL PACEMAKER

Fig. 10–18. Management of complete AV block.

Both isoproterenol (1.0 mg Isuprel, in 250 to 500 ml fluid, drip to effect) and dopamine (2 to 5 μg/kg/min of Intropin) have been used for this purpose. Although some clinicians have attempted long-term treatment of symptomatic bradycardia using high doses of oral or sublingual isoproterenol (Protenol), this type of treatment is usually ineffective and unnecessarily prolongs the period of time before implantation of a temporary and permanent pacemaker. Pacemaker therapy is described in Chapter 11 of this text.

Ventricular pre-excitation. Examples of ventricular pre-excitation include the Wolff-Parkinson-White and the Lown-Ganong-Levine syndromes. Both of these conditions are characterized by the presence of an accessory atrioventricular pathway that permits early depolarization (pre-excitation) of the ventricles. These accessory pathways predispose to supraventricular tachycardia by permitting a re-entry circuit to be formed using the atria, the AV node, the ventricle, and the anomalous AV connection (see Chapter 12). Although clinical experience with these arrhythmias in animals is sparse, successful management of associated supraventricular tachycardias could involve abrupt termination with vagal maneuvers, and acute and chronic suppression with antiarrhythmic drugs. Since the supraventricular tachycardia may be initiated by atrial premature complexes, one approach is to use drugs that suppress APCs. Such therapy is unlikely to be 100% successful; therefore, most efforts are directed to blocking conduction in either the AV node or the accessory pathway. A variety of drugs are used in man for these purposes, and there is some difference of opinion relative to the agents of choice.[119] Digitalis, propranolol, and verapamil have all been used to slow AV nodal conduction and thus abolish the circus movement. Verapamil, in particular, has been employed to acutely terminate episodes of supraventricular tachycardia. Other drugs, such as quinidine, procainamide, and amiodarone, have been given for their depressant effects on retrograde conduction across the accessory pathway. Greater experience in animals will be needed before firm recommendations can be offered for treatment. General aspects in the management of supraventricular tachycardias have been discussed previously.

SUMMARY OF THE THERAPY OF CARDIAC ARRHYTHMIAS

Multiple methods are available for the termination of cardiac arrhythmias in the dog and cat. More data are available, at this time, for the dog. *Tables 10–10 and 10–12 summarize our recommendations for the management of cardiac arrhythmias in the dog. Table 11–2 summarizes the drugs used in the management of cardiac resuscitation.* It is emphasized that these are general recommendations and that each patient must be approached and treated individually.

APPROACH TO THE PATIENT WITH REFRACTORY ARRHYTHMIAS

There are no simple methods that can be applied to every patient with a cardiac arrhythmia that is refractory to single-drug therapy. Although the majority of animals respond appropriately to antiarrhythmic therapy, a significant number of animals require multiple

Table 10–12. Treatment of cardiac arrhythmias in the dog

Rhythm	Acute therapy*	Chronic therapy†
SINUS RHYTHMS		
Sinus bradycardia	Atropine or glycopyrrolate Dopamine Epinephrine	Pacemaker
Sinus tachycardia	Treat underlying cause	Digitalis glycosides if CHF or SSS
Sinoatrial arrest and Sick sinus syndrome (SSS)	Atropine or glycopyrrolate Transvenous pacemaker	Pacemaker Oral anticholinergic therapy
SUPRAVENTRICULAR ARRHYTHMIAS		
Atrial and junctional premature complexes	Digitalis Propranolol Quinidine	Same
Atrial, junctional, supraventricular tachycardia	Vagal maneuver Digitalis Propranolol Verapamil Quinidine	Digitalis, propranolol, or quinidine (consider response to acute therapy) ?Verapamil
Atrial fibrillation or flutter	Quinidine if indicated (see text) Digitalis	Digitalis Propranolol ?Verapamil
VENTRICULAR ARRHYTHMIAS		
Ventricular premature complexes Ventricular tachycardia	Lidocaine Procainamide Propranolol Quinidine Investigational drug	Procainamide, quinidine, propranolol, phenytoin (consider response to acute therapy) Combination therapy
CONDUCTION DISTURBANCES		
Atrial standstill (hyperkalemia)	Sodium bicarbonate Intravenous saline Calcium gluconate R$_x$ primary disorder	Treat the primary disorder
Persistent atrial standstill	Atropine or glycopyrrolate Transvenous pacemaker	Pacemaker
Atrioventricular blocks	Transvenous pacemaker Atropine or glycopyrrolate Infusion of isoproterenol	Cardiac pacemaker Oral isoproterenol

*The usual "agent of choice" is listed first. See text for details
†Chronic therapy varies with etiology and response to acute therapy. CHF = congestive heart failure.
Modified from Bonagura, J.D.: Therapy of cardiac arrhythmias. In *Current Veterinary Therapy.* Volume 8. Edited by R.W. Kirk. Philadelphia, W.B. Saunders, 1983.

drugs, combination therapy, investigational agents, or other types of treatment. Significant emphasis has been directed to electrophysiologic testing in man in order to identify drugs that will repeatedly prevent the induction of arrhythmias under controlled circumstances.[120] At this time, there is no clinical information about the usefulness of this type of evaluation in clinical veterinary practice. Some principles applicable to the therapy of refractory arrhythmias can be enumerated:

1. The rhythm diagnosis must be correct; thus, all ECG traces should be re-evaluated and a current, complete 9- or 10-lead ECG obtained.

2. The predisposing or underlying condition must be identified and treated if possible. This point was emphasized in the previous section.

3. Acid-base and electrolyte status must be re-examined and corrected if abnormal.

4. The possibility that current drug therapy may be causing or aggravating the arrhythmia must be considered.

5. The possibility that the drug is not correctly administered or, in the case of oral medications, not absorbed must be considered.

6. Drug dosages must be re-evaluated with the intent of increasing the dosage, or preferably, determining serum drug concentrations to ensure that the drug has reached adequate blood levels.

7. When combination or additional drug therapy is indicated, the clinician must also consider agents that act by a different electrophysiologic mechanism than that of the current or previously administered, but unsuccessful, medications.

APPROACH TO SUPRAVENTRICULAR ARRHYTHMIAS

Supraventricular tachycardia (SVT) must be correctly identified as sinus, atrial, junctional, or re-entrant. Atrial fibrillation and atrial flutter must also be considered whenever a narrow QRS tachycardia is identified. *Sinus tachycardia* can be a particularly frustrating cause of persistent tachycardia, yet antiarrhythmic therapy is seldom indicated or useful for controlling this disturbance. Common causes of refractory sinus tachycardia are fever, shock, pain, anemia, sepsis, and administration of anticholinergic drugs such as atropine or isopropamide. These conditions can be overlooked or inapparent in some patients. particularly in postoperative animals. In each case, correction of the underlying problem is the only sure remedy for controlling compensatory sinus tachycardia. Less common causes of sinus tachycardia, such as severe thyrotoxicosis or catecholamine release from a pheochromocytoma, should respond to beta blockade with propranolol.

Narrow QRS tachycardia with a regular R-R interval can be difficult to diagnose, since atrial tachycardia with 1:1 conduction and first-degree AV block, atrial flutter with 1:1 or 2:1 AV conduction, and AV junctional tachycardias can all initially look the same. The critical element of rhythm identification is found in *identification of P waves* (or flutter waves), noting their configuration, and determining their relationship to P waves. P waves are invariably found in sinus and atrial tachycardia if the clinician evaluates multiple leads and scrutinizes the ST-T waves. Vagal maneuvers are particularly useful for identifying flutter waves when there is regular (1:1 or 2:1) AV conduction with a rapid ventricular response since a temporary degradation in AV conduction will result in irregular R-R intervals. When SVT is caused by re-entry using the AV node or an accessory pathway, the tachycardia often begins with a long P-R interval (often an APC or VPC initiates the SVT), is associated with a 1:1 QRS:P relationship, and ends with a retrograde P wave. Vagal maneuvers may terminate or slow these tachycardias. Again, all leads must be studied for buried P waves. On the other hand, automatic junctional tachycardias and tachycardias originating high in the ventricle (see Fig. 10–11) generally result in AV dissociation with a slower and independent atrial rate and fewer P waves than QRS complexes. Digitalis intoxication must always be ruled out whenever junctional tachycardia with AV dissociation is observed.

When SVT is caused by *atrial flutter* or *atrial tachycardia* and does not respond to initial therapy, which is usually digoxin, the clinician should attempt the following: (1) determine the serum digoxin concentration to ensure adequate blood levels, (2) add a beta-adrenergic blocker such as propranolol, administered by the intravenous or oral route (depending on how well the patient is tolerating the tachycardia), and (3) if the patient's status is critical and is not improved by these measures, consider the addition of verapamil (0.05 to 0.2 mg/kg IV or 0.5 mg/kg orally) to slow the ventricular rate. If the combination of digoxin-propranolol results in some slowing, the dose of the beta blocker can be gradually increased to further slow the ventricular rate. Therapy is then similar to that previously described for atrial fibrillation. Quinidine may convert atrial flutter or tachycardia to sinus rhythm, but it is safer to first block the AV node, since quinidine may result in an initial increase in ventricular rate. Pacing or cardioversion can be considered as last resorts.

When SVT is secondary to *AV nodal re-entry*, combination therapy with digoxin and propranolol may be effective in preventing circus movement. Additional agents to be considered are verapamil (0.5 to 1 mg/kg/orally, TID), quinidine, procainamide, and amiodarone. The latter three drugs may influence accessory pathways. More information is needed concerning the effectiveness of these drugs in animals.

Finally, when *junctional tachycardia with AV dissociation* is present and is refractory to digoxin and propranolol, consideration should be given to agents that both alter conduction and decrease automaticity. Lidocaine, quinidine, and procainamide have all been effective in individual patients. It is likely that some relatively narrow QRS tachycardias are actually originating from the uppermost portions of the ventricular conduction system; therefore, drugs typically used for ventricular tachycardia may be helpful in such cases.

APPROACH TO VENTRICULAR ARRHYTHMIAS

In the previous discussion of ventricular tachycardia, the use of "first- and second-line" drugs was described. In our experience, intravenous lidocaine is the agent of choice for acute ventricular tachycardia in the dog. Procainamide, propranolol, and quinidine are generally used as second-line drugs and are chosen when lidocaine is ineffective or when long-term antiarrhythmic therapy is indicated. On occasion, even the sequential use of lidocaine, procainamide, and propranolol fails to convert ventricular tachycardia to sinus rhythm. As each of these agents exhibit slightly different electrophysiologic and pharmacologic properties, an arrhythmia unresponsive to this combination of drugs is considered refractory.

The clinician, when confronted with refractory sustained ventricular tachycardia, should attempt the following: (1) Re-evaluate the ECG to completely rule out the possibility of SVT with aberrant ventricular conduction (see Chapter 12); if SVT with bundle branch block cannot be ruled out by identification of fusion complexes or atrioventricular dissociation, complete a vagal maneuver and observe its effect on the arrhythmia; (2) measure the serum potassium concentration; infuse KCl (0.5 mEq/kg/hour if the serum potassium is less than 3.0 mEq/dl or 0.25 mEq/kg/hour if the serum potassium is between 3 and 3.5 mEq/dl); (3) rule out digitalis toxicity as a cause of the arrhythmia; rule out quinidine, procainamide, or disopyramide toxicity if the ECG shows polymorphous ventricular tachycardia (torsade de pointes);[121,122] (4) consider the use of quinidine gluconate intravenously or intramuscularly; this must be given intravenously over a 5- to 10-minute period with monitoring of blood pressure; (5) initiate therapy with a group I antiarrhythmic drug (Table 10–2) combined with a beta-adrenergic blocker like propranolol; (6) consider obtaining and administering bretylium tosylate[123,124] (2 to 4 mg/kg IV), or an investigational drug that may be effective against ventricular tachycardia; (7) use high doses of the drug that had the greatest effect on the tachyarrhythmia and determine the plasma drug concentration at expected peak plasma concentration; this indicates whether "therapeutic" blood concentrations have been attained. (8) Consider DC cardioversion if available; (9) consider the intravenous infusion of isoproterenol if the ECG shows clear-cut evidence of polymorphous ventricular tachycardia;[112,121] (10) refer the patient for investigational drug therapy or ventricular pacing; or (11) do nothing but give supportive care if the patient is tolerating the arrhythmias. A brief discussion of investigational drugs follows.

NEWER ANTIARRHYTHMIC DRUGS

A number of new drugs have been released for clinical investigation for the control of cardiac arrhythmias in man (Table 10–11).[21] Many of these agents have been employed in human medical practice outside the United States, and in the case of some of these medications, there is extensive human experience. All of these agents have been tested in a variety of arrhythmia models using the dog, and, to a lesser degree, in the cat. Owing to the importance of myocardial ischemia in man, many of the experimental animal studies have involved arrhythmias produced by coronary occlusion. In addition, most studies use clinically normal dogs and employ these agents for relatively short periods of time. While it is difficult to extrapolate from laboratory studies to clinical situations, some potentially relevant aspects of these investigational drugs are described. Since we have had clinical and laboratory experience with some of these agents, this information is included here.

Aprindine

Aprindine is a local anesthetic agent that is highly effective in the control of refractory ventricular arrhythmias in the dog.[125–128] We have found that aprindine (0.5 to 2.0 mg/kg IV, or orally TID) will usually control ventricular tachycardia that is refractory to lidocaine, procainamide, and propranolol. Others have found this drug effective in the control of ventricular tachycardia associated with congestive cardiomyopathy in the dog.[127] Since the drug has a potential for ad-

verse effects, including leukopenia and hepatopathy, it should be reserved for refractory ventricular tachycardia. Both intravenous and oral routes of administration are effective in the dog. We have not used this drug in the cat.

Mexiletine

Mexiletine is an orally effective antiarrhythmic drug with electrophysiologic and toxic properties that are quite similar to those of lidocaine. The principal attraction of this drug has been its potential use in dogs who have responded to parenteral therapy with lidocaine and continue to need antiarrhythmic medication. Therapeutic plasma concentrations of this drug in man are approximately 0.5 to 2.0 μg/ml; however, toxicosis occurs at concentrations above 1.5 μg/ml.[21,129] The drug has been effective in dogs for the termination of VPCs caused by ouabain toxicity, halothane-epinephrine, and myocardial ischemia.[129] Parenteral doses of 0.25 to 8.0 mg/kg have been adequate in these studies. We have used this drug in a small number of dogs (1 to 2 mg/kg/day divided BID-TID) with limited success. Seizures occurred in one dog. Adequate clinical studies in dogs have not been conducted. Owing to its lidocaine-like effects, mexiletine should be administered with caution to cats.

Amiodarone

The prominent effect of amiodarone on isolated cardiac tissue is prolongation of the action potential duration with an associated increase in refractory period. Amiodarone increases the AH interval of the His electrogram, depresses AV nodal conduction and transmission across accessory pathways, and has variable effects on intra-atrial and intraventricular conduction.[21] The drug is effective for both atrial and ventricular arrhythmias in man and has been used for VPCs, ventricular tachycardia, paroxysmal atrial fibrillation, and SVT associated with the Wolff-Parkinson-White syndrome. We are unaware of adequate clinical studies with this drug in animals but initial experiences have been disappointing.[130] Toxicosis in man is a concern and involves the development of pulmonary fibrosis, corneal deposits, skin discoloration, thyroid dysfunction and hepatic enzyme abnormalities, and a drug interaction with digoxin.

Tocainide

Tocainide, a class I antiarrhythmic drug, is a synthetic analogue of lidocaine. Like mexiletine, tocainide was developed in an attempt to produce an orally active lidocaine-like preparation. The electrophysiologic, electrocardiographic, hemodynamic, and toxic effects of this drug are identical to those of lidocaine. Unlike lidocaine, tocainide is eliminated by both hepatic and renal mechanisms in the dog. The $t_{1/2\beta}$ following intravenous administration to dogs is approximately 5 hours; however, oral preparations may maintain plasma concentrations in the therapeutic range for as long as 12 hours.

Encainide and flecainide

Both encainide[131,132] and flecainide[133,134] are class I antiarrhythmic drugs with diverse pharmacologic and pharmacokinetic properties.

Both drugs were developed in an attempt to produce an antiarrhythmic agent that would be effective in treating arrhythmias refractory to conventional therapy. Their electrophysiologic effects differ somewhat, but both produce depression in conduction and increases in ventricular ERP. The hemodynamic effects of either drug have not been thoroughly investigated, although they can produce hypotension and decrease cardiac contractility. Pharmacokinetic studies of these compounds are incomplete, but both have a $t_{1/2\beta}$ in dogs that exceeds 6 hours. Active metabolites may be partially responsible for their antiarrhythmic actions.

These drugs are recommended as therapy for ventricular tachyarrhythmias of all types. Encainide is particularly effective in treating arrhythmias associated with the presence of an accessory pathway. A greater clinical experience is needed before specific recommendations can be made for their use in animals. Toxic effects of these drugs are similar to those of other class I drugs; consequently, similar precautions should be taken if these agents are used. Both encainide and flecainide cause or exaggerate ventricular arrhythmias and exacerbate signs of congestive heart failure. Depression, weakness, nausea, and emesis are signs of toxicosis in man.

REFERENCES

1. McIntosh, H.D., and Morris, J.J.: The hemodynamic consequences of arrhythmias. Prog. Cardiovasc. Dis., 8:330, 1966.
2. Resnekov, L.: Circulatory effects of cardiac dysrhythmias. Cardiovasc. Clin., 2:24, 1970.
3. Stewart, H.J., Crawford, J.H., and Hastings, A.B.: The effect of tachycardia on the blood flow in dogs. I. The effect of rapid irregular rhythms as seen in auricular fibrillation. J. Clin. Invest., 3:435, 1926.
4. Smirk, F.H., Nolla-Panades, J., and Wallis, T.: Experimental ventricular flutter and ventricular paroxysmal tachycardia. Am. J. Cardiol., 14:79, 1964.
5. Wegria, R., Frank, C.W., Wang, H.H., and Lammerant, J.: The effect of atrial and ventricular tachycardia on cardiac output, coronary blood flow and mean arterial blood pressure. Circ. Res., 6:624, 1958.
6. Ettinger, S.J.: Cardiac arrhythmias. In *Textbook of Veterinary Internal Medicine.* Edited by S.J. Ettinger. Philadelphia, W.B. Saunders, 1983.
7. Bonagura, J.D.: Therapy of cardiac arrhythmias. In *Current Veterinary Therapy VIII.* Edited by R.W. Kirk. Philadelphia, W.B. Saunders, 1983.
8. Hilwig, R.W.: Cardiac arrhythmias in the dog: Detection and treatment. J. Am. Vet. Med. Assoc., 168:789, 1976.
9. Singh, B.N., Collet, J.T., and Chew, C.Y.C.: New perspectives in the pharmacologic therapy of cardiac arrhythmias. Prog. Cardiovasc. Dis., 22:243, 1980.
10. Waxman, M.B., Wald, R.W., and Cameron, D.: Interactions between the autonomic nervous system and tachycardias in man. Cardiology Clin., 1:143, 1983.
11. Ten Eick, R.E., Baumgarten, C.M., and Singer, D.H.: Ventricular dysrhythmias: Membrane basis of currents, channels, gates, and cables. In *Cardiovascular Diseases.* Edited by E.H. Sonneblick. New York, Grune & Stratton, 1981.
12. Janse, M.J., and vanCapelle, F.J.L.: Electronic interactions across an inexcitable region as a cause of ectopic activity in acute regional myocardial ischemia. Circ. Res., 50:527, 1982.
13. Kuo, C., Munakata, K., Reddy, C.P., and Surawicz, B.: Characteristics and possible mechanism of ventricular arrhythmia dependent on the dispersion of action potential durations. Circulation, 67:1356, 1983.
14. Arnsdorf, M.F.: Electrophysiologic properties of antidysrhythmic drugs as a rational basis for therapy. Med. Clin. North Am., 60:213, 1976.
15. Bassett, A.L., and Wit, A.L.: Recent advances in electrophysiology of antiarrhythmic drugs. Prog. Drug. Res., 17:34, 1973.
16. Bigger, J.T., Jr., and Hoffman, B.F.: Antiarrhythmic Drugs. In *The Pharmacological Basis of Therapeutics.* 6th Edition. Edited by A.G. Gilman, L.S. Goodman, and A. Gilman. New York, Macmillan, 1980.
17. Malcolm, R., and Tozer, T.N.: *Clinical Pharmacokinetics: Concepts and Applications.* 1st Edition. Philadelphia, Lea & Febiger, 1980.
18. Singh, B.N., and Mandel, W.J.: Antiarrhythmic drugs: Basic concepts of their actions, pharmacokinetic characteristics, and clinical applications. In *Cardiac Arrhythmias.* Edited by W.J. Mandel. Philadelphia, J.B. Lippincott, 1980.
19. Woosley, R.L., and Shand, D.G.: Pharmacokinetics of antiarrhythmic drugs. Am. J. Cardiol., 41:986, 1978.
20. De Rick, A., Rosseel, M.T., Belpaire, F., and Bogaert, M.: Lidocaine plasma concentrations obtained with a standardized infusion in the awake and anaesthetized dog. J. Vet. Pharmacol. Therap., 4:129, 1981.
21. Heger, J.J., Prystowsky, E.N., and Zipes, D.P.: Drug therapy of cardiac arrhythmias. Cardiology Clin., 1:305, 1983.
22. Button, C., Gross, D.R., Johnston, J.T., and Yakatan, G.J.: Pharmacokinetics, bioavailability and dosage regimens of digoxin in dogs. Am. J. Vet. Res., 41:1230, 1980.
23. Carmeliet, E., and Saikawa, T.: Shortening of the action potential and reduction of pacemaker activity by lidocaine, quinidine, and procainamide in sheep cardiac Purkinje fibers. Circ. Res., 50:257, 1982.
24. Colatsky, T.J.: Mechanisms of action of lidocaine and quinidine on action potential duration in rabbit cardiac Purkinje fibers. Circ. Res., 50:17, 1982.
25. Nattel, S., and Bailey, J.C.: Time course of the electrophysiological effects of quinidine on canine cardiac Purkinje fibers: Concentration dependence and comparison with lidocaine and disopyramide. J. Pharmacol. Exp. Ther., 225:176, 1983.
26. Walsh, R.A., and Horwitz, L.D.: Adverse hemodynamic effects of intravenous disopyramide compared with quinidine in conscious dogs. Circulation, 60:1053, 1979.
27. Chassaing, C., Duchene-Marullas, P., and Paire, M.: Mechanism of action of quinidine on heart rate in the dog. J. Pharmacol. Exp. Ther., 222:688, 1982.
28. Clohiosy, D.R., and Gibson, T.P.: Comparison of pharmacokinetic parameters of intravenous quinidine in dogs. J. Cardiovasc. Pharmacol., 4:107, 1982.
29. Neff, C.A., Davis, L.E., and Baggot, J.D.: A comparative study of the pharmacokinetics of quinidine. Am. J. Vet. Res., 33:1521, 1972.
30. Warner, N.J., et al.: Tissue digoxin concentrations during the quinidine-digoxin interaction. Am. J. Cardiol., 51:1717, 1983.
31. Winkle, R.A., Glantz, S.A., and Harrison, D.C.: Pharmacologic therapy of ventricular arrhythmias. Am. J. Cardiol., 36:629, 1975.
32. Velebit, V., et al.: Aggravation and provocation of ventricular arrhythmias by antiarrhythmic drugs. Circulation, 65:886, 1982.
33. Singh, B.N., Cho, Y.W., and Kuemmerle, H.P.: Clinical pharmacology of antiarrhythmic drugs: a review and overview. Part I. Int. J. Clin. Pharm. Ther. Toxicol., 19:139, 1981.
34. Badke, F.R., et al.: Hemodynamic effects of N-acetylprocainamide compared with procainamide in conscious dogs. Circulation, 6:1142, 1981.
35. Schmid, P.G., et al.: Vascular effects of procaine amide in the dog. Circ. Res., 35:948, 1974.
36. Pearle, D.L., Souza, J.D., and Gillis, R.A.: Comparative vagolytic effects of procainamide and N-acetylprocainamide in the dog. J. Cardiovasc. Pharmacol., 5:450, 1983.
37. Mandel, W.J., et al.: Cardiorenal effects of lidocaine and procaineamide in the conscious dog. Am. J. Physiol., 228:1440, 1975.
38. Dreyfus, J., Ross, J.J., Jr., and Schreiber, E.C.: Absorption, excretion, and biotransformation of procainamide-C14 in the dog and Rhesus monkey. Arzneim.-Forsch., 21:948, 1971.
39. Kaufman, G.M., Weirich, W.E., and Mayer, P.R.: The pharmacokinetics of regular and sustained release procainamide in the dog. Abstract. Proceedings Am. Coll. Vet. Intern. Med., 1983, New York, p. 42.
40. Kus, T., and Sasyniuk, B.I.: Electrophysiological actions of disopyramide phosphate on canine ventricular muscle and Purkinje fibers. Circ. Res., 37:844, 1975.
41. Mirro, M.J., Watanabe, A.M., and Bailey, J.C.: Electrophysiological effects of the optical isomers of disopyramide and quinidine in the dog. Circ. Res., 48:867, 1981.

42. Ranney, R.E., Dean, R.R., Karim, A., and Radzialowski, F.M.: Disopyramide phosphate: pharmacokinetic and pharmacologic relationships of a new antiarrhythmic agent. Arch. Int. Pharmacodyn., *191*:162, 1971.

43. Rosen, M.R., Merker, C., and Pippenger, C.E.: The effects of lidocaine on the canine ECG and electrophysiologic properties of Purkinje fibers. Am. Heart J., *91*:191, 1976.

44. Obayashi, K., Hayakawa, H., and Mandel, W.J.: Interrelationships between external potassium concentration and lidocaine: Effects on canine Purkinje fiber. Am. Heart J., *89*:221, 1975.

45. Feely, J., et al.: Effect of hypotension on liver blood flow and lidocaine disposition. N. Engl. J. Med., *307*:866, 1982.

46. Wilcke, J.R., Davis, L.E., Neff-Davis, C.A., and Koritez, G.D.: Pharmacokinetics of lidocaine and its active metabolites in dogs. J. Vet. Pharmacol. Ther., *6*:49, 1983.

47. Handel, F., et al.: Lidocaine and its metabolites in canine plasma and myocardium. J. Cardiovasc. Pharmacol., *5*:44, 1983.

48. Branch, R.A., Shand, D.G., Wilkinson, G.R., and Nies, A.S.: The reduction of lidocaine clearance by dl-propranolol: An example of hemodynamic drug interaction. J. Pharmacol. Exp. Ther., *184*:515, 1973.

49. Ochs, H.R., Carstens, G., and Greenblatt, D.J.: Reduction in lidocaine clearance during continuous infusion and by coadministration of propranolol. N. Engl. J. Med., *303*:373, 1980.

50. Ikeda, M., Dohi, T., and Tsujimoto, A.: Inhibition of gamma-aminobutyric acid release from synaptosomes by local anesthetics. Am. Soc. Anesth., *38*:495, 1983.

51. Keene, B.W., and Hamlin, R.L.: Prophylaxis and treatment of digitalis-enhanced dysrhythmias with phenytoin in the dog. Abstract. Proceedings Am. Coll. Vet. Intern. Med., 1980, Washington, D.C., p. 118.

52. Sanders, J.E., and Yeary, R.A.: Serum concentrations of orally administered diphenylhydantoin in dogs. J. Am. Vet. Med. Assoc., *172*:153, 1978.

53. Conolly, M.E., Kersting, F., and Dollery, C.T.: The clinical pharmacology of Beta-adrenoceptor-blocking drugs. Prog. Cardiovasc. Dis., *19*:203, 1976.

54. Kates, R.E., Keene, B.W., and Hamlin, R.L.: Pharmacokinetics of propranolol in the dog. J. Vet. Pharmacol. Ther., *2*:21, 1979.

55. Weidler, D.J., Jallad, N.S., Garg, D.C., and Wagner, J.G.: Pharmacokinetics of propranolol in the cat and comparisons with three other species. Res. Comm. Chem. Path. Pharmacol., *26*:105, 1979.

56. Frishman, W.H.: Beta-adrenergic blockade in clinical practice. Hosp. Pract., *17*:57, 1982.

57. Frishman, W.: Clinical pharmacology of the new beta-adrenergic blocking drugs. Part 1. Pharmacodynamic and pharmacokinetic properties. Am. Heart J., *97*:663, 1979.

57a.Muir, W.W., and Sams, R.: Clinical pharmacodynamics and pharmacokinetics of beta-adrenoceptor blocking drugs in veterinary medicine. Comp. Cont. Educ., *6*:156, 1984.

58. Bigger, J.T., Jr., and Jaffe, C.C.: The effect of bretylium tosylate on the electrophysiologic properties of ventricular muscle and Purkinje fibers. Am. J. Cardiol., *27*:82, 1971.

59. Cardinal, R., and Sasyniuk, B.I.: Electrophysiological effects of bretylium tosylate on subendocardial Purkinje fibers from infarcted canine hearts. J. Pharmacol. Exp. Ther., *204*:159, 1978.

60. Bache, R.J., Cobb, F.R., and Greenfield, J.C.: Coronary and systemic haemodynamic effects of bretylium in the intact anesthetized dog. Cardiovasc. Res., *7*:755, 1973.

61. Breznock, E.M., Kagan, K., and Hibser, N.K.: Effects of bretylium tosylate on the in vivo fibrillating canine ventricle. Am. J. Vet. Res., *38*:89, 1977.

62. Gillis, R.A., Clancy, M.M., and Anderson, R.J.: Deleterious effects of bretylium in cats with digitalis induced ventricular tachycardia. Circulation, *47*:974, 1973.

63. Bacaner, M.B., Hoey, M., and Macres. M.G.: Suppression of ventricular fibrillation and positive inotropic action of bethanidine sulfate, a chemical analog of bretylium tosylate that is well absorbed orally. Am. J. Cardiol., *49*:45, 1982.

64. Antman, E.M., Stone, P.H., Muller, J.E., and Braunwald, E.: Calcium channel blocking agents in the treatment of cardiovascular disorders. Part I: Basic and clinical electrophysiologic effects. Ann. Intern. Med., *93*:875, 1980.

65. Kawai, C., Kanish, T., Matsuyama, E., and Okazaki, H.: Comparative effects of three calcium antagonists, diltiazem, verapamil, and nifedipine on the sinoatrial and atrioventricular nodes. Experimental and clinical studies. Circulation, *63*:1035, 1981.

66. McAllister, R.J., Jr.: Clinical pharmacology of slow channel blocking agents. Prog. Cardiovasc. Dis., *25*:83, 1982.

67. Nakaya, H., Schwartz, A., and Millard, R.W.: Reflex chronotropic and inotropic effects of calcium channel-blocking agents in conscious dogs. Diltiazem, verapamil, and nifedipine compared. Circ. Res., *52*:302, 1983.

68. Stone, P.H., Antman, E.M., Muller, J.E., and Braunwald, E.: Calcium channel blocking agents in the treatment of cardiovascular disorders. Part II: Hemodynamic effects and clinical applications. Ann. Intern. Med., *93*:886, 1980.

69. Keefe, D.L., and Kates, R.E.: Myocardial disposition and cardiac pharmacodynamics of verapamil in the dog. J. Pharmacol. Exp. Ther., *220*:91, 1982.

70. Klein, H.O., and Kaplinsky, E.: Verapamil and digoxin: Their respective effects on atrial fibrillation and their interaction. Am. J. Cardiol., *50*:894, 1982.

71. Hachisu, M., and Pappano, A.J.: A comparative study of the blockade of calcium-dependent action potentials by verapamil, nifedipine and nimodipine in ventricular muscle. J. Pharmacol. Exp. Ther., *225*:112, 1983.

72. Hoffman, B.F., and Bigger, J.T., Jr.: Digitalis and allied cardiac glycosides. In *The Pharmacological Basis of Therapeutics.* 6th Edition. Edited by A.G. Gilman, L.S. Goodman, and A. Gilman. New York, Macmillan, 1980.

73. Bolton, G.R., and Powell, W.: Plasma kinetics of digoxin in the cat. Am. J. Vet. Res., *43*:1994, 1982.

74. Gierke, K.D., Perrier, D., Mayersohn, M., and Marcus, F.I.: Digoxin disposition kinetics in dogs before and during azotemia. J. Pharmacol. Exp. Ther., *205*:459, 1978.

75. Bigger, J.T.: Pharmacologic and clinical control of antiarrhythmic drugs. Am. J. Med., *58*:479, 1975.

76. Greenblatt, D.J., and Koch-Weser, J.: Clinical pharmacokinetics. N. Engl. J. Med., *293*:702, 1975.

77. Loeb, J.M., Dalton, D.P., and Moran, J.M.: Sensitivity differences of SA and AV node to vagal stimulation: Attenuation of vagal effects at SA node. Am. J. Physiol., *241*:H684, 1981.

78. Schweitzer, P., and March, H.: The effect of atropine on cardiac arrhythmias and conduction. Am. Heart J., *100*:119, 1980.

79. Muir, W.W.: Effects of atropine on cardiac rate and rhythm in dogs. J. Am. Vet. Med. Assoc., *172*:917, 1978.

80. King, J.M., Roth, L., and Haschek, W.M.: Myocardial necrosis secondary to neural lesions in domestic animals. J. Am. Vet. Med. Assoc., *180*:144, 1982.

81. Ferrer, M.I.: The sick sinus syndrome. Circulation, *47*:635, 1973.

82. Mandel, W.J.: *Cardiac Arrhythmias.* Philadelphia, J.B. Lippincott, 1980.

83. Hamlin, R.L., Smetzer, D.L., and Breznock, E.M.: Sinoatrial syncope in Miniature Schnauzers. J. Am. Vet. Med. Assoc., *161*:1022, 1972.

84. Lombard, C.M., Tilley, L.P., and Yoshioka, M.M.: Pacemaker implantation in the dog. J. Am. Anim. Hosp. Assoc., *17*:751, 1981.

85. Boyden, P.A., et al.: Effects of left atrial enlargement on atrial transmembrane potentials and structure in dogs with mitral valve fibrosis. Am. J. Cardiol., *49*:1896, 1982.

86. Truccone, N.J., and Krangrad, E.: Hemodynamic effects of rapid atrial stimulation in adult and young dogs. Circ. Res., *4*:130, 1977.

87. Wildenthal, K., and Atkins, J.M.: Use of the "diving reflex" for the treatment of paroxysmal supraventricular tachycardia. Am. Heart J., *98*:536, 1979.

88. Hayes, A., and Cooper, R.G.: Studies on the absorption, distribution and excretion of propranolol in rat, dog, and monkey. J. Pharmacol. Exp. Ther., *176*:302, 1971.

89. Webb, J.G., Newman, W.H., Walle, T., and Daniell, H.B.: Myocardial sensitivity to isoproterenol following abrupt propranolol withdrawal in conscious dogs. J. Cardiovasc. Pharmacol., *3*:622, 1981.

90. Tse, F.L.S., Sanders, T.M., and Reo, J.P.: Bioavailability of propranolol in the dog. Arch. Int. Pharmacodyn., *248*:180, 1980.

91. Goad, D.L.: Calcium entry blockers: A review. J. Vet. Pharmacol. Ther., *5*:233, 1982.

92. Bohn, F.K., Patterson, D.F., and Pyle, R.L.: Atrial fibrillation in dogs. Br. Vet. J., *127*:485, 1971.

93. Bolton, G.R., and Ettinger, S.: Paroxysmal atrial fibrillation in the dog. J. Am. Vet. Med. Assoc., *158*:64, 1971.

94. Saito, D., et al.: Effect of atrial fibrillation on coronary circulation and blood flow distribution across the left ventricular wall in anesthetized open-chest dogs. Jap. Circ. J., *42*:417, 1978.

95. Hilwig, R.W.: Hemodynamic relationships in dogs with sinus arrhythmia and atrial fibrillation. Am. J. Vet. Res., *33*:475, 1972.

96. Brorson, L., et al.: Effects of concentration and steric configuration of propranolol on AV conduction and ventricular repolarization in the dog. J. Cardiovasc. Pharmacol., *3*:692, 1981.

97. D'Agrasa, L.S.: Cardiac arrhythmias of sympathetic origin in the dog. Am. J. Physiol., *233*:H535, 1977.

98. Vassalle, M., Greenspan, K., and Hoffman, B.K.: An analysis of arrhythmias induced by ouabain in intact dogs. Circ. Res., *13*:132, 1963.

99. Muir, W.W.: Electrocardiographic interpretation of thiobarbiturate-induced dysrhythmias in dogs. J. Am. Vet. Med. Assoc., *170*:1419, 1977.

100. Muir, W.W.: Gastric dilatation-volvulus in the dog, with emphasis on cardiac dysrhythmias. J. Am. Vet. Med. Assoc., *180*:739, 1982.

101. Zenoble, R.D., and Hill, B.L.: Hypothermia and associated cardiac arrhythmias in two dogs. J. Am. Vet. Med. Assoc., *175*:840, 1979.

102. Buss, D.D., Hess, R.E., Webb, A.I., and Spencer, K.R.: Incidence of postanaesthetic arrhythmias in the dog. J. Small Anim. Pract., *23*:399, 1982.

103. Lister, J.W., et al.: Effect of pacemaker site on cardiac output and ventricular activation in dogs with complete heart block. Am. J. Cardiol., *14*:494, 1964.

104. Lown, B., and Graboys, T.B.: Management of patients with malignant ventricular arrhythmias. Am. J. Cardiol., *39*:910, 1977.

105. Vlay, S.C., and Reid, P.R.: Ventricular ectopy: Etiology, evaluation, and therapy. Am. J. Med., *73*:899, 1982.

106. Whiting, R.B.: Ventricular premature contractions: Which should be treated? Arch. Intern. Med., *140*:1423, 1980.

107. Vassalle, M., et al.: An analysis of fast idioventricular rhythm in the dog. Circ. Res., *13*:218, 1977.

108. Hordof, A.J., Rose, E., Danilo, P., Jr., and Rosen, M.R.: Alpha and beta-adrenergic effects of epinephrine on ventricular pacemakers in dogs. Am. J. Physiol., *242*:H677, 1982.

109. Collinsworth, K.A., Sumner, M.K., and Harrison, D.C.: The clinical pharmacology of lidocaine as an antiarrhythmic drug. Circulation, *50*:1217, 1974.

110. LeLorier, J., Moisan, R., Gagne, J., and Caille, G.: Effect of the duration of infusion on the disposition of lidocaine in dogs. J. Pharmacol. Exp. Ther., *203*:507, 1977.

111. Carson, D.L., and Dresel, P.E.: Effects of lidocaine on conduction of extrasystoles in the normal canine heart. J. Cardiovasc. Pharmacol., *3*:924, 1981.

112. Lamanna, V., Antzelev, C., and Moe, G.K.: Effects of lidocaine on conduction through depolarized canine false tendons and on a model of reflected reentry. J. Pharmacol. Exp. Ther., *221*:353, 1982.

113. Muir, W.W., and Lipowitz, A.J.: Cardiac dysrhythmias associated with gastric dilatation-volvulus in the dog. J. Am. Vet. Med. Assoc., *172*:683, 1978.

114. Difazio, C.A., and Brown, R.E.: Lidocaine metabolism in normal and phenobarbital pre-treated dogs. Anesthesiology, *36*:238, 1972.

114a. Muir, W.W., and Bonagura, J.D.: Treatment of cardiac arrhythmias in dogs with gastric distention-volvulus. J. Am. Vet. Med. Assoc., *184*:1366, 1984.

115. Lown, B., et al.: Effect of a digitalis drug on ventricular premature beats. N. Engl. J. Med., *296*:301, 1977.

116. Stargel, W.W., et al.: Clinical comparison of rapid infusion and multiple injection methods for lidocaine loading. Am. Heart J., *102*:872, 1981.

117. Davison, R., Parker, M., and Atkinson, A.J.: Excessive serum lidocaine levels during maintenance infusions: Mechanisms and prevention. Am. Heart J., *104*:203, 1982.

118. Bonagura, J.D., Helphrey, M.L., and Muir, W.W.: Complications associated with permanent pacemaker implantation in the dog. J. Am. Vet. Med. Assoc., *182*:149, 1983.

119. Wellens, H.J.J., Farre, J., and Bar, F.W.H.M.: The Wolff-Parkinson-White syndrome. In *Cardiac Arrhythmias.* Edited by W.J. Mandel. Philadelphia, J.B. Lippincott, 1980.

120. Josephson, M.E., and Horowitz, L.N.: Electrophysiologic approach to therapy of recurrent sustained ventricular tachycardia. Am. J. Cardiol., *43*:631, 1979.

121. Sclarovsky, S., Strasberg, B., Lewin, R.F., and Agman, J.: Polymorphous ventricular tachycardia: Clinical feature and treatment. Am. J. Cardiol., *44*:339, 1979.

122. Keren, A., et al.: Etiology, warning signs and therapy of torsade de pointes. A study in 10 patients. Circulation, *64*:1167, 1981.

123. Patterson, E., Gibson, J.K., and Lucchesi, B.R.: Prevention of chronic ventricular tachyarrhythmias with bretylium tosylate. Circulation, *64*:1045, 1981.

124. Anderson, J.L., et al.: Kinetics of antifibrillatory effects of bretylium: Correlation with myocardial drug concentrations. Am. J. Cardiol., *46*:583, 1980.

125. Danilo, P., Jr.: Aprindine. Am. Heart J., *97*:119, 1979.

126. Muir, W.W., and Bonagura, J.D.: Aprindine for treatment of ventricular arrhythmias in the dog. Am. J. Vet. Res., *43*:1815, 1982.

127. Calvert, C.A., Chapman, W.L., and Toal, R.L.: Congestive cardiomyopathy in Doberman Pinscher dogs. J. Am. Vet. Med. Assoc., *181*:598, 1982.

128. DeSurray, J.M., and Breekpot, F.: Pharmacokinetic study of aprindine and moxaprindine in dogs. Int. J. Clin. Pharmacol. Ther. Toxicol., *19*:209, 1981.

129. Danilo, P., Jr.: Mexiletine. Am. Heart J., *97*:399, 1979.

130. Latini, R., Connolly, S.J., and Kates, R.E.: Myocardial disposition of amiodarone in the dog. J. Pharmacol. Exp. Ther., *224*:603, 1983.

131. Sami, M., Mason, J.W., Oh, G., and Harrison, D.C.: Canine electrophysiology of encainide, a new antiarrhythmic drug. Am. J. Cardiol., *43*:1149, 1979.

132. Elharrar, V., and Zipes, D.P.: Effects of encainide and metabolites (MJ14030 and MJ9444) on canine cardiac Purkinje and ventricular fibers. J. Pharmacol. Exp. Ther., *220*:440, 1982.

133. Hodges, M., et al.: Suppression of ventricular ectopic depolarizations by flecainide acetate, a new antiarrhythmic agent. Circulation, *65*:879, 1982.

134. Legrand, V., Vandormael, M., Collignon, P., and Kulbertus, H.E.: Hemodynamic effects of a new antiarrhythmic agent, Flecainide (R-818), in coronary heart disease. Am. J. Cardiol., *51*:422, 1983.

11 Special methods for analyzing and treating arrhythmias

The office of medicine is but to tune this curious harp of man's (the animal's) body and to reduce it to harmony.

SIR FRANCIS BACON, 1605

I cannot state with certainty whether this bundle actually conducts the impulse from the auricle to the ventricle . . . . Its presence, in all events, is contrary to the opinion of those, who, in the absence of such a muscular connection between the auricle and ventricle, attempt to prove the necessary presence of a nerve conduction.[1]

WILHELM HIS, JR., 1893

The single-channel electrocardiograph is the mainstay of electrocardiography and has provided the foundation for our better understanding of cardiac arrhythmias. For the animal who is brought to a cardiovascular clinic with fainting episodes, the single-channel electrocardiograph is usually adequate to diagnose the arrhythmia if it is the underlying disorder. The use of various vagal maneuvers, or the administration of intravenous cardiac drugs while continuously maintaining the electrocardiogram is usually sufficient to diagnose the arrhythmia in question. On occasion, more advanced methods are needed to analyze and treat the arrhythmia.

The diagnosis and treatment of arrhythmias can sometimes be difficult. Certain techniques, some more advanced than others, are required to analyze and treat some arrhythmias. The clinical evaluation of the electrical activity of the heart has advanced significantly during the past 10 to 15 years. The mechanisms for certain arrhythmias have been more clearly defined, the nature and site of various forms of heart block have been found, and methods for assessing function of the rest of the conduction system have been developed. These advances in both the human field and in veterinary medicine have led to the use of pacemaker therapy as well as to new approaches to the diagnosis and treatment of life-threatening arrhythmias.

In this chapter, the following methods for analyzing and treating arrhythmias will be discussed: use of calipers or blank card in arrhythmia analysis, noncompensatory versus compensatory pause, vagal stimulation, use of precordial chest leads, use of the multichannel electrocardiograph, chest "thump" method, computerized electrocardiography, long-term monitoring, intracardiac electrocardiography, His bundle electrocardiography, epicardial pacemaker implantation, cardiopulmonary resuscitation, and electrical cardioversion and defibrillation. Table 10–1 in the previous chapter summarizes the methods available for terminating arrhythmia. The various methods cannot all be discussed in detail, nor can the literature be reviewed exhaustively. The reader should consult those books and journal articles that I have found particularly helpful and significant.

USE OF CALIPERS OR A BLANK CARD IN ARRHYTHMIA ANALYSIS

If the initial inspection of the electrocardiogram suggests that there is an arrhythmia, a long strip should be taken. The analysis of arrhythmias can also be facilitated by consulting an electrocardiogram obtained prior to the onset of the arrhythmia. The morphology of the P waves and of the QRS complexes can then be compared.

The clinician can also use electrocardiographic calipers for plotting intervals. If calipers are not available, a simple method is to place a blank card immediately beneath the apex of the recognizable P waves (or QRS complexes) (Fig. 11–1); a vertical line is drawn immediately under the apex of each P wave (or R wave if that is being examined) that can be definitely recognized; the card can then be shifted to the right or left so that the marks fall under other P waves. If the rhythm is regular, all marks will fall under the appropriate complexes. The lines on the card can now be used to indicate or predict the location of all P waves. For example, this method can be used to find P waves in arrhythmias with P waves hidden in the QRS complexes.

NONCOMPENSATORY PAUSE VERSUS COMPENSATORY PAUSE— DIFFERENTIATING PREMATURE COMPLEXES

The calipers or the blank card are essential in measuring the length of the pause after premature complexes. The duration of the pause in the electrocardiogram may be helpful in distinguishing atrial premature complexes from those of ventricular origin. The length of this pause depends on whether the SA node is also depolarized prematurely by the ectopic stimulus. Premature complexes are usually followed by a pause, termed noncompensatory or compensatory according to its duration (Fig. 11–2).

With an APC (atrial premature complex) the ectopic impulse usually depolarizes the SA node as well as the atrial myocardium. The basic rhythm of the SA node is then disturbed, and the node resumes its normal pacemaker activity at an earlier time than would have been expected from the normal R-R interval. In this case, the interval from the premature complex to the next normal SA node impulse is called a *noncompensatory pause* (or less than compensatory pause) (Fig. 11–2). The R-R interval of the two normal SA impulses enclosing the early

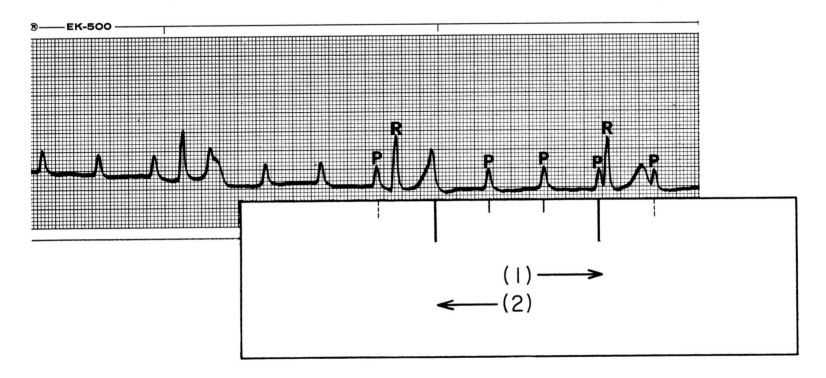

Fig. 11–1. Card method for examining arrhythmias. A card has been marked at two places (small dark lines) beneath the apex of two waves. By moving the card to the right (1), the examiner can see that a P wave (heavy dark line) falls within an R wave. By moving the card to the left (2), he determines that a P wave (heavy dark line) falls within a T wave (explaining its increased amplitude). This electrocardiogram is an example of complete heart block.

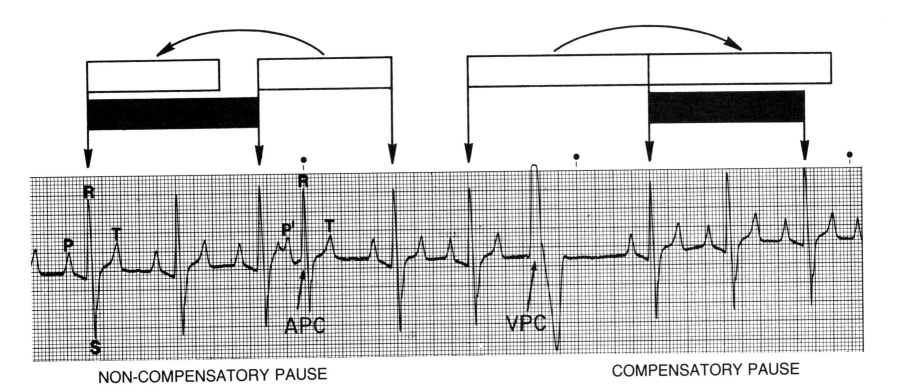

NON-COMPENSATORY PAUSE   COMPENSATORY PAUSE

Fig. 11–2. Noncompensatory pause versus compensatory pause, differentiating an atrial premature complex (APC) from a ventricular premature complex (VPC). P', Atrial premature complex.

complex is less than twice the normal R-R interval. Atrial and AV junctional premature complexes are generally followed by a noncompensatory pause.

VPCs (ventricular premature complexes) are usually conducted retrograde to the AV junction but not across into the atria and SA node. The SA node, which is not depolarized, continues its own rhythmic activity and depolarizes the atria. The P wave, occurring just before, during, or just after the ventricular premature complexes and thus falling within the refractory period of the ventricle, cannot therefore elicit a ventricular response. In this case, the interval from the VPC to the next normal SA node impulse is called a *compensatory pause* (Fig. 11–2).

The pause following the VPC is long enough to make the R-R interval between the two normal SA impulses that flank the premature complex equal to or slightly greater than the sum of two normal R-R intervals. VPCs are generally followed by a compensatory pause, unless they are interpolated or retrograde atrial activation resets the SA node.

When the pause after a premature complex is absent, the complex is termed *interpolated*. The ectopic impulse is interposed between two sinus impulses, with little or no effect on the dominant rhythm.

VAGAL STIMULATION

Vagal stimulation involves the mechanical application of pressure to receptors that cause a reflex increase in vagal tone. The vagus nerve innervates the SA node, atria, AV node, and ventricles. The effects of increasing vagal tone are mainly supraventricular, causing a slowing of the heart rate and a decrease in conduction through the AV junction. Vagal stimulation serves as a method for both analyzing and treating an arrhythmia.[2] The decreased conduction rate through the AV junction causes the ventricular rate to be so reduced that supraventricular rhythms are more easily interpreted. The use of vagal stimulation as a temporary means to break a supraventricular tachycardia and to identify discrete P waves is demonstrated in Figures 11–3 and 11–4 (see also Figs. 10–10 and 10–11). When the heart rate of an ectopic focus is slowed, the hemodynamic consequences of the supraventricular arrhythmias can also be temporarily eliminated.

Vagal tone can be increased by two methods: by ocular pressure or by carotid sinus massage. In the first technique, gentle pressure is applied to one or both eyeballs. In the second, a gentle massaging motion of the fingers below the bifurcation of the carotid arteries or just below the angle of the mandible is done. The electrocardiograph

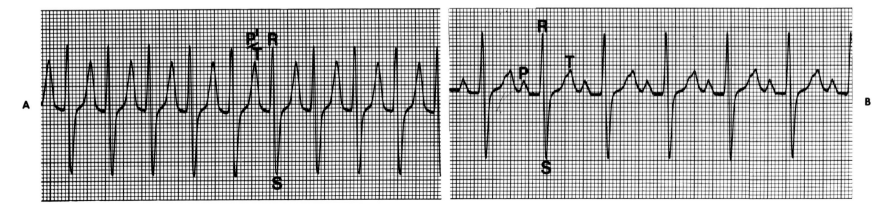

Fig. 11–3. Value of vagal stimulation by ocular pressure for the analysis and temporary treatment of a tachycardia in a dog. **A,** Before ocular pressure; **B,** after ocular pressure. The P and T waves can be easily seen. This response most often favors a diagnosis of supraventricular tachycardia. The atrial ectopic complexes (P′) are superimposed on the T waves of the previous complexes (P′/T) in **A.**

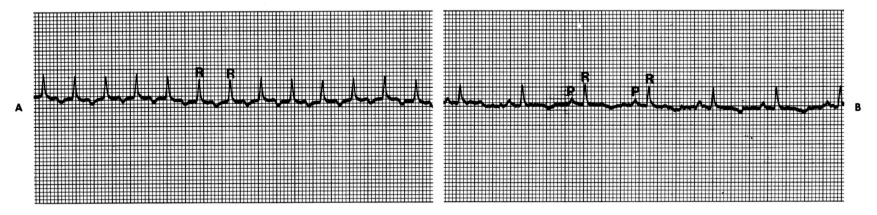

Fig. 11–4. Value of vagal stimulation by ocular pressure for the analysis and temporary treatment of a tachycardia in a cat. **A,** Before ocular pressure. The ventricular rate is very rapid (350 beats/min) with P waves not visible. **B,** Following ocular pressure, the tachycardia is eliminated. The P waves can now be easily seen. This response most often favors a diagnosis of supraventricular tachycardia. (Note: The use of ocular pressure in the cat to terminate a supraventricular tachycardia is often not so successful as in the dog.)

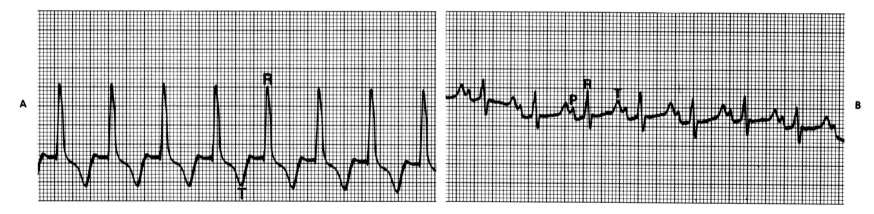

Fig. 11–5. Use of the precordial chest leads for P wave identification. **A,** Lead II rhythm strip in a cat with hypertrophic cardiomyopathy. Differential diagnosis must include ventricular tachycardia (right ventricular focus) because of the large QRS-T complexes and the lack of distinct P waves. **B,** The use of the precordial chest lead, CV_6LL, allowed the P wave to be easily seen. A supraventricular tachycardia is present with P waves hidden in the previous T waves. An intraventricular conduction defect and/or ventricular enlargement are also present.

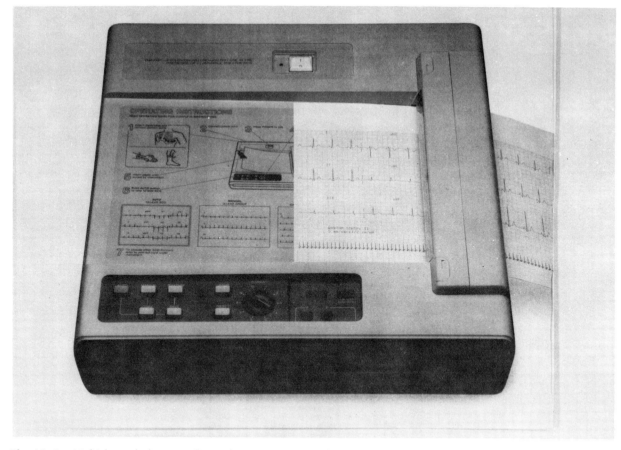

Fig. 11–6. Multichannel electrocardiograph (Page Writer Cardiograph, model 4700A), which records diagnostic electrocardiographic tracings and data on a single, standard size page. A number of electrocardiographic formats can be recorded, at the touch of the button. (Courtesy of Hewlett Packard, Waltham, MA.)

should always be running at the time of vagal stimulation so that any response will be noted. Pressure should be released when a positive effect is observed on the electrocardiogram (Figs. 11–3 and 11–4). In man, vagal stimulation can sometimes result in cardiac systole, ventricular tachycardia, and ventricular fibrillation.[2] I have not seen these complications in animals, but serious effects must always be considered.

USE OF PRECORDIAL CHEST LEADS

The precordial chest leads are exploring electrodes that can record electrical activity from the dorsal and ventral surfaces of the heart. When the lead selection is set at the V position, the electrocardiograph can measure the voltage from the heart to the selected location of the chest electrodes (Fig. 4–86). The precordial chest leads can be valuable for diagnosing cardiac arrhythmias, since P waves are often better visualized in the precordial leads (Fig. 11–5).

MULTICHANNEL ELECTROCARDIOGRAPH

New multichannel electrocardiographs are available now that record diagnostic electrocardiographic tracings and data on a single, standard size page (Fig. 11–6). When selected, a set of formats can be used simply, at the touch of a button. The type of records that can be made include automatic multichannel electrocardiograms, a 12-lead electrocardiogram with rhythm strip, or a simultaneous-lead electrocardiogram from various leads (Figs. 11–7 and 11–8), for extended periods of time. Lead notations are marked automatically at normal paper speed or up to speeds of 100 to 200 mm/sec. The one-page electrocardiogram is convenient for filing and also has room for important animal history information as well as the final interpretation.

The multichannel electrocardiograph obviously has many advantages. Arrhythmias and conduction disturbances can be accurately evaluated when multiple leads are acquired simultaneously. Figures

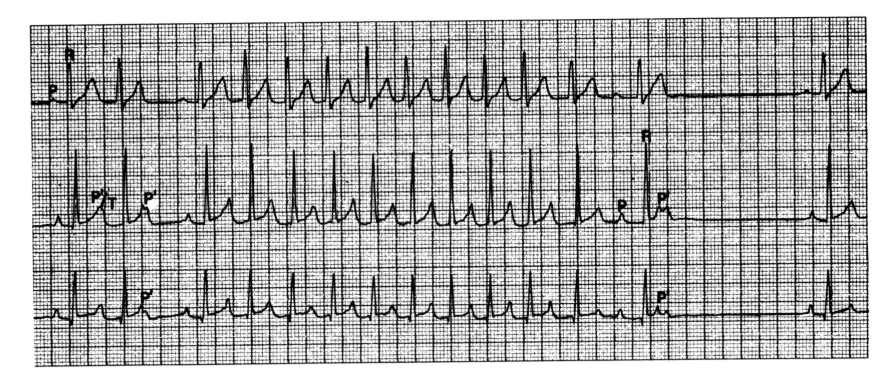

Fig. 11–7. Multichannel electrocardiograph recorded from a Boxer being evaluated for surgery. A simultaneous three-lead electrocardiogram is recorded; CV₅RL, CV₆LL, and CV₆LU. Paroxysmal atrial tachycardia is present after the third QRS complex. Nonconducted atrial premature complexes (P′) occurs after the second QRS complex and also at the end of the atrial tachycardia (after the sinus P-QRS complex that breaks the rhythm). It is obvious that the nonconducted atrial premature complexes (P′) are more well-defined in certain leads, as they deform the T wave of the preceding QRS complex. The P′ waves are not seen on the top rhythm strip. A conducted atrial premature complex (P′/T) is present after the first sinus P-QRS complex. The arrhythmia can be accurately evaluated by using the simultaneous lead recording. (Courtesy of Dr. Anna Tidholm, Stockholm, Sweden.)

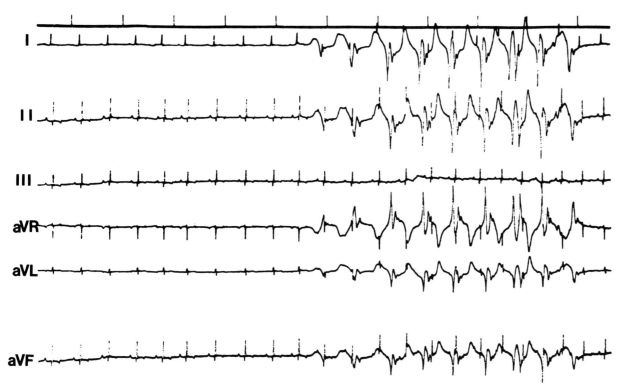

Fig. 11–8. A simultaneous six-lead electrocardiogram recorded from a puppy with suspected parvovirus myocarditis. An arrhythmia (possibly ventricular tachycardia) is demonstrated in all leads except lead III. When the puppy ceased wagging its tail, the suspected arrhythmia disappeared. The motion artifact was not found on lead III since those lead electrodes were not interfered with. Without the simultaneous lead recording, a serious cardiac arrhythmia would have been diagnosed. (From Fisher, E.W.: Electrocardiogram of a tail wag. Vet. Rec., *111*:461, 1982, with permission.)

11–7 and 11–8 illustrate how an abnormality in rhythm can be misdiagnosed if a multichannel electrocardiograph were not available. Recording the paper speed up to 200 mm/sec can also provide a more detailed examination of the waveforms.

Chest "thump" technique

A "thump" or blow over the left precordial area has been shown to be successful in terminating ventricular tachycardia[3] and atrial tachycardia;[4] especially in an emergency when resuscitative drugs and equipment are unavailable (Fig. 11–9). Pennington reported termination of 12 episodes of paroxysmal ventricular tachycardia occurring in five patients by using the "thump" method.[5] The sharp thump to the chest provides a low-energy depolarization current to the heart through electromechanical transduction, probably disrupting the re-entry pathway.[6]

COMPUTERIZED ELECTROCARDIOGRAPHY

In humans, computerized electrocardiographic interpretation is a rapidly progressing field. In veterinary medicine, the technique has been used by some laboratories for the evaluation of cardiotoxicity.[7] The cost of computerized analysis of electrocardiograms is volume dependent because it involves substantial fixed costs, such as transmitting carts and computer systems. The minimum number of electrocardiograms needed at one location to justify a three-channel transmitting cart is about three to ten per day, at a cost of about $3.50 per electrocardiogram for the cart and analysis. The number of electrocardiograms needed to justify a computer facility is in excess of 50 per day, at a processing cost of $2.00 per electrocardiogram.[8,9]

It is important that all electrocardiograms be over-read by an electrocardiographer and that the computer interpretation not be the final analysis. Computer analysis of electrocardiograms in humans has accomplished the following: (1) improved the technical quality of the electrocardiogram, (2) improved the technician's efficiency, (3) been a stimulus for the improvement of diagnostic criteria, (4) enhanced the teaching of electrocardiographic interpretation, and (5) reduced the amount of time required of the clinician for interpretation of the electrocardiograms.[8,10]

The most important variable in the evaluation of the potential ben-

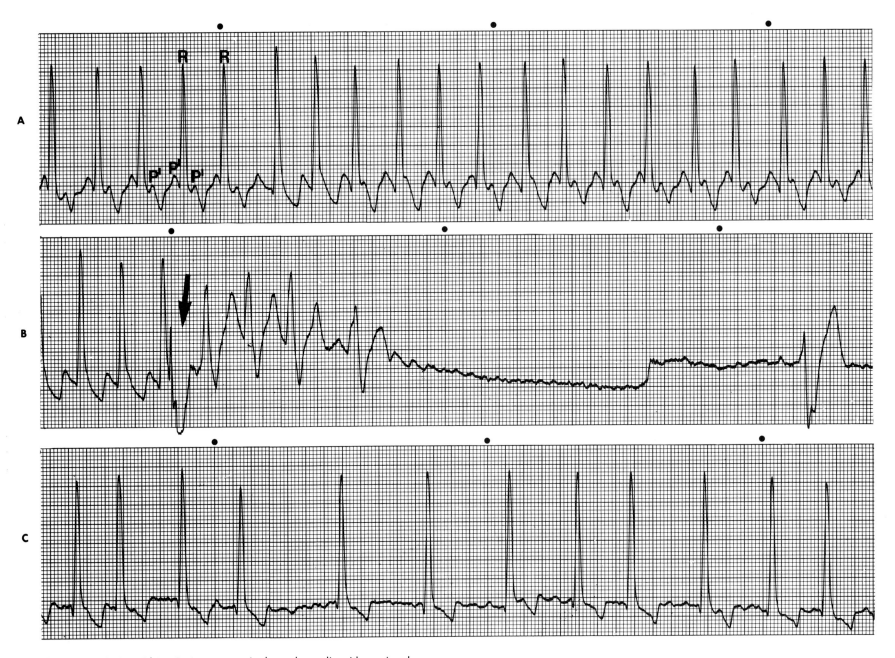

Fig. 11–9. **A,** A rapid (canine) supraventricular tachycardia with varying degrees of atrial conduction (primarily 2:1). Drugs were unsuccessful in converting the arrhythmia. Because direct-current cardioversion equipment was unavailable and the dog was in a crisis, a blow (chest thump) to the left precordial area was given. **B,** A premature depolarization complex created by the chest thump (arrow) was successful in converting the rapid heart rate. Ventricular asystole occurs for approximately 2 seconds. **C,** A strip recorded seconds later reveals atrial fibrillation; the heart rate is now greatly decreased. This technique probably represents the first step in treatment, especially in an emergency when drugs and equipment are not available.

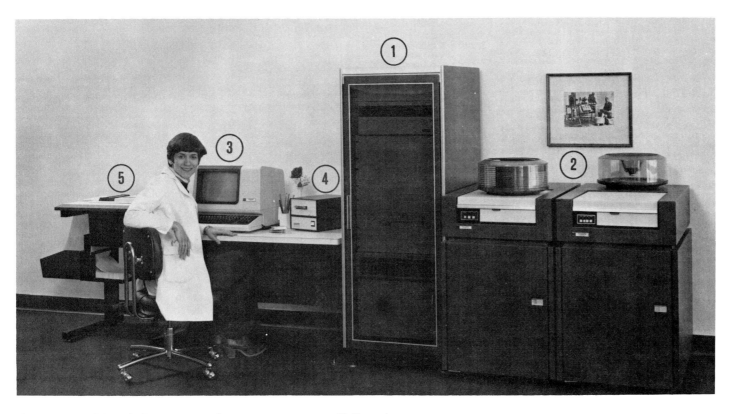

Fig. 11–10. ECG analysis, storage, and management system. (1) Central processing unit, acquisition interface, and communications chassis; (2) Disc drives (300 Mbytes each); (3) CRT for ECG report editing; (4) Acquisition interface (tape cassettes); and (5) Writer/printer (12 lines/3 channels). (Courtesy of Marquette Electronics Inc., Milwaukee, WI.)

efit of computerized analysis of electrocardiograms is the diagnostic accuracy of the computer programs. In humans, most programs can analyze normal electrocardiograms with an overall accuracy of greater than 98%. Abnormal electrocardiograms can be analyzed with a degree of accuracy of 80 to 90% depending on the specific abnormality.[8,11] One of the major causes of difficulty in computerized rhythm analysis is the occasional inability to obtain artifact-free tracings. Also, irregular rhythms (such as atrial fibrillation) with wide QRS complexes secondary to bundle branch block make it difficult to detect ventricular premature complexes.[7]

The use of computer systems to analyze and store the standard electrocardiograms has increased dramatically in recent years. In man, there are continued new developments in hardware as well as improved software programs for electrocardiographic analysis, record keeping, storage, and on-line service to peripheral hospitals. Figure 11–10 shows an example of an electrocardiographic analysis, storage, and management system.

Figure 11–11 illustrates the basic mechanics of how the computer processes and interprets the electrocardiogram. The electrocardiographic signal is received by a standard electrocardiograph and transmitted to the computer, usually by a telephone line. The transmitted signal includes the unprocessed signal along with the coded information such as the animal's case number, clinician, medication, and diagnosis.[12]

Once the quality of the incoming data has been approved, the computer passes the digitalized signal to the "measurement matrix," which identifies according to program instructions all identifiable waveforms and then makes all of the measurements. The data are then transferred to the "criteria matrix," which contains previously agreed upon diagnostic criteria. Once all possible diagnostic criteria have been applied, the diagnoses along with standard measurements, such as heart rate and intervals, and identification data are printed out on a report (Figs. 11–12 and 11–13). The report is attached to the electrocardiogram and given to the electrocardiographer for review.[7,10]

With the rapid development of new computer technology, the costs of computer systems will probably decline. For major institutions and

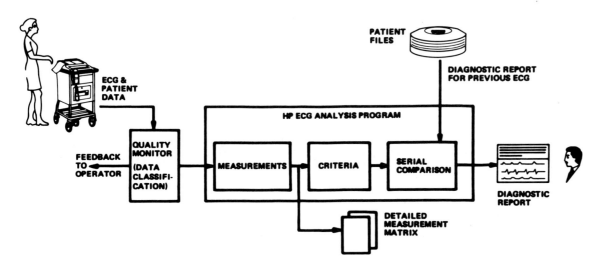

Fig. 11–11. Analysis program module of an ECG management system, illustrating the basic mechanics of how the computer processes and interprets the ECG. The system is composed of three subsections that act sequentially on the ECG data. After passing through the Quality Monitor, the ECG waveforms are first processed by the *Measurements* section of the program. Here all the various waveforms components are identified and measured. The next phase of analysis is testing the measurements against an extensive set of medical criteria for the interpretation of the ECG. This *Criteria* section yields all the pertinent diagnostic statements characterizing the ECG. A final diagnostic report is completed after the ECG has been compared with the recent previous ECG. (From Hewlett Packard ECG Analysis Program-Physicians Guide. Andover, Massachusetts, Hewlett-Packard Company, 1979; reproduced with permission.)

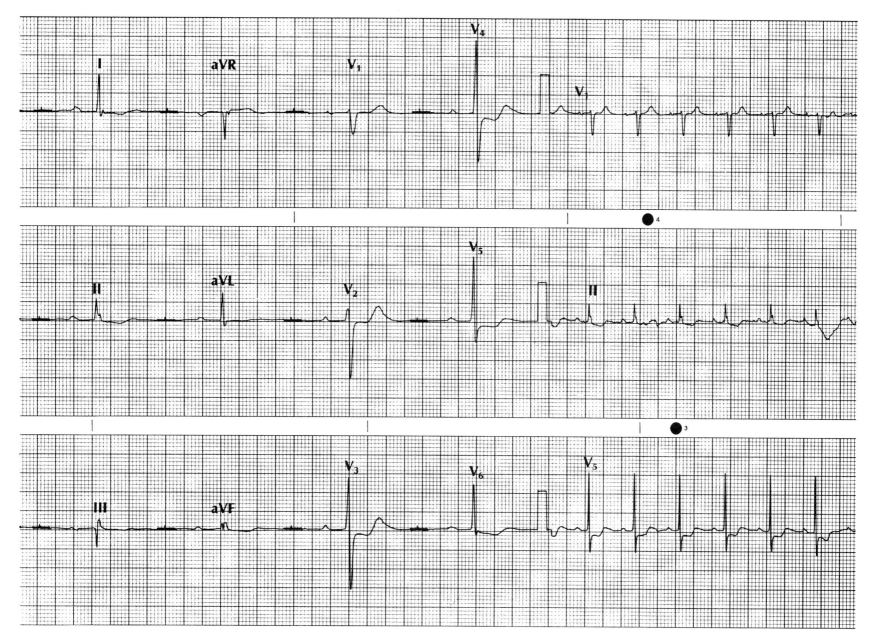

Fig. 11–12. A 12-simultaneous-lead graphic record from the computerized ECG analysis, storage, and management system in Figure 11–10. The complete ECG record and analysis is on a single page. Simultaneous time-aligned cycles of all 12 leads for morphologic analysis and an unswitched 10-second rhythm strip of 3 leads (V_1, II, and V_5) for arrhythmia recognition are included. The P waves are detected with much greater reliability when all the leads are evaluated. (Courtesy of Marquette Electronics Inc., Milwaukee, WI.)

```
** ELECTROCARDIOGRAM ANALYSIS RESULTS **

HEART RATE
97 BEATS/MINUTE


AXIS
P   46              QRS   67              T   68              (DEGREES)


AMPLITUDES
LEAD         P        Q        R        S        T       S-T    (ALL AMPLITUDES IN MV)
I           .05     -.04      .52       0       .23      .04
II          .05     -.09     1.06     -.08      .35      .01
III         .02     -.07      .81       0       .24      .01
AVR        -.05      .03     -.59       0      -.24     -.03
AVL         .02      .04     -.15      .05     -.02      .02
AVF         .06     -.01      .75     -.02      .29      .03


DURATIONS
LEAD          P      QRS      T      P-R      Q-T     (ALL TIMES IN MSEC)
I, II, & III  94     46     104     131     287
AVR, AVL, & AVF 47    31     123     127     289
ALL LEADS     70     38     113     129     288


RHYTHM ANALYSIS

ATRIAL FLUTTER
IRREGULAR R-R INTERVAL
IRREGULAR P-R INTERVAL
FIRST DEGREE HEART BLOCK
LEFT VENTRICULAR HYPERTROPHY
```

Fig. 11–13. Example of an electrocardiographic computer analysis of a monkey. The diagnosis and standard measurements are printed. (From Tilley, L.P.: Advanced electrocardiographic techniques. Vet. Clin. North Am., *13*:365, 1983, with permission.)

laboratories, it should also be realized that the computer also performs ancillary cost-saving services, such as statistical analysis and book-keeping functions.[8,10]

LONG-TERM ELECTROCARDIOGRAPHIC MONITORING

The resting surface electrocardiogram has the disadvantage in that it only records a brief period of heart rhythm. Many rhythm abnormalities are precipitated by activity and are not reproduced on the resting tracing. The standard electrocardiogram also represents only a small sample (60 to 70 beats) of the animal's daily average (greater than 100,000 beats). A 24-hour tape recording of cardiac electrical activity undoubtedly reveals more arrhythmias than would be shown by routine clinical electrocardiograms (Figs. 11–14 and 11–15). The portable tape recording system is now small enough that almost any dog or cat can wear one (Fig. 11–15B).[7]

High-speed playback and, more recently, computer techniques allow this electrocardiographic information to be analyzed rapidly. These monitoring techniques have allowed an opportunity to correlate symptoms with the concomitant recorded rhythm. Several ambulatory electrocardiographic recording systems are now available.

Most of them consist of a small electrocardiographic amplifier and precision amplitude and frequency modulation recorder capable of recording 24 or more hours of electrocardiographic readings from electrodes attached to the animal's chest. In the past, the time and technology necessary to analyze the recordings have made ambulatory electrocardiography an expensive technique. At present, the costs are lower, and some services have rental equipment. Large teaching institutions and research laboratories have found this diagnostic technique useful and practical.[7,13]

An example of an ambulatory electrocardiographic system is shown in Figure 11–14. Printouts of each of the displayed time segments of an arrhythmia are illustrated in Figure 11–15.

Long-term monitoring may be helpful for the following problems:[14,15]

1. Determining the etiology of syncope (Fig. 11–15C) when a cardiac origin is suspected;
2. Assessing the effectiveness of antiarrhythmic therapy;
3. Evaluating animals with chronic bifascicular or complete heart block for asymptomatic but potentially life-threatening arrhythmias. A pacemaker or antiarrhythmic therapy may be indicated, even in the absence of symptoms.

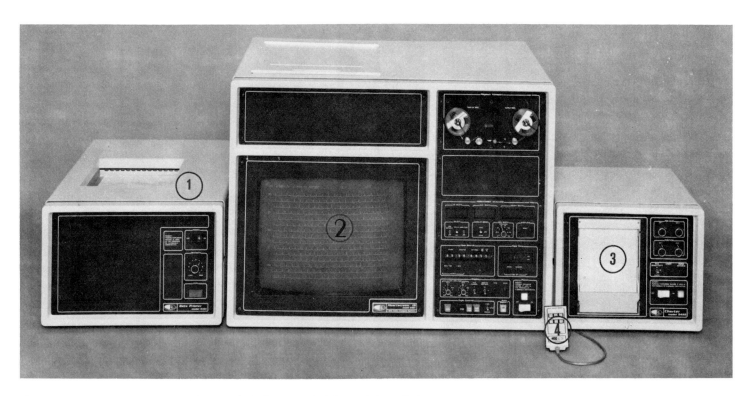

Fig. 11–14. Heartscreen DCG Video Analysis System (Model 9401) from Del Mar Avionics. This system lets you visually scan a 24-hour ambulatory electrocardiographic recording by displaying 60-, 10-, 5-minute or 15-second segments (see Fig. 11–15) on a large 19-inch screen. Front-panel control switches allow enlargement of the displayed electrocardiogram for more detailed review. **(1)** External printer that copies any display on the scope; **(2)** ECG display scope; **(3)** an external chart printer module; and **(4)** hand control for scanning and documentation. The control panel to the right of the display scope has a number of possible functions, including a computer for screening arrhythmias automatically. (Courtesy of Del Mar Avionics, Irvine, California.)

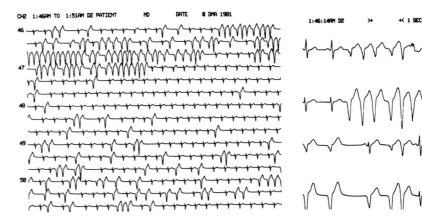

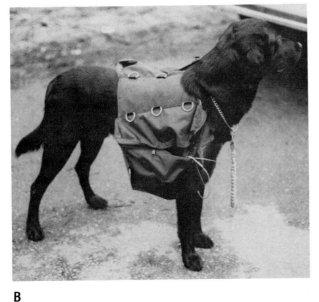

B

C

Fig. 11–15. **A.** Print-outs of three of the displayed time segments from system shown in Figure 11–14. As can be noted, the period of ventricular tachycardia can be easily recognized and correlated with the times of occurrence by referring to digital time entries displayed adjacent to the electrocardiographic data. Detected ventricular ectopic activity can be efficiently recognized and also enlarged, especially on the 15-second time segment for complete analysis and documentation. (Courtesy of Del Mar Avionics, Irvine, California.) **B.** Dog with portable tape recording system (Holter monitor). (Courtesy of Dr. T. Bauer.) **C.** Segment of a 24-hour recording of a patient in atrial fibrillation with unexplained syncope. Note the long period of sinus arrest. (Courtesy of Dr. T. Bauer.)

INTRACARDIAC ELECTROPHYSIOLOGIC STUDIES

Various intracardiac electrophysiologic techniques can be used for the clinical evaluations of the electrical activity of the heart.[16–18,18a] These tests can provide a basis for the management of animals with cardiac arrhythmias; especially to the possible arrhythmic causes of syncope.[15,19] Many clinically significant cardiac arrhythmias can be reproduced under controlled conditions. A comprehensive evaluation usually includes assessment of sinoatrial node function, AV conduction, and responses to programmed atrial and ventricular stimulation. The electrophysiologic techniques will not be discussed in complete detail. The interested reader should consult the selected references. An electrophysiologic study consists of the recording of intracardiac electrical activity and the recording of responses to programmed stimulation. Intracavitary electrocardiography, including the recording of His bundle electrical potentials, will be discussed.

Programmed stimulation includes a variety of pacing techniques: extra beats added during the patient's underlying rhythm, regular pacing followed by single or multiple premature stimuli, and pacing at rapid rates.[18] Programmed stimulation can be used for the induction of ventricular or supraventricular tachycardias, for the electrical termination of such tachycardias, and to restudy tachycardias after various drugs are given.

For example, atrial pacing can be used in dogs with suspected "sick sinus" syndrome so as to measure sinus node recovery time. Recording sinus node recovery time is based on the phenomenon of overdrive suppression. The automaticity of the sinoatrial node can be suppressed by rapid pacing at a site close to, or in electrical connection with, the sinoatrial pacemaker. The ability of the pacemaker to recover upon abruptly terminating the stimulation is related to its functional status.[16,19] Other indications for programmed stimulation include supraventricular tachycardia, tachyarrhythmias due to accessory bypass tracts, and recurrent ventricular tachycardia.[20] The results of an electrophysiologic study are most useful when a specific arrhythmic mechanism is found. In most cases, a trial of specific antiarrhythmic therapy can be outlined.

INTRACARDIAC ELECTROCARDIOGRAPHY

Intracardiac electrophysiologic studies have led to considerable advances in the understanding of cardiac arrhythmias. The majority of arrhythmias can be diagnosed by the standard electrocardiographic leads in the dog and cat. Many times, however, the P waves are hidden in the QRS, S-T, or T wave complexes. Without the accurate identification of the P waves, the determination of the arrhythmia is often impossible. Esophageal lead recordings over the heart and intracardiac recordings can so magnify the P waves that a previously obscured atrial deflection can be identified. For example, the recording of intraatrial electrical activity during paroxysmal tachycardia helps to differentiate between a ventricular and supraventricular tachycardia. These invasive leads have been described in both the dog and the cat.[7,21] The intracardiac leads can also be used for pacing the heart for diagnostic and therapeutic purposes.

To record the electrical activity of the heart, electrode catheters are introduced into different locations in the heart, including the right atrium (Fig. 11–16), area of the tricuspid valve (His bundle), right ventricle (see Fig. 11–19) and sometimes the left ventricle. The main advantage of an intracavitary recording is the demonstration of atrial activity in complex arrhythmias (see Figs. 11–21 to 11–23). The procedure is also useful in establishing a medical regimen. For symptomatic supraventricular arrhythmias or conduction disturbances, the right atrium or right ventricle can be paced by attaching the electrode wire to a temporary artificial pacemaker. It has been well described in the literature.[2,22–24]

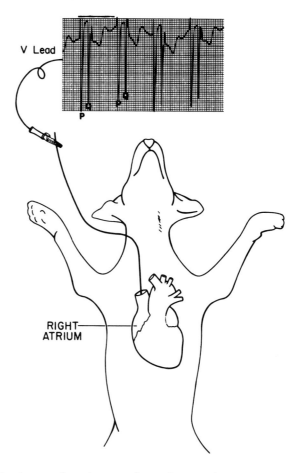

Fig. 11–16. Intracardiac electrocardiography. An electrode catheter is passed through a jugular venipuncture. The wire is then attached to the exploring electrode (V lead) of the electrocardiograph by an alligator clip. The nature of the P waves and the QRS complexes gives the location of the catheter tip. In this case, the recording is from high in the right atrium. The P waves can now easily be identified. The Q wave represents ventricular activity.

Some of the equipment required to carry out intracavitary electrocardiography includes a unipolar or bipolar electrode catheter (semifloating 003992, 4F-USCI, Billerica, Mass.), a 15- or 16-gauge needle, a short length of shielded wire with alligator clamps at each end, and an electrocardiograph. A pacing kit and pacing probe can also be used (KBE Balectrode pacing kit and 0530 Balectrode pacing probe, Elecath, Rahway, NJ).

The dog is preanesthetized with diazepam (0.1 to 0.25 mg/kg) and the skin over the jugular vein is blocked with 2% lidocaine. A jugular venipuncture is performed and the wire passed through the needle. Aseptic technique is important. The wire is then attached to the exploring electrode (C lead) of the electrocardiograph by the alligator clips (Fig. 11–16). The electrocardiograph is run continuously while the wire is advanced. The machine must be properly grounded. A sequence of P wave configurations occurs that represents the location of the electrode catheter tips (Figs. 11–17 and 11–18). The P waves gradually enlarge as the right atrium is entered. It is also possible to get the wire into the ventricle and obtain a right ventricular tracing (Fig. 11–19). After the tracings have been obtained, the wire is gently withdrawn.

Intracardiac electrode catheters can be uni-, bi-, tri-, quadri-, or hexapolar. A record of electrical activity of the heart taken with the electrode(s) within a cavity of the heart is called a *cardiac electrogram.* Cardiac electrograms can be further defined according to the position of the recording electrodes. For example, an electrogram from the area of the AV junction and bundle of His with a His bundle deflection is termed a *His bundle electrogram.* The accurate localization of impulse formation and disorders of conduction has been made possible by recording His bundle activity.

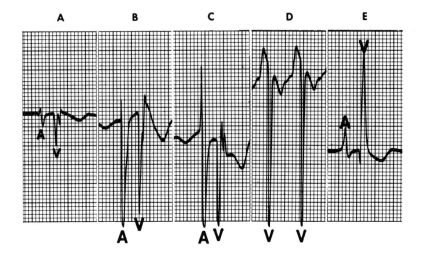

Fig. 11–17. Intracavitary electrogram recorded from various positions of the electrode catheter tip in a normal dog. **A,** Anterior vena cava; **B,** junction of the anterior vena cava and right atrium (note the increased size of the complexes); **C,** in the middle of the right atrium; **D,** right ventricle (0.5 cm = 1 mv; paper speed, 25 mm/sec); deflections are very large; **E,** posterior vena cava; tracings look like those from lead II. A, Atrial complexes; V, ventricular complexes.

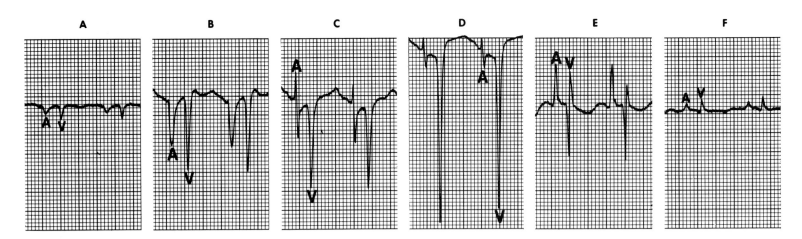

Fig. 11–18. Intracavitary electrogram recorded from various positions of the electrode catheter tip in a normal cat. **A,** Anterior vena cava; **B,** junction of the anterior vena cava and the right atrium; **C,** in the middle of the right atrium; **D,** right ventricle (deflections are very large); **E,** junction of the posterior vena cava and the right atrium; **F,** posterior vena cava (tracing looks like that from lead II). A, Atrial; V, ventricular.

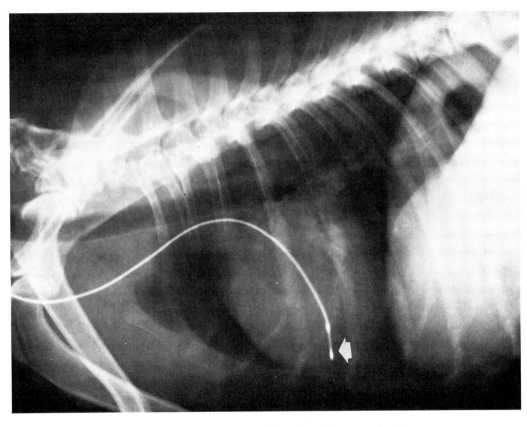

Fig. 11–19. Bipolar electrode catheter positioned in the right ventricle. The catheter was blindly passed (without fluoroscopy) into the right ventricle, the electrogram being used as an indicator of the position of the catheter tip (arrow) (see Fig. 11–17).

HIS BUNDLE ELECTROCARDIOGRAPHY

The electrical potentials of the specialized conducting tissues are too small to be recorded by the surface electrocardiogram. For example, the P-R interval can suggest the presence of a conduction delay but not its exact site. To obtain more detailed electrophysiologic data, direct recordings from the His bundle can be obtained.[25] This is accomplished by using intracardiac electrode catheters that can record His bundle electrical activity. His bundle electrocardiographic studies in the dog have been reported.[13,22,26–29]

The His bundle catheter is usually inserted percutaneously into the jugular vein and advanced under fluoroscopic control across the tricuspid valve (Fig. 11–24). The recording electrodes are located on the distal portion of the catheter in such a way that His bundle electrograms can be recorded when the catheter is properly positioned (Figs. 11–25 and 11–26). The His bundle electrogram is recognized as a small, biphasic or triphasic deflection between the atrial (A) and ventricular (V) electrogram. The His bundle electrogram divides the PR interval into three components defined by the P-A, A-H, and H-V intervals. The P-A interval is an approximate measurement of intra-atrial conduction time from the area around the SA node to the low right atrium. The A-H interval is the conduction time from the low right atrium near the AV node to the His bundle. This interval is an approximation of AV nodal conduction time. The H-V interval measures the conduction time from the proximal His bundle to depolarization of the ventricular myocardium.

A method for locating an electrode catheter for observing electrical activity of the bundle of His without fluoroscopic guidance has been described.[27,28] A catheter containing four electrodes and two internal capillary tubes was developed. The catheter has two distal orifices 18 mm apart (Fig. 11–27). The position of the catheter tip is determined by observing blood pressure recordings from the two internal capillary tubes (Fig. 11–28). When the tip is positioned properly, the proximal orifice will monitor atrial pressure, and the distal orifice will detect ventricular pressure.

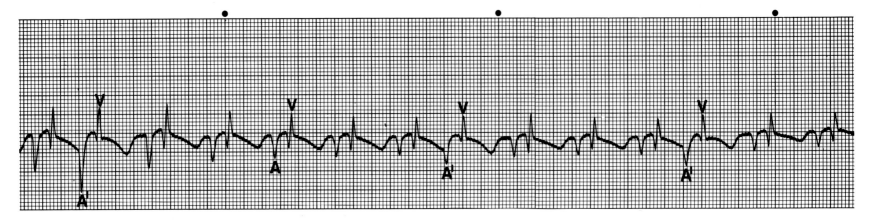

Fig. 11–20. Intracavitary electrogram recorded from the right atrium in a normal cat. APCs (A'V) are present, probably owing to the intermittent touching of the catheter tip on the atrial endocardial surface. A, Atrial; V, ventricular.

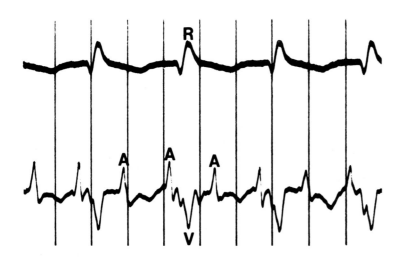

Fig. 11–21. Simultaneous lead II electrocardiogram (top strip) and intra-atrial electrogram (bottom strip). Supraventricular tachycardia, 2:1 AV conduction (every other atrial impulse conducted). Note that the P waves cannot be identified on the lead II electrocardiogram. Time lines, 0.1 sec; 0.5 cm = 1 mv, A, Atrial complexes; V, ventricular complexes.

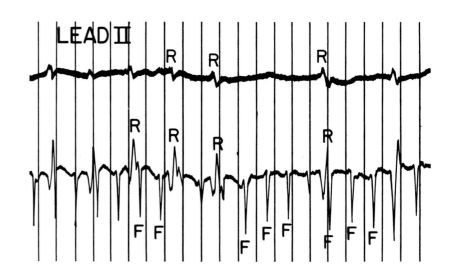

Fig. 11–22. Intracavitary electrogram (bottom tracing) recorded from the right atrium in a cat with atrial fibrillation. The top tracing represents a lead II electrocardiogram. The heart rate is rapid and irregular, with P waves absent. The fibrillatory waves (F) are prominent on the electrogram, occurring at a rapid irregular rate. (From Tilley, L.P.: Pharmacologic and other forms of medical therapy in feline cardiac disease. Vet. Clin. North Am., 7:273, 1977; reprinted with permission.)

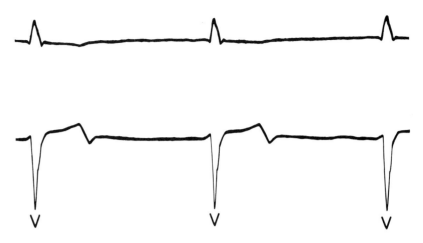

Fig. 11–23. Atrial standstill due to hyperkalemia in a cat with a urethral obstruction. No P waves can be seen in the top (lead II) rhythm strip. This is confirmed on the intra-atrial recording; only ventricular complexes (V) occur. There are no atrial complexes because the atrial myocardium is not activated owing to the high serum potassium. The rhythm is termed sinoventricular since the SA node continues to fire with impulses transmitted via the internodal pathways. (From Tilley, L.P., and Weitz, J.: Pharmacologic and other forms of medical therapy in feline cardiac disease. Vet. Clin. North Am., 7:425, 1977; reprinted with permission.)

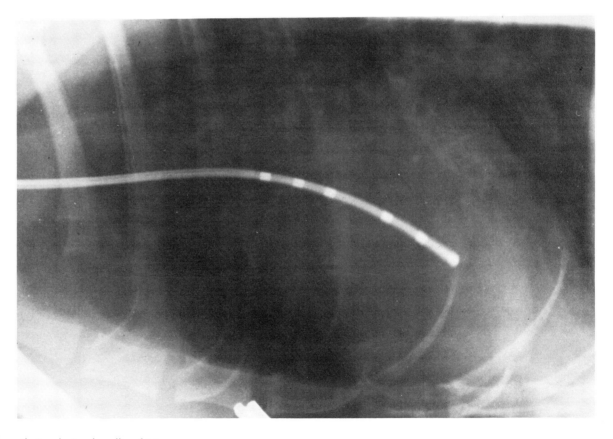

Fig. 11–24. Position of a multipolar electrode catheter during bundle of His recordings. The tip of the catheter is positioned in the right ventricle, with proximal electrodes lying adjacent to the right bundle, the His bundle, and the atrial wall. By means of a switch box, electrical activity can be recorded from the bundle of His. Records from this electrode catheter will look like those in Figures 11–25 and 11–26.

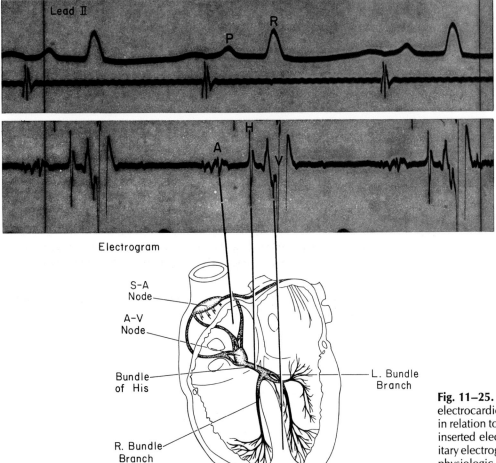

Lead II

P R

Electrogram

A H V

S-A
Node

A-V
Node

Bundle
of His

R. Bundle
Branch

L. Bundle
Branch

Fig. 11–25. Bundle of His electrogram recorded simultaneously with a lead II electrocardiogram. The various portions of the conduction system are illustrated in relation to the events observed in an electrogram recorded from a transvenously inserted electrode catheter positioned close to the conduction system. Intracavitary electrograms represent a relatively new technique for obtaining more detailed physiologic as well as diagnostic information on the electrical activity of the conduction system. A, Atrial deflection; H, His bundle deflection; V, ventricular deflection. A right atrial electrogram is recorded below lead II.

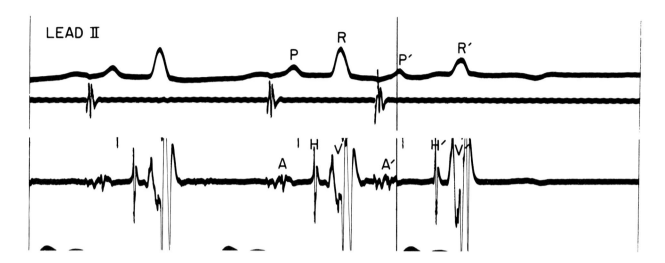

Fig. 11–26. Canine bundle of His electrogram recorded simultaneously with a lead II electrocardiogram (top tracing). Events recorded from the intracardiac electrode catheter: A, atrial deflection; H, His bundle deflection; V, ventricular deflection. His bundle recordings can be useful in determining the origin of aberrant ventricular complexes. The third complex (P'R') is slightly aberrant because an early premature impulse has not given a portion of the bundle branches enough time to fully recover. The premature impulse is supraventricular since the electrogram shows a prolonged A'-H' interval. The H'-V' interval of the premature complex is normal. With ventricular ectopic complexes, the H' spikes follow, are buried in, or precede V' by less than the normal H-V interval. The middle tracing is a right atrial electrogram.

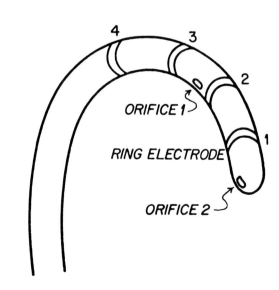

Fig. 11–27. Configuration and drawing of the electrode catheter used to record records in Figure 11–28. (From Ishijima, M., and Hembrough, F.B.: Electrode catheterization for recording electrical activity of fasciculus atrioventricularis (Bundle of His). Am. J. Vet. Res., 40:1800, 1979, with permission.)

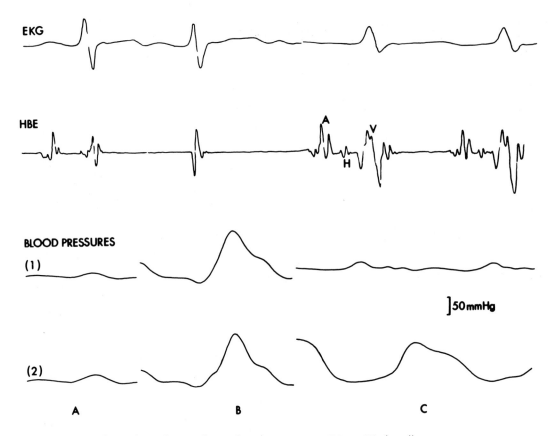

Fig. 11–28. Relationship of EKG, fascicular electrogram (HBE = His bundle electrogram), and blood pressures. Blood pressure 1 indicates the pressure at an orifice 18 mm above the distal and end of the catheter; 2 is taken at the very distal end of the catheter. **A,** The catheter tip is in the atrium. **B,** The ring electrodes are both in the ventricle. **C,** The catheter is in the vicinity of the atrioventricular fascicle. The gain of the EKG amplifier is small and the gain of the fascicular amplifier is larger than those recorded in **A** and **B.** (From Ishijima, M., and Hembrough, F.B.: Electrode catheterization for recording electrical activity of fasciculus atrioventricularis (Bundle of His). Am. J. Vet. Res., *40*:1800, 1979, with permission.)

Methods are also now in use, and some being evaluated, to record the His potential by noninvasive means.[29–31] The most commonly used method is the signal-averaging technique. As the equipment and methods are perfected, this technique may be clinically useful.

The indications for His bundle electrocardiography are numerous. Some of the indications include: supraventricular versus ventricular tachycardia, second-degree AV block, pre-excitation, concealed conduction, bundle branch block (bifascicular) with symptoms, and syncope (if neurologic evaluation and electrocardiographic monitoring are negative).

CARDIAC PACING

Pacemakers have now been used for years in veterinary medi-

cine.[32–35,35a,36,36a] A survey of 6 veterinary institutions reported a total of 31 cases.[37] It is estimated that approximately 30 to 60 pacemakers are implanted each year in small animals.[36a] Artificial pacemaker rhythms are produced by electrical devices that create electrical stimuli for initiating cardiac contractions.

Pacemakers consist of two major components: the pulse generator and the "electrode wire (lead)," which connects the pulse generator to the heart (Fig. 11–29). The electrode may be inserted transvenously (usually the external jugular vein), to pace the right ventricular or atrial endocardium, or transthoracically, being sutured to the left ventricular myocardium. There is a greater chance of dislodgements following placement of some endocardial leads. A sutureless "corkscrew" electrode (Medtronics sutureless myocardial pacing lead, model 6917, Medtronics, Inc., Minneapolis) is presently being used

338

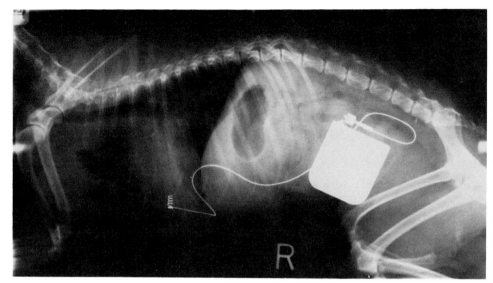
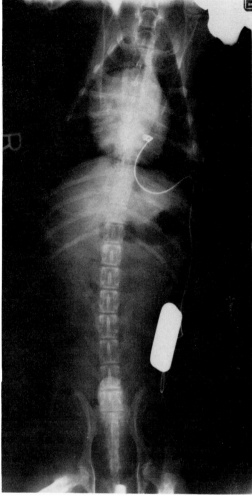

Fig. 11–29. Postoperative lateral (left photo) and dorsoventral (right photo) radiograph from a dog, after implantation of a permanent pacemaker and epicardial lead electrode. The pulse generator is situated in the left side of the abdomen. The corkscrew epicardial electrode is on the apex of the left ventricle.

at The Animal Medical Center (see Fig. 11–29). The electrode twists into the myocardium and is held in place by fibrous attachments to a polyester netting on the electrode above the tip.

Pacemaker generators

There are over 30 types of pacemakers manufactured. Two types, also commonly used in man, have been used by our institution: an asynchronous (fixed-rate) pacemaker and a synchronous (noncompetitive) pacemaker. Synchronous pacemakers are further subdivided into ventricular inhibited (demand) pacemakers and ventricular triggered (standby) pacemakers. Asynchronous pacemakers put out a continuous pulse at a fixed rate and are not synchronized with the underlying intrinsic rate of the heart. Most modern pulse generators are synchronous with the intrinsic cardiac rhythm. The synchronous pacemaker has a sensing circuit that detects spontaneous electrical ventricular activity via the electrode lead. If ventricular activity is sensed, the generators pulsing circuit does not discharge. The demand

pacemaker fires only if the pulsing circuit does not sense ventricular activity within a specific period of time. This advancement in pacemaker technology has increased the longevity of the pacemaker by decreasing the current drain from the batteries.[36a]

Pacemakers are given a three-letter code to identify the mode of operation of a pulse generator. The first letter represents the chamber paced (A = atrium, V = ventricle, and D = both); the second letter represents the chamber sensed, if any (A = atrium, V = ventricle, and O = not applicable), and the third letter represents the mode of response (I = inhibited, T = triggered, and O = not applicable).[35a,36a] Thus, VVI (a demand synchronous pacemaker) units sense intrinsic R waves and inhibit the pacemaker from discharging an electrical impulse. VOO units pace the ventricle at a fixed rate without any sensing activity.

Modern pacemakers are now quite complex, as major advances have been made in power source technology, circuit design, encapsulation technique, and pacing electrode design and technology.[38] A "typical"

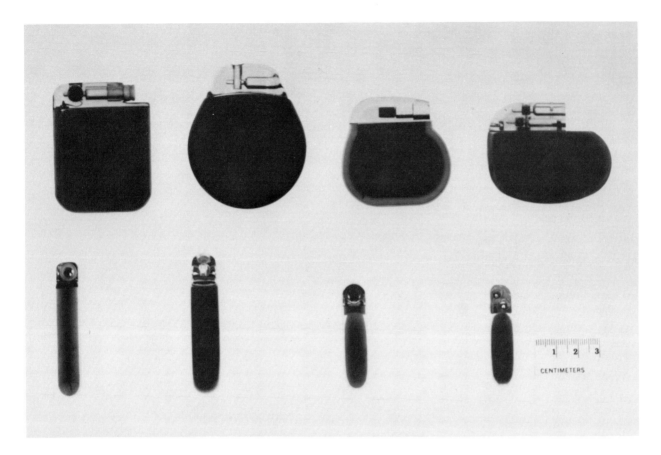

Fig. 11–30. Commonly used modern pacemakers. From left to right: Intermedics Cyber Lith, Cordis Onmi-Stanicor Theta, CPI Microthin and Medtronic Spectrax. The upper panel shows the pacemakers in the lateral view, the lower panel in the frontal view. The translucent plastic portion of each pacemaker contains the connection for the pacing electrode; the larger portion of the pacemaker consists of a metal can that contains the battery and electronic components. The battery, most often a lithium type, powers the circuitry, which converts the battery's electricity into a pulse. The duration (milliseconds), voltage (millivolts), and amperage (milliamps) of the generated pulse may be varied to provide the desired stimulus. (From Belic, N., and Gardic, J.M.: Implantable cardiac pacemakers—An overview. Int. J. Dermatol., *21*:543, 1982, with permission.)

new generation pacemaker (Fig. 11–30) is light-weight (40- to 80-g range), encapsulated in a metal container, powered by a lithium battery (expected service life of 5 to 10 years at least), contains hybrid circuitry, and allows noninvasive programming of pacing parameters.[38,38a]

Electrocardiographic features (cardiac pacing)[39,40] (*Figs. 11–31 to 11–38*)

Each time the pacemaker gives off an electrical signal (a sharp deflection on the electrocardiogram called a pacemaker spike), the signal is conducted down the wire to the heart. The pacemaker impulse then spreads into the His-Purkinje system and is conducted into the left and right ventricles, causing the heart to contract. If the pacemaker fires 90 times a minute, the heart will beat 90 times a minute. It has been recently reported in the literature that ventricular pacing does not always result in the highest possible cardiac output for a given pacing rate. It has been suggested that atrial pacing be used as the first choice, especially in the situation in which cardiac output is crucial and when complete heart block is not present.[40a] To complete the circuit in an unipolar system, the electrical impulse travels back through the body to reach the opposite terminal, a metal plate on the pacemaker itself or a second wire attached to the skin. For the bipolar system, positive and negative electrodes are on the same lead if endocardial or on two different leads if epicardial.

1. Heart rate and rhythm: The pacemaker pulse rate is regular with a fixed-rate asynchronous pacemaker. A ventricular inhibited (demand) pacemaker's rate is irregular, producing a pulse only when an intrinsic R-wave is not sensed during a given timing sequence.

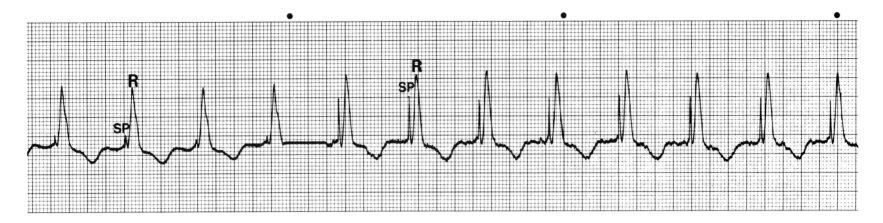

Fig. 11–31. Left bundle branch block pattern in a cat with a transvenous electrode wire in the right ventricle. In right ventricular stimulation, the left ventricle is activated late. The QRS complex width is increased to 0.06 second (3 boxes) and is positive. The first four complexes are lead I; the rest of the strip is lead II. SP, Pacemaker spike, electrical impulse delivered by the artificial pacemaker.

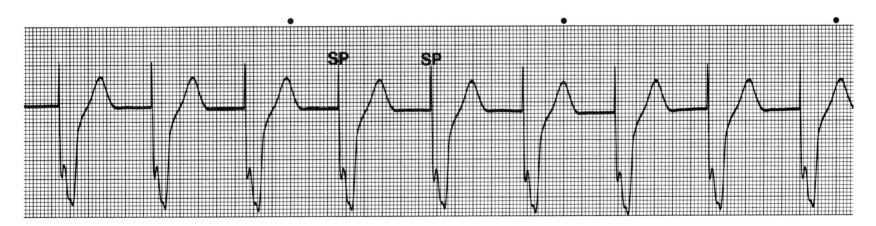

Fig. 11–32. A fixed-rate artificial pacemaker rhythm with electrode attached to the left ventricle. SP, Pacemaker spike or electrical impulse from the artificial pacemaker. A wide and bizarre QRS complex follows each spike, representing ventricular activation.

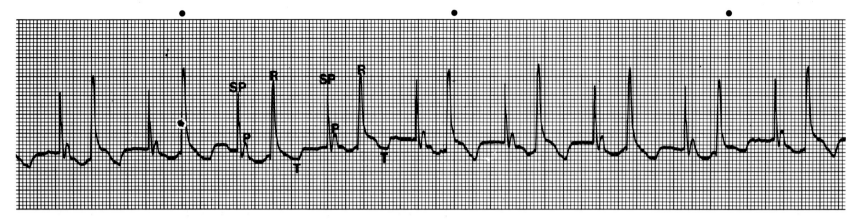

Fig. 11–33. A fixed-rate artificial pacemaker rhythm with electrode in the atrium. Each stimulus artifact (SP) is followed by a P wave and QRS-T complex.

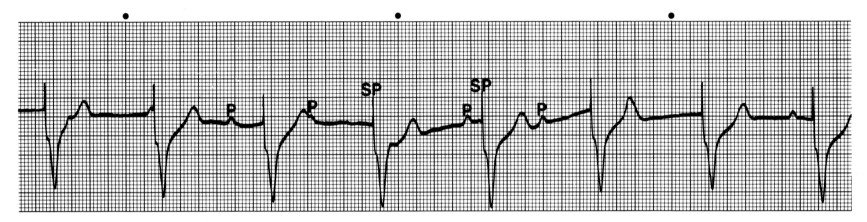

Fig. 11–34. Fixed-rate artificial pacemaker rhythm in a dog with complete heart block. The blocked P waves can still be seen. When the ventricular rate was increased with a pacemaker, this dog's fainting episodes were eliminated.

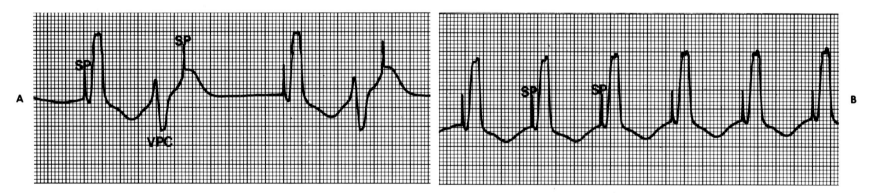

Fig. 11–35. Fixed-rate pacemaker. **A,** Spontaneous VPCs are ignored by the pacemaker, and ineffective spikes (competition) fall on the T wave during the refractory period of the ventricles. This type of pacemaker can be hazardous, especially if the spikes fall during the vulnerable period of the T wave and cause ventricular fibrillation. **B,** The pacemaker's rate was increased, and all pacemaker spikes are now effective.

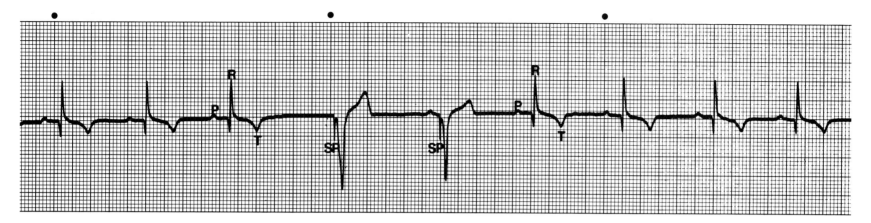

Fig. 11–36. Normal response of a demand (ventricular inhibited) pacemaker. Spontaneous sinus complexes at first are sensed and temporarily inhibit the pacemaker activity. The pacemaker unit fires when spontaneous ventricular complexes fail to occur. The pacemaker stops firing when the rate of spontaneous complexes becomes faster than the pacing rate. The "ventricular demand" pacemaker has a special switch by which the sensing function is rendered inoperative when a magnet is placed over the pacemaker. The stimulating function, however, is not affected. An analysis of pacemaker output is thus possible even when the animal's spontaneous rhythm exceeds the pacemaker rate.

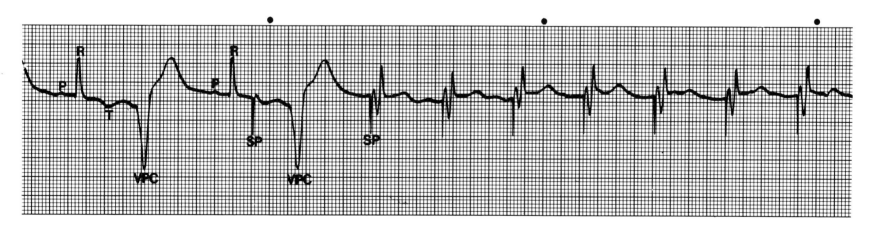

Fig. 11–37. Fixed-rate artificial pacemaker used in a dog with numerous ventricular premature complexes that were resistant to antiarrhythmic drugs. As pacemaker is turned on, the first spike is ineffective because it happens to fall on the T wave. The pacemaker rhythm rescues the heart from a potentially serious arrhythmia. Paper speed, 25 mm/sec; 0.5 cm = 1 mv.

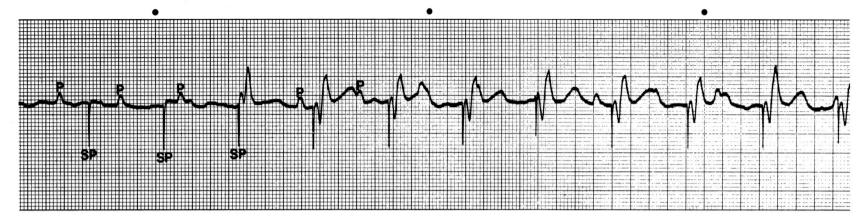

Fig. 11–38. Failure of a fixed-rate pacemaker in a dog with complete AV block. The first two spikes fail to activate the ventricles, even though the ventricles have recovered. The pacemaker unit was later changed. Paper speed, 25 mm/sec; 0.5 cm = 1 mv.

2. Pacemaker spike: A stimulus artifact or spike is followed by a P wave and QRS complex if atrial pacing, and by a QRS complex if ventricular pacing.
3. QRS complex: The QRS complex from right ventricular pacing produces a pattern of left bundle branch block. Left ventricular pacing produces a QRS pattern of right bundle branch block.
4. Pacemaker spike-QRS relationship: In fixed-rate (asynchronous) pacemakers, the spikes may fall on the QRS, ST segment, or T wave of spontaneous beats. Spikes on the T wave could cause ventricular fibrillation. In demand (synchronous) pacemakers, premature contractions as well as conducted beats can temporarily turn the pacemaker off.

Indications for cardiac pacing

Electronic pacemakers are used on a temporary or permanent basis for treating symptomatic bradycardia and occasionally for controlling a tachycardia resistant to drug therapy. As of 1979, The Animal Medical Center has implanted 13 permanent pacemakers—6 for AV block, 2 for persistent atrial standstill, and 5 for sick sinus syndrome. A 15-year-old Yorkshire Terrier (that recently died) with complete AV block had a pacemaker for 6 years.

Many conduction abnormalities that might require pacemaker insertion are acute and transient. These include infectious processes, inflammatory processes, pharmacologic effects (e.g., digoxin, propranolol), and electrolyte abnormalities (potassium).[39] Temporary pacemaker management may be needed in some cases, but permanent pacemakers should be used only for persistent defects.

Table 11–1 outlines adapted recommendations for permanent pacemaker implantations of a committee reported in the Journal of the American Medical Association, August 14, 1981.[36a,40]

Table 11–1. Guidelines for permanent pacemaker implantations*

I. Complete heart block, acquired, symptomatic
II. Congenital complete heart block, symptomatic
III. Mobitz type II block (second degree AV block), symptomatic
IV. Bifascicular block (right bundle branch block plus left anterior fascicular block) and syncopal spells not due to other central nervous system or vascular disorders
V. Sick sinus syndrome (bradycardia-tachycardia syndrome)—with periods of asystole clearly documented on EKG recording to correlate with clinical signs of severe syncope or facilitate medication treatment of tachyarrhythmia
VI. Carotid sinus hypersensitivity (sensitive carotid sinus with stimulation of vagal nerve and syncope as a result; may not be sick sinus syndrome)
VII. Overdrive for arrhythmia control (In rare cases, "overdrive" can be used to control a tachyarrhythmia)
VIII. Persistent atrial standstill, symptomatic

*Adapted from recommendations of a committee reported in the Journal of the American Medical Association, August 14, 1981.[40] These guidelines were drawn up by a committee of cardiologists and cardiac surgeons to review the adequacy of pacemaker insertions at a large teaching center. The criteria for implantation of a permanent pacemaker are not rigid and should be individualized. Symptoms such as syncope and heart failure accompanying certain arrhythmias generally indicate definitive therapy.

Pacemaker implantation

A *permanent* pacemaker is implanted in the body, either between the abdominal oblique muscles or in the abdominal cavity. A *temporary* pacemaker (Fig. 11–39) remains outside the body, with the wire coming out through the jugular vein and skin to be connected to the temporary pacemaker (Fig. 11–40). Temporary pacing is used only for a few days. The indications for temporary pacing are (1) to correct the rhythm before a permanent pacemaker is implanted, (2) to treat an arrhythmia that is not expected to last long, and (3) to see whether pacing is successful before implanting a permanent pacemaker.[41] The

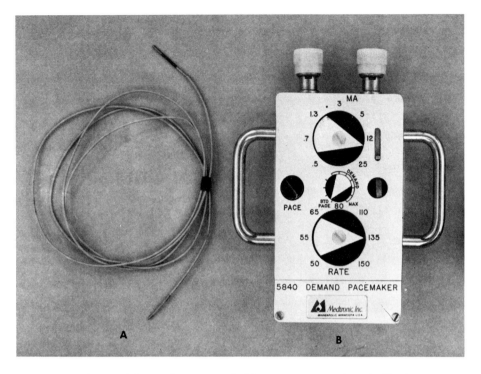

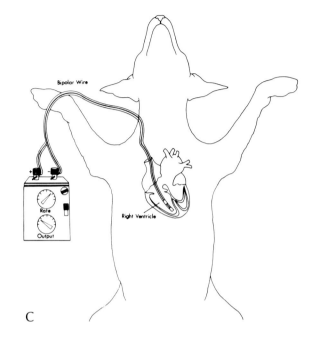

Fig. 11–39. Some of the equipment needed for temporary pacing. **A,** Bipolar electrode catheter; **B,** Medtronics external (model 5840) pacemaker for temporary pacing. **C,** Illustration of a temporary pacemaker with the electrode wire in the right ventricle for proper temporary pacing.

technique for noninvasive cardiac pacing in man has just recently been described, since temporary transvenous pacing requires skill and time for electrode insertion and at some risk.[41a]

Temporary pacing technique. An electrode for temporary pacing is placed by the same technique discussed in the previous section on intracavitary electrocardiography. An Elecath semifloating electrode or a Cordis electrode set-up is usually used, but any combination of a large-bore needle and pacing catheter that will fit through it may be used. If the procedure is done under fluoroscopic control, the position of the catheter can be observed as it passes down the anterior vena cava, into the atrium, and through the tricuspid valve into the ventricle. If fluoroscopy is not available, one of two methods can be used to determine the position of the catheter. First, the catheter can be attached to the V lead of a grounded electrocardiograph machine and the configuration of the tracing on the electrocardiographic paper observed until a large ventricular complex is seen (see Figure 11–17). Another method is to attach the catheter to a battery-operated pacemaker set at approximately 5mA with an impulse rate of approximately 10 to 15 beats greater than that of the patient's own heart rate (Fig. 11–39).[42] An electrocardiographic tracing can be observed for pacing of the heart at the atrial (see Fig. 11–33) or ventricular level (see Fig. 11–31). In most cases, the animals are paced 24 to 48 hours prior to surgery.

Epicardial pacemaker implantation.[42,43] Once the animal is stabilized with the temporary pacemaker, general anesthesia can be administered. With temporary pacing during surgery and close monitoring of the electrocardiogram, complications are kept at a minimum.

The combination of narcotics, benzodiazepines, and thiobarbiturates is preferred since the induction period is rapid, safe, and excitement-free. Drugs that cause potent direct depressant effects on Purkinje fiber automaticity or upon ventricular contractility, such as halothane or pentobarbital, should be avoided.[36,36a] Anesthesia can also be induced with low doses of thiobarbiturates (3 to 6 mg/kg, IV) and inhalation anesthetics. Inhalation anesthetics in combination with potent narcotic analgesics (fentanyl) can be used to maintain general anesthesia.[36a]

The surgical approach can include a left lateral thoracotomy or caudal one third median sternotomy and a ventral midline abdominal approach.[36,36a] The linea alba is opened to the umbilicus and carried through the caudal third of the sternum. The lateral thoracotomy is performed at the left, fifth or sixth intercostal space (Fig. 11–41). With the left ventricle exposed, a 2- to 3-cm incision is made into the pericardium to allow observation of the coronary vessels. The tip of the lead, located on the insertion tool, is placed against the epicardium and screwed with a clockwise rotation into the myocardium, with special attention to avoid the coronary vessels (Fig. 11–42). The elec-

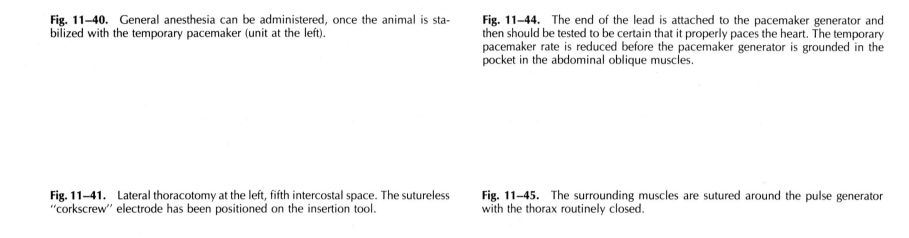

Fig. 11–40. General anesthesia can be administered, once the animal is stabilized with the temporary pacemaker (unit at the left).

Fig. 11–44. The end of the lead is attached to the pacemaker generator and then should be tested to be certain that it properly paces the heart. The temporary pacemaker rate is reduced before the pacemaker generator is grounded in the pocket in the abdominal oblique muscles.

Fig. 11–41. Lateral thoracotomy at the left, fifth intercostal space. The sutureless "corkscrew" electrode has been positioned on the insertion tool.

Fig. 11–45. The surrounding muscles are sutured around the pulse generator with the thorax routinely closed.

Fig. 11–42. The electrode is placed against the epicardium and screwed with a clockwise rotation into the myocardium, with special attention to avoid the coronary vessels. The sutureless electrode is held in place by fibrous attachments to a polyester netting on the electrode above the tip.

Fig. 11–46. Ventral midline abdominal and caudal median sternotomy approach (different dog from other figures). The lead wire can be seen passing from the heart around the diaphragm and through the peritoneum caudal to the left lobe of the liver. The generator is then placed in a mesh pouch and sutured to the left lateral peritoneal surface.

Fig. 11–43. The lead is attached to the tunneler and then passed subcutaneously from the seventh intercostal space to a subcutaneous pocket located between the external and internal abdominal oblique muscles.

Fig. 11–47. Postoperative care includes continuous electrocardiographic monitoring. A thoracic radiograph should be taken.

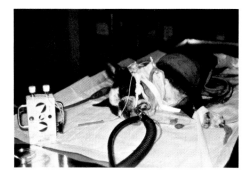

Fig. 11-40

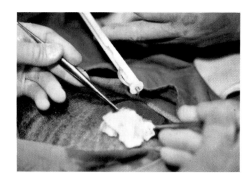

Fig. 11-41

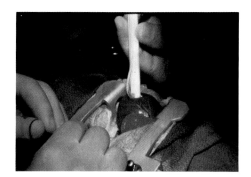

Fig. 11-42

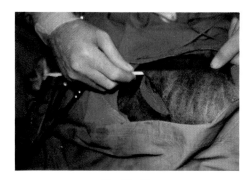

Fig. 11-43

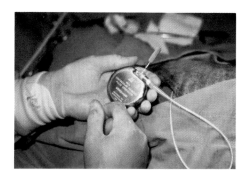

Fig. 11-44

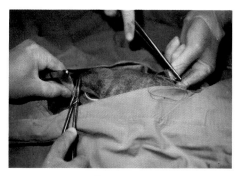

Fig. 11-45

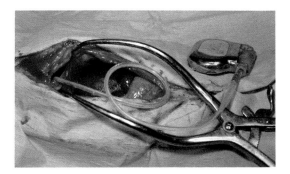

Fig. 11-46

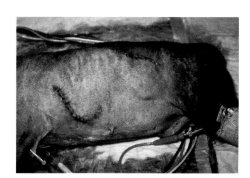

Fig. 11-47

trode is then gently released from the handle with care taken not to damage the myocardial wall. The pericardium is then loosely covered over the electrode tip. The Dacron collar should fit tightly against the ventricle. Scar tissue will form under the lead if it is too loose. The number of turns on the corkscrew indicate the number of turns necessary to properly insert the lead (usually 3 turns).

An incision in the left flank just posterior to the last rib is made to create a pocket for the pulse generator. The pocket is located between the external and internal abdominal oblique muscles. Placement between muscle layers can cause muscle stimulation in unipolar systems. The generator can also be placed against the peritoneal surface when the abdominal approach is used. A device (tunneler) is then passed subcutaneously from the pocket to the seventh intercostal space (Fig. 11–43). The lead is attached to the tunneler and pulled from the chest and attached to the pulse generator (Fig. 11–44). For the ventral midline approach, the lead wire is passed around the diaphragm and through the peritoneum caudal to the left lobe of the liver. The unit is tested to be certain that it properly paces the heart. The ground plate of the generator (+ charge) must be placed against the tissue surface. The rate of the temporary pacemaker is decreased to prevent a competitive rhythm. The electrocardiogram should show that the permanent pacemaker is discharging at its programmed rate (usually 80 to 100 beats/min) with pacemaker spike–QRS complexes present. Redundant wire cable is left in the thoracic cavity to avoid undue tension on the lead wire. The surrounding muscles are sutured around the pulse generator with the thorax closed routinely (Fig. 11–45). A polypropylene mesh pouch (Prolene mesh, Ethicon, Summit, N.J.) is recommended for storing the generator, especially to prevent migration of the generator.[36a] For the ventral approach, the mesh pouch is sutured with nonabsorbable material to the left lateral peritoneal surface caudal to the liver (Fig. 11–46). A chest tube is inserted, or thoracentesis performed following closure. Postoperative care includes continuous electrocardiographic monitoring (Fig. 11–47) and the administration of antibiotics. Radiographs are taken to confirm the location of the generator and lead wire. Most dogs can be sent home on strict confinement after 3 to 4 days. The electrocardiogram should be evaluated in 2 weeks, 1 month, and then approximately every 3 months to determine the integrity of the electrode and pulse generator. The pacemaker rate and stimulus artifact should be evaluated each time on the electrocardiogram.

Pacemaker complications in veterinary medicine have been reported.[36,37] In 11 dogs, serious complications resulted from underlying heart disease, cardiac arrhythmias, drugs and anesthetic agents, surgery, pulse generator and pacemaker lead malfunction, and infection.[36,36a] Many of these complications can be anticipated and successfully treated. Based on our experience as well as that of others,[44,45] long-term transvenous cardiac pacemakers are often accompanied by electrode displacement and secondary morphologic changes in the heart.

MANAGEMENT OF CARDIAC ARREST

Cardiac arrest is an emergency situation in which there is a sudden lack of effective myocardial contractions. The ventricles are no longer able to pump enough blood to maintain perfusion of the body's vital organs. Cardiac arrest can be correlated electrocardiographically with (1) ventricular flutter or fibrillation, (2) ventricular asystole, or (3) electrical-mechanical dissociation. (See respective sections in Chapters 6 and 7.)

Many factors can predispose an animal to cardiac arrest, including a wide variety of chronic and acute cardiovascular conditions.[46,47] Electrolyte abnormalities in animals with chronic renal disease (hyperkalemia) may result in cardiac arrest. A number of drugs, including anesthetic agents, can cause cardiac arrest. Cardiac arrest may also occur secondary to respiratory arrest. It is important to understand the causes of cardiac arrest, since prevention of the cardiopulmonary arrest is truly the basis of sound critical patient care.

The signs of cardiac arrest include: no auscultatable heart beat, no palpable arterial pulse, gray or cyanotic discoloration of the mucous membranes, dilated pupils, and no ventilatory attempts.[48,48a] The sud-

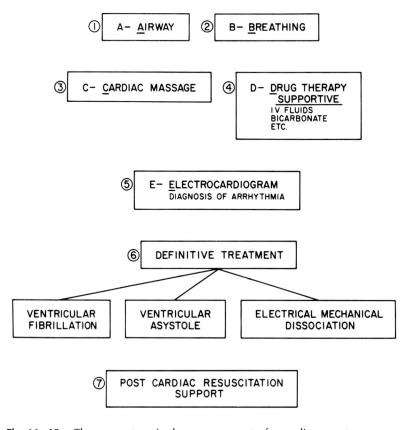

Fig. 11–48. The seven steps in the management of a cardiac arrest.

den collapse of any animal must be considered a cardiac arrest until proved otherwise. Successful treatment is vitally dependent on the immediate diagnosis of cardiac arrest. Cerebral tissue may be irreversibly damaged if totally anoxic for longer than 3 to 4 minutes. Emergency cardiopulmonary resuscitation should be instituted in the absence of a pulse in a collapsed animal, even if respiration continues.

The basic principles for the management of cardiac arrest are illustrated as a flow chart in Figure 11–48. The steps outlined are discussed only briefly. Pertinent references should be consulted for further information.[2,46,48–53] To effectively manage a cardiac arrest, the clinician must follow seven steps, but before he does this, he must first establish the diagnosis of cardiac arrest and decide whether the animal should be resuscitated. Necessary equipment and drugs should be organized and set up in advance. Drug dosages (Table 11–2) and protocols should be posted in plain view. Successful resuscitation is usually accomplished within 5 to 10 minutes of the arrest, but as long as 30 to 40 minutes may be needed.[48a]

Seven steps in resuscitation

The first five steps in the management of cardiac arrest represent the "A-B-C-D-E" of resuscitation (Fig. 11–48). The sixth step is treating the arrhythmia. The seventh and final step is managing the animal after resuscitation.

Step 1. A—Airway

The first and perhaps most important maneuver during resuscitation is establishing an open airway. An open airway should be established and maintained by endotracheal intubation.

Step 2. B—Breathing

Artificial ventilation should be supplied, preferably with 100% oxygen. Intermittent positive-pressure ventilation at one ventilation every 5 seconds or approximately every fifth chest compression should be done. If there is no tracheal tube, mouth-to-nostril breathing will allow some air exchange.

Step 3. C—Cardiac massage or circulation

External cardiac compression is done by placing the animal in right lateral recumbency. The heel of one hand is placed under the thorax at the level of the fifth rib interspace. The heel of the other hand is brought vertically downward over the first at the rate of 60 to 80 cycles per minute. A general rule is to compress the heart for about one third of a cycle and release for about two thirds of a cycle. A recent study demonstrated that cardiac stroke volume and coronary blood flow was maximized with manual chest compression performed with moderate force and brief duration.[48b] It is important to restore cardiac action as soon as possible. In large or barrel-chested breeds, external cardiac compression may not be effective.

Adjunctive procedures that increase intrathoracic pressure during chest compression such as simultaneous ventilation[48,48a,54] and/or ab-

dominal binding[55] can possibly be used. Simultaneous compression ventilation consists of chest compressions administered simultaneously with ventilations at a high airway pressure. Simultaneous ventilation and/or abdominal binding should probably be avoided until evidence is found that proves that these techniques improve survival.[56] A recent article reports that coronary blood flow is not improved despite increased carotid blood flow.[56a]

Internal cardiac compression is indicated whenever it is determined that the external technique is ineffective. If the artificial circulation procedure is effective, there will be an improvement in mucous membrane color and a reduction in pupil size. A common misconception is that the technique of cardiopulmonary resuscitation is adequate if external chest compression results in a strong palpable arterial pulse. It should be understood that successful cardiopulmonary resuscitation is independent of the systolic arterial pressure generated during chest compression but instead depends upon an adequate aortic diastolic pressure.[56] Drugs and techniques that increase diastolic and mean blood pressure during the resuscitation procedure improve survival.

Step 4. D—Drug therapy

Rapid establishment of an intravenous line is an important aspect of cardiac resuscitation. A rapid infusion of lactated Ringer's solution (or equivalent solution) should be given to fill the increasing capacity of the vascular compartment.[48] The objectives of drug therapy during cardiac arrest are, first, to increase blood flow to the coronary arteries, and, second, to minimize the adverse effects of metabolic acidosis secondary to inadequate tissue perfusion.[52] Epinephrine can be effective by its action of increasing peripheral vascular resistance, while also increasing aortic diastolic pressure.[56] Increased coronary blood flow is the result.[56b] Epinephrine is also useful for the conversion of "fine" to "coarse" fibrillation, which is necessary for successful electrical defibrillation. There should be no delay in using a vasoconstrictor such as epinephrine during cardiac arrest.[56] Drugs that have their principal effect by cardiac stimulation, such as isoproterenol, may be useful in supporting circulation after the heart is restarted, but are not effective during cardiac arrest.[56] Dopamine, dobutamine, or mephentermine for hypotension are also used in the postresuscitation period because of their ability to support myocardial contractility and blood pressure.

Sodium bicarbonate is used to prevent metabolic acidosis from lowering the threshold of the heart to ventricular fibrillation. Sodium bicarbonate is often used in excess during attempted cardiopulmonary resuscitation. When resuscitation with adequate ventilation is started within 3 minutes of cardiac arrest, the arterial pH increases progressively, and for the first 5 minutes the animal becomes alkalotic.[56] Just after defibrillation and/or restoration of an adequate perfusion pressure, there is a marked drop in arterial pH. This is the time for bicarbonate therapy, since lactic acidosis should be treated.[56]

Lidocaine has been shown to increase the threshold for ventricular fibrillation.[53] It is also useful for suppressing ventricular ectopic ac-

Table 11–2. Drugs used in the management of cardiac resuscitation*[48a,49]

Generic name	Trade name	Major indications	Dosage and route of administration
Cardiostimulatory and vasoactive agents			
Epinephrine	Adrenalin	Cardiac arrest	IC: 6–10 µg/kg IV: 0.05–0.5 mg (0.5–5 ml 1:10,000 dilution) for average-sized dog (15 kg)
Isoproterenol	Isuprel	Sinus bradycardia, complete AV block, cardiac stimulation	IV: 0.4 mg in 250 ml of 5% dextrose/water and titrate to effect
Dopamine	Intropin	Increases heart rate, cardiac output, and mean arterial blood pressure. Improves blood flow to coronary, renal, and mesenteric circulation	IV: 80–200 mg in 500 ml of 5% dextrose/water. Drip slowly at rate of 2–10 µg/kg/min to effect
Mephentermine	Wyamine	Blood pressure support	IV: 0.1–0.5 mg/kg
Dobutamine	Dobutrex	Blood pressure support	IV: 100–400 mg in 500 ml 5% dextrose/water to effect, start 5 µg/kg/min (10–20 µg/kg/min as maximum)
Calcium		Increases cardiac output, ventricular asystole, and electrical-mechanical dissociation	IV., IC: 0.05–0.10 ml/kg of the 10% solution
Sodium bicarbonate		Buffers acidosis	IV: 0.5–1.0 mEq/kg
Isotonic intravenous fluids		Expand the blood volume. Treat hypotension. Increase tissue perfusion	IV: 40 ml/kg (dog); 20 ml/kg (cat) of lactated Ringer's or equivalent solution
Atropine		Parasympatholytic effects	IV: 0.01–0.02 mg/kg
Lidocaine	Xylocaine (without epinephrine)	Ventricular premature complexes, ventricular tachycardia	IV: 2–4 mg/kg, repeat to maximum of 8 mg/kg. CRI (dog): 25–75 µg/kg/min. For the cat 0.25 to 1 mg/kg over 5 min
Procainamide	Pronestyl	Ventricular premature complexes, ventricular tachycardia	IV: 6–8 mg/kg over 5 min, 25–40 µg/kg/min (to effect), CRI: 25–40 µg/kg/min
Propranolol	Inderal	Supraventricular tachyarrhythmias, ventricular premature complexes	IV: 0.04–0.06 mg/kg slowly
Mannitol		Osmotic diuretic: reduces cerebral edema	IV: 1–2 g/kg

IC = intracardiac
IV = intravenously
Formula for CRI (constant-rate infusion): Body weight (in kg) × dose (in µg/kg/min) × 0.36 = total dose in mg to administer intravenously over 6 hours
*Antiarrhythmic agents are discussed in detail in Chapter 10.

tivity. Calcium in cardiac arrest provides increased myocardial contractility and the enhancement of ventricular excitability. It is primarily indicated for the "flabby" or weakly beating heart with a restoration of electrical rhythm in asystole.[53]

The essential drugs utilized in cardiac arrest include oxygen, sodium bicarbonate, epinephrine, atropine sulfate, lidocaine, and calcium chloride. Other useful drugs include vasoactive drugs (e.g., levarterenol), isoproterenol, propranolol, corticosteroids, dopamine, diuretics, and procainamide.[53] Cardiotonic drugs like catecholamines and calcium should be administered directly into the left ventricle. Drugs can be given intravenously when the desired effect is peripheral or when large volumes of drugs are to be administered.[48a] Table 11–2 summarizes the drugs used during and after cardiac resuscitation.[48a,49]

Step 5. E—Electrocardiogram

An electrocardiogram should be obtained to diagnose the arrhythmia responsible for the cardiac arrest—usually ventricular fibrillation, asystole, or electrical-mechanical dissociation.

Step 6. Treatment of the Arrhythmia

This subject is covered in the respective sections of Chapters 6 and 7, and discussed in detail in Chapter 10 on antiarrhythmic therapy. The following is a summary of the management of three cardiac arrhythmias associated with cardiac arrest (Fig. 11–48).

Electromechanical dissociation. Electromechanical dissociation is uncommon, with very guarded prognosis. Treatment includes the use of sodium bicarbonate, epinephrine, calcium chloride, and isoproterenol. Adequate electrical stimulation without adequate mechanical response on occasion may be due to massive acute hypovolemia, instead of a severely failing myocardial muscle. In these cases, fluid therapy may be helpful.[52]

Ventricular asystole. Ventricular asystole may be either a primary asystolic arrest or may be a result of degeneration of another arrest rhythm. Treatment protocols involve the use of sodium bicarbonate, epinephrine, calcium chloride, atropine sulfate, and dopamine hydrochloride. Atropine may be very effective, especially when the asystole is due to marked increases in vagal tone.

Ventricular fibrillation. Ventricular fibrillation is the most common rhythm in cardiac arrest and is the arrhythmia most likely to respond to therapy. Just recently, the American Heart Association has changed its position and now suggests immediate defibrillation for any patient with ventricular fibrillation.[57] In the past, it has always been suggested that the acidosis and hypoxia be corrected before defibrillation is attempted. If defibrillation is unsuccessful, the animal should receive sodium bicarbonate, epinephrine, and lidocaine therapy. This should be followed by a second attempt at defibrillation. Other antiarrhythmic agents such as procainamide may also be used. Before further defibrillation attempts, the protocol should be proper oxygenation, correction of severe acidosis and electrolyte abnormalities, and attempts to determine and correct any other possible underlying cause.[48,48a,57] Pharmacologic defibrillation may be effective: a mixture of 1.0 mEq potassium/kg body weight and 6.0 mg acetylcholine/kg body weight by intracardiac injection.

Step 7. Postcardiac resuscitation support

The seventh step in the management of a cardiac arrest involves stabilizing the condition of the cardiac arrest case. Follow-up support involves: ensuring effective ventilation, establishing and maintaining an effective cardiac rhythm and circulation, maintaining effective electrocardiographic monitoring, and maintaining an intravenous fluid drip for administering appropriate drugs.

CARDIOVERSION AND DEFIBRILLATION

Cardioversion is the method of electrically converting arrhythmias to a sinus rhythm by a timed delivery of direct current shock. Defibrillation is the electrical conversion of fibrillation to a sinus rhythm without a timed delivery. The technique of electrical cardioversion and defibrillation is described in various reports.[46-51,58-62] Electroshock therapy is used as an emergency procedure during ventricular fibrillation and also for the conversion of certain fast cardiac rhythms. An electrical shock causes instant depolarization of an ectopic rhythm, often re-establishing the sinoatrial pacemaker.

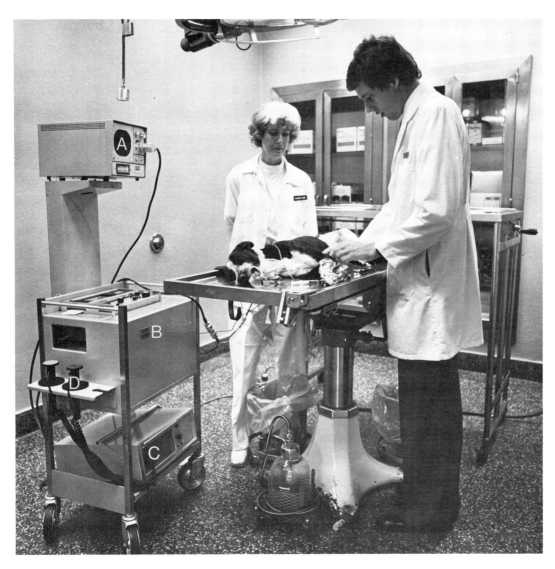

Fig. 11–49. An oscilloscope (A) can be used to continually monitor the electrocardiogram (B). A unit for cardioversion or defibrillation (C) converts certain arrhythmias unresponsive to drugs. The paddles (D) for cardioversion or defibrillation are applied to each side of the thorax. (Courtesy of Burdick Corp., Milton, Wis.)

Cardioversion

Equipment (Fig. 11–49) currently available is capable of delivering up to 400 watt-seconds of direct current by means of paddles applied to the animal's skin. The delivered current can be programmed to be triggered by the R waves of the electrocardiogram, thereby avoiding the apex of the T wave (the vulnerable phase of ventricular excitability) (Fig. 11–50). The vulnerable phase of ventricular excitability has been shown to occur 27 msec before the end of ventricular systole (or just before the end of the T wave) in the dog.[60] Synchronization with the R wave is ideal in the electrical cardioversion of the rapid cardiac rhythm disturbances. If no synchronizer is available, an unsynchronized direct current shock can still be used since the chance of ventricular fibrillation is only 2%.[60] It is important, however, that a higher-energy level setting be used in this situation. For ventricular fibrillation, a nonprogrammed shock only is needed.

Cardioversion may be recommended for the following rapid cardiac rhythm disturbances: (1) atrial fibrillation, such as found with patent ductus arteriosus, in which the underlying cause has been corrected, (2) atrial flutter, (3) ventricular tachycardia that is not responsive to drugs, and (4) atrial tachycardia that does not respond to routine measures and when the animal is being affected hemodynamically.

In general, the following measures for cardioversion should be taken:

1. Digoxin should be withheld for 1 to 2 days if possible. Electrical stimulation can potentiate the effects of digoxin. A short-acting barbiturate or diazepam (Valium) intravenously administered may be needed for the awake animal with a rapid cardiac rhythm.[63]
2. The electrocardiographic electrodes are attached to the animal and the cardiac rhythm analyzed. The paddles are well lubricated with electrode paste and positioned with one paddle over the apex and the other over the base of the heart.
3. The cardioverter is synchronized with the R wave of the QRS complex for cardioversion of a tachyarrhythmia.
4. When the energy setting is established, all persons are to stand clear of the table. The discharge is fired, and the electrocardiogram is immediately checked. The initial energy settings for the supraventricular and ventricular tachycardias are 10 to 50 watt-seconds, followed as necessary by 25 to 50 watt-second increments.
5. If the animal does not convert, the procedure is repeated at a higher energy level.

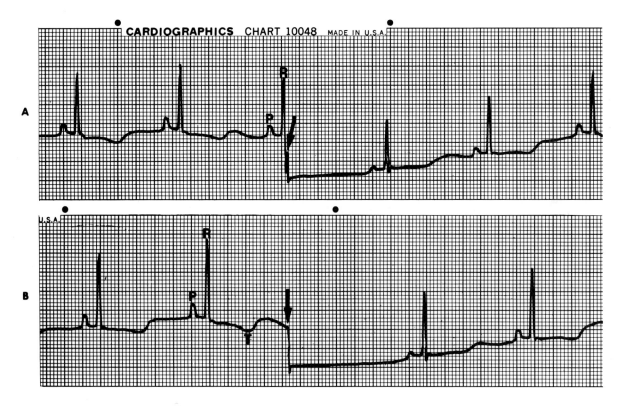

Fig. 11–50. Test electrical shock (arrow) (defibrillation paddles held together). **A,** Synchronization with the R wave of the QRS, ideal for the electrical conversion of rapid cardiac rhythm disturbances. **B,** No synchronization, for the electrical conversion of ventricular fibrillation.

Defibrillation

With ventricular fibrillation, the initial dose of 0.5 to 10 watt-sec/kg is advised. If this has no effect, the energy dose should be doubled. For internal defibrillation (spoon-shaped paddles), 0.2 to 0.4 watt-sec/kg is advisable.[60] The factors that determine the shock strength for defibrillation and cardioversion should be known—body weight, electrolyte imbalances, myocardial ischemia, drug actions, and body temperature.[64,65] The size and frequency of the waves in ventricular fibrillation are also related to the success of defibrillation. Epinephrine, adequate oxygenation, calcium, and bicarbonate will restore a coarse fibrillation and make the heart more susceptible to electrical defibrillation. The incidence of myocardial damage increases directly with the increases in voltage applied.[57,58,66] Multiple low-energy shocks and intravenous verapamil have recently been shown to reduce cardiac damage.[67] After adequate support therapy has been provided, the lubricated paddles are applied firmly to the chest wall or heart. When the energy setting is established, the discharge is fired after all personnel are clear of the animal, the table, and accompanying equipment. The electrocardiogram is immediately checked for cardioversion. Cardiopulmonary support therapy is re-instituted. If the heart did not defibrillate the first time, the procedure is repeated at a higher power setting.

REFERENCES

1. His, W., Jr.: Die Thätigkeit des embryonalen Herzens und deren Bedeutung für die Lehre von der Herzbewegung beim Erwachsenen, *Arbeiten aus der med. Klin. zu Leipzig,* 1893, pp. 14–50.
2. Bilitch, M.: *A Manual of Cardiac Arrhythmias.* Boston, Little, Brown, 1971.
3. Lynfield, J.: Paroxysmal atrial tachycardia in infants and children. Lancet, *1*:1235, 1971.
4. Befeler, B.: Mechanical stimulation of the heart, its therapeutic value in tachyarrhythmias. Chest, *73*:832, 1978.
5. Pennington, J.E., Taylor, J., and Lown, B.: Chest thump for reverting ventricular tachycardia. N. Engl. J. Med., *283*:1192, 1970.
6. Banka, V.S., and Helfant, R.H.: Ventricular arrhythmias. In *Bellet's Essentials of Cardiac Arrhythmias.* Edited by R.H. Helfant. 2nd Edition. Philadelphia, W.B. Saunders, 1980.
7. Tilley, L.P.: Advanced electrocardiographic techniques. Vet. Clin. North Am., *13*:365, 1983.
8. Ariet, M., and Crevasse, L.E.: Status report on computerized ECG analysis. JAMA, *239*:1201, 1978.
9. Jenkins, J.M.: Automated electrocardiography and arrhythmia monitoring. Prog. Cardiovasc. Dis., *25*:367, 1983.
10. Anderson, G.J.: Computerized electrocardiographic systems in the 1980's. In *New Diagnostic Techniques. Proceedings from the 55th Hahneman Symposium.* Edited by H.A. Miller et al. New York, Grune & Stratton, 1982.
11. Bernard, P., et al.: Comparative diagnostic performance of the Telamed computer ECG program. J. Electrocardiol., *16*:97, 1983.
12. Rautaharju, P.M., et al.: Task Force III: Computers in diagnostic electrocardiography. Am. J. Cardiol., *41*:158, 1978.
13. Kehoe, R., et al.: Adriamycin-induced cardiac dysrhythmias in an experimental dog model. Cancer Treat. Rep., *62*:963, 1978.
14. Branch, C.E., Beckett, S.D., and Robertson, B.T.: Spontaneous syncopal attacks in dogs: a method of documentation. J. Am. Anim. Hosp. Assoc., *13*:673, 1977.
15. Klein, G.J., and Gulamhusein, S.S.: Undiagnosed syncope: search for an arrhythmic etiology. Stroke, *13*:746, 1982.
16. Fisher, J.D.: Role of electrophysiologic testing in the diagnosis and treatment of patients with known and suspected bradycardias and tachycardias. Prog. Cardiovasc. Dis., *24*:25, 1981.
17. Michelson, E.L., and Dreifus, L.S.: The diagnosis of arrhythmias—the relative roles of the ECG, Holter monitoring, exercise stress testing, and electrophysiologic studies. Med. Times, *108*:35, 1980.
18. Wiener, I.: Current applications of clinical electrophysiologic study in the diagnosis and treatment of cardiac arrhythmias. Am. J. Cardiol., *49*:1287, 1982.
18a.Scheinman, M.M., and Morady, F.: Invasive cardiac electrophysiologic testing: the current state of the art. Circulation, *67*:1169, 1983.
19. DiMarco, J.P., Garan, H., and Ruskin, J.N.: Approach to the patient with recurrent syncope of unknown cause. Mod. Concepts Cardiovasc. Dis., *52*:11, 1983.
20. Wellens, H.J.J.: Value and limitations of programmed electrical stimulation of the heart in the study and treatment of tachycardias. Circulation, *57*:845, 1978.
21. Tilley, L.P., and Weitz, J.: Pharmacologic and other forms of medical therapy in feline cardiac disease. Vet. Clin. North Am., *7*:425, 1977.
22. Muir, W.W.: Electrocardiographic interpretation of thiobarbiturate-induced dysrhythmias in dogs. J. Am. Vet. Med. Assoc., *170*:1419, 1977.
23. Pittman, D.E., and Gay, T.C.: Diagnostic uses of intraatrial electrocardiography. Angiology, *28*:599, 1977.
24. Vogel, J.K., et al.: A simple technique for identifying P waves in complex arrhythmias. Am. Heart J., *67*:158, 1964.
25. Damato, A.N., et al.: Study of atrioventricular conduction in man using electrode catheter recording of His bundle activity. Circulation, *39*:287, 1969.
26. Scherlag, B.J., Helfant, R.H., and Damato, A.N.: A catheterization technique for His bundle stimulation and recording in the intact dog. J. Appl. Physiol., *25*:425, 1968.
27. Scherlag, B.J., Kosowsky, B.D., and Damato, A.N.: Technique for ventricular pacing from the His bundle of the intact heart. J. Appl. Physiol., *22*:584, 1967.
28. Ishijima, M., and Hembrough, F.B.: Electrode catheterization for recording electrical activity of fasciculus atrioventricularis (Bundle of His). Am. J. Vet. Res., *40*:1800, 1979.
29. Allor, D.R.: A non-invasive method of recording a serial His-Purkinje study in man. J. Cardiovasc. Pulm. Technology, *8*:16, 1980.
30. Flowers, N.C., et al.: Surface recording of electrical activity from the region of the bundle of His. Am. J. Cardiol., *33*:384, 1974.
31. Beribari, E.J., et al.: Noninvasive technique for detection of electrical activity during the P-R segment. Circulation, *48*:1005, 1973.
32. Brown, K.K.: Bradyarrhythmias and pacemaker therapy. In *Current Veterinary Therapy: Small Animal Practice.* Volume 6. Edited by R.W. Kirk. Philadelphia, W.B. Saunders, 1977.
33. Buchanan, J.W., Dear, M.G., Pyle, R.L., and Berg, P.: Medical and pacemaker therapy of complete heart block and congestive heart failure in a dog. J. Am. Vet. Med. Assoc., *152*:1099, 1968.
34. Clark, D.R., et al.: Artificial pacemaker implantation for control of sinoatrial syncope in a miniature Schnauzer. Southwest. Vet., *28*:101, 1975.
35. Webb, T.J., Clark, D.R., and McCrady, J.D.: Artificial cardiac pacemakers and some clinical indications for pacemaking. Southwest. Vet., *28*:91, 1975.
35a.Kimm, S.M., and Hill, B.L.: Indications and technique for permanent cardiac pacemaker implantation in the dog. Iowa State Veterinarian, *45*:37, 1983.
36. Bonagura, J.D., Helphrey, M.L., and Muir, W.W.: Complications associated with permanent pacemaker implantation in the dog. J. Am. Vet. Med. Assoc., *182*:149, 1983.
36a.Helphrey, M.L., and Schollmeyer, M.: Pacemaker therapy. In *Current Veterinary Therapy: Small Animal Practice.* Volume 8. Edited by R.W. Kirk. Philadelphia, W.B. Saunders, 1983.
37. Lombard, C., Tilley, L.P., and Yoshioka, M.: Pacemaker implantation in the dog: Survey and literature review. Am. Hosp. Assoc. J., *17*:751, 1981.
38. Belic, N., and Gardin, J.M.: Implantable cardiac pacemakers—an overview. Int. J. Dermatol., *21*:543, 1982.
38a.Parsonnet, V. (Chairman), Furman, S., Smyth, N.P.D., and Bilitch, M.: Optimal resources for implantable cardiac pacemakers. Pacemaker study group. Circulation, *68*:227A, 1983.
39. Foster, P.R., and Zipes, D.P.: Pacing and cardiac arrhythmias. In *Cardiac Arrhythmias—Their Mechanisms, Diagnosis, and Management.* Edited by W.J. Mandel. Philadelphia, J.B. Lippincott Co., 1980.
40. Chokshi, A.B., et al.: Impact of peer review in reduction of permanent pacemaker implantations. JAMA, *246*:754, 1981.
40a.Zaidan, J.R.: Pacemakers. Anesthesiology, *60*:319, 1984.
41. Furman, S.: Cardiac pacing and pacemakers. I. Indications for pacing bradyarrhythmias. Am. Heart J., *93*:523, 1977.

41a. Falk, R.H., Zoll, P.M., and Zoll, R.H.: Safety and efficacy of noninvasive cardiac pacing. N. Engl. J. Med., *309*:1166, 1983.
42. Mansour, K.A., Dorney, E.R., and King III, S.B.: Techniques for insertion of pervenous and epicardial pacemakers. In *The Heart.* J.W. Hurst, Editor-in-chief. 5th Edition. New York, McGraw-Hill, 1982.
43. Yoshioka, M.M., et al.: Permanent pacemaker implantation in the dog. J. Am. Anim. Hosp. Assoc., *17*:746, 1981.
44. Cummings, J.R., et al.: Long term evaluation in large dogs and sheep of a series of new fixed-rate and ventricular synchronous pacemakers. J. Thorac. Cardiovasc. Surg., *66*:645, 1973.
45. Fishbein, M.C., et al.: Cardiac pathology of transvenous pacemakers in dogs. Am. Heart J., *93*:73, 1977.
46. Morgan, R.V.: Cardiac emergencies—Part II. Compend. Contin. Educ. Pract Vet., *3*:838, 1981.
47. Ross, J.N., and Breznock, E.M.: Resuscitation. In *Veterinary Critical Care.* Edited by F.P. Sattler, R.P. Knowles, and W.G. Whittick. Philadelphia, Lea & Febiger, 1981.
48. Haskins, S.C.: Cardiopulmonary resuscitation. Compend. Contin. Educ. Pract. Vet., *3*:170, 1982.
48a. Haskins, S.C.: Cardiopulmonary resuscitation. In *Current Veterinary Therapy: Small Animal Practice.* Volume 8. Edited by R.W. Kirk. Philadelphia, W.B. Saunders, 1983.
48b. Maier, G.W., et al.: The physiology of external cardiac massage: high impulse cardiopulmonary resuscitation. Circulation, *70*:86, 1984.
49. Bonagura, J.D.: Feline cardiovascular emergencies. Vet. Clin. North Am., 7:385, 1977.
50. Paddleford, R., and Short, C.E.: Cardiopulmonary resuscitation in the small animal patient. Canine Pract., *4*:63, 1977.
51. Clark, D.R.: Recognition and treatment of cardiac emergencies. J. Am. Vet. Med. Assoc., *171*:98, 1977.
52. DeBard, M.C.: Cardiopulmonary resuscitation: Analysis of six years experience and review of the literature. Ann. Emerg. Med., *10*:408, 1981.
53. Adams, H.R.: Cardiovascular emergencies—drugs and resuscitative principles. Vet. Clin. North Am., *11*:77, 1981.
54. Luce, J.M., et al.: Regional blood flow during cardiopulmonary resuscitation in dogs using simultaneous and nonsimultaneous compression and ventilation. Circulation, *67*:258, 1983.
55. Koehler, R.C., et al.: Augmentation of cerebral perfusion by simultaneous chest compression and lung inflation with abdominal binding after cardiac arrest in dogs. Circulation, *67*:266, 1983.
56. Ewy, G.A.: Cardiopulmonary resuscitation: 1983. Medical Times, *111*:60, 1983.
56a. Nieman, J.T., Rosborough, J.P., Ung, S., and Criley, J.M.: Hemodynamic effects of continuous abdominal binding during cardiac arrest and resuscitation. Am. J. Cardiol., *53*:269, 1984.
56b. Michael, J.R., et al.: Mechanisms by which epinephrine augments cerebral and myocardial perfusion during cardiopulmonary resuscitation in dogs. Circulation, *69*:822, 1984.
57. Standards and guidelines for cardiopulmonary resuscitation (CPR) and emergency cardiac care (ECC). JAMA, *244*:453, 1980.
58. Chameides, L., et al.: Guidelines for defibrillation in infants and children. Report of the American Heart Association target activity group, Circulation, *56*:502A, 1977.
59. Ettinger, S.J.: Conversion of spontaneous atrial fibrillation in dogs, using direct current synchronized shock. J. Am. Vet. Med. Assoc., *152*:41, 1968.
60. Resenkov, L.: Present status of electroversion in the management of cardiac dysrhythmias. Circulation, *47*:1356, 1973.
61. Resnekov, L.: High-energy electrical current in the management of cardiac dysrhythmias. In *Cardiac Arrhythmias.* Edited by W.J. Mandel. Philadelphia, J.B. Lippincott, 1980.
62. Lown, B., and DeSilva, R.A.: The technique of cardioversion. In *The Heart.* Edited by J.W. Hurst. 5th Edition. New York, McGraw-Hill, 1982.
63. Muenster, J.J., Rosenburg, M.S., Carleton, R.H., and Graettinger, J.S.: Comparison between diazepam and sodium thiopental during DC countershock. JAMA, *10*:168, 1967.
64. Babbs, C.F.: Effect of pentobarbital anesthesia on ventricular defibrillation threshold in dogs. Am. Heart J., *95*:331, 1978.
65. Geddes, L.A., et al.: Electrical dose for ventricular defibrillation of large and small animals using precordial electrodes. J. Clin. Invest., *53*:310, 1974.
66. Van Vleet, J.F., Tacker, W.A., Geddes, L.A., and Ferrans, V.J.: Sequential cardiac morphologic alternations induced in dogs by single transthoracic dampened sinusoidal waveform defibrillator shocks. Am. J. Vet. Res., *39*:271, 1978.
67. Patton, J.N., Allen, J.D., and Pantridge, J.F.: The effects of shock energy, propranolol, and verapamil on cardiac damage caused by transthoracic countershock. Circulation, *69*:357, 1984.

Section Six

Interpretation of Complex Arrhythmias

12 Uncommon complex arrhythmias

Because they were human men. They were trying to write down the heart's truth out of the heart's driving complexity, for all the complex and troubled hearts which would beat after them.*

WILLIAM FAULKNER, 1942

The diagnosis of some arrhythmias can be difficult because the routine surface electrocardiogram provides only a superficial understanding of the electrophysiologic events. Electrophysiologic studies discussed in Chapter 11, such as the recording of His bundle electrograms have been helpful in clarifying certain of these arrhythmias in the dog.[1-4] Many complex arrhythmias are subject to multiple interpretations, and cardiologists often disagree as to which is correct. The diagnosis of complex arrhythmias and an understanding of their mechanisms constitute an added stimulation as well as a frustration to clinicians proficient in electrocardiography.

Many abnormalities of impulse formation and/or conduction require a knowledge of electrophysiologic principles. These principles are discussed in detail in Chapter 9. The concept of arrhythmias in man has undergone many changes during the last several years. The knowledge and clinical application of electrophysiologic principles are extensive and well established in man. Understanding these principles is essential to the explanation of arrhythmias in dogs and cats.

It is beyond the scope of this section to provide a detailed discussion of complex arrhythmias. The literature on the subject can be consulted to enhance the reader's knowledge.[5-8a] The mechanisms of some of these arrhythmias will be discussed briefly, and examples of several will be presented.

LADDER DIAGRAMS

The ladder diagram technique, which is used commonly in man, enhances the clinician's understanding of arrhythmias.[9] It has not been described in the veterinary literature. Ladder diagrams are a valuable teaching and interpretive tool and should be applied to the field of veterinary cardiology. They are used in this section only to explain the more complex arrhythmias, when illustrating the underlying mechanisms would otherwise be difficult. To further clarify the mechanism outlined, the clinician should feel free to apply the ladder diagram technique to any other arrhythmia.

The technique (Figs. 12–1 and 12–2)

The electrocardiogram is first mounted on a piece of paper. The AV ladder diagram is then drawn or placed beneath the electrocardiogram. (*A*, Atrial conduction; *V*, ventricular conduction: *A-V*, conduction in the AV junction.) A ruler is used to line up the beginning of the P waves with a subsequent line drawn at the A level. The ventricular complexes are then drawn in the V level, a line coinciding with the beginning of the ventricular complexes. The last step consists of indicating AV conduction by connecting the bottom of the atrial line with the top of the ventricular line. A dot is used to indicate the site of impulse formation.

Representative examples of the AV ladder diagram in various arrhythmias are illustrated in Figure 12–1. This simple teaching tool is surprisingly useful for understanding many of the complex arrhythmias.

---

*Faulkner, W.: "The Bear." *The Saturday Evening Post.* Volume CCXIV, May 9, 1942.

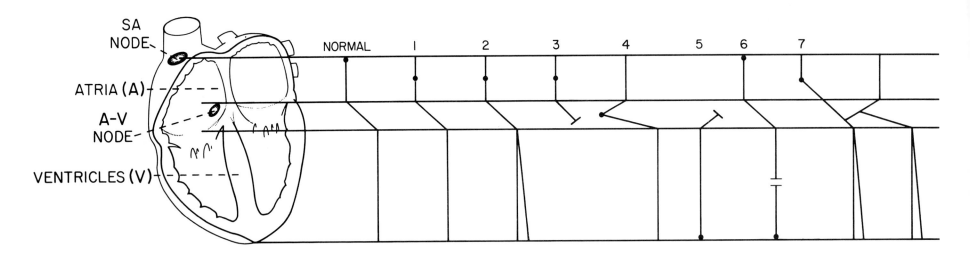

Fig. 12–1. Representative examples of the AV ladder diagram: **1,** Atrial premature complex (APC) with normal conduction; **2,** APC with aberrant ventricular conduction (also used to illustrate left and right bundle branches); **3,** APC not conducted; **4,** AV junctional premature complex with anterograde ventricular and retrograde atrial conduction; **5,** ventricular premature complex (VPC) with partial penetration of the AV junction; **6,** ventricular fusion complex between a sinus impulse and an ectopic ventricular impulse; **7,** APC and one reciprocal complex (re-entry) with aberrant ventricular conduction.

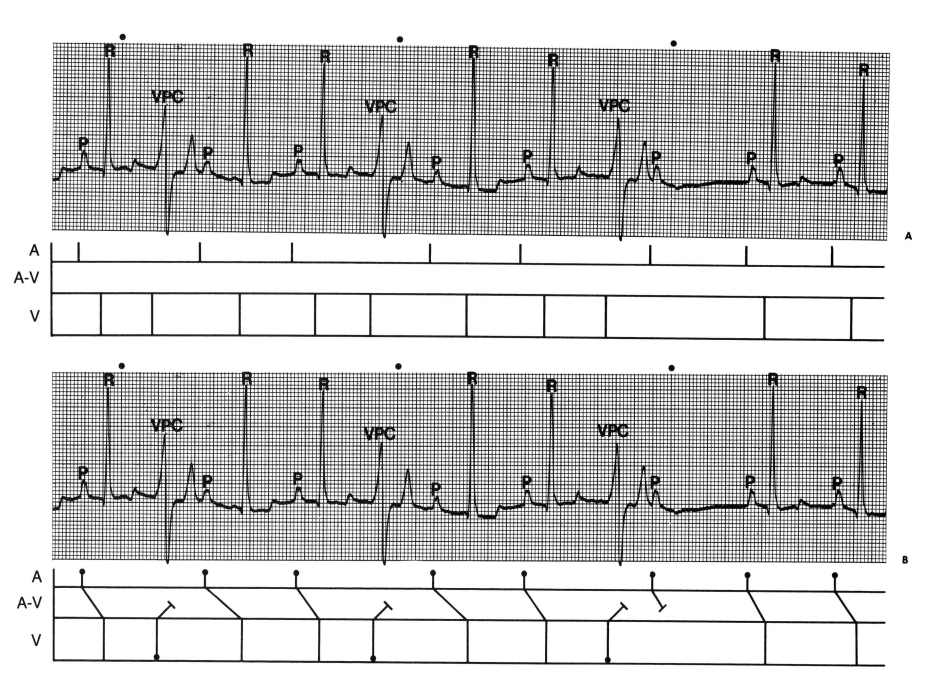

Fig. 12–2. How to use the AV ladder diagram. **A,** First draw the lines for the P waves (A level) and QRS complexes (V level); the lines should coincide with the beginning of the P wave and the QRS complex, respectively. **B,** Then draw a line between the A and V levels to indicate AV conduction. The site of impulse formation can be represented by a dot.

The ladder diagram easily explains the prolonged P-R interval after the first two VPCs, as well as the blocked P wave after the third VPC. The first two interpolated VPCs have penetrated the AV junction and caused the subsequent P-R interval to be prolonged. The third VPC has rendered the AV junction completely refractory, blocking the next sinus P wave. A compensatory pause exists after the third VPC.

ABERRANT VENTRICULAR CONDUCTION (Figs. 12–3, 12–11, 12–14, 12–15, 12–33, 12–34, 12–36, 12–37)

In aberrant ventricular conduction (ventricular aberration), a supraventricular impulse encounters parts of the intraventricular conduction system that are refractory to normal conduction. Such impulses often are "early" with respect to the preceding cycle, leading to phasic aberrant ventricular conduction. A bundle branch block pattern is usually the result. Aberrant ventricular conduction may occur during sinus rhythm and during various supraventricular arrhythmias (e.g., atrial and AV junctional premature complexes, atrial and AV junctional tachycardia, atrial flutter, and atrial fibrillation).

Bundle branch block or aberrant ventricular conduction can occur during a series of consecutive complexes, being dependent on the heart rate[10,11] (Figs. 12–15 and 12–34). Above a critical heart rate, impulses reach the bundle branch during its prolonged refractory period, causing a conduction block. Below the critical rate, conduction becomes normal since impulses now reach the affected bundle after recovery is completed. Bundle branch block can also be bradycardia-dependent.[7,12]

Electrocardiographic features[7,12]

1. A right bundle branch block pattern is observed in 80% of the cases in man and appears frequently in the dog and cat as well. Recovery normally takes longer in the right bundle branch.

2. A P wave usually precedes each aberrantly conducted complex.

3. The aberrant complexes generally resemble normally conducted complexes in the same lead, especially the initial portion of the QRS complex.

4. The aberrant complexes sometimes vary slightly from complex to complex, being similar to previously observed aberrancy.

5. The coupling intervals of the aberrant beat to the preceding conducted beat may vary.

6. Aberrant conduction is more likely when long cardiac cycles precede short cycles. A direct relationship exists between cycle length and refractoriness in the intraventricular conduction system. This long-short cycle sequence often occurs in atrial fibrillation and is called the Ashman phenomenon in man.

It is important to differentiate aberrant complexes from ventricular ectopic complexes (VPCs), since they are usually treated differently. For example, an incorrect diagnosis of VPCs during supraventricular rhythm with aberrant conduction may lead to the use of quinidine, when digitalis should be given. Electrograms of the His bundle can be used to differentiate aberrant ventricular conducted complexes from VPCs. Other data, derived from deductive interpretation of the electrocardiogram, may lead the clinician to a proper diagnosis.

The differential diagnosis of a tachycardia with abnormal QRS complexes without obvious P waves (Fig. 12–36) should always include either ventricular ectopic tachycardia or a supraventricular tachycardia with aberrant ventricular conduction. The following factors pertain:

1. The diagnosis of a supraventricular tachycardia with a pre-existing intraventricular conduction defect can be established if electrocardiograms prior or subsequent to the tachycardia demonstrate the same intraventricular conduction defect during sinus rhythm.
2. Ocular pressure sometimes will terminate a supraventricular tachycardia.
3. The diagnosis of ventricular tachycardia is supported by the presence of ventricular capture complexes, with the configuration of the capture complexes normal and that of the ectopic complexes abnormal.
4. The presence of ventricular fusion complexes essentially proves that a tachycardia with abnormal QRS complexes is of ventricular origin.

CONCEALED CONDUCTION

Concealed conduction may be defined as the partial penetration of a sinus or ectopic impulse into the AV junction. It can also occur within the bundle branches[7,12] (Fig. 12–15). In a surface electrocardiogram (as opposed to a His bundle electrogram) the penetration of an impulse into a specific structure can be deduced only from the effect on subsequent complexes. The classic example of concealed conduction occurs when an interpolated VPC has been conducted retrograde or upward into the AV junction. A prolonged P-R interval or a block of the next sinus P wave follows the VPC (Fig. 12–2).

Concealed conduction explains the various degrees of AV block in atrial tachycardia and especially in atrial flutter. The numerous supraventricular impulses partially invade the AV junction, causing the block of subsequent impulses.

The irregular ventricular rate in atrial fibrillation is due to concealed conduction at different levels in the AV junction. The aberrant ven-

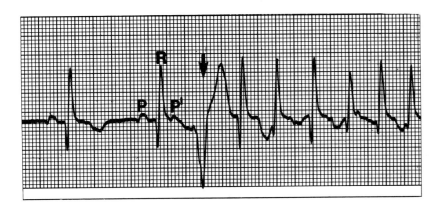

Fig. 12–3. Aberrant ventricular conduction (canine). An atrial tachycardia is introduced by an APC (after the second sinus complex) that contains a long P'-R interval with aberration of the first complex (arrow). This aberrancy is probably secondary to Ashman's phenomenon, owing to the long cardiac cycle preceding the short cycle. Secondary ST-T changes also are noted.

tricular complexes in atrial fibrillation could also represent concealed conduction into one of the bundle branches (Fig. 12–14).

RECIPROCAL COMPLEXES AND RHYTHM (RE-ENTRY) *(Figs. 12–4, 12–6, 12–16, 12–26, 12–31)*

Re-entry, the mechanism reponsible for the production of reciprocal complexes and rhythm, is discussed in detail in Chapter 9. Reciprocal arrhythmias have been discussed in some clinical reports in the veterinary literature.[1,3,13]

As the normal cardiac impulse spreads from the SA node through the atria and ventricles, the entire heart becomes activated. Refractory tissue (which cannot be re-excited) is the result; the cardiac impulse eventually dies out as it finds itself surrounded by refractory fibers into which it cannot conduct. The heart slowly recovers excitability with a new impulse starting from the SA node. This sequence of events is repeated 70 to 240 times per minute in the normal dog or cat heart.

In certain conditions, the impulse may not die out after the heart has been excited once. A pathway of excitable fibers may be found over which the original impulse can return to re-excite part or all of the heart. This concept, termed *re-entry*,[14] has been used to explain almost every known arrhythmia of the heart. Reciprocal complexes and rhythm (re-entry) occur when an impulse originating in the SA node, atria, AV junction, or ventricles is conducted in one direction through one pathway and then returns through another pathway. The impulse therefore returns to (or toward) its area of origin.

Re-entry may result in one (reciprocal complex) or more (reciprocal rhythm) activations of the heart or part of it. The requirements for reciprocal conduction to occur between atria and ventricles are that (1) there must be at least *two* conduction pathways (either both present in the AV junction [Figs. 12–4 and 12–6A] or one present in the normal AV conduction pathway and the other in an accessory pathway [Fig. 12–5]), (2) the pathways must have *different* conduction rates,

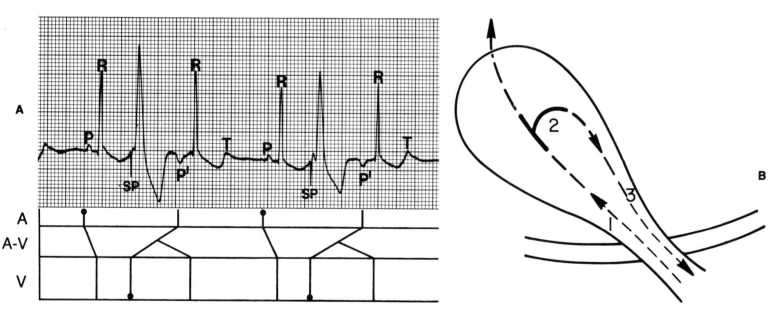

Fig. 12–4. A, Ventricular reciprocal complexes produced by an artificial pacemaker. Normal sinus complexes are followed each time by a pacemaker stimulus or spike *(SP)* and a ventricular response. These pacemaker impulses are transmitted forward into the ventricles and retrograde into the AV junction and atria. The inverted P′ waves indicate retrograde atrial conduction. The QRS complex following indicates that the inverted P′ wave has re-entered the AV junction to be conducted into the ventricles. **B,** Possible mechanism of a ventricular reciprocal complex. The paced ventricular complex enters the AV junction *(1)* by retrograde conduction. The conduction velocity decreases as the impulse rises in the AV junction (thickening larger lines). If the conduction is decreased sufficiently, the impulse may turn about *(2)* and conduct back to the ventricles (anterograde) over a pathway *(3)* that is no longer refractory. This property, whereby one pathway is refractory when an adjacent pathway can conduct, is known as unidirectional block. (From Kastor, J.A., Goldreyer, B.N., Moore, N.E., and Spear, J.F.: Cardiovasc. Clin., 6:111, 1974; reprinted with permission.)

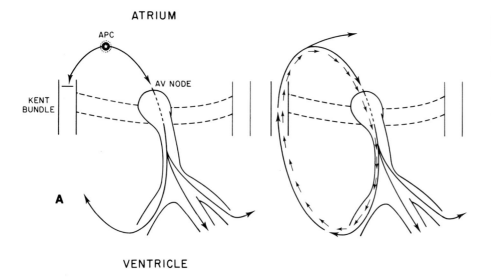

ATRIUM

APC

KENT
BUNDLE

AV NODE

A

VENTRICLE

Fig. 12–5. Reciprocal rhythm. A, Mechanisms of paroxysmal supraventricular tachycardia associated with ventricular pre-excitation. The Wolff-Parkinson-White syndrome provides a classic example of macro-re-entry (re-entrant pathways that are utilized are long). The atrial ectopic impulse *(APC)* is conducted down the AV node and His-Purkinje network but not the accessory bundle of Kent. After reaching the ventricles, the impulse re-enters the atria by passing up through the bypass tract (Kent bundle shown here). This sequence is repeated, causing a reciprocal tachycardia. **B,** Wolff-Parkinson-White syndrome (canine). Ventricular pre-excitation is represented by the short P-R interval, wide QRS complex, and delta wave (arrow) in *CV₆LU*. Paroxysms of supraventricular tachycardia in this same case are represented in the long lead *II* rhythm strip. The QRS complexes during tachycardia have a different configuration because the impulse travels anterograde over the AV node. **C,** Wolff-Parkinson-White syndrome (feline). Intermittent pre-excitation pattern due to brief 2:1 block in the bypass tract. Normally conducted sinus complexes alternate at first with pre-excitation complexes (arrows). A run of supraventricular tachycardia (a reciprocal rhythm) occurs after the fourth complex. Intermittent pre-excitation then follows the tachycardia.

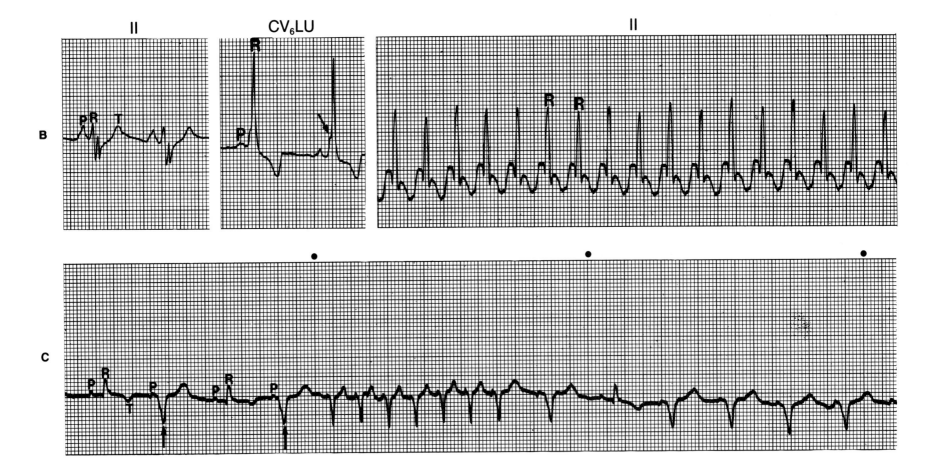

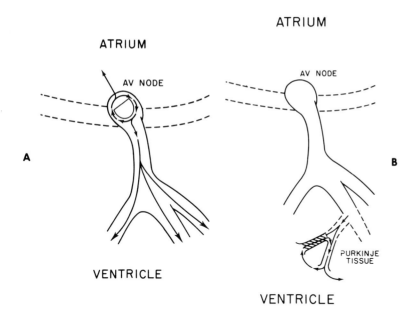

ATRIUM

ATRIUM

AV NODE

AV NODE

A

B

PURKINJE
TISSUE

VENTRICLE

VENTRICLE

Fig. 12–6. **Reciprocal rhythm;** other anatomic sites for re-entry. **A,** The re-entrant pathway for supraventricular tachycardia can occur within the AV junction *(AV node)*. It has been postulated that dual pathways for impulse transmission can exist in the AV junction, as diagrammed in Figure 12–4. Unidirectional block in one of the pathways will set the stage for re-entry. **B,** Ventricular tachycardia can be the result of a re-entrant circuit localized within the myocardium or Purkinje network.

and (3) *block* must occur in one direction at some time during the reciprocal sequence.

The mechanism for most cases of supraventricular tachycardia is probably AV nodal re-entry.[14] With re-entrant supraventricular tachycardia, AV nodal conduction delay is usually required for initiation of the tachycardia. The P wave morphology (when seen) is inverted except for the first premature complex, and ocular or carotid sinus pressure often terminates the tachycardia without the production of AV block (Fig. 12–26).

On an electrophysiologic basis, high degrees of AV block cannot occur when the mechanism for supraventricular tachycardia is AV nodal re-entry. Then a re-entry mechanism is unlikely because (1) ventricular depolarization is necessary for the impulse to reach the ventricular portion of the bypass tract, and (2) it is difficult for re-entry to be maintained in the AV node with AV nodal block.[7,15]

The supraventricular tachycardias that occur frequently in animals with ventricular pre-excitation (Wolff-Parkinson-White syndrome) provide the prototype for re-entrant mechanisms[16] (Fig. 12–5). If an APC is properly timed, it is conducted down the normal AV junction pathway but not down the Kent bundle pathway. After conduction through the bundle branches, it reaches the ventricular end of the Kent pathway and is conducted back (retrograde) into the atrium. Th retrograde impulse reaches the AV junction as soon as the junction is ready to conduct. A second cycle is then established.

This circuit can repeat itself, creating a continuous circus movement (Fig. 12–5) between the atria and the ventricles, and is responsible for the supraventricular tachycardia often associated with the Wolff-Parkinson-White syndrome. Continued re-entry can also occur within the AV junction (Fig. 12–6A). Evidence indicates that re-entrant tachycardias can also occur within the ventricles, without involvement of the A-V junction[17] (Fig. 12–6B). Ventricular tachycardia can then result.

The mechanism of re-entry explains many arrhythmias, e.g., the supraventricular tachycardias, VPCs in a bigeminal rhythm, and some ventricular tachycardias. By appreciating the mechanisms of re-entry, one can easily understand why drugs that alter conduction can be used for treatment.

For example, the use of digitalis for the treatment of atrial fibrillation in Wolff-Parkinson-White syndrome with rapid conduction via the accessory pathway can be dangerous. Digitalis glycosides may actually shorten the antegrade refractory period of the accessory pathway and thereby accelerate AV conduction.[18] Verapamil and propranolol would also be contraindicated, since they also reduce the refractoriness of the accessory pathway. The treatment of choice in such cases is either lidocaine or procainamide. Propranolol and digitalis glycosides are the drugs of choice in the therapy of regular reciprocating supraventricular tachycardia.[19] The safest policy is to give neither digoxin nor verapamil to animals with WPW syndrome without a prior electrophysiologic evaluation of the risk of antero-grade conduction.

ATRIOVENTRICULAR DISSOCIATION[7,20,21] (Figs. 12–7, 12–17, and 12–35)

AV dissociation implies that the atria and ventricles are discharged by two independent foci of impulse formation. The SA node or an atrial focus controls the atria; an AV junctional or ventricular focus controls the ventricles. Under certain circumstances, these pacemakers can exist together without discharging each other. This phenomenon can be produced by many different mechanisms and is present in a number of arrhythmias. The clinician should remember that AV dissociation is never a primary disturbance of rhythm but rather the result of a basic abnormality of impulse formation and/or conduction.

AV dissociation was not discussed in connection with canine and feline arrhythmias because it is *not* an electrocardiographic diagnosis, any more than fever is a clinical diagnosis. AV dissociation can be caused by one or a combination of the following mechanisms:

1. Depressed SA node automaticity, allowing an AV junctional or a ventricular focus to escape and control the ventricles
2. Increased AV junctional or ventricular automaticity (An ectopic focus assumes control of the ventricles while the SA node continues to activate the atria.)
3. Disturbed AV conduction (The slower ventricular rate may allow an AV junctional focus [below the area of the block] or a ventricular focus to control the ventricles. Two independent rhythms are then established, one in the atria and the other below the area of conduction delay.)

It is often difficult to determine which of the three mechanisms is playing a major role in producing AV dissociation. A combination of two or even three mechanisms can be suggested.

The most frequent form of AV dissociation occurs between the SA node and the AV junction (Figs. 12–7 and 12–17). The two independent pacemaking foci can exist together because their discharge rates are nearly identical or because there is a stoppage or delay in conduction between them. The sinus P waves have no constant relationship to the QRS complexes of AV junctional origin. The P waves may precede the QRS, be in the middle of it, or follow it without changing their form. The configuration of the QRS complexes is usually normal.

For example, when the AV junction discharges before the sinus impulse arrives, the sinus impulse finds the AV junctional tissues refractory. The refractory junctional tissues thereby interfere with the conduction of the normal sinus impulse through the AV junction. When the AV junctional pacemaker is discharging at about the same rate as the SA node, each SA impulse encounters refractory tissue caused by the discharge of the AV junctional pacemaker; and during this period no SA impulses reach the ventricles. In simple terms, the AV junctional pacemaker "gets in the way" of the SA complexes.

The term *AV dissociation* therefore is general, meaning simply that the atrial and ventricular rhythms are independent of each other. With complete pathologic interruption of conduction between the atria and ventricles, the atria and the ventricles also beat independently but the mechanisms are not identical. To avoid confusion, this arrhythmia should be called complete AV block and not AV dissociation.[21]

Complete AV block produces AV dissociation, but the presence of

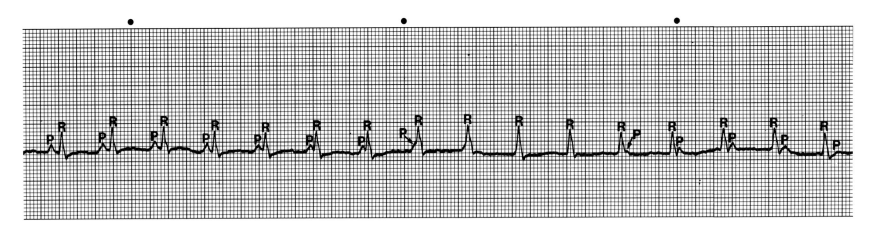

Fig. 12–7. AV dissociation (feline), probably caused by a combination of two mechanisms: an increased automaticity in the AV junction and a disturbance in AV conduction. This electrocardiogram was recorded from a cat with the dilated form of cardiomyopathy.

Two independent pacemaker foci coexist: one in the SA node and one in the AV junction. The P waves travel toward, inside, and beyond the QRS complexes. The sinus impulses spread through the atria, creating normal P waves, but cannot reach the ventricles because the AV junctional impulses reach the P waves first and render them refractory. The AV junctional impulses, on their part, spread to the ventricles but cannot reach the atria (rendered refractory by the sinus impulses).

AV dissociation does not mean that complete AV block is present. The major difference between AV dissociation and complete AV block is the rate of the two pacemakers. In complete AV block, the atrial rate is more rapid than the AV junctional or ventricular rate. In AV dissociation the atrial rate is slower than the AV junctional rate.

In AV dissociation, the atria and ventricles beat independently of each other under the control of separate pacemaking foci. This can be termed *complete AV dissociation* (Figs. 12–7 and 12–17). Impulses from the SA node can occasionally be conducted to the ventricle during AV dissociation, causing ventricular capture and ventricular fusion complexes. This, then, is termed *incomplete AV dissociation* (see Fig. 12–35).

Ventricular capture and ventricular fusion complexes occur whenever a sinus or ectopic supraventricular impulse arrives at a time when the AV junctional and/or ventricular pathways have recovered from the preceding impulse.

Ventricular capture complex. If the timing is right, a normal sinus impulse may reach the AV junction while the junction is in a recovered state. The impulse can then be conducted normally and capture the ventricles for one complex. A ventricular capture appears as a premature complex during AV dissociation. A capture complex consists of a P wave and a QRS complex that resembles the conducted sinus complexes during regular sinus rhythm.

Ventricular fusion complex. This results from the simultaneous activation of the ventricles by both a supraventricular and a ventricular focus. Each fusion complex appears as a premature complex during AV dissociation and is always preceded by a P wave. The QRS complex of the fusion complex has a configuration intermediate to that of a normal sinus complex and a ventricular ectopic complex.

Summary. The term AV dissociation should not be used to describe an electrocardiogram. If it is used in this regard, it reveals an ignorance of electrocardiographic interpretation. It is descriptive only of a phenomenon secondary to various types of electrical abnormalities requiring different types of treatment. For example, if AV dissociation is due to AV block, treatment may be a pacemaker; if it is due to an accelerated junctional rhythm, the animal may be toxic to digoxin or may have myocarditis.

VENTRICULAR PARASYSTOLE

Parasystole is an automatic, ectopic rhythm that functions alongside the underlying dominant rhythm. The dominant rhythm is usually normal sinus rhythm, but could be another rhythm such as atrial fibrillation. The features of ventricular parasystole are illustrated in Figure 12–8. The independent focus is "protected" from being discharged by the normal excitation of the heart. This phenomenon is known as *"entrance block."* [22,23] The exact nature of this protection is unknown. The diagnosis of ventricular parasystole can be made on the basis of varying coupling intervals (interval from an ectopic beat to the preceding beat of the basic rhythm) with constant shortest interectopic intervals (interval between two ectopic beats). *"Exit block"* will take place when the expected parasystolic impulse is not conducted to the heart, so that a longer interectopic interval will be produced. Thus, a long interectopic interval shows multiples of the shortest interectopic interval. Fusion beats also frequently occur, when the cardiac chamber is activated by two or more different foci simultaneously leading to a mixed beat.

The diagnostic criteria of parasystole can be summarized as follows: (1) varying coupling intervals, (2) constant shortest interectopic interval, (3) long interectopic interval, a multiple of the shortest interectopic interval (some slight variations may be present) and (4) frequent fusion beats (this criterion not necessary in every case).

If understanding ventricular parasystole is difficult, think in terms of a fixed-rate electronic pacemaker. It is the perfect artificial analogue of a naturally occurring parasystole. The fixed-rate pacemaker is not influenced by the natural beats of a competitive rhythm. It continues to function at its own rate without interruption. A QRS complex is produced, however, only when the pacemaker spike lands at a point when the ventricles are responsive. The pacemaker is "protected" in the sense that nothing can shut it off. All the interectopic intervals are multiples of a common denominator (the pacing rate), and whenever the two rhythms coincide, a fusion beat results. An example of a fixed-rate pacemaker rhythm is shown in Figure 12–9. Figure 12–10 is an example of parasystolic tachycardia in a dog.[22]

On a clinical basis, ventricular parasystole is more commonly found in cardiac patients than in healthy patients, but the arrhythmia is usually benign. Treatment is usually not indicated. In fact, the parasystolic focus is often very difficult to eliminate with antiarrhythmic drugs. The parasystolic focus is in essence "living on its island."[23] Thus, identification of parasystole may be important so that the veterinarian does not prescribe increasing doses of potentially toxic drugs to suppress the arrhythmia.[23]

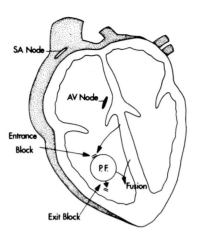

Fig. 12–8. Ventricular parasystole. This diagram depicts how two pacemakers coexist. The parasystolic focus (PF) maintains its own rate of discharge, is protected by entrance block, may be unable to emerge because of exit block and, by coincidence, may participate with the sinus-conducted impulse, resulting in a fusion beat. A clue to diagnosis is a lack of "fixed coupling," in sharp contrast to the usual ventricular premature complex. (From Nelson, W.P.: Parasystole— "one heart beating as two!" Medical Times, *108*:141, 1980, with permission.)

Fig. 12–9. A fixed-rate pacemaker illustrating **the parasystolic principle**—the longer interectopic intervals are multiples of the basic pacer cycle (0.56 sec or approximately 107 beats/min). The artificial pacemaker is not influenced by the intrinsic excitation of the heart, which, in this case, is complete AV block (note nonconducted P waves) and an escape rhythm (R waves) probably above the bifurcation of the bundle of His. In the top and bottom strips, stimulus artifacts are noted by arrows. Paced beats are seen after the first R wave. After a fusion complex (F), the intrinsic junctional escape rhythm takes over and the pacemaker stimulus is seen to march through the normal complexes. Ventricular activation does not take place after pacemaker stimuli because of their timing in the refractory period of the conducted impulses. The continuous bottom strip shows a similar pattern of normal excitation impulses, paced impulses, and fusion complexes. The second electronic stimulus on the bottom strip finds just the right moment for "capture," and a paced impulse occurs and begins another period of pacemaker rhythm.[23]

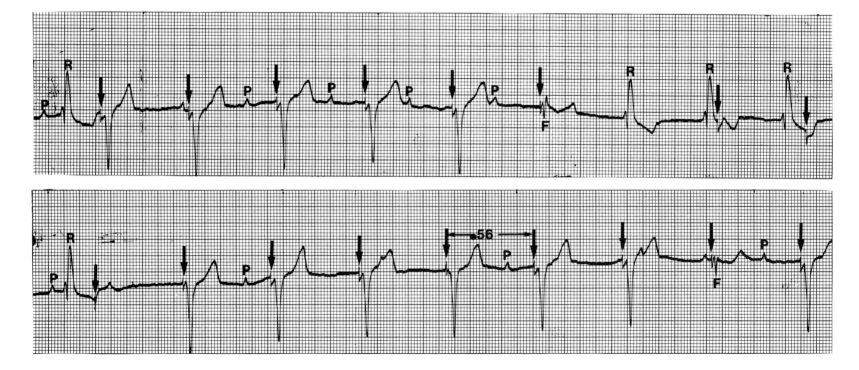

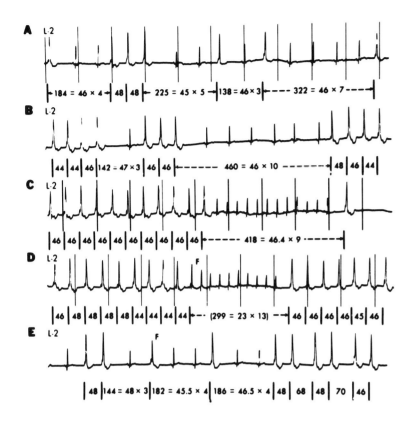

Fig. 12–10. Experimental **parasystolic tachycardia** recordings from a dog. Note the presence of marked variation of the coupling intervals and presence of fusion beats (F). The ectopic cycle length during the parasystolic tachycardia is 0.44 to 0.48 second (average rate 130/min). Some of the long interectopic intervals, however, are multiples of one half the ectopic cycle length (in D). This suggests that the inherent ectopic cycle length is 0.23 second (rate 260/min) and that the apparent rate of the parasystolic tachycardia represents a 2:1 exit block. The group beating during the parasystolic tachycardia seen in E is explained by alternating 2:1 and 3:1 exit block from a fast ectopic center. Note that the parasystolic discharge could be overdriven by atrial pacing at rates higher than the apparent ectopic rate but significantly lower than the fast inherent rate of the ectopic center (in C and D). The numbers represent hundredths of a second. (From El-Sherif, N.: The ventricular premature complex: mechanisms and significance. In *Cardiac Arrhythmias.* Edited by W.J. Mandel. Philadelphia, J.B. Lippincott, 1980, with permission.)

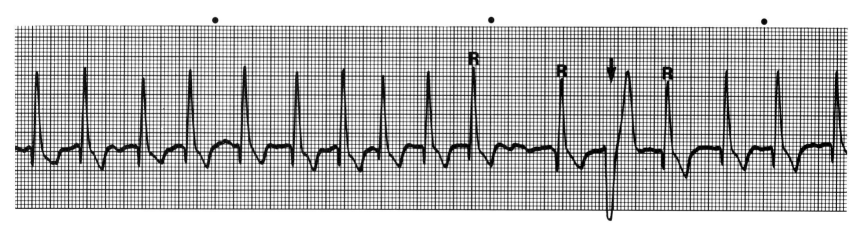

Fig. 12–11. Atrial fibrillation (canine) with a rapid ventricular rate. The abnormal ventricular complex (arrow) probably represents **aberrant ventricular conduction.** The aberrant complex shows a right bundle branch block configuration without the compensatory pause, typical of VPCs. The aberrant complex also terminates a short cycle preceded by a longer cycle (Ashman's phenomenon). Remember also, however, that a long ventricular cycle tends to precipitate a VPC. Aberrant ventricular complexes can easily be confused with VPCs in atrial fibrillation.

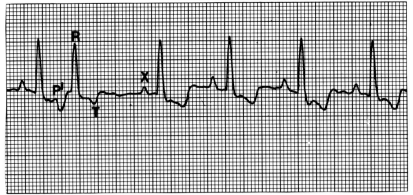

Fig. 12–12. Aberrant atrial conduction in two different dogs. There are atrial premature complexes (P'), each followed by bizarre P waves (marked x) of the sinus beats. The bizarre P wave of a sinus beat following any ectopic beat (usually an atrial premature complex) is termed "aberrant atrial conduction" or "Chung's phenomenon." This phenomenon is considered to be due to a change of the refractoriness in the atria soon after any ectopic beat. The finding is nonspecific, with no clinical significance.[24]

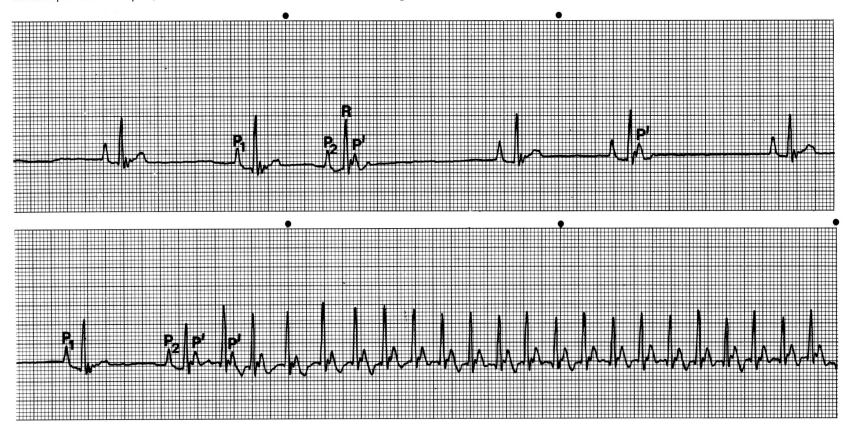

Fig. 12–13. Nonconducted atrial premature complexes (top strip) leading to atrial tachycardia (bottom strip). The premature P' wave discharges early in the cycle, with the impulse finding the AV node and the ventricles still refractory. The P' waves are not followed by a QRS complex and are termed nonconducted atrial premature complexes. Frequent atrial premature complexes (APC) may lead to atrial tachycardia, flutter, or fibrillation if the premature impulse fires during the vulnerable period of the atria. In man, a formula has been developed for determining whether the P' wave falls in this vulnerable period. The prematurity of an individual APC is expressed as the ratio of the coupling interval to the preceding cycle length, or

$$\text{coupling index} = \frac{\text{coupling interval}}{\text{preceding cycle length}} = \frac{P_2 - P'}{P_1 - P_2}$$

where P' represents the APC, P_2 the immediately preceding atrial discharge, and P_1 the atrial discharge immediately preceding P_2. If the coupling index is less than 0.50, the chance of an atrial tachyarrhythmia is high. When it is greater than 0.60, the chance of an atrial tachyarrhythmia following that particular premature P' is small.[25,26] The coupling index for the first premature P' wave that starts the atrial tachycardia is 0.25. Obviously, the fact that these APCs are not conducted because of their prematurity indicates a likely chance of atrial tachycardia. This formula can be especially useful for cases with numerous APCs that are conducted.

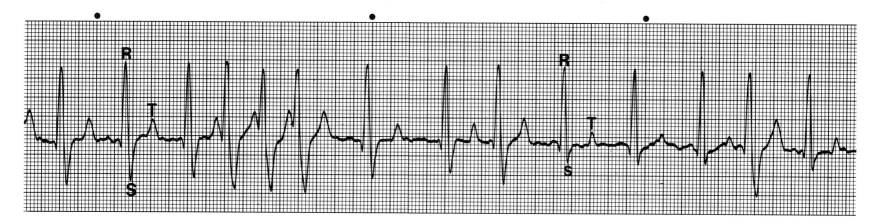

Fig. 12–14. Atrial fibrillation (canine) and **intermittent aberrant ventricular conduction** that can easily be confused with VPCs. Support for ventricular aberration includes a right bundle branch block-like configuration, initial portion of the QRS complexes the same, different degrees of aberration, and varying intervals between the aberrant complexes.

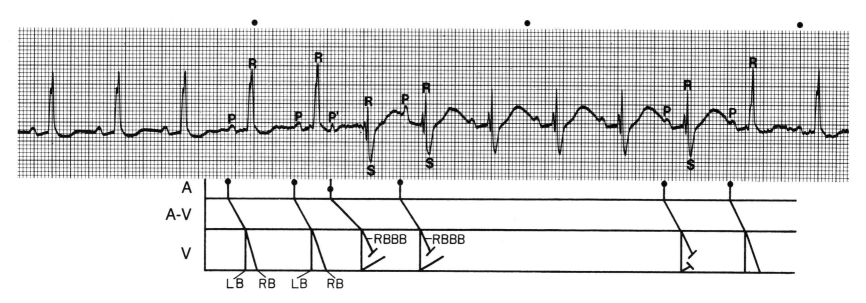

Fig. 12–15. **Aberrant ventricular conduction** (canine) due to concealed retrograde invasion of the right bundle branch after an atrial premature complex *(P')* (sixth complex). The refractory period of the right bundle branch is longer than that of the left. The right bundle branch block pattern persists for six complexes, and then the retrograde conduction finally blocks for some reason.

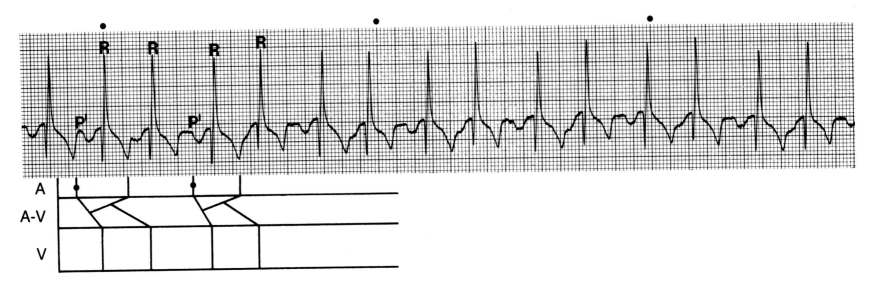

Fig. 12–16. Bigeminal rhythm (canine) in which each ectopic atrial or junctional impulse *(P')* is followed by a reciprocal complex. This sequence continues throughout the strip.

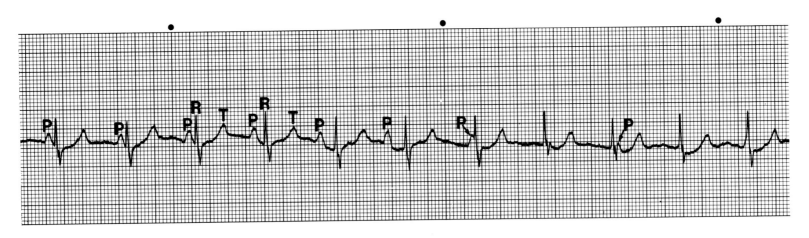

Fig. 12–17. **AV dissociation** (canine) between the SA node and the AV junction, probably due to an accelerated AV junctional focus. The P waves travel away from and then toward and finally merge with the QRS complexes. This dog had severe digitalis intoxication.

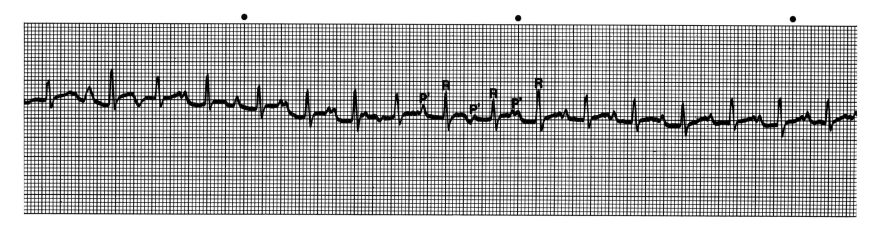

Fig. 12–18. **Multifocal atrial tachycardia** (chaotic atrial rhythm) (canine) due to the repetitive and rapid firing of two or more ectopic atrial foci. The atrial rhythm is irregular, and the P' waves and P'-R intervals vary in configuration. In man, this arrhythmia generally occurs in pulmonary disease or after major surgery and does not respond to digoxin. The treatment is usually directed to the underlying pulmonary disease.[12]

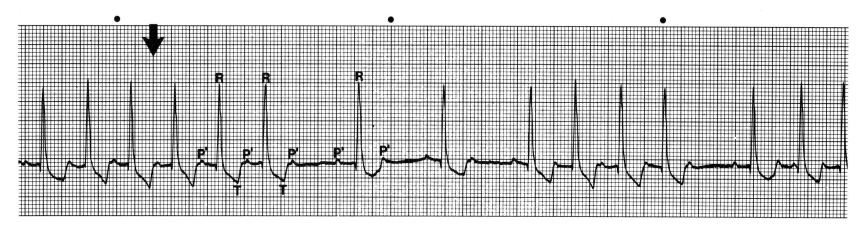

Fig. 12–19. **Automatic atrial tachycardia** (canine) secondary to digitalis toxicity. During the initial supraventricular tachycardia, ocular pressure (arrow) is applied to explain the underlying mechanism. The presence of automatic atrial tachycardia is revealed as the AV junctional block appears and the P' waves continue at the same rapid rate. Automatic atrial tachycardia should be differentiated from a tachycardia due to AV nodal re-entry.

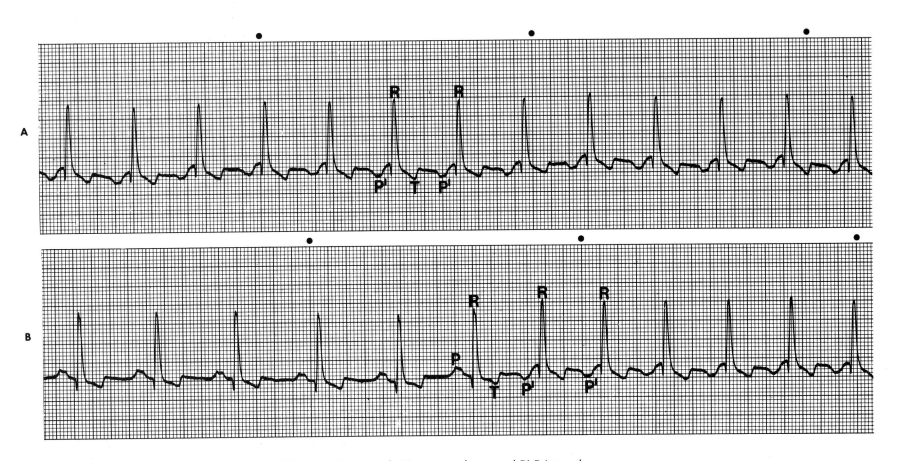

Fig. 12–20. Continuous tachycardia (canine) with inverted retrograde P' waves and a normal P'-R interval. **A,** It is impossible to determine from this strip alone whether the tachycardia is atrial, AV junctional, or re-entrant.[12] A strip recording the onset of this rhythm is needed for differentiating the probable mechanism: (1) If the tachycardia begins with an inverted P' wave-QRS complex, a normal to prolonged P'-R interval, and subsequent P' waves of the same configuration, the focus for the tachycardia is low in the atria. (2) If the tachycardia starts with an inverted P' wave and short P'-R interval, an inverted P' wave following the QRS complex, or no P' wave, the tachycardia is AV junctional in origin. (3) If the tachycardia begins with an atrial (P') premature complex, a prolonged P'-R interval, and subsequent P' waves being inverted, the tachycardia is re-entrant. **B,** The onset (after the sixth complex) of the paroxysmal tachycardia has been recorded. The tachycardia begins with an inverted P' wave and a normal P'-R interval. The subsequent P waves all have the same basic configuration. The diagnosis for both strips is either an atrial tachycardia (low in the atrium) or an AV junctional tachycardia with delayed conduction into the ventricles.[12]

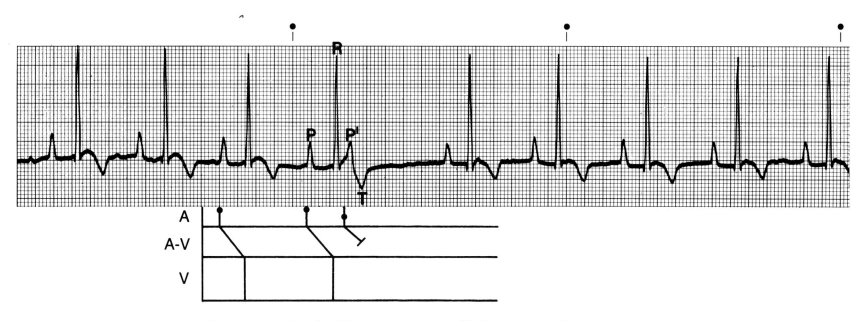

Fig. 12–21.   Sinus rhythm (canine) with one **nonconducted atrial premature complex** *(P′)*. The premature P′ wave is so early that the AV junction has not totally recovered; the impulse is not conducted to the ventricles. It has deformed the T wave of the preceding complex. The pause after the atrial ectopic impulse is noncompensatory.

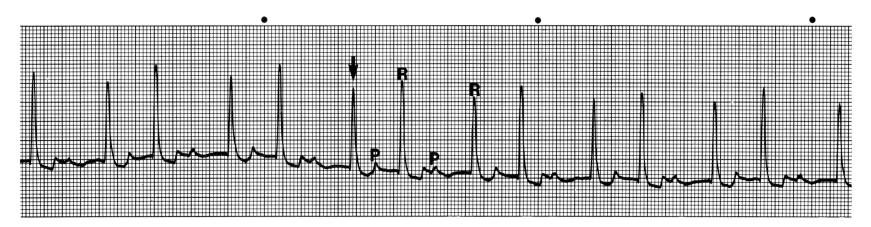

Fig. 12–22.   A number of mechanisms can be used to explain this unusual (canine) arrhythmia. Two possible mechanisms are as follows: (1) A regular supraventricular tachycardia is conducted over two different pathways, one being slow (the longer P-R interval) and the other fast (the shorter P-R interval) in the AV junction. (2) Second-degree AV block has developed, with junctional escape (arrow)—capture bigeminy (a 2:1 block). The escape complex occurs because of the pause created by the previously blocked P wave. The P wave after the escape beat is then conducted, a capture complex.

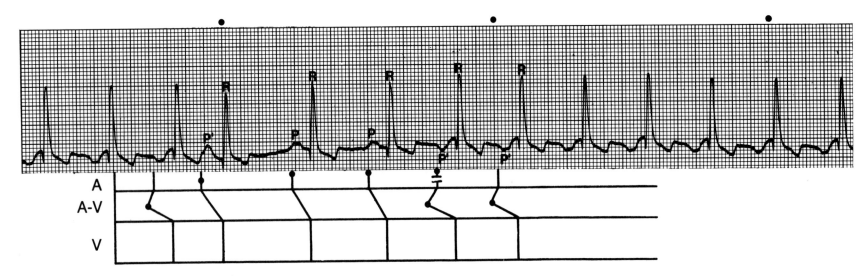

Fig. 12–23. An atrial premature complex (canine) (fourth complex) has suppressed the AV junctional focus enough to allow the SA node to conduct normally for two sinus complexes. The AV junctional focus then "warms" up to a faster than SA-node rate to assume control (an accelerated AV junctional rhythm) beginning with an **atrial fusion complex.** An atrial fusion complex occurs when the AV junction activates the atria simultaneously with the discharge of the sinus pacemaker. The morphology of the P wave is intermediate between that of the sinus P wave and that of the AV junctional P wave.

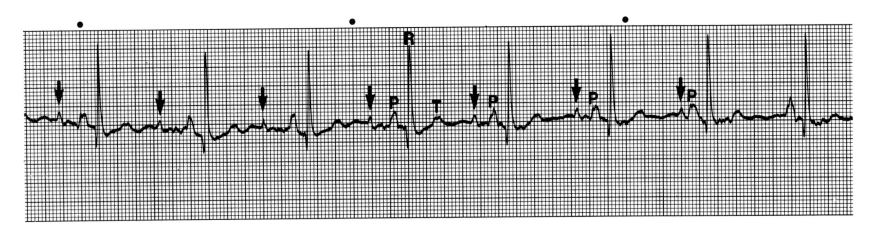

Fig. 12–24. **Atrial dissociation** in a dog with severe congestive heart failure. There are two independent atrial rhythms, one sinoatrial (P waves) and the other ectopic atrial (arrows). Both the sinus and the interectopic intervals are constant. The ectopic atrial focus is never conducted to the ventricles; it controls only a part of the atrium because of a probable intra-atrial block in that region. The sinus complexes cannot interfere with the ectopic rhythm, and vice-versa. In man, this arrhythmia is often seen with advanced congestive heart failure.

  Such an atrial focus could be confused with an artifact, a possible consideration. In this case, however, the arrhythmia was found on repeat electrocardiograms. Most of these independent P waves in man are actually artifacts produced by the accessory muscles of respiration.[22]

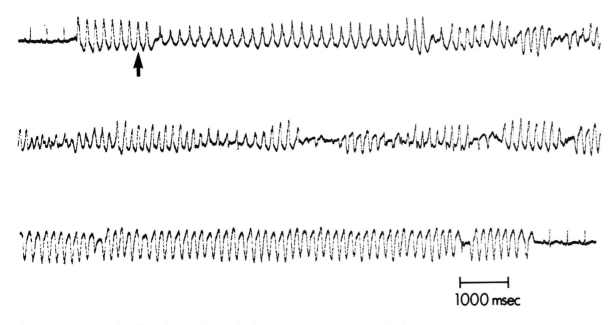

|———————|
1000 msec

Fig. 12–25. Torsades de pointes. This arrhythmia represents a form of polymorphous ventricular tachycardia in which the polarity of the QRS complex exhibits phasic alterations in both axis and rate. The arrhythmia is associated with a variety of congenital and acquired (including drug and metabolic) causes of Q-T prolongation.[27] The name of this arrhythmia implies a continual change in the amplitude of the tachycardia complexes, which appear to twist around the isoelectric line. Ventricular tachycardia can be distinguished from torsades de pointes by the ventricular complexes, which are generally stable from beat to beat except when there is a transient capture. Also, ventricular tachycardia occurs with an underlying basal rhythm that has a normal Q-T interval. The distinction from ventricular fibrillation is not absolute, but with torsades de pointes, there is the reappearance of individual QRS complexes and a return to sinus rhythm.[28] The exact mechanism is unknown, but electrophysiologic studies so far favor a reentrant cause.[28,29] The most common causes of torsades de pointes include myocarditis, complete AV block, extreme sinus bradycardia, numerous drugs (e.g., quinidine, procainamide, disopyramide), central nervous system disorders, hypothermia, and electrolyte disturbances such as hypokalemia.[27] The diagnosis of torsades de pointes has therapeutic implications; antiarrhythmic drugs such as quinidine should be avoided, with cardiac pacing usually indicated.[27] It is extremely important to correct or to eliminate the underlying cause if recognized. Antiarrhythmic agents that do not prolong the Q-T interval such as propranolol, lidocaine, or phenytoin can be tried, but are not always predictable. Artificial pacing or magnesium sulfate[29a] is more reliable.

This figure illustrates a limb lead II recording from a dog with a run of torsades de pointes induced with an eight-beat salvo of rapid ventricular pacing (cycle length, 165 msec). The Q-T interval was first prolonged with quinidine. The arrow designates the last paced beat. The three strips are continuous. Note how the ventricular complexes change in amplitude and shape, continuously and progressively varying so that there is a twisting appearance. Note also the reappearance of some QRS complexes and the return to sinus rhythm. (From Bardy, G.H., et al.: A mechanism of torsades de pointes in a canine model. Circulation, 67:52, 1983, with permission of the American Heart Assoc. Inc.)[30]

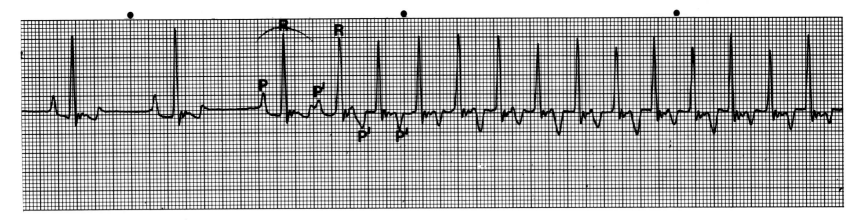

Fig. 12–26. Paroxysmal re-entrant supraventricular tachycardia. The mechanism for most cases of supraventricular tachycardia is probably AV nodal re-entry, but ectopic automatic atrial tachycardias may also occur. In re-entrant tachycardia, the P' wave morphology is retrograde (inverted) except for the initiating atrial premature complex (arrow), which is upright. The initiating beat is also associated with AV nodal conduction delay. Abrupt termination of a supraventricular tachycardia by carotid massage or other vagal maneuvers favors a re-entrant mechanism.[26] This does not prove re-entry if triggered activity due to delayed afterdepolarization is accepted as a possibility (see Chapter 9). This strip is consistent with and suggestive of re-entry. Note also the electrical alternans during the tachycardia; the QRS-T complexes alternate in amplitude and configuration. This is usually of no significance in a tachycardia, as it is probably secondary to alternating prolongation of the refractory phase of the heart.

Fig. 12–27. Right atrial pacing from a dog with Wolff-Parkinson-White syndrome. A, Lead II rhythm strip showing ventricular pre-excitation. The P-R interval is short and the QRS complex wide. **B,** Attempt at right atrial pacing. At first, stimulus artifacts (SP) are not all followed by P waves. The first three QRS complexes represent a spontaneous ventricular pre-excitation rhythm. After the pacemaker mA is increased, the stimulus artifacts (SP) are followed by P waves and QRS complexes with no pre-excitation present. **C,** The atrial pacing wire has probably been moved closer to the accessory pathway, resulting in ventricular pre-excitation. **D,** The atrial pacing wire has again been moved, away from the accessory pathway; resulting in each stimulus artifact (SP) followed by a P wave and QRS complex. Strips **B**, **C**, and **D** are at ½ cm = 1 mv.

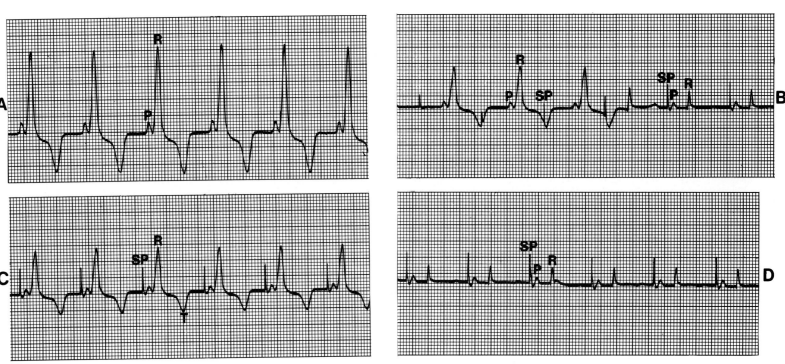

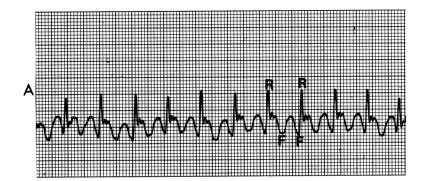
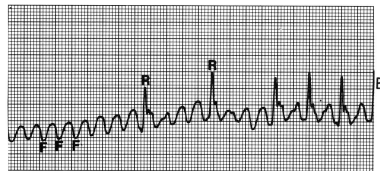

Fig. 12–28. A, Atrial flutter with a 2:1 response. The ventricular heart rate is 300 beats/min. In any rhythm in which the ventricular rate is 300 beats/min or above and regular, the possibility of atrial flutter should be part of the differential diagnosis. The term "response" is sometimes used instead of "block" because the 2:1 AV conduction in atrial flutter is due to a longer physiologic refractory period in the AV junction.

B, With ocular pressure, the increased vagal activity increases the degree of response in the AV node and the flutter waves (F) are more easily identified with their characteristic sawtooth pattern as well as rate. The atrial rate is 600 beats/ min. The therapeutic approach can be pharmacologic (e.g., digitalis, propranolol, and quinidine) and/or electrical (e.g., cardioversion or right atrial pacing). Cardioversion is the treatment of choice if the animal is critical. Atrial flutter may reduce cerebral circulation, producing clinical signs of weakness and syncope. Digitalis is the drug of choice for decreasing the ventricular rate by increasing the AV response.

Fig. 12–29. Atrial tachycardia with alternating 2:1 block at level 1 (upper portion) in the AV junction and 3:2 block at level 2 (lower portion) in the AV junction.[8] The grouping of complexes results from these two levels of block. Since the refractory period of the AV junction is longer than that of the atria, all the atrial impulses cannot be conducted to the ventricles. There is usually 2:1 AV conduction, not due to block but to physiologic interference in the AV junction. Atrioventricular conduction ratios greater than 2:1 are indicative of AV block.[12] Two regions of block are most likely present with conduction ratios greater than 2:1. All impulses penetrate for same distance into the upper portion of the AV junction, but only alternate impulses are transmitted to the lower portion. In the lower portion, another region of block may cause some of the arriving impulses to be dropped in a sequence. This block is usually with the Wenckebach phenomenon.[12] Even-numbered conduction ratios such as 2:1 are more common with atrial flutter or tachycardia, whereas odd-numbered conduction ratios are rare and suggest the presence of a pathologic conduction disturbance in the AV junction.[21] Electrophysiologic studies are indicated for confirming these two regions of atrioventricular block. Paroxysmal atrial tachycardia with varying block at one level should also be considered.

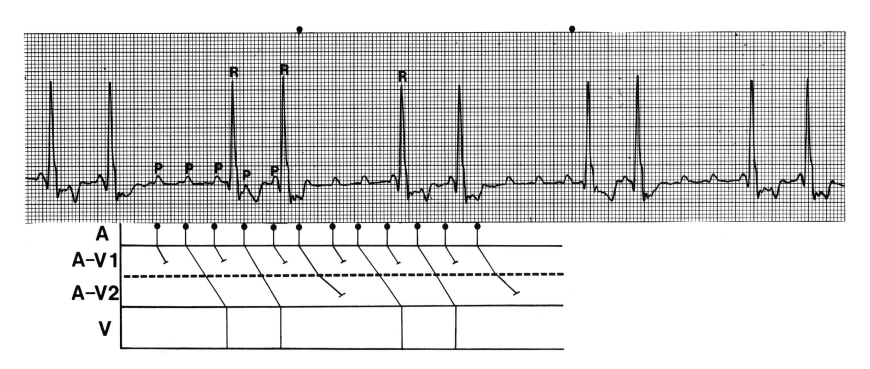

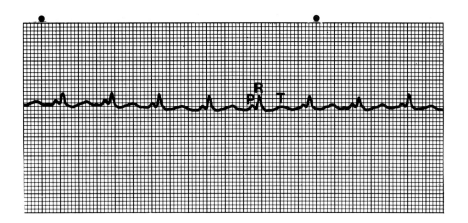

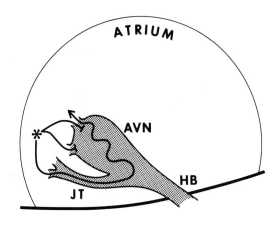

Fig. 12–30. Lown-Ganong-Levine (LGL) syndrome. This electrocardiogram recorded from a cat with syncope has a short P-R interval with a normal QRS complex and no delta wave. Thus, Wolff-Parkinson-White syndrome cannot be diagnosed. LGL syndrome is usually a variant of the WPW syndrome in many cases, since the delta wave is not obvious because the anomalous pathway is close to the normal AV conduction pathway. LGL syndrome can be diagnosed when the electrocardiographic findings consist of a short P-R interval and normal QRS complex associated with paroxysmal supraventricular tachycardia.[31] It should also be noted that the P-R interval is frequently short when there is a stressful situation such as with severe pain, anxiety, etc. The P-R interval is also short with various high-output states such as anemia or hyperthyroidism.

The diagram on the right illustrates the James tract (JT) inserting at the junction of the AV node (AVN) and His bundle (HB). The James fibers have been speculated as the possible pathway for LGL syndrome. A more descriptive term for LGL syndrome is "short-PR-normal-QRS syndrome" since the anatomic and physiologic correlations are controversial. An impulse originating in the atrium is shown to follow a re-entrant circuit by blocking initially at the input to the AV node and conducting down the bypass tract and retrogradely up the node to the atrium. A re-entrant circuit in this location can lead to regular supraventricular tachyarrhythmias. (From Lazzara, R.: Anomalous atrioventricular conduction and the pre-excitation syndrome. In *Bellet's Essentials of Cardiac Arrhythmias*. Edited by R.H. Helfant. 2nd Edition. Philadelphia, W.B. Saunders, 1980, with permission.)[18]

Fig. 12–31. Ventricular premature complex followed by a **reciprocal beat** (re-entrant beat or echo beat—marked x). The arrow indicates a retrograde P wave. The QRS complex following the inverted P wave (x) indicates that the inverted P wave has re-entered the AV junction to be conducted into the ventricles. The mechanism is explained in Figure 12–4. Once a reciprocal beat is produced, the re-entry cycle may repeat consecutively, leading to a reciprocal rhythm or tachycardia.

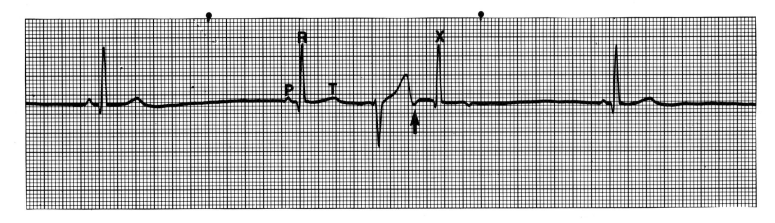

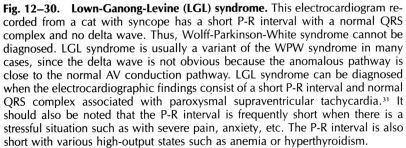

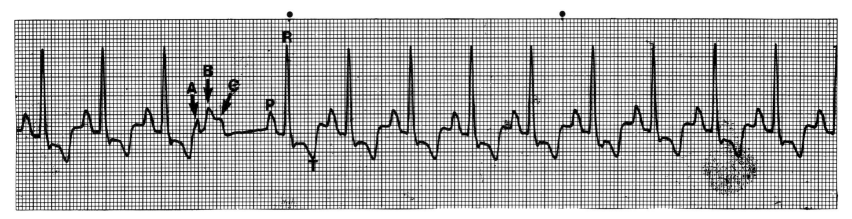

Fig. 12–32. The pause in this lead II rhythm strip is due to a premature complex. **B** represents the normal atrial P wave (from the sinoatrial node) that does not conduct to the ventricle because either the AV node or ventricle is refractory to the event labeled **A**. Since **A** does not activate the atria but we see it, it must represent ventricular activation. Since it does not look the same as conducted sinus beats, it must be a ventricular premature complex. Thus, **A** is the QRS and **C** is the T wave of the ventricular premature complex.

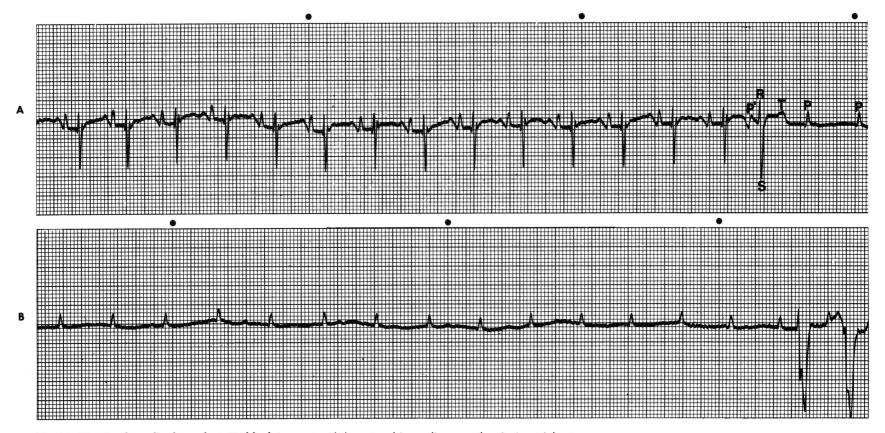

Fig. 12–33. **Bradycardia-dependent AV block** in a cat with hypertrophic cardiomyopathy. **A,** An atrial premature complex *(P′)* with aberrant ventricular conduction has created a long enough pause that sequential P waves are blocked. In man, the first P wave is blocked because the previous pause has allowed time for spontaneous phase 4 depolarization to occur in the area of the bundle of His.[33] The P wave is not conducted because this area has been partially depolarized. The area remains depolarized, so sequential P waves are blocked. **B,** Two ventricular escape complexes occur at the end of the strip. If the escape complex to the next P wave interval is short enough, the P waves may have time to be conducted (not enough of a pause for spontaneous depolarization to take place in the His bundle).

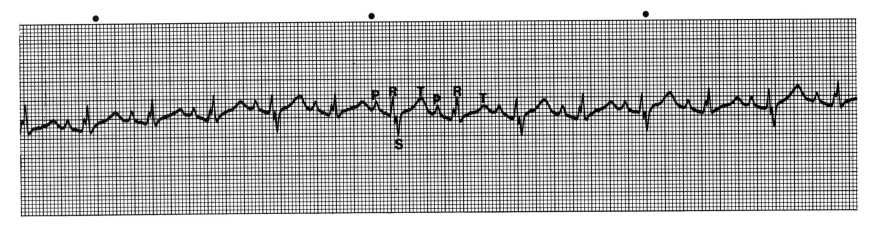

Fig. 12–34. **2:1 Conduction block** (feline) in some portion of the ventricular specialized conduction system after the first three sinus complexes. The duration of the refractory periods of the conduction tissue is often influenced by the heart rate. This phenomenon is sometimes termed rate-related aberrant ventricular conduction.[11]

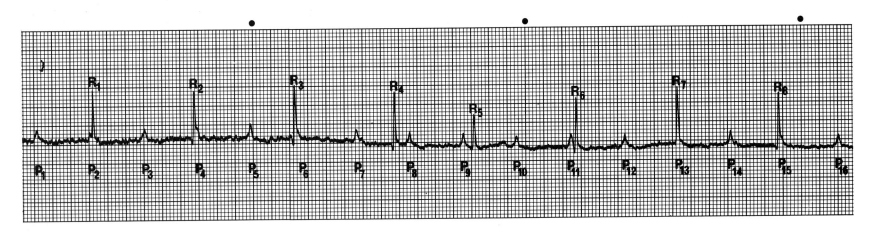

Fig. 12–35. Diagnosis: "sinus rhythm with an AV conduction disturbance and junctional escape complexes" or "AV dissociation due to sinus rhythm with an AV conduction disturbance and junctional escape complexes." The term AV dissociation should not be used alone. The electrocardiogram was recorded from a cat with AV block due to myocarditis.

This electrocardiogram actually shows **incomplete AV dissociation** due to a disturbance in AV conduction. The only thing that makes it incomplete is R_5, which is early; all R-R intervals are equal except R_4-R_5, which is shorter. P_9 must then conduct to R_5.

If we left out that complex, we would have *complete* AV dissociation due to a disturbance in AV conduction. We cannot call it complete AV block because the first P wave in each series of two P waves never has the opportunity to show us that it would block; i.e., P_1, P_3, P_5, P_7, P_8, P_{10}, P_{12}, P_{14}, and P_{16} all block; P_9 conducts with a P-R interval of 0.06 second. The alternate Ps (P_2, P_4, P_6, P_{11}, P_{13}, and P_{15}) precede (or fall within) the next QRS complexes by less than 0.06 second so they do not have the opportunity of conducting to the ventricles before a junctional escape complex occurs.

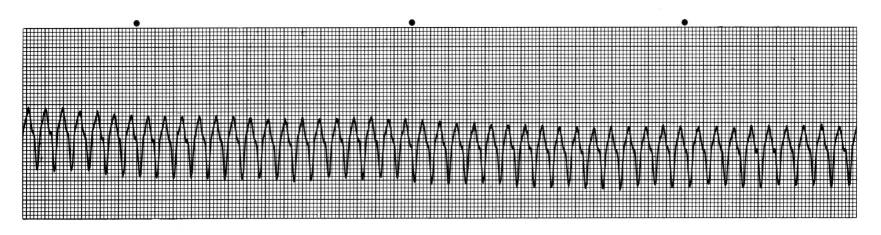

Fig. 12–36. Supraventricular tachycardia (feline) with aberrant ventricular conduction (atrial tachycardia, atrial flutter, Wolff-Parkinson-White syndrome) versus ventricular tachycardia. Paper speed, 25 mm/sec. The P waves could not be distinguished, even when the paper speed was increased to 50 mm/sec (not shown). It is usually helpful to compare this tracing with previous tracings and rhythm strips. If major clinical signs are present, electrical cardioversion is often successful.

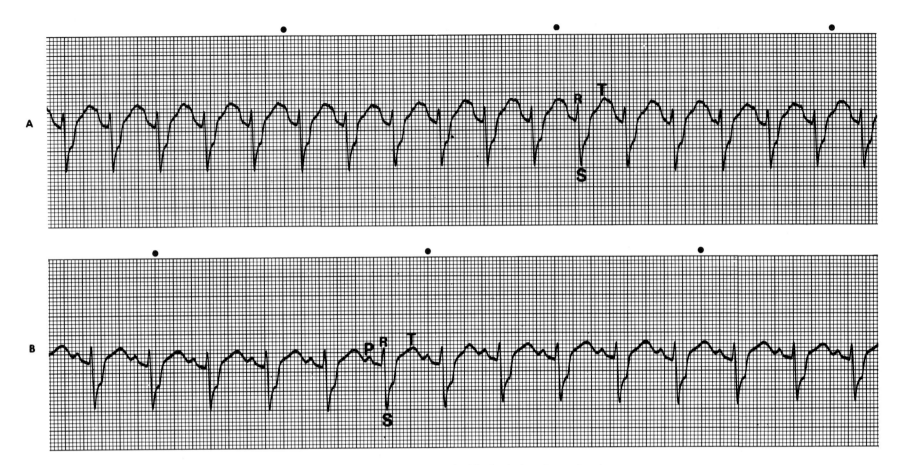

Fig. 12–37. Supraventricular tachycardia (feline) with pre-existing intraventricular block. **A,** A tachycardia of 230 beats/min with abnormal and widened QRS complexes is present. P waves are not distinct. Differential diagnosis must include both ventricular tachycardia and supraventricular tachycardia with pre-existing intraventricular conduction block or aberrant ventricular conduction. **B,** Normal sinus rhythm. Vagal stimulation by ocular pressure has terminated the tachycardia. The QRS complexes are identical in both strips, which indicates that the tachycardia in **A** is supraventricular in origin.

A dangerous arrhythmia (ventricular tachycardia) has thus been eliminated from the differential diagnosis. The other limb leads were also compatible with an intraventricular block (a right bundle branch block pattern).

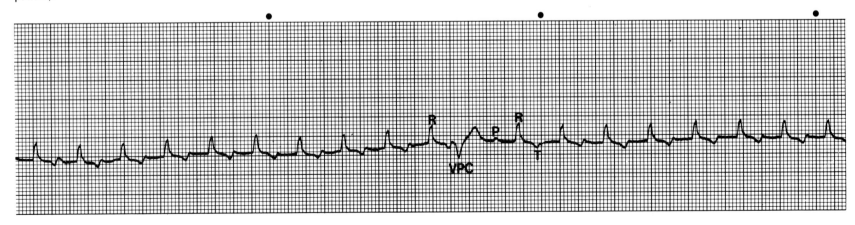

Fig. 12–38. Supraventricular tachycardia (feline) at 250 beats/min. It is difficult to diagnose the rhythm before the VPC, since the P wave is difficult to differentiate from the T wave. The T wave also could be just biphasic, without a P wave. The VPC with the compensatory pause allows the following P wave to be seen. The P waves are all sinus, superimposed on the previous T wave.

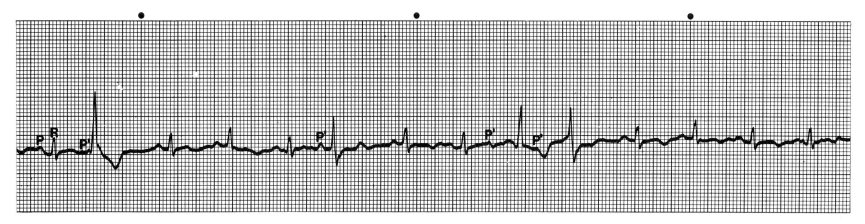

Fig. 12–39. Atrial premature complexes (feline) with **aberrant ventricular conduction** occurring in the second, sixth, ninth, and tenth complexes. The complexes are all preceded by premature P′ waves, with noncompensatory pauses.

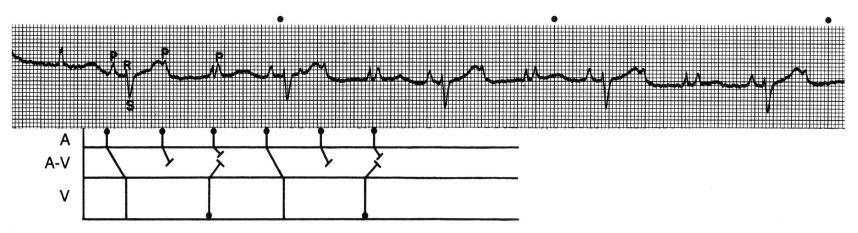

Fig. 12–40. 2:1 AV block (feline) (two P waves for every conducted QRS complex) with ventricular escape complexes (causing physiologic block of the third P wave in each series). This is an example of **escape-capture bigeminy** in the presence of AV block.

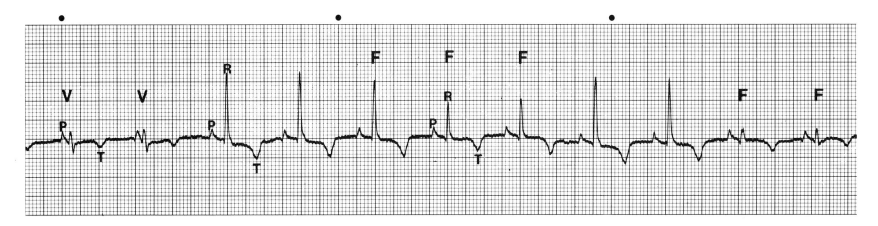

Fig. 12–41. Accelerated ventricular rhythm (feline). The third, fourth, eighth, and ninth complexes appear to be normal sinus complexes. The rest of the QRS complexes are from the ventricular focus or are fusion complexes. *F,* Fusion complex; *V,* pure ventricular focus. The ventricular focus appears to be reset each time. The dilated form of cardiomyopathy was diagnosed in this cat.

383

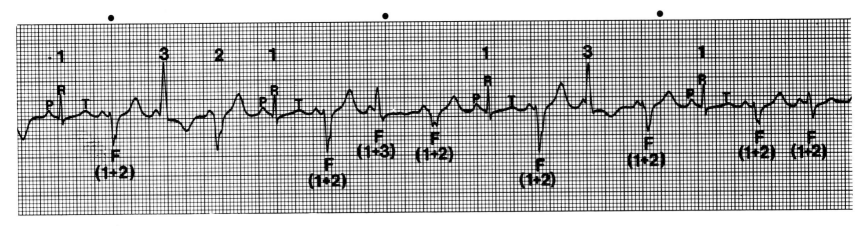

Fig. 12–42. Three different foci are probably present in this cat with dilated cardiomyopathy. The three foci include *(1)* a normal sinus complex, *(2)* a ventricular premature complex (VPC), and *(3)* another VPC. The simultaneous activation of the ventricles by the sinus complex and one of the other two ventricular foci creates **ventricular fusion complexes** *(F)*. Some fusion complexes may represent fusion of all three foci.

REFERENCES

1. Moore, E.N., Morse, H.T., and Price, H.L.: Cardiac arrhythmias produced by catecholamines in anesthetized dogs. Circ. Res., *15*:77, 1964.
2. Muir, W.W.: Electrocardiographic interpretation of thiobarbiturate-induced dysrhythmias in dogs. J. Am. Vet. Med. Assoc., *170*:1419, 1977.
3. Muir, W.W., Werner, L.L., and Hamlin, R.L.: Antiarrhythmic effects of diazepam during coronary artery occlusion in dogs. Am. J. Vet. Res., *36*:1203, 1975.
4. Scherlag, B.H., Helfant, R.H., and Donato, A.N.: A catheterization technique for His bundle stimulation and recording in the intact dog. J. Appl. Physiol., *25*:425, 1968.
5. Cranefield, P.F.: *The Conduction of the Cardiac Impulse.* Mt. Kisco, NY, Futura Publishing Co., 1975.
6. Kastor, J.A., Goldreyer, B.N., Moore, E.N., and Spear, J.F.: Re-entry: an important mechanism of cardiac arrhythmias. Cardiovasc. Clin., *6*:111, 1974.
7. Mandel, W.J.: *Cardiac Arrhythmias—Their Mechanisms, Diagnosis, and Management.* Philadelphia, J.B. Lippincott, 1980.
8. Pick, A., and Langendorf, R.: *Interpretation of Complex Arrhythmias.* Philadelphia, Lea & Febiger, 1979.
8a. Marriott, H.J.L., and Conover, M.H.B.: *Advanced Concepts in Arrhythmias.* St. Louis, C.V. Mosby, 1983.
9. Conover, M.H., and Zalis, E.G.: *Understanding Electrocardiography, Physiological and Interpretive Concepts.* 2nd Edition. St. Louis, C.V. Mosby, 1976.
10. Jalife, J., Antzelevitch, C., Lamanna, V., and Moe, G.K.: Rate-dependent changes in excitability of depressed cardiac Purkinje fibers as a mechanism of intermittent bundle branch block. Circulation, *67*:912, 1983.
11. Cohen, H.C., et al.: Tachycardia and bradycardia-dependent bundle branch block alternans. Circulation, *55*:242, 1977.
12. Friedman, H.H.: *Diagnostic Electrocardiography and Vectorcardiography.* 2nd Edition. New York, McGraw-Hill, 1977.
13. Muir, W.W.: Thiobarbiturate-induced dysrhythmias: the role of heart rate and autonomic imbalance. Am. J. Vet. Res., *38*:1377, 1977.
14. Wit, A.L., and Cranefield, P.F.: Reentrant excitation as a cause of cardiac arrhythmias. Am. J. Physiol., *235*:H1, 1978.
15. Josephson, M.E.: Paroxysmal supraventricular tachycardia: an electrophysiologic approach. Am. J. Cardiol., *41*:1123, 1978.
16. Moore, E.N., Spear, J.F., and Boineau, J.P.: Arrhythmias and conduction disturbances in simulated Wolff-Parkinson-White syndrome in the dog. Am. J. Cardiol., *26*:650, 1971.
17. Wit, A.L., Rosen, M.R., and Hoffman, B.F.: Electrophysiology and pharmacology of cardiac arrhythmias. II. Relationship of normal and abnormal electrical activity of cardiac fibers to the genesis of arrhythmias. B. Re-entry. Section 2, Am. Heart J., *88*:798, 1974.
18. Lazzara, R.: Anomalous atrioventricular conduction and the pre-excitation syndrome. In *Bellet's Essentials of Cardiac Arrhythmias.* Edited by R.H. Helfant. 2nd Edition. Philadelphia, W.B. Saunders, 1980.
19. Gunnar, R.M. (Chairman), et al.: Task Force IV: Pharmacologic interventions. Am. J. Cardiol., *50*:393, 1982.
20. Ettinger, S.J., and Buergelt, C.D.: Atrioventricular dissociation with accrochage in a dog with ruptured chordae tendineae. Am. J. Vet. Res., *29*:1499, 1968.
21. Watanabe, Y., and Dreifus, L.S.: *Cardiac Arrhythmias, Electrophysiologic Basis for Clinical Interpretation.* New York, Grune & Stratton, 1977.
22. El-Sherif, N.: The ventricular premature complex: mechanisms and significance. In *Cardiac Arrhythmias.* Edited by W.J. Mandel. Philadelphia, J.B. Lippincott, 1980.
23. Nelson, W.P.: Parasystole—"One heart beating as two!" Medical Times, *108*:141, 1980.
24. Chung, E.K.: Cardiac arrhythmias: diagnostic approach. In *Quick Reference to Cardiovascular Diseases.* 2nd Edition. Philadelphia, J.B. Lippincott, 1983.
25. Killip, T., and Gault, J.H.: Mode of onset of atrial fibrillation in man. Am. Heart J., *70*:172, 1965.
26. Friedman, H.H.: *Diagnostic Electrocardiography and Vectorcardiography.* 2nd Edition. New York, McGraw-Hill, 1977, p. 408.
27. Soffer, J., Dreifus, L.S., and Michelson, E.L.: Polymorphous ventricular tachycardia associated with normal and long Q-T intervals. Am. J. Cardiol., *49*:2021, 1982.
28. Smith, W.M., and Gallagher, J.J.: "Les Torsades de Pointes": an unusual ventricular arrhythmia. Ann. Intern. Med., *93*:578, 1980.
29. Tzivoni, D., Keren, A., and Stern, S.: Torsades de Pointes versus polymorphous ventricular tachycardia. Am. J. Cardiol., *52*:639, 1983.
29a. Tzivoni, D., et al.: Magnesium therapy for Torsades de Pointes. Am. J. Cardiol., *53*:528, 1984.
30. Bardy, G.H., Ungerleider, R.M., Smith, W.M., and Ideker, R.E.: A mechanism of Torsades de Pointes in a canine model. Circulation, *67*:52, 1983.
31. Lown, B., Ganong, W.F., and Levine, S.A.: The syndrome of short P-R interval, normal QRS complex and paroxysmal rapid heart action. Circulation, *5*:693, 1952.
32. Wiener, I.: Syndromes of Lown-Ganong-Levine and enhanced atrioventricular nodal conduction. Am. J. Cardiol., *52*:637, 1983.
33. Rosenbaum, M.B., and Elizari, M.V.: Mechanisms of intermittent bundle-branch block and paroxysmal atrioventricular block. Postgrad. Med., *53*(5):87, 1973.

Section Seven

Self-assessment Tracings

Canine (1–47)

Feline (48–71)

To make no mistakes is not in the power of man; but from their errors and mistakes the wise and good learn wisdom for the future.*

PLUTARCH

This self-assessment section is aimed at providing the reader with additional opportunities to evaluate his own understanding by interpreting electrocardiograms and solving arrhythmia problems as they occur clinically. Each tracing is accompanied by a short case history and question on interpretation. The tracing is then again shown on the reverse side of the page with appropriate labeling and interpretation. Consult Chapter 10, on the use of antiarrhythmic drugs in the dog and cat, for a complete discussion on the respective drug being recommended. As a study aid, each answer has been referenced to direct the reader to the appropriate section of the book if further clarification is needed.

Before evaluating the electrocardiographic tracings in this self-assessment section, the systematic approach to the electrocardiogram should first be reviewed. In general, the person best qualified to read the electrocardiogram is the clinician who is taking care of the animal. If someone else reads the electrocardiogram, he should become a consultant and should discuss the clinical picture with the clinician before the first interpretation is made.

The electrocardiogram must be evaluated in conjunction with a complete data base. The ideal data base for the cardiovascular system consists of history, physical examination, and laboratory profile. The history includes age, breed, weight, medication (especially digitalis), and associated diseases. The laboratory examination includes thoracic radiography, and an analysis of blood, urine, and extravascular fluids.

Before the electrocardiogram is examined, it is preferable to read the tracing before it is cut and mounted. It is important to study long strips of one lead (usually lead II) for the accurate analysis of rhythm and heart rate. Lead II is usually used for the analysis of heart rate, heart rhythm, and measuring complexes and intervals. Following are the steps in analysis:

1. **Calculate the heart rate.**
2. **Determine the rhythm.**

---

*Edwards, T. (Ed.): *The New Dictionary of Thoughts: A Cyclopedia of Quotations*. Standard Book Co., 1957.

3. **Measure the complexes and intervals:**
   P wave, P-R interval, QRS complex
   S-T segment, T wave, and Q-T interval.
4. **Examine the basic limb leads** (I, II, III, aVR, aVL, and aVF).
5. **Determine the mean electrical axis.**

A systematic method for an accurate electrocardiographic analysis of a rhythm strip (usually lead II) for arrhythmias includes the following steps:

Step 1. General inspection of the rhythm strip.
   Is the rhythm normal sinus or characteristic of a type of cardiac arrhythmia? The heart rate should also be classified as rapid, slow, or normal.

Step 2. Identification of P waves.
   Is the atrial activity regular and the shape uniform?

Step 3. Recognition of QRS complexes.
   The QRS complexes should be characterized as to their morphology, uniformity, and regularity.

Step 4. Relationship between P waves and QRS complexes.

Step 5. Summary of findings and final classification of the arrhythmia.
   What is the predominant rhythm? Is the arrhythmia an abnormality of impulse formation or of impulse conduction or both? If either or both, what is the site of the abnormality?

The final interpretation can include the following possibilities:
1. The tracing is normal.
2. Borderline record; there are minor changes, the significance of which will depend on the clinical findings and serial electrocardiogram.
3. Abnormal tracing typical of (name of condition).
4. Abnormal tracing consistent with (name of conditions).
5. Abnormal tracing not characteristic of any specific entity.

When an arrhythmia is diagnosed; the following questions should be asked:
1. What caused the rhythm and/or conduction disturbances?
2. How will the abnormality affect the hemodynamic aspect of the animal's clinical picture?
3. How can progressive complications be anticipated and prevented?
4. What is the therapeutic regimen?

Case 1

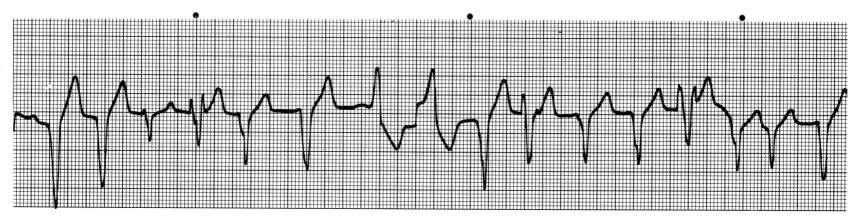

Question. This tracing was recorded from a dog with generalized weakness, 2 days after having been hit by a car. What is your interpretation? How should it be treated?

Case 2

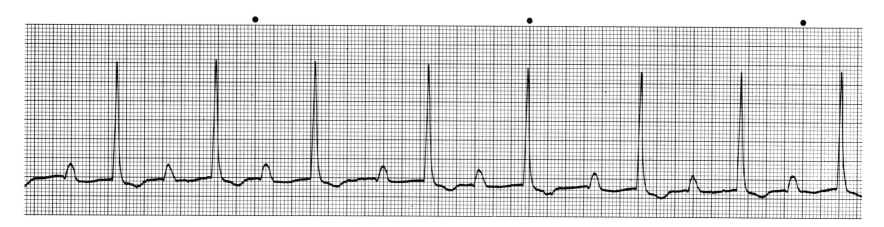

Question. This rhythm strip was obtained from a dog with chronic mitral valvular insufficiency on treatment with digoxin. Severe vomiting and diarrhea were present for 2 days. What is your interpretation? How should it be treated?

Case 1

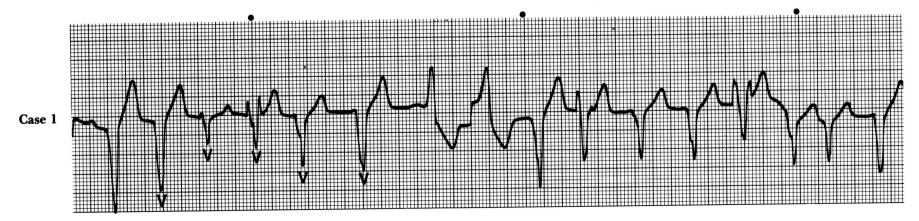

Answer. Ventricular tachycardia, a continuous series of VPCs (ventricular premature complexes) of variable shape (multiform) (V). (Refer to Chapter 6.) Ventricular tachycardia should be treated as soon as possible since ventricular fibrillation can easily follow. Cases with ventricular tachycardia must be continuously monitored. The drug of choice is lidocaine via continuous drip or intravenous bolus, or both. Electrical cardioversion is indicated if the animal is in a hemodynamic crisis and lidocaine fails. Any underlying acid-base and electrolyte abnormalities must be corrected. Oral antiarrhythmic therapy (quinidine or procainamide, drugs of choice) is used to prevent recurrent ventricular tachycardia. Ventricular tachycardia is generally considered the most serious of all tachyarrhythmias. There is usually a marked fall in cardiac output and consequently in cerebral as well as renal blood flow, especially when there is myocardial disease.

Case 2

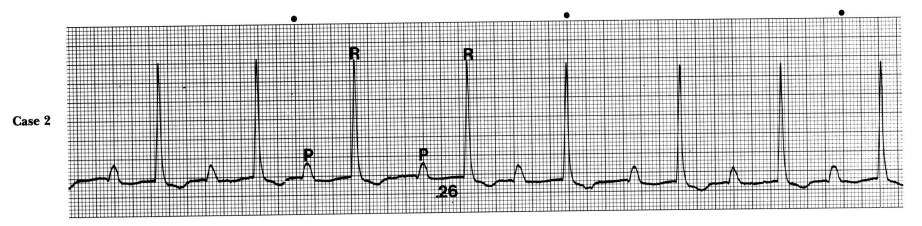

Answer. Sinus rhythm at a rate of 110 beats/min with severe first-degree AV block. (Refer to Chapter 6.) The P-R interval is 0.26 second (13 boxes, normal not greater than 0.13 sec or 6½ boxes). The wide P waves (0.06 sec) indicate probable left atrial enlargement. (Refer to Chapter 4.) Digoxin toxicity is the most common cause of first-degree AV block. Prevention of digoxin toxicity is the safest approach. Discontinuation of the drug is the treatment of choice until all toxic signs are resolved, which may take a number of days. The dosage of digoxin should then be reduced, especially if there is reduced renal function and lowered body weight. The dose of digoxin should always be calculated on the basis of lean body weight (usually by subtracting 10% to 15% of the actual weight).

Case 3

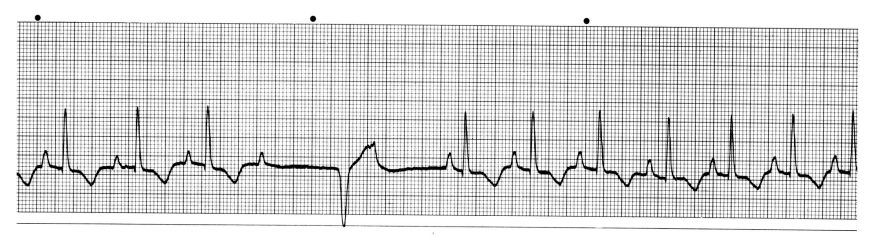

Question. This rhythm strip was recorded from a dog with episodes of fainting. What is your interpretation? How should it be treated?

Case 4

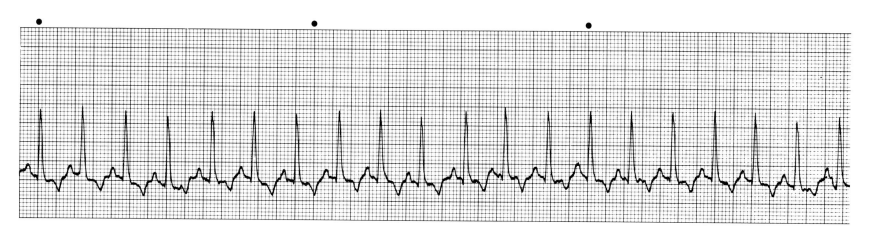

Question. This rhythm strip was recorded from a dog with a fever. What is your interpretation? How should it be treated?

Case 3

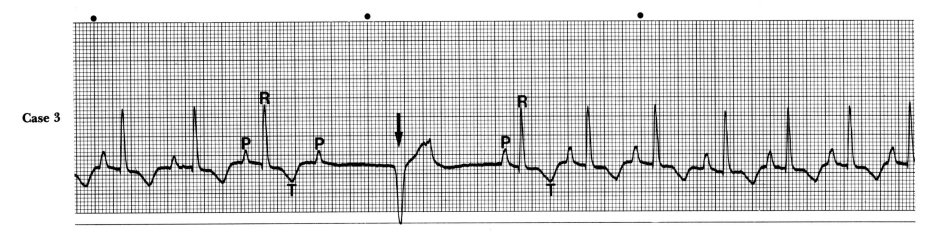

Answer. Ventricular escape complex (arrow) following second-degree AV block. (Refer to Chapter 6.) The P wave preceding the escape complex is blocked, causing a marked pause in the rhythm. The ventricle rescues the heart rhythm after the pause for one complex. The rhythm then returns to normal sinus. The actual ventricular escape complex should not be suppressed with quinidine, a common mistake. Treatment may include atropine, glycopyrrolate, isoproterenol, or artificial pacing. In an asymptomatic dog, second-degree AV block (P waves not followed by QRS-T complexes, a fixed P-R interval) may be a normal finding. Escape complexes are usually not present.

Case 4

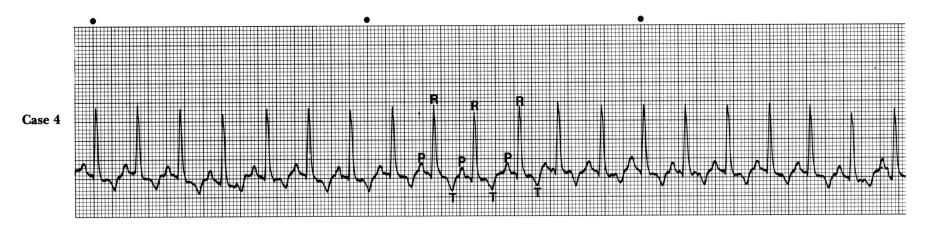

Answer. Sinus tachycardia at a rate of 260 beats/min (approximate rate determined by counting R-R intervals between two sets of dots and multiplying by 20; i.e., 13 × 20 = 260). (Refer to Chapter 6.) This arrhythmia should be approached by simply identifying and eliminating the underlying factor. For example, antibiotics were administered to the dog for a bacterial infection that was causing the fever. The infection and accompanying sinus tachycardia eventually were eliminated. If the sinus tachycardia is due to congestive heart failure, digoxin for the underlying cardiac insufficiency is indicated. The short P-R interval can be a normal variant in fever, anemia, hyperthyroidism, and other heightened adrenergic states.

Case 5

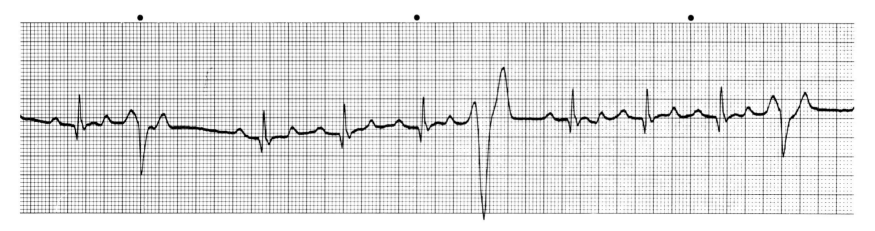

Question. This rhythm strip was obtained from a Great Dane with a gastric torsion. What is your interpretation? How should it be treated?

Case 6

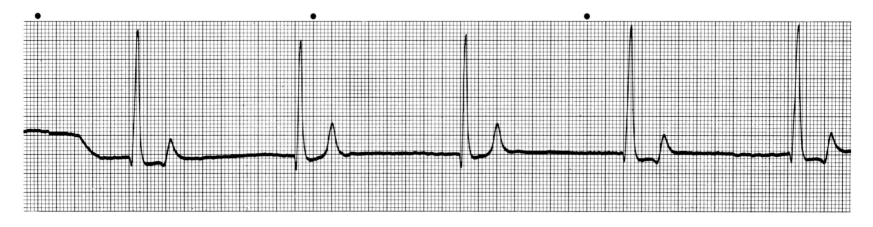

Question. This rhythm strip was recorded from a dog with an acute onset of diarrhea and weakness. What is your interpretation? How should it be treated?

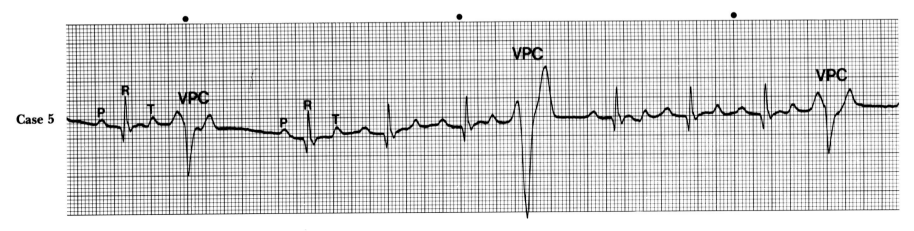

Case 5

Answer. Sinus rhythm at a rate of 140 beats/min with three multiform VPCs. (Refer to Chapter 6.) The low-voltage QRS complexes are usually normal in dogs with large thoracic cavities. In addition to relieving the gastic torsion, therapy would include lidocaine, quinidine, or procainamide. Close monitoring of the electrocardiogram is important during surgery. Supportive measures are important; acid-base and electrolyte abnormalities should be corrected. It is important to remember that ventricular arrhythmias may not occur until 12 to 36 hours after the gastric torsion.

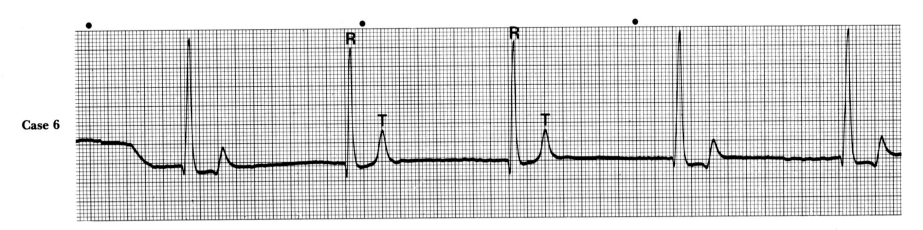

Case 6

Answer. Atrial standstill with a sinoventricular rhythm and rate of 65 beats/min in a dog with Addison's disease. (Refer to Chapter 6.) No P waves are visible, and the T waves are tall and peaked. Renal insufficiency (usually from oliguric renal failure or obstructive uropathy) is another cause of hyperkalemia. Lowering the serum potassium (9.8 mEq/L in this case) involves administration of fluids, sodium bicarbonate, intravenous glucocorticoids, regular insulin and dextrose (for emergency treatment), and mineralocorticoids.

Case 7

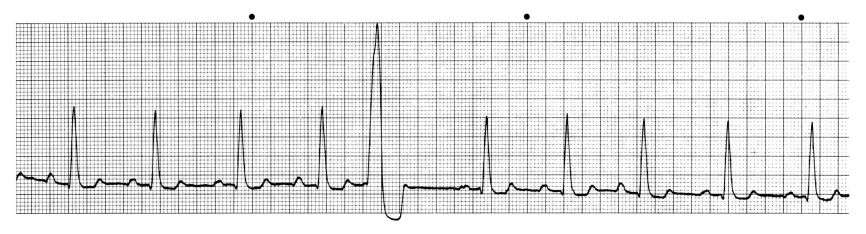

Question. This rhythm strip was recorded from a dog with chronic mitral insufficiency receiving treatment with digoxin. What is your interpretation? What treatment would you recommend?

Case 8

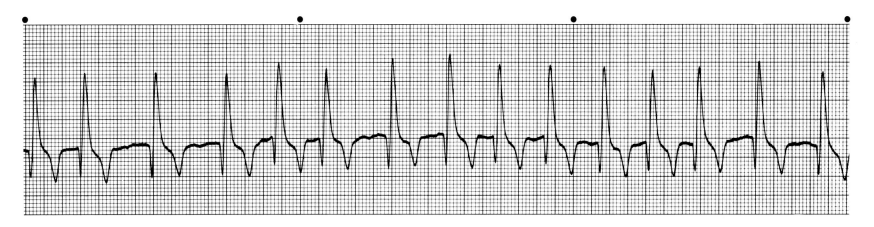

Question. This rhythm strip was recorded from a Great Dane with heart failure. What two conditions are commonly associated with this arrhythmia? What treatment would you recommend?

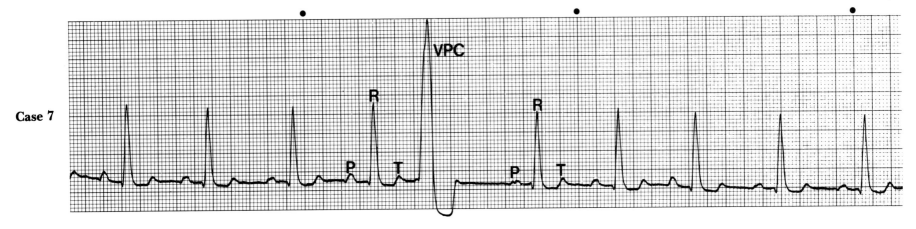

Case 7

Answer. Sinus rhythm at a rate of 140 beats/min with one VPC originating in the right ventricle (positive QRS). (Refer to Chapter 6.) The wide P wave (0.05 sec) and the wide QRS complex (0.07 sec) indicate probable left atrial and left ventricular enlargement. The change in the configuration of the P waves indicates a wandering sinus pacemaker. An occasional single VPC is usually not significant. Digoxin toxicity should be considered. The dog's weight should be rechecked, and laboratory tests for renal insufficiency done.

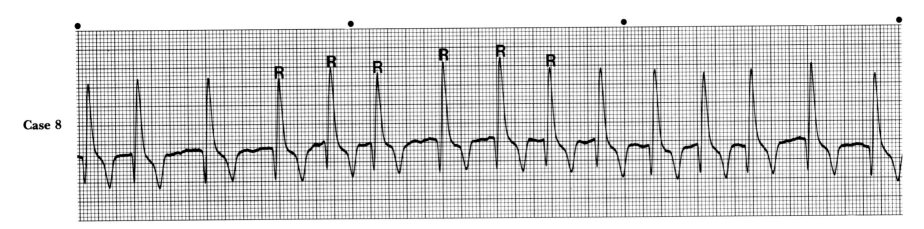

Case 8

Answer. Atrial fibrillation with a ventricular rate averaging 200 beats/min. (Refer to Chapter 6.) The ventricular rhythm is irregular with absent P waves. The wide QRS complexes (0.08 sec) and S-T segment coving probably indicate left ventricular enlargement (refer to Chapter 4). Chronic atrioventricular valvular insufficiency (small breeds) and the dilated form of cardiomyopathy (this dog) often are associated with atrial fibrillation. Digitalization to reduce the heart rate to less than 160 beats/min is the treatment of choice. Propranolol is usually necessary as an additional drug for slowing the ventricular rate.

Case 9

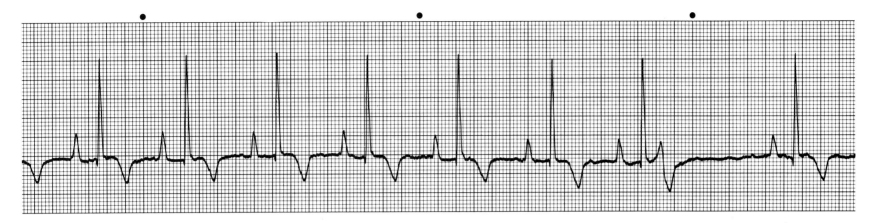

Question. This rhythm strip was recorded from a dog with a chronic cough. The dog had been given digoxin for a suspected cardiac insufficiency. What is your interpretation?

Case 10

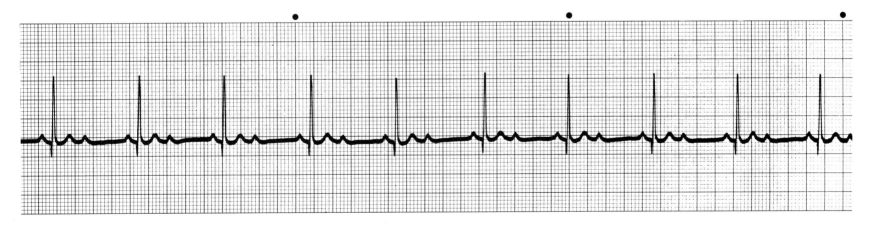

Question. This tracing was recorded from an 8-year-old Standard Poodle with episodes of syncope (paper speed, 25 mm/sec). What is your interpretation? How should it be treated?

Case 9

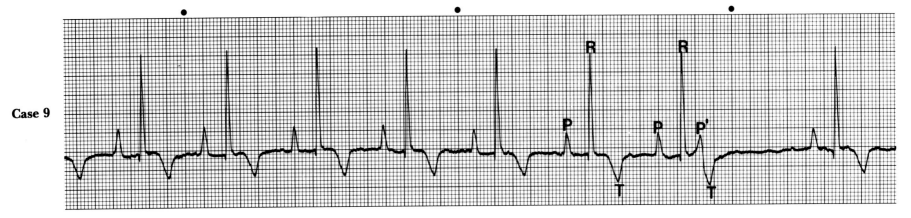

Answer. Sinus rhythm at a rate of 120 beats/min. P′ represents a nonconducted APC (atrial premature complex). (Refer to Chapter 6.) The premature P′ wave is so early that the AV junction has not totally recovered; i.e., the impulse is not conducted to the ventricles. The premature P′ wave is superimposed on the T wave of the QRS complex. The tall peaked P waves, indicative of right atrial enlargement, were compatible with secondary pulmonary hypertension from a collapsed trachea on thoracic radiographs. (Refer to Chapter 4.) Digoxin should not be given for this condition. By way of review, the following steps should be used to analyze any rhythm strip: (1) general inspection of the electrocardiogram—heart rate (normal on this strip), rhythm (regular with a pause on this strip), (2) identification of the P waves (P′-shaped complex deforming the T wave of the QRS complex before the pause), (3) recognition of the QRS complexes (normal-appearing), (4) the relationship between P waves and QRS complexes (no QRS complex following the P′ wave, explaining the noncompensatory pause in rhythm; other P waves associated with the QRS complexes), and (5) summary of findings with final classification of the arrhythmia (sinus rhythm with a nonconducted APC).

Case 10

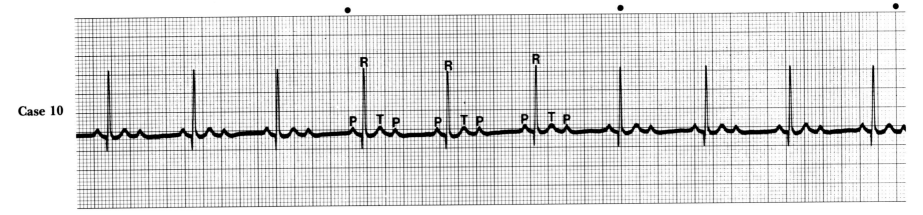

Answer. Ventricular rate (QRS complexes) of 65 beats/min and 2:1 second-degree AV block. (Refer to Chapter 6.) The atrial rate (P waves) is 130 beats/min, every other P wave being blocked. The blocked P waves could be mistaken for T waves, but the P-P intervals are essentially constant throughout the strip. The QRS configurations are normal, an indication that the bundle branches are probably not affected. Choices of therapy could include atropine, glycopyrrolate, isoproterenol, or pacemaker insertion.

Case 11

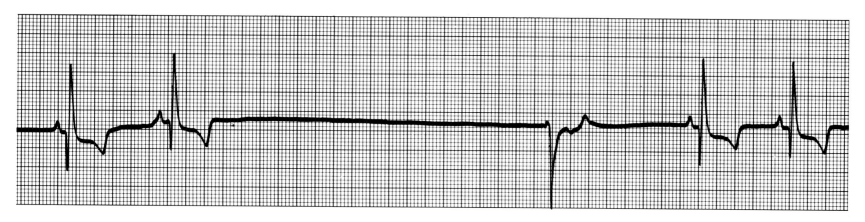

Question. This strip was recorded from a dog with a reaction to acetylpromazine as a preanesthetic medication. What is your interpretation of the rhythm? How should it be treated?

Case 12

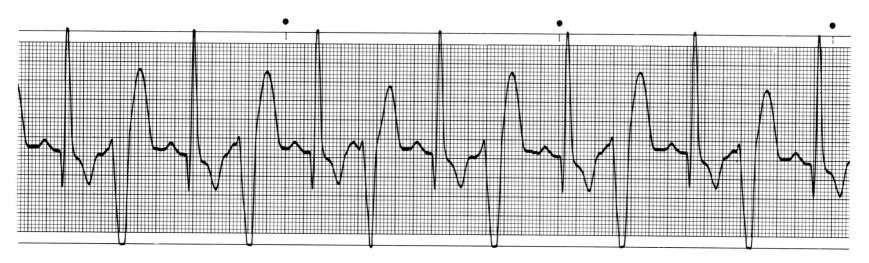

Question. This rhythm strip was recorded from an 8-month-old Collie with congestive heart failure and a machinery murmur on auscultation. What is your interpretation? How should it be treated?

Case 11

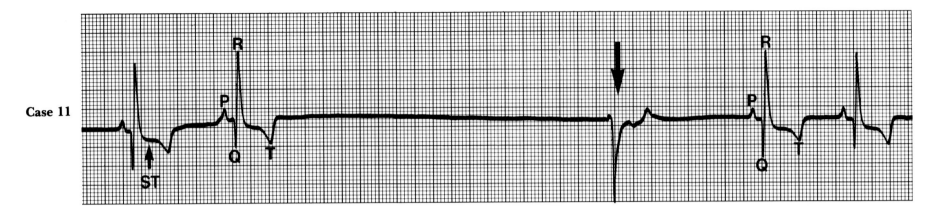

Answer. Sinoatrial (SA) arrest with a ventricular escape complex (arrow) occurring after a long pause (1.5 sec). (Refer to Chapter 6.) This ventricular escape complex represents a rescuing mechanism for the heart. The SA node soon takes over.

Treatment of the animal involves correction of the underlying ar-

rhythmia. Atropine was used in this case to eliminate the high vagal tone and subsequent SA arrest from the tranquilizer reaction. The S-T segment depression indicates probable myocardial hypoxia. The large Q waves can be normal, especially in young and thin-chested large breeds. (Refer to Chapter 4.)

Case 12

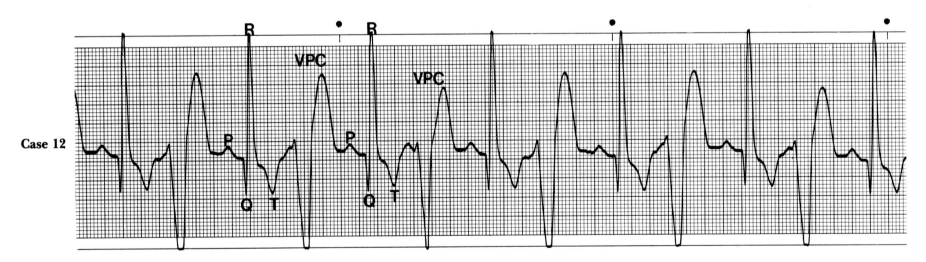

Answer. Ventricular bigeminy, left VPCs alternating with a normal sinus complex. (Refer to Chapter 6.) The wide P waves and the tall and wide QRS complexes indicate left atrial and left ventricular enlargement. (Refer to Chapter 4.) Thoracic radiographs were compatible with a patent ductus arteriosus and left-sided heart failure.

Digoxin and diuretics were later used to treat the heart failure. Lidocaine followed by procainamide was used to control the ventricular arrhythmia. Surgical correction of the defect was later performed.

Case 13

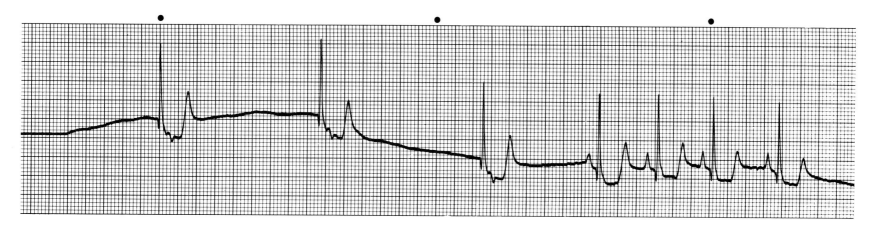

Question. This rhythm strip was recorded from a Miniature Schnauzer with episodes of syncope. What is your interpretation? How should it be treated?

Case 14

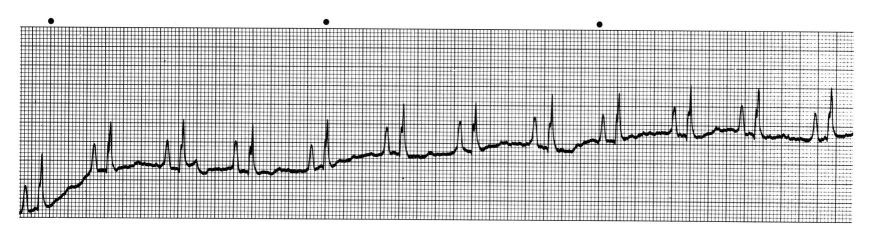

Question. This electrocardiogram was recorded from an obese Toy Poodle with a chronic cough. What is your interpretation? What underlying condition should you first consider?

Case 13

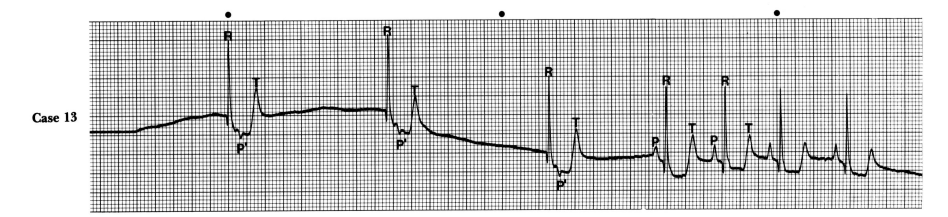

Answer. Junctional escape rhythm (the first three complexes) representing a safety or rescuing mechanism that operates when a pause occurs in the heart rhythm. (Refer to Chapter 6.) Inverted P' waves follow each of the three QRS complexes. The negative P' waves in junctional complexes may precede, be superimposed on, or follow the QRS. The rhythm returns to a normal sinus rhythm at the end of the strip. The electrocardiographic pattern is compatible with sick sinus syndrome. Large T waves and S-T segment depression may indicate myocardial hypoxia. This SA abnormality is frequently found in Miniature Schnauzers. Drugs such as atropine are usually of no value, even as a temporary measure. Insertion of an artificial pacemaker is probably the only guaranteed therapy for symptomatic sick sinus syndrome.

Case 14

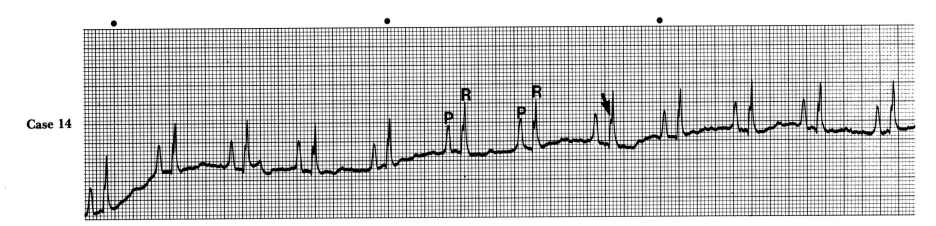

Answer. Normal sinus rhythm at a rate of 140 beats/min. The P waves are tall (0.7 or 7 boxes), slender, and peaked, indicating right atrial enlargement. (Refer to Chapter 4.) This is often seen in dogs with a chronic collapsed trachea. The notched QRS complex (arrow) may be a normal finding, or it may represent a minor intraventricular conduction defect since the QRS duration is normal. The wandering baseline is the result of movement of the animal during the recording.

Case 15

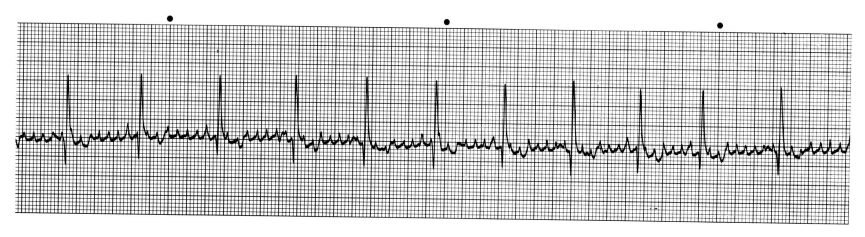

Question. This rhythm strip was recorded from a dog with a history of vomiting. What is your interpretation?

Case 16

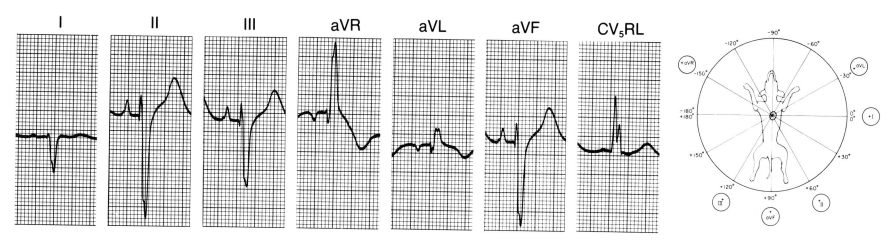

Question. These electrocardiographic leads were recorded from a dog after a right ventricular catheterization and angiocardiogram. The electrocardiogram was normal before the study. What is your interpretation? How should it be treated?

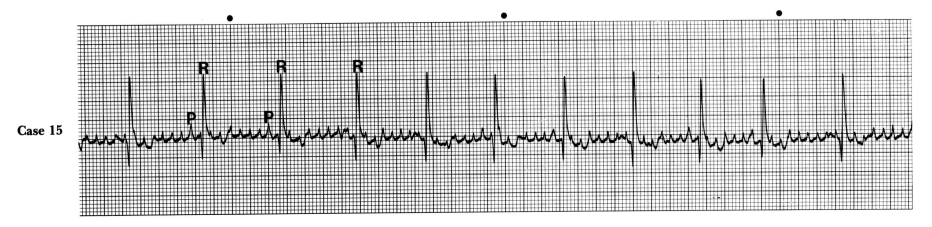

Case 15

Answer. Sinus rhythm at a rate of 140 beats/min and artifacts due to muscle tremor. (Refer to Chapter 2.) The P waves are difficult to identify and the ventricular rhythm is regular. The rapid and irregular vibrations of the baseline resemble atrial ectopic waves. The artifacts disappeared (not shown) after the dog relaxed.

I	II	III	aVR	aVL	aVF	CV₅RL

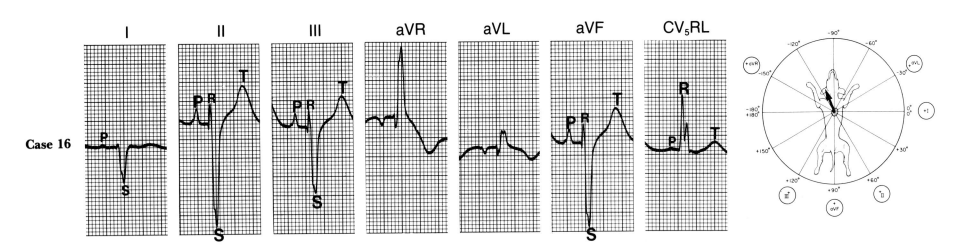

Case 16

Answer. Right bundle branch block. (Refer to Chapter 4.) The electrocardiographic features include QRS duration of 0.08 second; positive QRS complex in aVR, aVL, and CV₅RL (M shaped); and large wide S waves in leads I, II, III, and aVF. There is a right axis deviation (approximately − 110°; lead aVL the closest isoelectric lead, with lead II perpendicular and negative). The right bundle branch is vulnerable to injury. The right bundle was assumed to have been injured during the cardiac catheterization. This conduction defect disappeared in 2 days. Right bundle branch block, in and of itself, does not cause hemodynamic problems. It cannot be differentiated from right ventricular hypertrophy on the electrocardiogram. A thoracic radiograph is necessary to rule out right ventricular enlargement.

Case 17

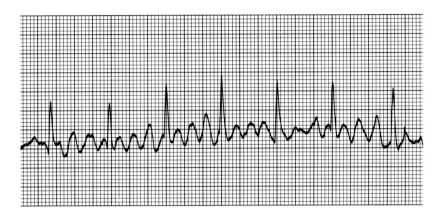 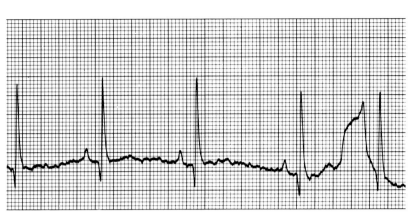

Question. These two tracings were recorded from different dogs. What is your interpretation?

Case 18

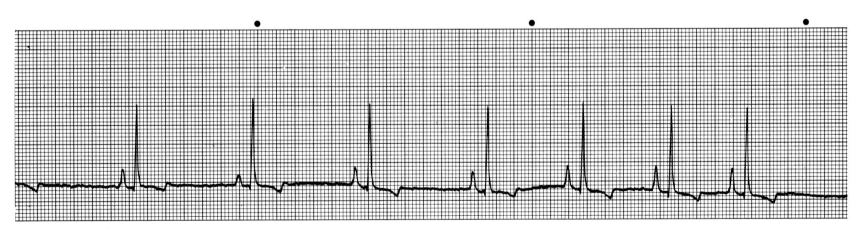

Question. This tracing was recorded from a dog with a chronic respiratory condition. What is your interpretation?

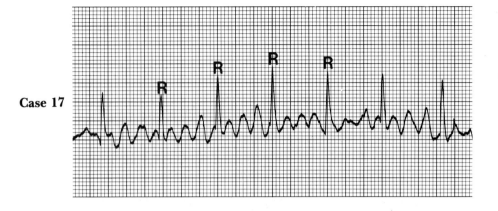

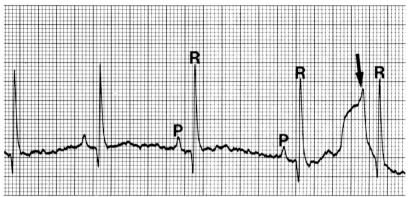

Case 17

Answer. Artifact. (Refer to Chapter 6.) The strip on the left was recorded from a nervous dog. The rapid and irregular vibrations of the baseline resemble atrial ectopic waves. The ventricular rhythm (R) is regular with the rate of vibrations irregular. If the rhythm were atrial, the ventricular rate would probably be more rapid with the rhythm irregular. The artifact (arrow) on the right strip was created when the dog jerked its leg. The artifact simulates a VPC, but the ventricular rhythm is not interrupted.

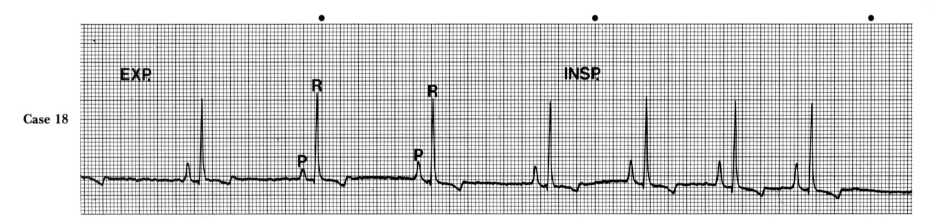

Case 18

Answer. Respiratory sinus arrhythmia with an average rate of 120 beats/min. (Refer to Chapter 6.) The variations in heart rate are usually related to respiration, the rate increasing with inspiration *(INSP)* and decreasing with expiration *(EXP)*. The normal SA pacemaker is under the continuous monitoring influence of the autonomic nervous system. The configuration of the P waves during inspiration is different from that of the P waves during expiration (a wandering sinus pacemaker). The tall peaked P waves during inspiration may indicate right atrial enlargement.

Case 19

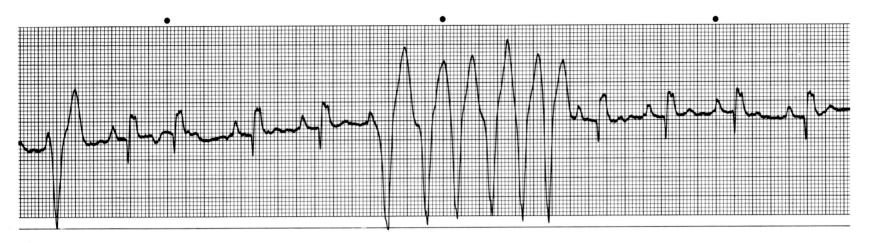

Question. This rhythm strip was recorded from a dog with mitral insufficiency and pulmonary edema. What are your interpretations and recommendations for treatment?

Case 20

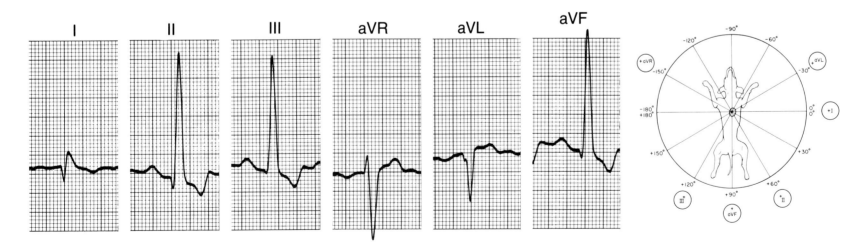

Question. These electrocardiographic strips were recorded from a Collie puppy with a cardiac murmur. What is your interpretation? What advice should you give the owner?

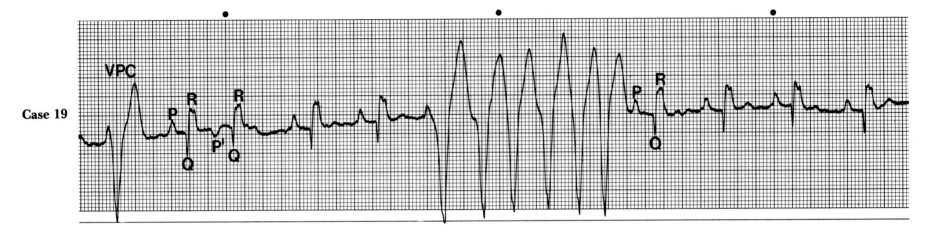

Case 19

Answer. Paroxysmal ventricular tachycardia (midsection of strip) with one VPC and one supraventricular ectopic complex (P'-QR) at the first portion of the strip. (Refer to Chapter 6.) The ectopic P' wave is inverted, indicating that the atrial focus is in the lower portion of the atria near the AV junction. Supraventricular complexes commonly occur in severe mitral valvular insufficiency. The ventricular tachycardia is most likely due to severe heart failure and secondary myocardial hypoxia. Cage rest, digoxin, diuretics, and oxygen eliminated the ventricular arrhythmia. If paroxysms of ventricular tachycardia persist, lidocaine should be used since it is most effective and safest. Procainamide or quinidine may also be needed. Ventricular tachycardia can cause a marked fall in cardiac output. The low-voltage sinus complexes are probably caused by the pulmonary edema.

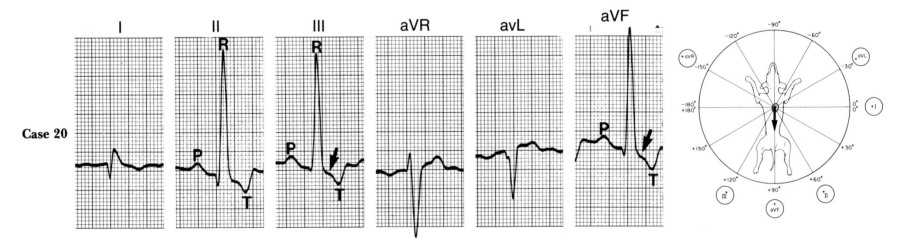

Case 20

Answer. Left ventricular and left atrial enlargement. (Refer to Chapter 4.) The electrocardiographic features for left ventricular enlargement include tall R waves in leads II, III, and aVF (averaging 3.0 mv), wide QRS complexes (0.08 sec), and S-T segment coving (arrows). The electrical axis is normal; +90° (lead I isoelectric). The P waves are wide (0.06 sec), an indication of probable left atrial enlargement. Congenital cardiac defects causing left heart enlargement should be considered—e.g., patent ductus arteriosus, congenital mitral valvular insufficiency, and aortic stenosis (electrocardiograms often normal). A thoracic radiograph should be the next step because of these marked electrocardiographic changes. A patent ductus arteriosus was confirmed on thoracic radiographs.

Case 21

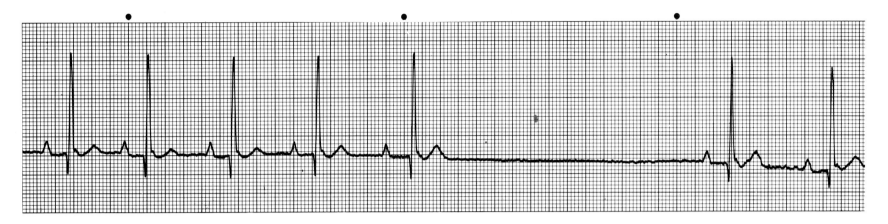

Question. This tracing was recorded from a dog with chronic mitral insufficiency that was being treated with digoxin and diuretics. The dog was doing well clinically on a recheck visit. What is your interpretation of the rhythm?

Case 22

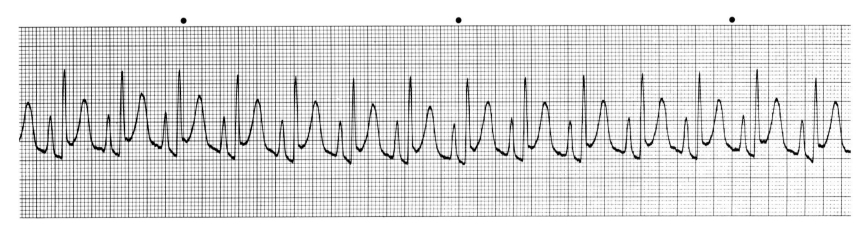

Question. This tracing was obtained from a Yorkshire Terrier with a chronic cough for 9 months. The dog was admitted to the hospital with severe dyspnea. What is your interpretation? What condition is most likely associated with this electrocardiogram?

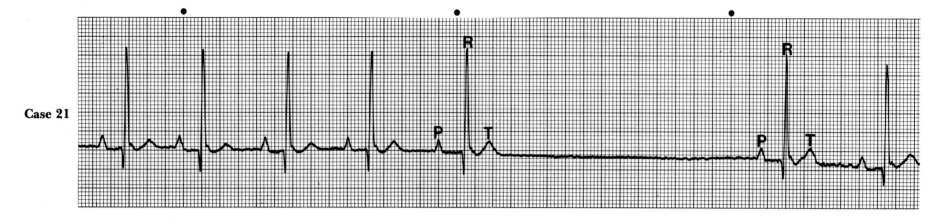

Case 21

Answer. SA arrest. (Refer to Chapter 6.) The pause that occurs is longer than two of the normal R-R intervals. Early digoxin toxicity, causing an increased vagal tone, is a possibility in this case. Digoxin acts directly on the vagus nerve. The P-R intervals are of varying duration (P-R interval prolonged in the complex before the pause, 0.15 sec), probably secondary to the increased vagal tone. Both the digoxin and the diuretic should be temporarily stopped for 1 or 2 days, and a second electrocardiogram obtained. Renal function tests should be evaluated.

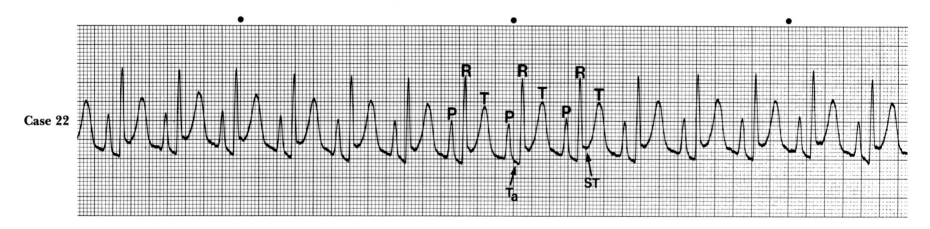

Case 22

Answer. Sinus tachycardia at a rate of 190 beats/min, right atrial enlargement (tall peaked P waves), S-T segment elevation, an increased amplitude of the T wave, and a T_a wave (depression of the baseline following the P wave). (Refer to Chapter 4.) The S-T segment elevation and large T waves are compatible with myocardial hypoxia. The T_a wave is often seen with atrial enlargement. All these electrocardiographic changes are commonly seen in dogs with severe respiratory signs from a collapsed trachea. This diagnosis was later confirmed on thoracic radiographs.

Case 23

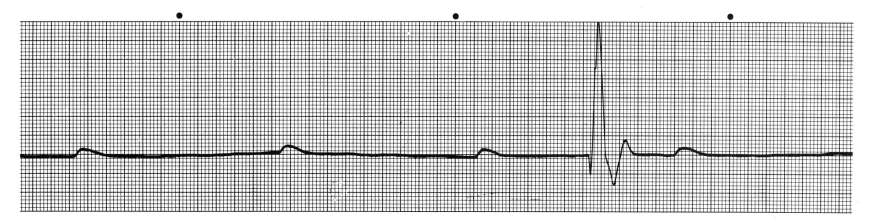

Question. This rhythm strip was recorded from a dog in cardiac arrest. What is your interpretation? What treatment would you institute?

Case 24

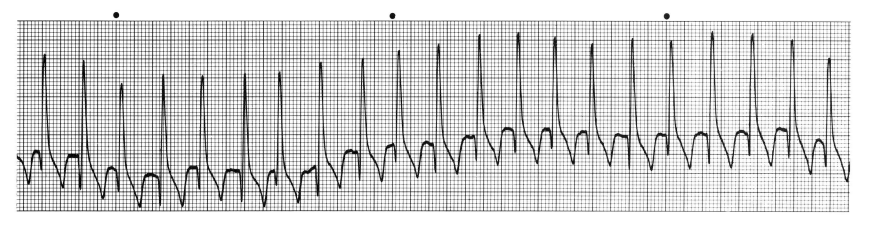

Question. This rhythm strip was recorded from a dog with chronic mitral valvular insufficiency. What is your interpretation? What treatment would you recommend? What is the prognosis?

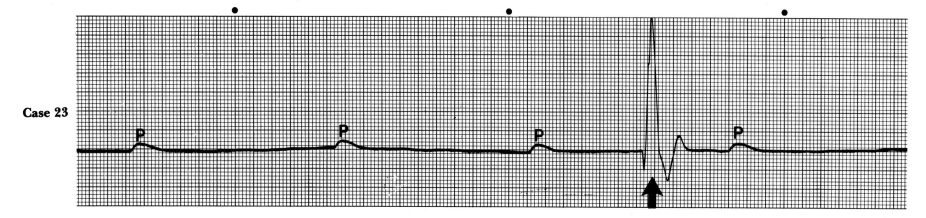

Case 23

Answer. Third-degree AV block (ventricular asystole) with one ventricular escape complex (arrow) attempting to rescue the heart. (Refer to Chapter 6.) The atrial rate (P waves) is extremely slow with a marked interatrial conduction delay (P waves 0.12 sec or six boxes in duration). The wide P waves represent false-positive left atrial enlargement. This is the electrocardiogram of a dying heart with probable *final* cardiac arrest. Cardiac resuscitation is usually not successful. Isoproterenol is one of the drugs indicated, especially for the AV block. Artificial pacing is necessary.

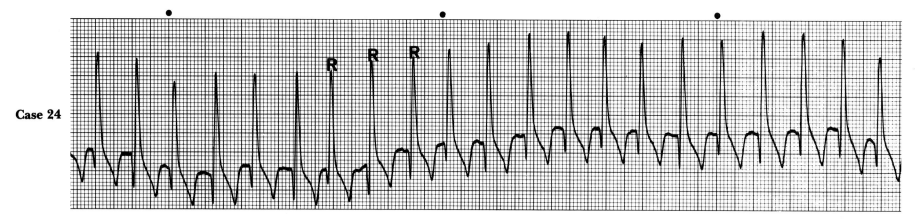

Case 24

Answer. Atrial fibrillation with an average ventricular rate of 300 beats/min. (Refer to Chapter 6.) The ventricular rhythm appears less irregular at rapid ventricular rates. Atrial activity is chaotic and uncoordinated, with atrial function essentially lost. In dogs the condition most often associated with atrial fibrillation is chronic mitral valvular insufficiency. The rapid irregular heart rate makes some ventricular beats ineffective, producing a pulse deficit. The onset of atrial fibrillation in a dog with mitral valvular insufficiency usually brings about marked clinical deterioration. The prognosis is guarded. Digitalization is indicated first, with propranolol often needed to further slow the ventricular rate.

Case 25

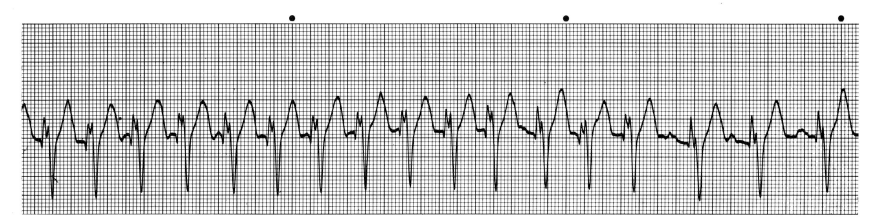

Question. This tracing was recorded from a 10-year-old dog with mitral valvular insufficiency and episodes of fainting. Ocular pressure was applied during the recording. What is your interpretation? What treatment would you recommend?

Case 26

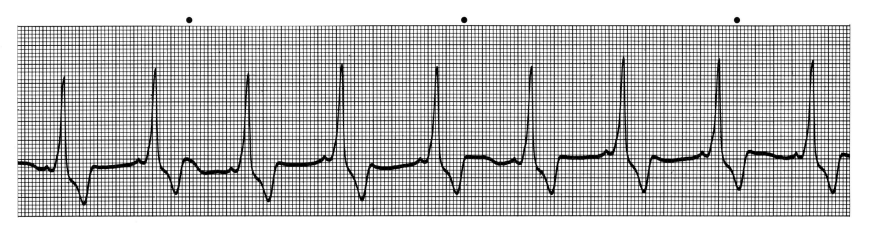

Question. This tracing was obtained from a dog undergoing evaluation for surgery. There were no signs of cardiac disease. What is your interpretation, and what treatment would you recommend?

Case 25

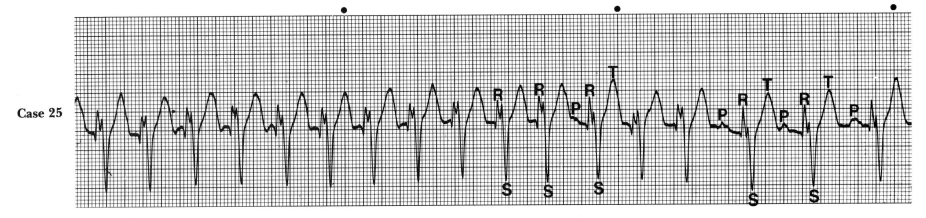

Answer. Supraventricular tachycardia (Refer to Chapter 6.) with a pre-existing intraventricular block (right bundle branch block) at a rate of 250 beats/min. Whether the tachycardia in the first part of the tracing is ventricular cannot be determined. P waves are not visible. Vagal stimulation by ocular pressure eventually terminated the tachycardia. The last three complexes and the sixth complex from the end are sinus in origin with QRS complexes identical to those present during the tachycardia. These sinus ventricular complexes are the result of atrial activity (P waves). The P waves are wide and notched, an indication of left atrial enlargement that may explain the source of the supraventricular tachycardia. Digoxin can be used to prevent the attacks of tachycardia.

Case 26

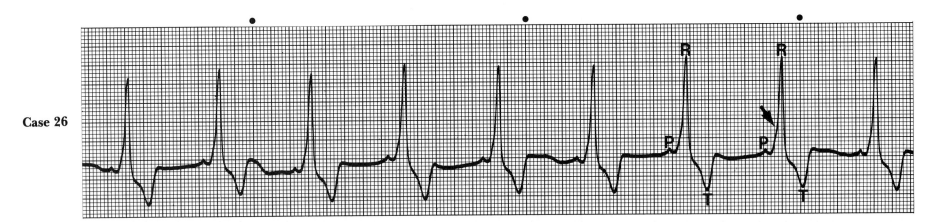

Answer. Ventricular pre-excitation (Wolff-Parkinson-White syndrome if paroxysms of supraventricular tachycardia are present in other strips). (Refer to Chapter 6.) Ventricular pre-excitation occurs when impulses originating in the SA node or atrium activate a portion of the ventricles prematurely through an accessory pathway around the AV node. Electrocardiographic features include a shortened P-R interval and a widened QRS complex with slurring or notching (arrow) (delta wave) of the upstroke of the R wave. Ventricular pre-excitation without tachycardia requires no therapy. The dog should be closely monitored during surgery, and atropine should not be given.

Case 27

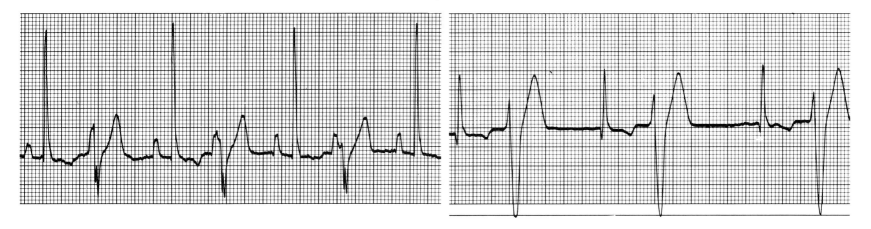

Question. These two strips were recorded from different dogs. The strip on the left was recorded from a normal dog during anesthesia, that on the right from a dog with atrial fibrillation being treated with digoxin and diuretics for a chronic heart condition. What is your interpretation? What two drugs can often cause these undesirable arrhythmias?

Case 28

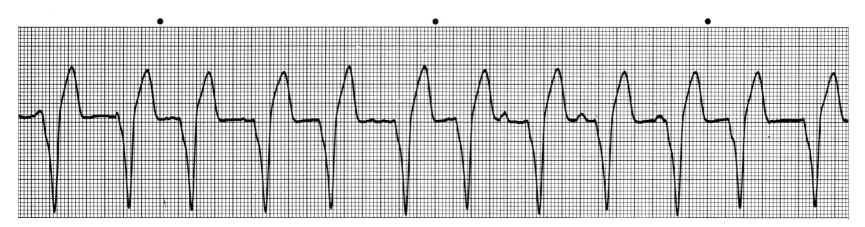

Question. This tracing was recorded from a Boxer with reduced exercise tolerance. The heart was of normal size on thoracic radiographs. What is your interpretation, and what treatment would you recommend?

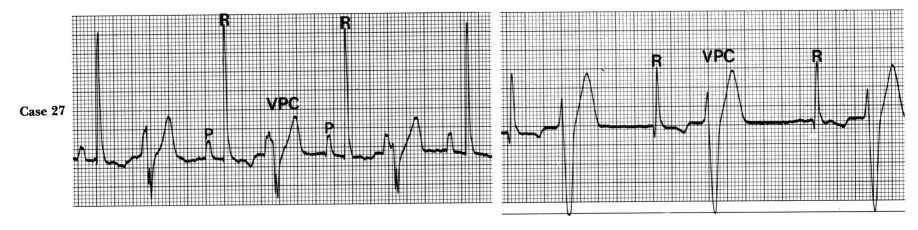

Case 27

Answer. Ventricular bigeminy is evident in both strips. (Refer to Chapter 6.) The strip on the left has VPCs alternating with sinus complexes. Barbiturate anesthetics can often cause this arrhythmia. The strip on the right is atrial fibrillation and ventricular bigeminy.

No P waves are present. The slow regular ventricular rate (R) indicates a probable block in the AV junction. When such a cardiac rhythm disorder is encountered during digoxin therapy, the diagnosis of digoxin toxicity is likely.

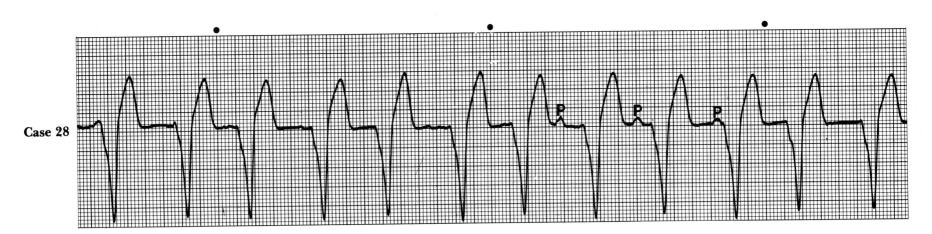

Case 28

Answer. Ventricular tachycardia. (Refer to Chapter 6.) The wide and bizarre QRS complexes occur at a rate of 160 beats/min, with no relationship to the P waves. There are more QRS complexes than P waves. Ventricular tachycardia should be treated as soon as possible. Acid-base and electrolyte abnormalities should always be corrected. The Boxer breed appears to be very susceptible to myocarditis; the etiology is unknown. The drug of choice is lidocaine administered intravenously. Procainamide is the second drug of choice, if lidocaine is ineffective. For maintenance or long-term therapy, oral quinidine or procainamide is effective. A "thump" on the chest can be used, especially in an emergency when drugs are ineffective.

Case 29

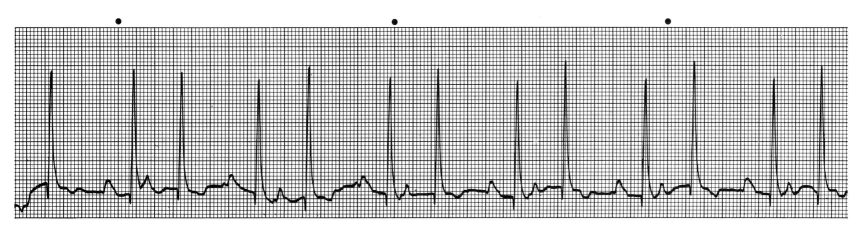

Question. This rhythm strip was recorded from a 12-year-old dog with chronic mitral valvular insufficiency. What is your interpretation? What treatment would you recommend?

Case 30

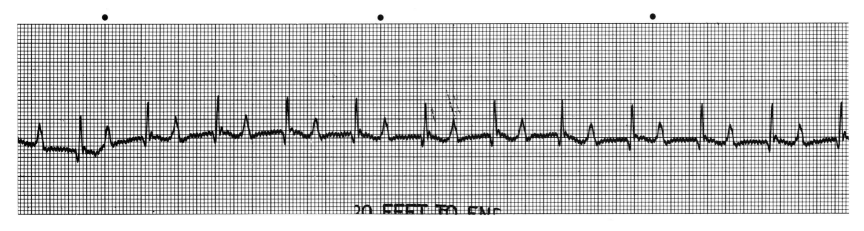

Question. This tracing was recorded from a dog with vomiting and diarrhea for 4 days. Digoxin was being given for a cardiac problem. What is your interpretation? What treatment would you recommend?

Case 29

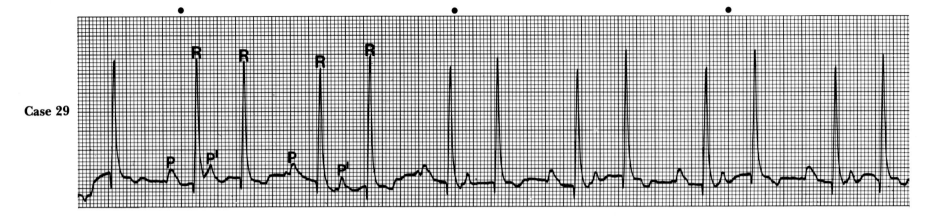

Answer. The rhythm is sinus with frequent APCs producing atrial bigeminy. (Refer to Chapter 6.) The second complex of each pair is an APC. The ectopic positive P′ wave is premature (superimposed on the T wave of the preceding complex) with the configuration of the P′ wave different from that of the sinus P waves. The sinus P waves are wide and notched, indicating left atrial enlargement. Digoxin is the treatment of choice for APCs as well as for the cardiac decompensation usually present.

Case 30

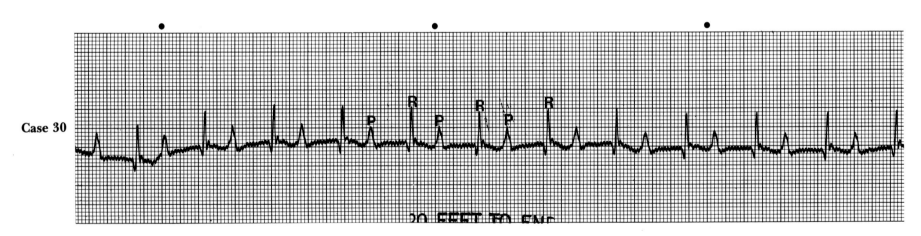

Answer. Severe first-degree AV block (P-R interval prolonged to 0.22 sec or 11 boxes) with a ventricular rate of 160 beats/min. (Refer to Chapter 6.) Because of the very long P-R interval, the P wave could easily be confused with a T wave. If this were a T wave, however, the rhythm would have to be atrial standstill or AV junctional. The ventricular rates should be much slower for these two arrhythmias. Electrical interference (60-cycle) is indicated by the jagged baseline. Digoxin toxicity is present. The gastrointestinal signs usually occur before the electrocardiographic signs. Discontinuation of the drug is the safest action. Signs of digoxin toxicity may persist for days, during which time careful supervision of the patient is necessary.

Case 31

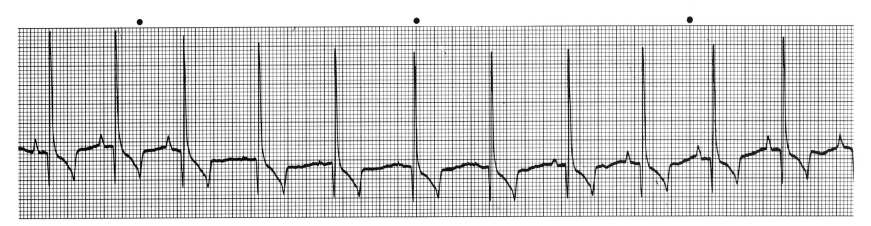

Question. This tracing was recorded from a 1-year-old Collie undergoing evaluation for surgery. What is your interpretation? What is your recommendation for treatment?

Case 32

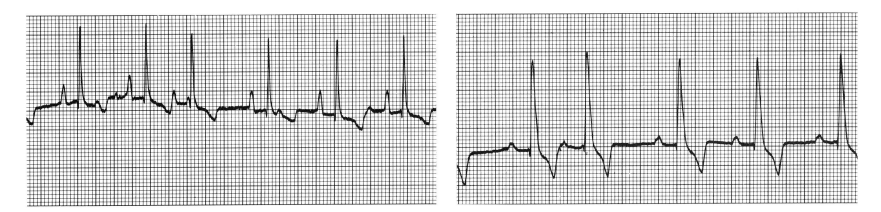

Question. These two strips were obtained from different dogs each having mitral valvular insufficiency and a history of coughing. The dog with the recording on the left was being treated with digitalis. What arrhythmia is present in both strips? What are the conditions associated with this arrhythmia? What are your recommendations for treatment?

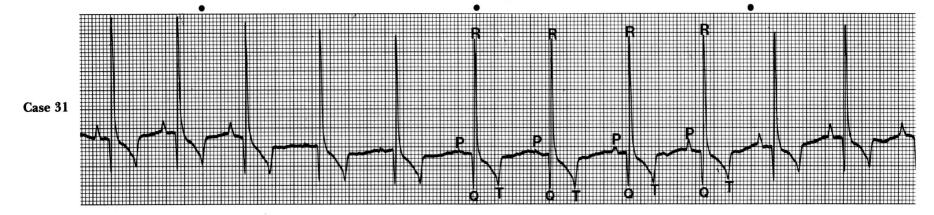

Case 31

Answer. Wandering sinus pacemaker. (Refer to Chapter 6.) This represents a shift of the pacemaker within the SA node and/or AV junction. The configuration of the P wave gradually changes, becoming isoelectric and then back to positive, a frequent normal finding in dogs. No specific therapy is required. A wandering sinus pacemaker should be differentiated from other atrial arrhythmias. The tall R waves (3.0 mv or 30 boxes) and deep Q waves (0.8 mv or 8 boxes) are also normal. Thin deep-chested dogs under 2 years of age can have high-amplitude R waves and deep Q waves.

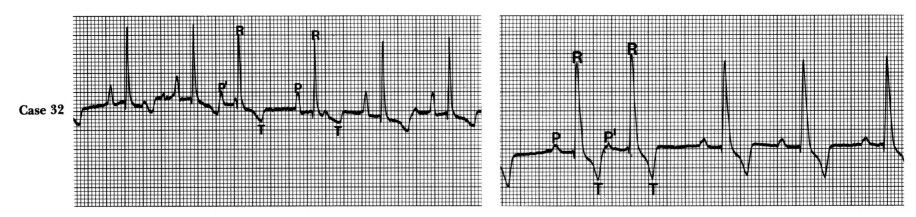

Case 32

Answer. APCs. (Refer to Chapter 6.) Atrial premature QRS complexes usually have a QRS configuration similar to that of sinus complexes, and the P′ waves are premature with a different configuration from sinus P waves. The strip on the left has tall peaked sinus P waves, indicating probable right atrial enlargement. Digoxin was discontinued since it contributed to the origin of the arrhythmia. The coughing was due to a chronic respiratory condition and not to cardiac failure. The APC on the right was caused by left atrial enlargement secondary to the mitral valvular insufficiency. Digoxin is indicated in this case. If digoxin was being given to this dog, a reaction to the drug should also be considered.

Case 33

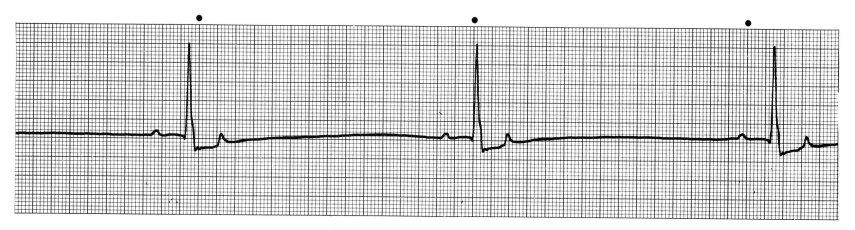

Question. This tracing was recorded from a 15-year-old Schnauzer with numerous episodes of syncope. A biochemistry blood profile was found to be normal. What is your interpretation? How should it be treated?

Case 34

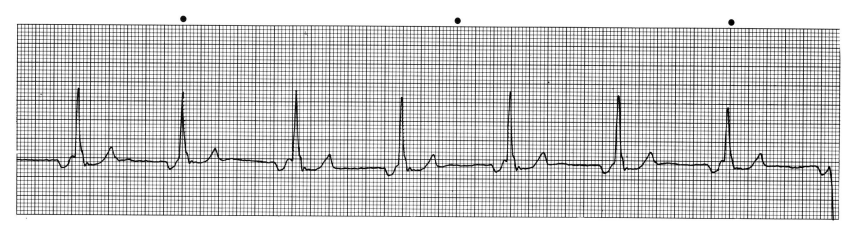

Question. This rhythm strip was recorded from a 9-year-old dog with chronic mitral valvular insufficiency, receiving treatment with digoxin. Anorexia and vomiting were present. What is your interpretation and what treatment would you recommend?

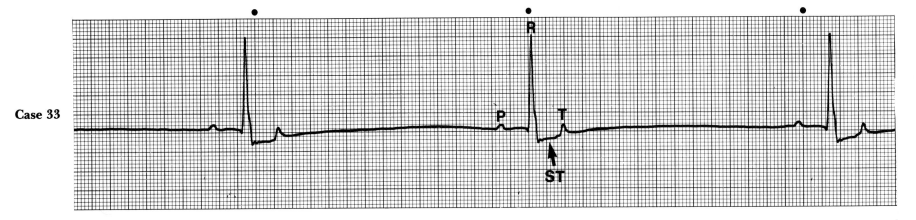

Case 33

Answer. Sinus bradycardia at a rate of 40 beats/min with first-degree AV block (P-R is 0.17 sec or 8½ boxes) and S-T segment depression. Atropine was given intravenously and failed to cause a marked increase in heart rate, indicating that the SA node dysfunction is not due to excessive vagal tone. Sick sinus syndrome (refer to Chapter 6) is most likely present, a term given to a number of abnormalities of the SA node and probably of a genetic inheritance in the Miniature Schnauzer. The treatment of choice is a permanent artificial pacemaker. The S-T segment depression may represent myocardial hypoxia, while the AV block may represent AV nodal degenerative changes common in aged dogs.

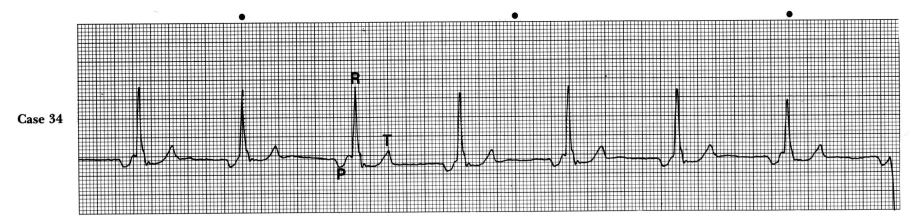

Case 34

Answer. Atrioventricular junctional tachycardia (refer to Chapter 6) at a heart rate of 100 beats/min. The heart rate is faster than the AV junctional inherent rate of 40 to 60 beats/min, indicating a tachycardia. Negative P waves precede each of the QRS complexes. Digitalis toxicity is present. The digitalis should be stopped with an electrocardiogram obtained at least three or four times a day during the toxicity. This abnormality could progress to life-threatening arrhythmias. Specific therapy may include intravenous potassium, phenytoin, and a temporary transvenous pacemaker.

Case 35

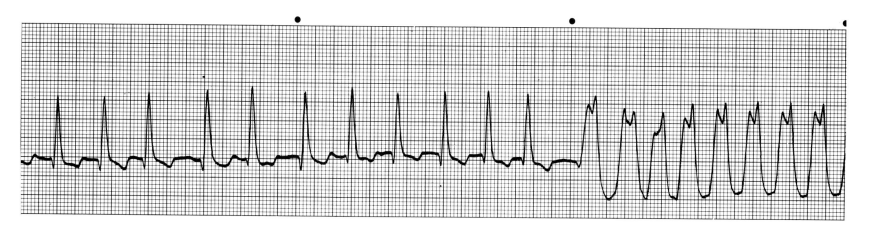

Question. This rhythm strip was recorded from an 8-year-old Boxer with ascites and marked lethargy. What is your interpretation? How should it be treated?

Case 36

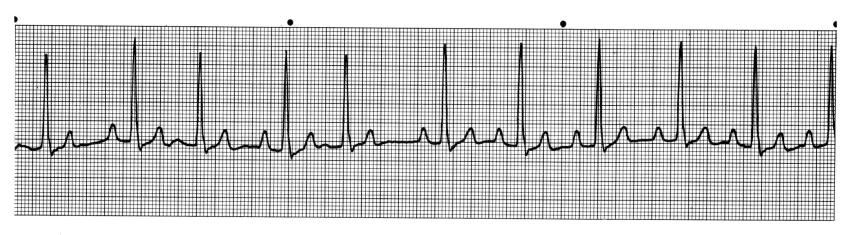

Question. This tracing was recorded from a 9-year-old German Shepherd with mitral valvular insufficiency and pulmonary edema. What is your interpretation and recommendation for treatment?

Case 35

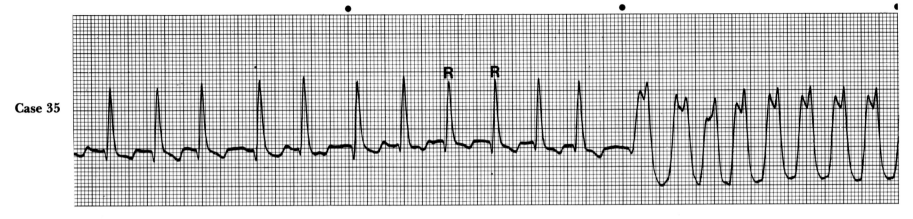

Answer. Atrial fibrillation with paroxysmal ventricular tachycardia (refer to Chapter 6) at the end of the strip. Ventricular premature complexes are commonly associated with atrial fibrillation. They can occur occasionally or frequently and are often seen in the Boxer breed. The ventricular rhythm should be differentiated from aberrant conduction (refer to Chapter 12). To reduce the atrial fibrillation rate, digoxin is indicated, followed by propranolol. Quinidine or procainamide is also indicated for the ventricular arrhythmia, which in some cases can convert atrial fibrillation to a normal sinus rhythm. Atrial fibrillation is associated with marked hemodynamic changes, especially because of the failure of the atria to contract as well as because of the irregular ventricular rhythm.

Case 36

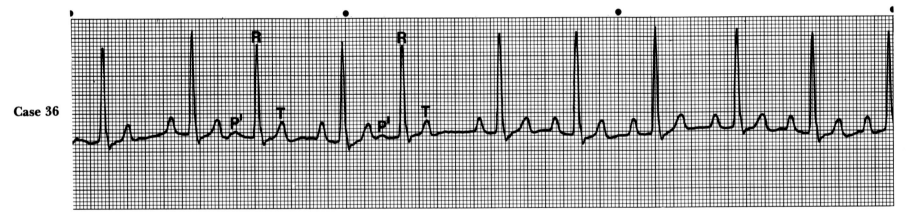

Answer. The rhythm is sinus with two atrial premature complexes (refer to Chapter 6). The ectopic P′-QRS complexes are premature, with the configuration of the P′ wave different from that of the sinus P wave. Digoxin is the treatment of choice as well as for the heart failure usually present. Atrial premature complexes are usually associated with atrial enlargement secondary to chronic AV valvular insufficiency. In very aged dogs, atrial premature complexes can be of normal variation.

Case 37

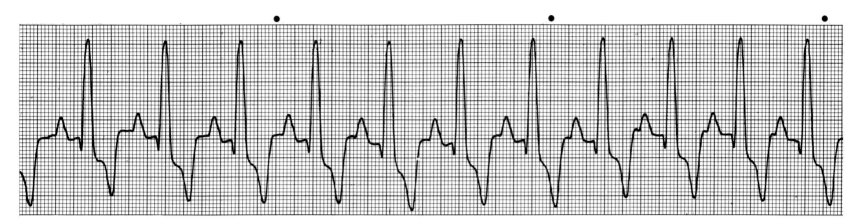

Question. This rhythm strip was recorded from a 35-pound mixed 10-year-old dog with a chronic history of coughing and occasional fainting episodes. Mitral valvular insufficiency was auscultated. What is your interpretation? What other tests may be needed?

Case 38

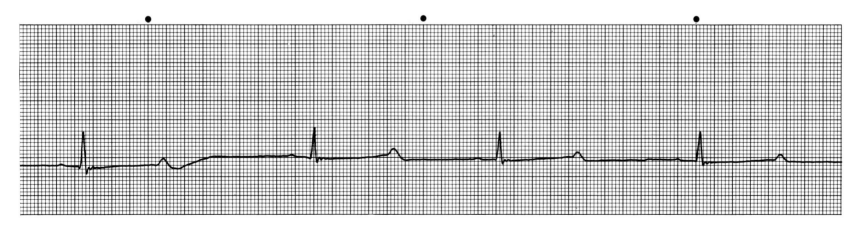

Question. This tracing was recorded from a 7-year-old Great Dane with severe vomiting and diarrhea secondary to pancreatitis. What is your interpretation, and to what serious arrhythmia is this animal prone?

Case 37

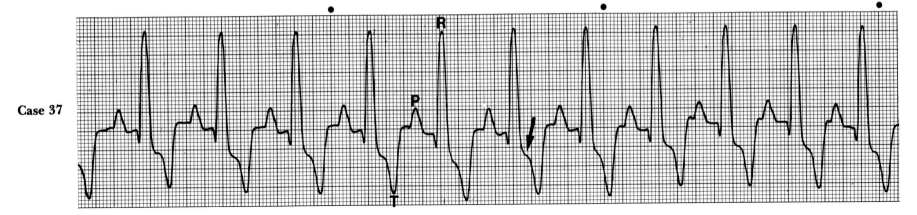

Answer. Biatrial and left ventricular enlargement (refer to Chapter 4). The QRS duration is wide (0.08 sec or 4 boxes). The S-T segment depression or coving (arrow) supports the diagnosis of left ventricular enlargement. The P waves are wide (0.07 sec or 3½ boxes) and tall (0.5 mv or 5 boxes), suggesting biatrial enlargement. The rhythm is sinus with a rate of 150 beats/min. A thoracic radiograph should be taken to substantiate the cardiac chamber enlargement and evaluate the degree of congestive heart failure. Digoxin is most likely indicated. The fainting episodes could be secondary to atrial arrhythmias commonly associated with the marked atrial enlargement.

Case 38

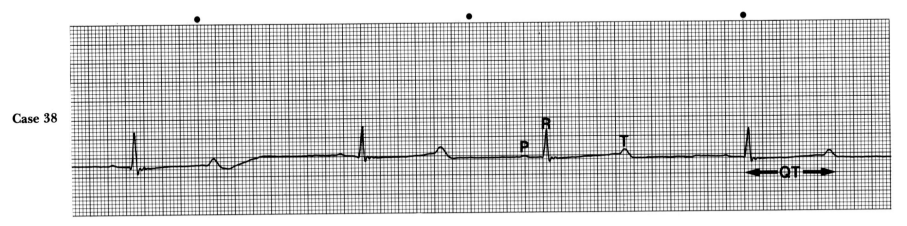

Answer. Sinus bradycardia (heart rate approximately 50 beats/min, which can be of normal variation in large breeds) and prolongation of the Q-T interval (0.50 sec or 25 boxes) (refer to Chapter 4). Despite the slow heart rate, the Q-T interval is prolonged (refer to tables in various electrocardiographic textbooks in man). Corrections of the Q-T interval for heart rate appear to be applicable under circumstances such as exercise. Severe hypocalcemia (serum calcium: 1.9 mg/dl) was present; probably secondary to metabolic and respiratory alkalosis and accompanying hypokalemia. The vulnerable period of the ventricles is increased, so that ventricular premature complexes falling within that period can result in ventricular fibrillation. The Q-T interval will return to normal when the underlying disorder is controlled.

Case 39

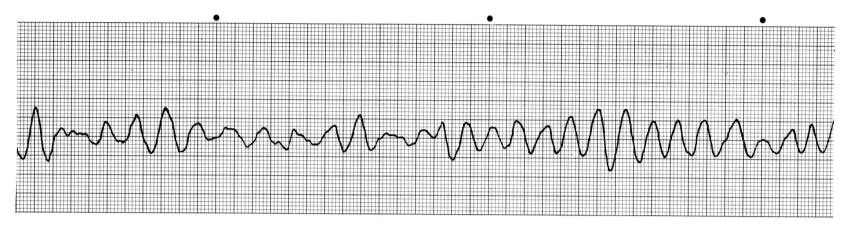

Question. This tracing was recorded from a dog in cardiac arrest during a surgical procedure. What is your interpretation and approach to treatment?

Case 40

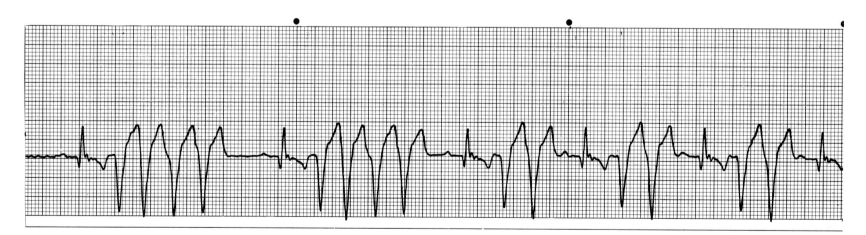

Question. This rhythm strip was recorded from a 7-year-old Collie with a persistent fever, shifting leg lameness, and dyspnea. What is your interpretation of the arrhythmia present? What is your diagnostic plan and therapeutic regimen? What are the hemodynamic consequences?

425

Case 39

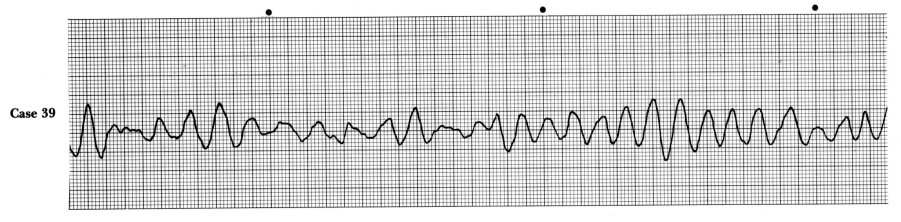

Answer. Ventricular flutter—fibrillation (refer to Chapter 6). The cardiac rhythm reveals a chaotic and grossly irregular ventricular rhythm. This rhythm is often fatal despite all available cardiopulmonary resuscitative measures. The ventricular fibrillatory waves may be relatively large (coarse fibrillation) as seen in this tracing, or the fibrillatory waves may be very small (fine fibrillation). In general, coarse ventricular fibrillation has a better prognosis. With monitoring devices, the *prevention* of ventricular fibrillation is crucial. Treatment consists of cardiopulmonary resuscitation, direct current countershock, and drugs (refer to Chapter 11).

Case 40

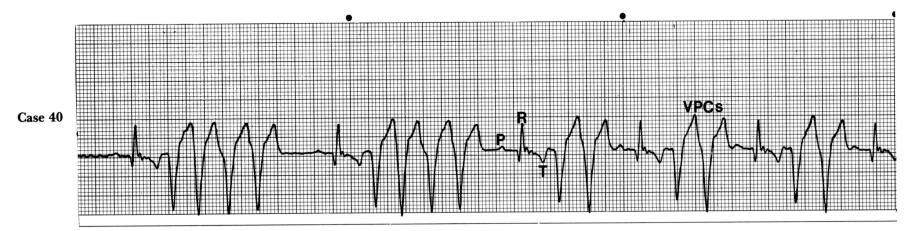

Answer. Frequent ventricular premature complexes (refer to Chapter 6) producing paroxysmal ventricular tachycardia (three or more VPCs in a row) are present. This ventricular arrhythmia no doubt could lead to ventricular tachycardia of a longer duration or even ventricular fibrillation. Septicemia-endomyocarditis should first be considered, with blood cultures and a complete blood profile indicated. Congestive heart failure may also be present. The underlying disorder should be treated as well as giving lidocaine and procainamide. Physical examination usually reveals a pulse deficit during each of the VPCs, as the cardiac output is temporarily decreased. The reduction in output is more significant when there is pre-existing cardiac disease.

Case 41

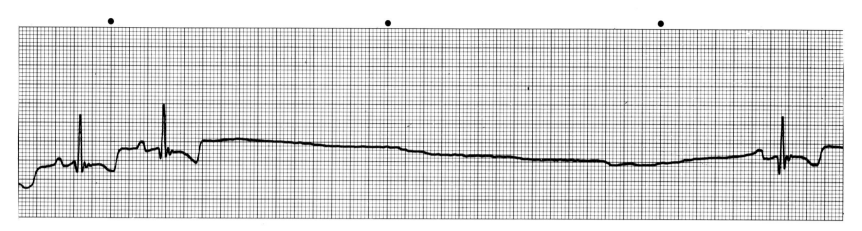

Question. This transtelephonic tracing was recorded from a Miniature Schnauzer with numerous episodes of syncope. What is your interpretation and your therapeutic regimen? Palpation of the femoral pulse will reveal what abnormalities?

Case 42

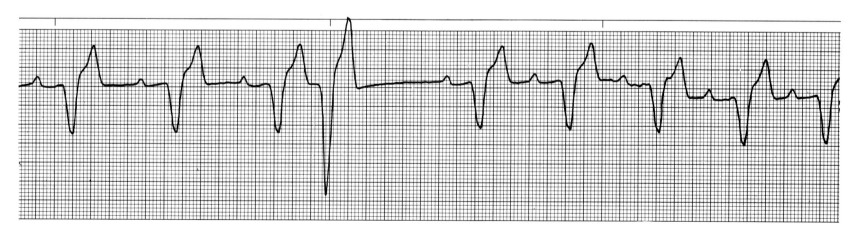

Question. This rhythm strip was recorded from a 10-year-old German Shepherd with clinical signs of lethargy. What three abnormalities are present and what are the possible causes?

Case 41

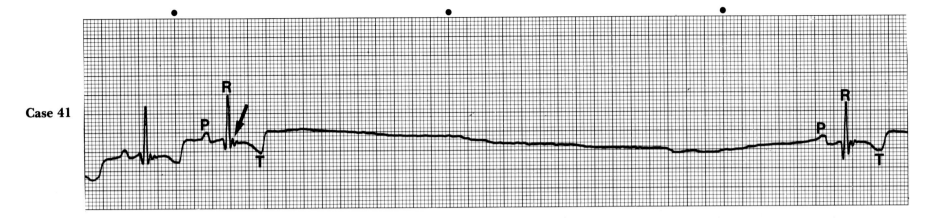

Answer. Sinoatrial block (sinus arrest), associated with sick sinus syndrome commonly seen with this breed (refer to Chapter 6). Baseline movement artifact is present from animal movement. After the second sinus complex, P-QRS-T complexes fail to occur for over 3 seconds. The S-T segment artifact (arrow) is due to an inadequate low-frequency response of the telephone transmitter. Atropine may have an effect on increasing the rate. Insertion of an artificial pacemaker is usually indicated. Palpation of the femoral pulse will reveal a normal but occasionally slower heart rate that is regular in rhythm but periodically interrupted by a pause.

Case 42

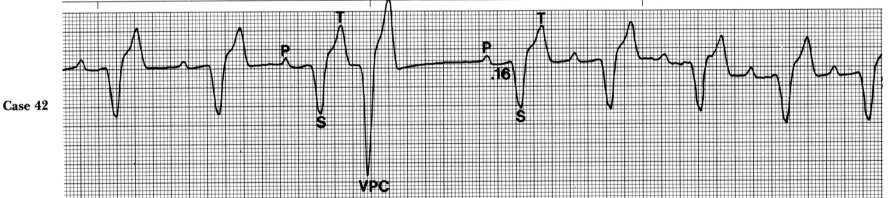

Answer. First-degree AV block (P-R interval 0.16 seconds or 8 boxes); one ventricular premature complex (VPC); and right ventricular enlargement and/or right bundle branch block (if large S waves are found in leads I, III, and aVF). A chest radiograph should be taken to document right heart enlargement; if not present, right bundle branch block is most likely present. Right bundle branch block and first-degree AV block (refer to Chapter 4) can indicate a large lesion that could progress to complete AV block. First-degree AV block and occasional VPCs can be of normal variation in aged dogs.

Case 43

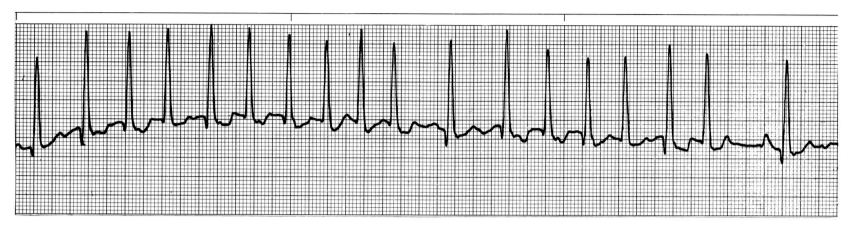

Question. This electrocardiogram was recorded from an Irish Wolfhound with episodes of collapse and weight loss over the last 2 weeks. What is your interpretation and therapeutic plan?

Case 44

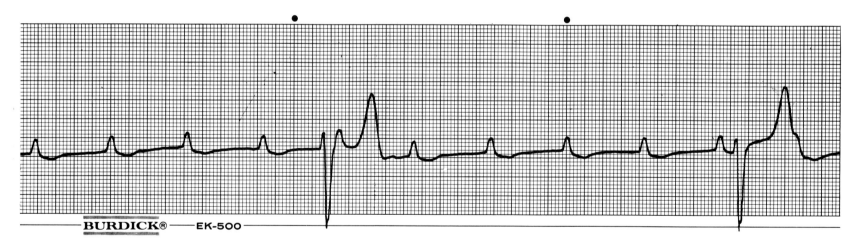

BURDICK® —EK-500

Question. This rhythm strip was recorded from a 9-year-old mixed canine with clinical signs of syncope and severe ascites. Mammary tumors were removed surgically 3 months ago. What is your interpretation? What is the probable underlying disorder and the hemodynamic consequences of the arrhythmia?

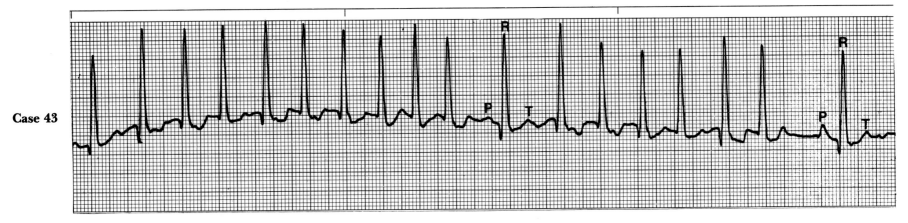

Case 43

Answer. This uncommon abnormality in rhythm is paroxysmal atrial fibrillation (refer to Chapter 6). Atrial fibrillation may resemble multifocal atrial tachycardia because of the rapid and irregular ventricular response. Well-defined P' waves before each QRS complex are present in multifocal atrial tachycardia. Atrial flutter with varying ventricular response may also appear like atrial fibrillation. A careful search for flutter waves or P' waves on other leads is essential. Note the two well-defined sinus complexes. The dilated form of cardiomyopathy should first be considered with digoxin, the drug of choice. This dog eventually had atrial fibrillation throughout the strip, despite the use of digoxin. Blood flow in the coronary arteries and in the cerebral circulation is markedly reduced with rapid atrial fibrillation. Clinical signs can include heart failure, weakness, and syncope.

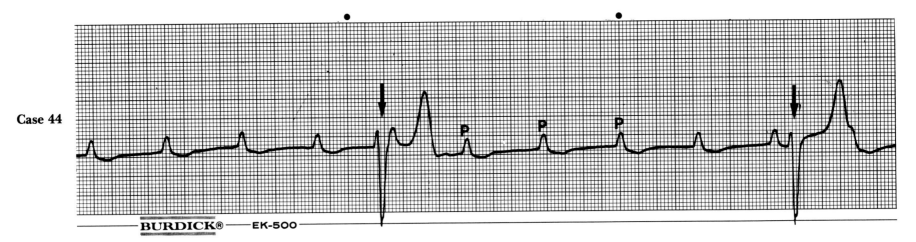

Case 44

Answer. Complete heart block with an idioventricular escape rhythm of 30 beats/min (refer to Chapter 6). The P waves bear no constant relationship to the QRS complexes. The bizarre QRS-T complexes (arrows) are from a focus below the bundle of His. A neoplasm involving the heart secondary to the metastasis of the mammary tumor was found at necropsy. On auscultation, the classic sign of complete heart block is a change of intensity in the first heart sound, owing to the variation in relationship between atrial and ventricular contractions. The venous pressure is elevated since the right atrium often contracts against a closed tricuspid valve.

Case 45

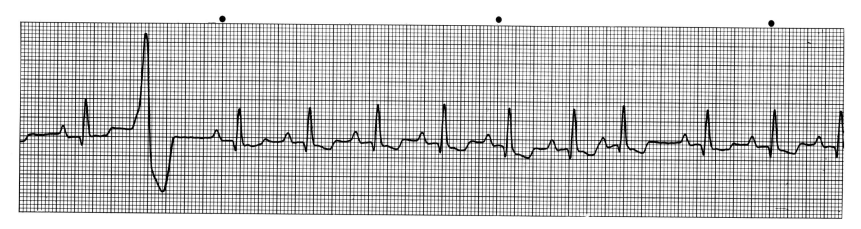

Question. This tracing was recorded from a canine with a history of being hit by a car 2 days ago. What is your interpretation? The different pauses in this strip are for what reason?

Case 46

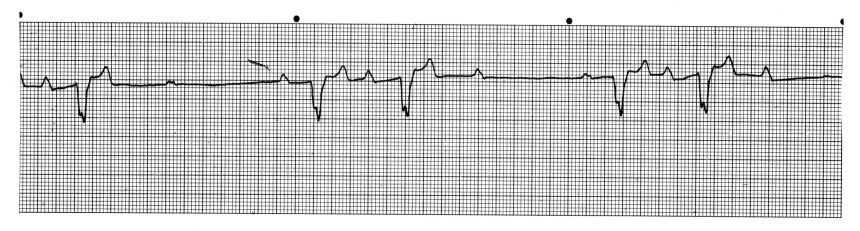

Question. This electrocardiogram was recorded from a dog with no clinical signs, but an arrhythmia with varying intensity to the first heart sound was heard. What is your interpretation and treatment?

Case 45

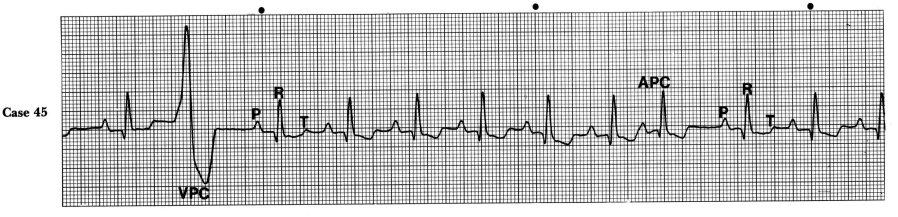

Answer. Sinus rhythm at a heart rate of 165 beats/min with one ventricular premature complex (VPC) and one atrial premature complex (APC) (refer to Chapter 6). Premature complexes are usually followed by a pause, termed noncompensatory or compensatory according to its duration. With a VPC, the ectopic impulse generally cannot penetrate through the AV junction and disturb the normal SA rhythm. A compensatory pause usually follows a VPC, as the next sinus impulse after the VPC occurs on time. A noncompensatory pause (or less-than-compensatory pause) occurs with an APC. The ectopic atrial impulse discharges the SA node and resets its cycle.

Case 46

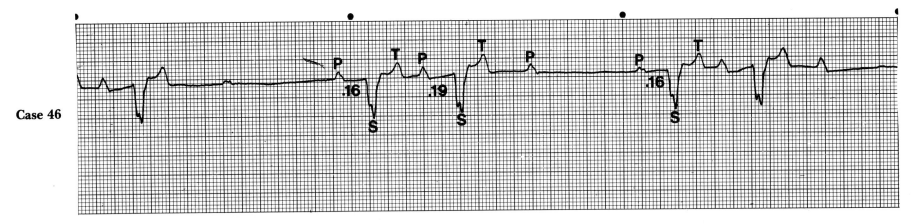

Answer. Mobitz type I AV block with a 3:2 ventricular response (refer to Chapter 6). This Wenckebach type of AV block is characterized by progressive lengthening of the P-R interval until a point is reached at which no ventricular complex follows the P wave. Following the blocked atrial impulse, the P-R interval shortens to its original value (0.16 sec or 8 boxes), and the sequence is repeated. First-degree AV block is also present as the P-R interval is prolonged. The changing configuration of the P wave represents a wandering pacemaker. The wide and negative QRS complex may indicate that the conduction defect is below the AV node. An artificial pacemaker may be indicated if clinical signs (syncope, lethargy) would occur or if the rhythm progresses to complete AV block.

Case 47

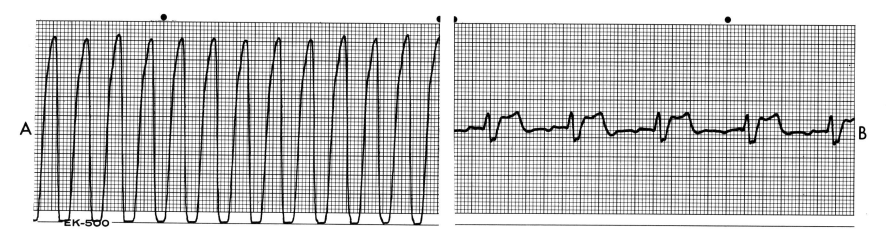

Question. Strip A was recorded from a dog with an acute onset of collapse preceded by 2 days of vomiting and diarrhea. Strip B was recorded after an intravenous cardiac drug was given. What are the differentials for the tachycardia in strip A and what drug was given? What are the abnormalities in strip B?

Case 48

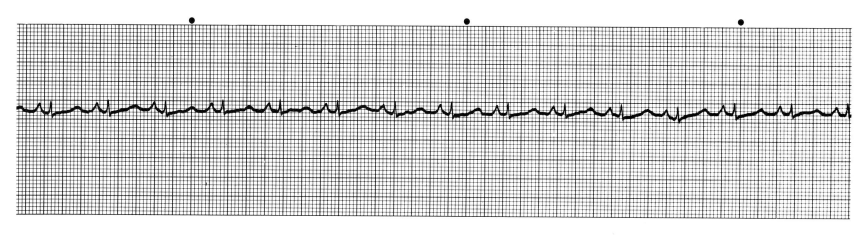

Question. This tracing was recorded from a cat undergoing evaluation for surgery. What is your interpretation?

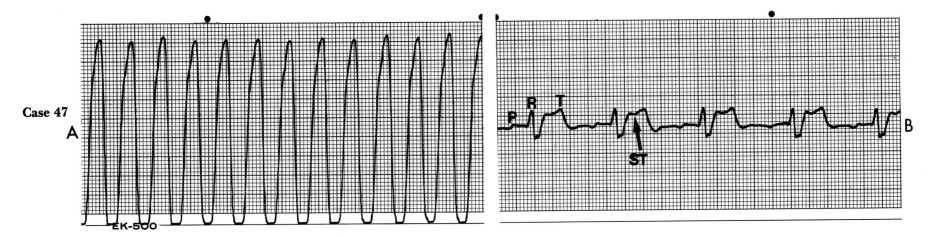

Case 47

A

EK-500

B

P R T
P R T

ST

Answer. A. Ventricular flutter (refer to Chapter 6). The rhythm is regular and rapid with extremely bizarre QRS complexes. No P waves can be seen. The boundary between the QRS complexes, S-T segment, and T wave is unclear so that the entire complexes appear to be a continuous loopform. Differential diagnosis should also include supraventricular tachycardia (e.g., atrial tachycardia); with bundle branch block, aberrant QRS complex, Wolff-Parkinson-White syndrome, or nonspecific QRS widening (hyperkalemia/acidosis, or severe left heart enlargement). Ventricular flutter has almost the same clinical significance as ventricular fibrillation. The first treatment of choice for ventricular flutter is direct current shock and intravenous infusion of lidocaine.

B. After lidocaine injection. Normal sinus rhythm is present. The small P waves and S-T segment elevation probably represent secondary electrolyte abnormalities and/or hypoxia. The increased duration of the QRS complex may represent an intraventricular conduction defect. An intravenous drip of lidocaine should be continued.

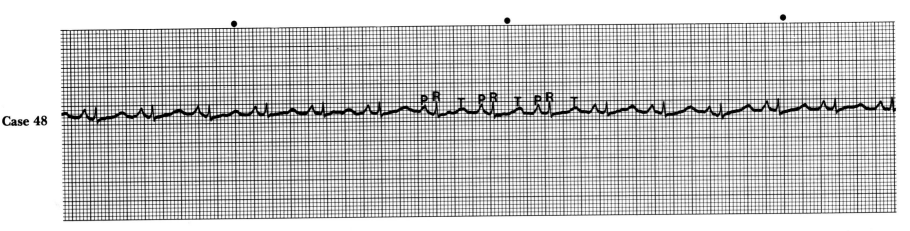

Case 48

PR I PR I PR I

Answer. Normal sinus rhythm (refer to Chapter 7) at a rate of 195 beats/min (9½ R-R intervals between two sets of dots × 20 = 190). By way of review, the following steps should be used for analyzing any rhythm strip: (1) general inspection of the electrocardiogram—heart rate (normal on this strip), rhythm (regular on this strip; sinus arrhythmia rare in cats), (2) identification of the P waves, (3) recognition of the QRS complexes (R normally small), (4) the relationship between P waves and QRS complexes (constant in this strip), and (5) summary of findings with final classification of the arrhythmia.

Case 49

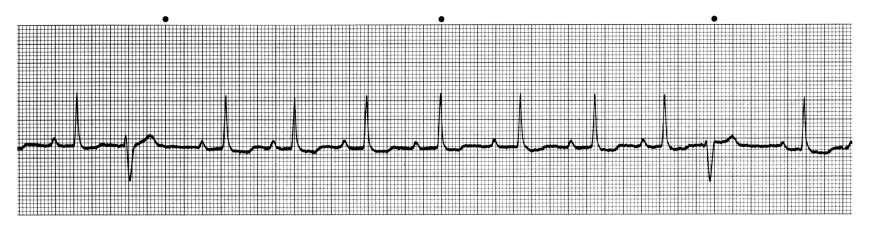

Question. This rhythm strip was obtained from a cat with the dilated form of cardiomyopathy. The cat was being treated with digoxin; its appetite had decreased and it was not as active. What is your interpretation of the rhythm, and what treatment would you recommend?

Case 50

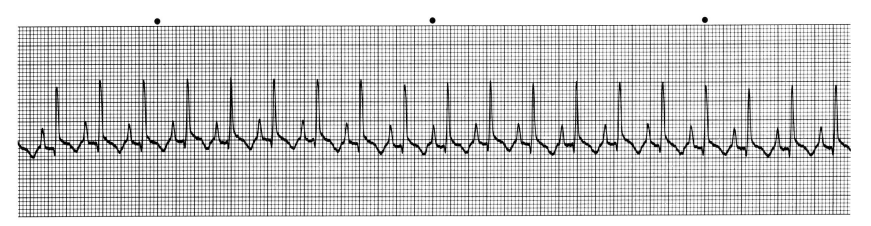

Question. This rhythm strip was recorded from a cat with hypertrophic cardiomyopathy and congestive heart failure. What is your interpretation?

Case 49

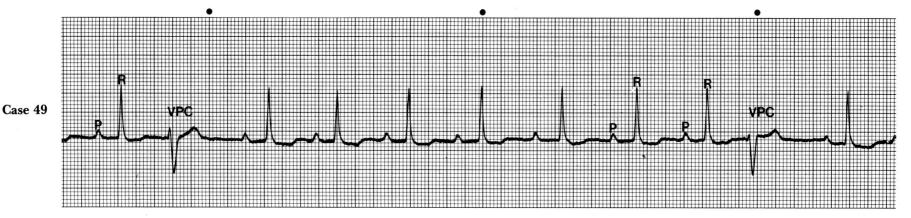

Answer. The strip shows sinus rhythm with two VPCs (ventricular premature complexes). (Refer to Chapter 7.) First-degree AV block is also present, the P-R interval prolonged to 0.14 second or 7 boxes (normal not greater than 0.09 sec or 4½ boxes). The tall R waves of 1.4 mv or 14 boxes (normal not greater than 0.9 mv or 9 boxes) indicates left ventricular enlargement. (Refer to Chapter 5.) Digoxin toxicity is the likely diagnosis. The VPCs disappeared, the P-R interval returned to normal, and the cat improved clinically after the digoxin was temporarily stopped. Physical examination usually reveals a pulse deficit during a VPC, as the cardiac output is temporarily decreased. A reduction in cardiac output is of greater significance when the cat has pre-existing heart disease.

Case 50

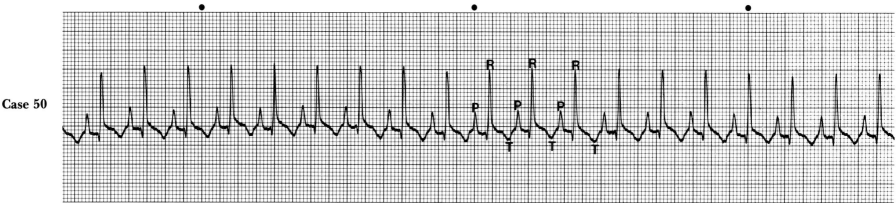

Answer. Sinus tachycardia at a rate of 250 beats/min. (Refer to Chapter 7.) The P wave is touching the T wave of the preceding complex. The tall (1.6 mv or 16 boxes) and wide (0.05 sec) R waves indicate left ventricular enlargement. The tall (0.5 mv or 5 boxes) P waves indicate right atrial enlargement. (Refer to Chapter 5.) The amplitude of the P wave can also be increased with a rapid heart rate. The heart rate was reduced to normal (below 240 beats/min) (strip not shown) after cage rest, and diuretics were prescribed. Propranolol was later used for the prevention of the stress-induced sinus tachycardia, which could precipitate heart failure again. Hyperthyroidism should also be considered.

Case 51

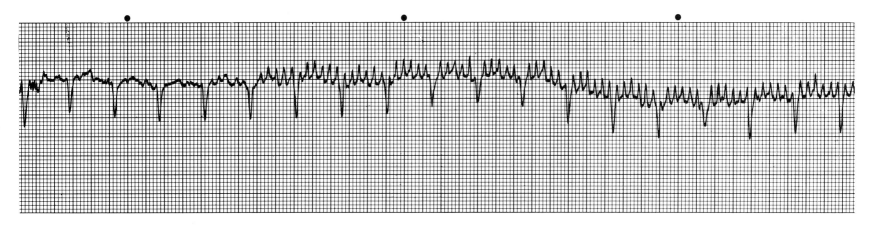

Question. This strip was recorded from a cat with suspected heart disease. What is your interpretation of the rhythm?

Case 52

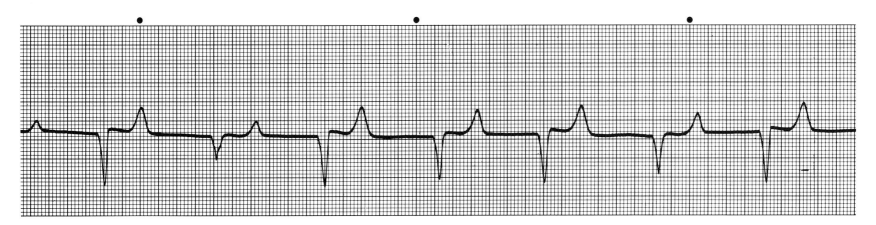

Question. This electrocardiogram was recorded from a male cat with an urethral obstruction. What is your interpretation of the rhythm? What treatment do you recommend?

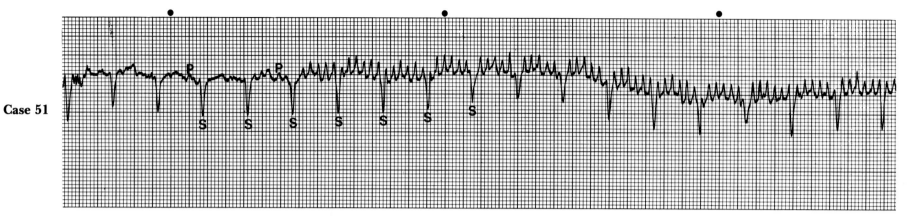

Case 51

Answer. Sinus tachycardia at the rate of 250 beats/min. Gross artifacts (caused by purring) mimic an atrial arrhythmia: some of the normal sinus P waves, however, can be identified among the artifacts. (Refer to Chapter 7.) The ventricular rhythm (S waves) is also regular. If an atrial arrhythmia were present, the ventricular rate would be very rapid with the rhythm often irregular. The large S waves are the only clue to possible heart disease. The other leads will have to be studied.

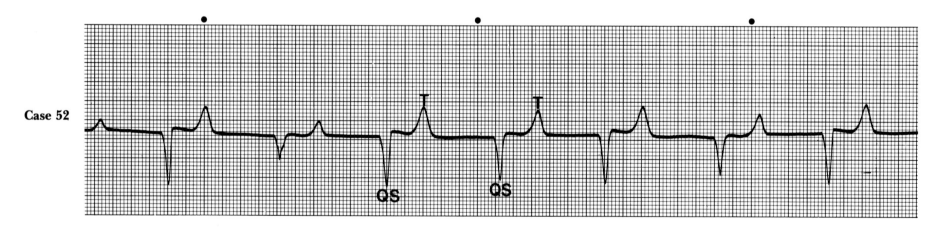

Case 52

Answer. The tracing shows atrial standstill (no visible P waves) with a sinoventricular rhythm. (Refer to Chapter 7.) Severe hyperkalemia (serum potassium, 9.5 mEq/L) was present. The wide and bizarre QS-T complexes (ventricular rate, 100 beats/min) represent the effect of hyperkalemia on intraventricular conduction. Treatment includes relief of the urethral obstruction, intravenous fluids, sodium bicarbonate, and calcium gluconate. Regular insulin with dextrose is indicated if the arrhythmia persists and the cat remains in a crisis.

438

Case 53

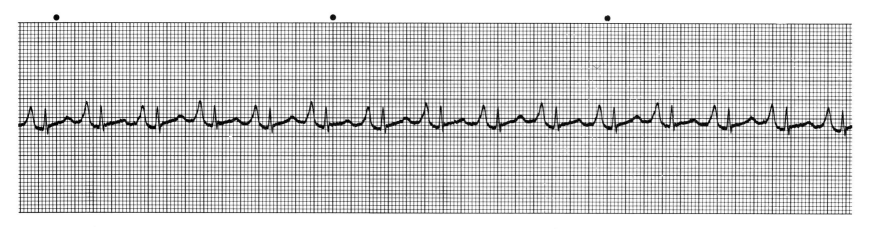

Question. This electrocardiogram was recorded from a kitten with a cardiac murmur at auscultation. What is your interpretation? What advice should you give the owner?

Case 54

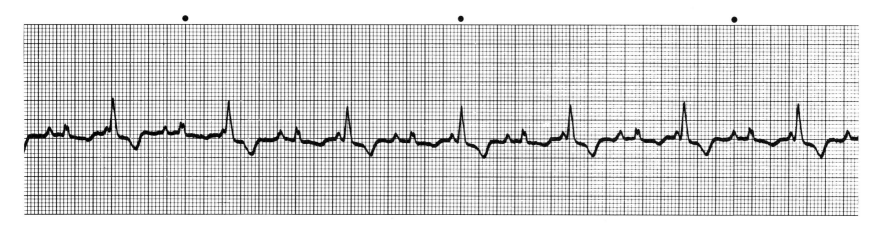

Question. This rhythm strip was recorded from a cat while it was under anesthesia. What is your interpretation of the rhythm? What treatment would you recommend?

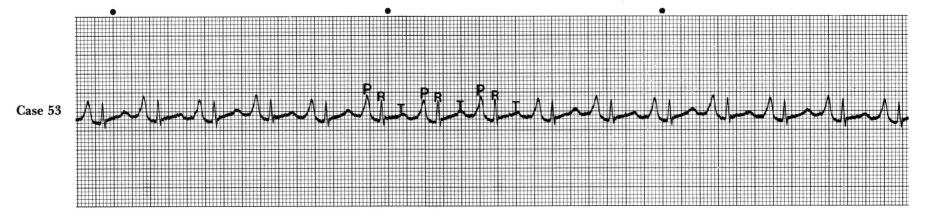

Case 53

Answer. Sinus rhythm at a rate of 190 beats/min. The P waves are both abnormally wide (0.05 sec or 2½ boxes) and abnormally tall (approaching 0.5 mv or 5 boxes). (Refer to Chapter 5.) They should not be wider than 0.04 second (2 boxes) or taller than 0.2 mv (2 boxes). Biatrial enlargement is most likely present. Clinical signs of cardiac disease are probably impending, making a complete evaluation (including thoracic radiographs and angiocardiography) advisable. A common AV canal (AV septal defect) was later found.

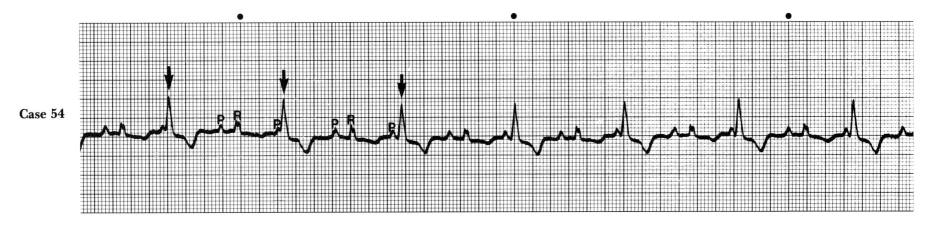

Case 54

Answer. Ventricular bigeminy, right VPCs alternating with a normal sinus complex. (Refer to Chapter 7.) The VPCs (arrows) are not associated with the P waves (no constant P-R interval). The independent normal P waves just precede or are just within each VPC. This arrhythmia was eliminated after the anesthetic level was reduced. Alterations in vagal and sympathetic tone as well as electrolyte and acid-base disturbances that occur during anesthesia and surgery should also be considered. The notch in the sinus R wave is often seen in normal cats.

Case 55

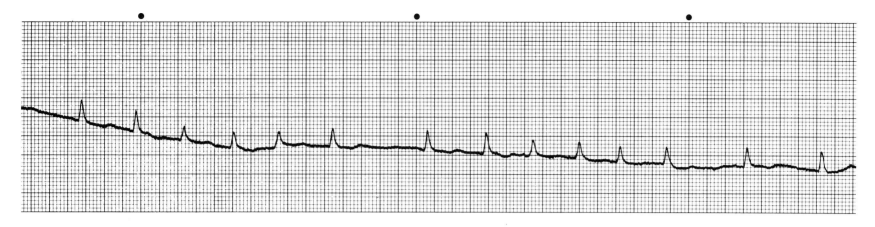

Question. This strip was obtained from a cat with previous episodes of dyspnea and a femoral pulse deficit on physical examination. What is your interpretation of the rhythm? What common cardiac disease is often found accompanying the condition?

Case 56

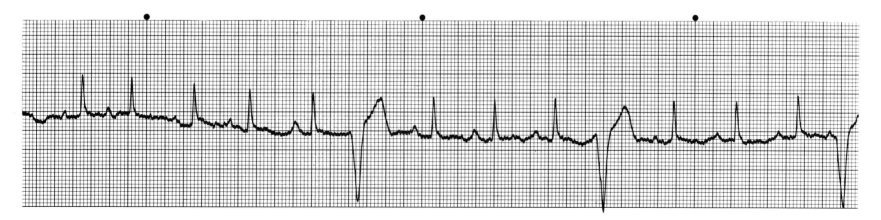

Question. This rhythm strip was recorded from a cat with hypertrophic cardiomyopathy and heart failure. What is your interpretation of the rhythm?

Case 55

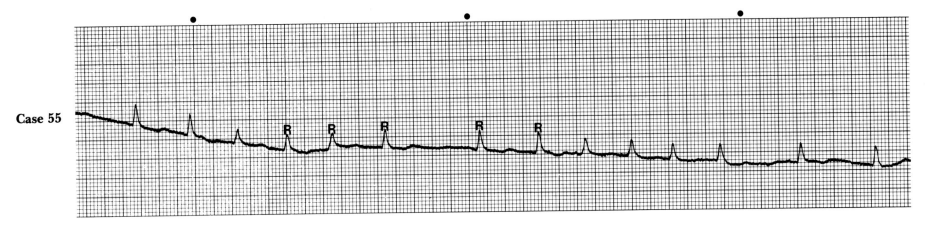

Answer. This strip shows atrial fibrillation with an average ventricular rate of 200 beats/min. (Refer to Chapter 7.) Note the total irregularity of the R waves and the absence of P waves. Hypertrophic cardiomyopathy with severe left atrial enlargement is the most common associated condition. Digoxin and propranolol were given together for this condition and were the reason for the normal ventricular rate. The loss of the "atrial kick" combined with the rapid heart rate may substantially reduce cardiac output and cause congestive heart failure.

Case 56

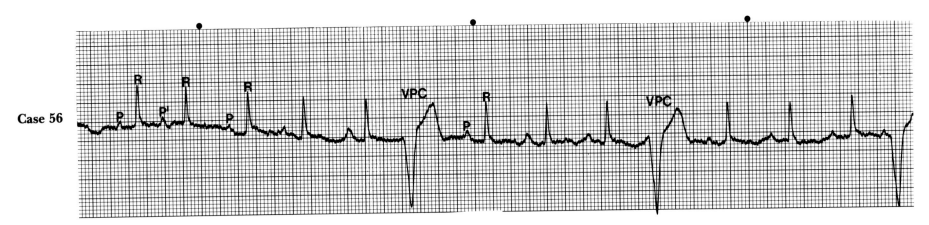

Answer. Normal sinus rhythm with three VPCs of left ventricular origin (right bundle branch block-like pattern). Another type of premature complex is also present on this strip. A rhythm strip should always be evaluated from left to right, always looking for premature complexes or pauses in the rhythm. The second complex is an APC. (Refer to Chapter 7.) The P' wave and the QRS complex are both premature. These arrhythmias disappeared after the heart failure was treated with simple cage rest and diuretics. Some minor artifact is present, indicated by the jagged baseline. Good electrode contact was probably not obtained.

Case 57

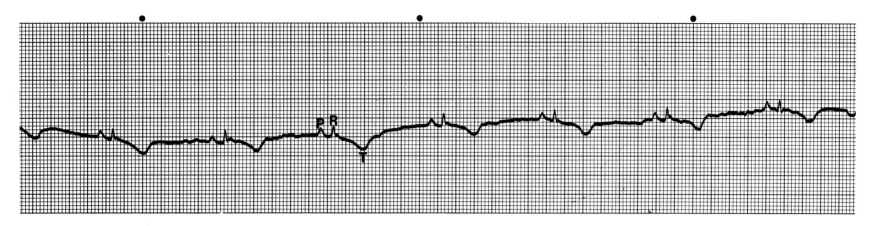

Question. This tracing from a cat was observed on an electrocardiographic monitor during surgery. What is your interpretation of the rhythm? What treatment would you recommend?

Case 58

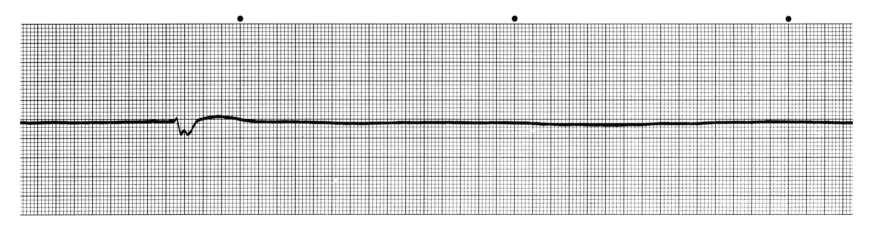

Question. This tracing was recorded from a cat after therapy (intravenous fluids and bicarbonate) for hyperkalemia (serum potassium, 11 mEq/L) due to urethral obstruction. What is your interpretation, and what treatment would you recommend?

Case 57

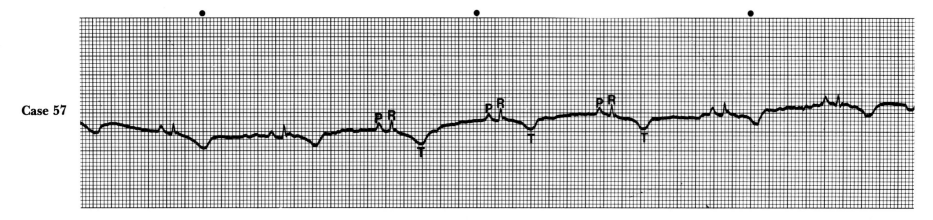

Answer. Sinus bradycardia at a rate of 100 beats/min. (Refer to Chapter 7.) The large T waves may indicate myocardial hypoxia. Slight baseline movement (artifact) is present between some of the P-QRS complexes. Sinus bradycardia usually signifies a serious under-lying disorder that needs immediate attention. Ventricular fibrillation could easily follow. Termination of anesthesia, administration of oxygen and atropine, and close monitoring are immediately indicated. Acid-base and electrolyte abnormalities should be corrected.

Case 58

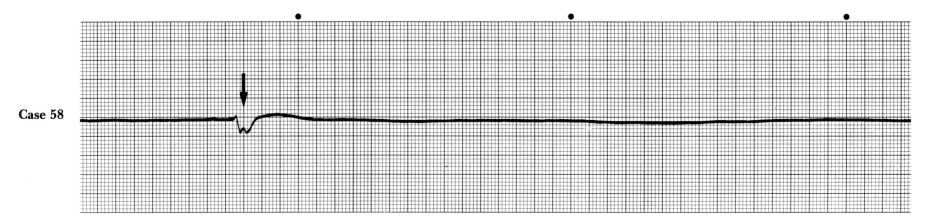

Answer. Ventricular asystole (cardiac arrest) with one bizarre ventricular escape complex (arrow) attempting to rescue the heart. The "A-B-C-D-E" of cardiac resuscitation should be followed immediately. (Refer to Chapter 11.) Cardiac resuscitation failed in this case, and the animal died. Regular insulin and dextrose would be indicated as part of the therapeutic regimen.

Case 59

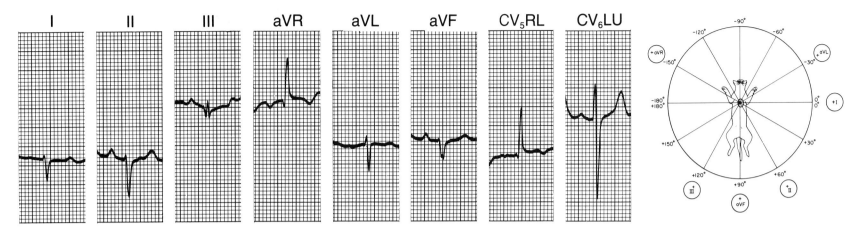

Question. These electrocardiographic strips were recorded from an asymptomatic kitten with a cardiac murmur on routine physical examination. What is your interpretation? What condition is most likely associated with this electrocardiogram?

Case 60

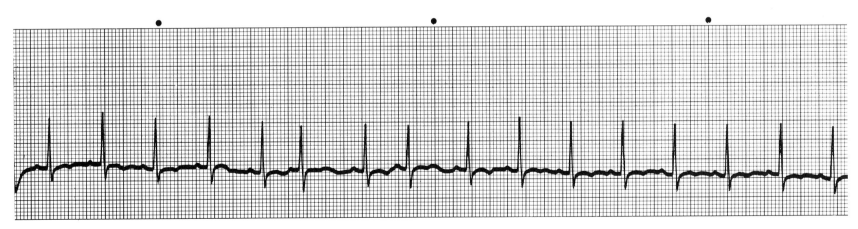

Question. This tracing was obtained from a cat with episodes of fainting. What is your interpretation of the rhythm? What treatment would you recommend?

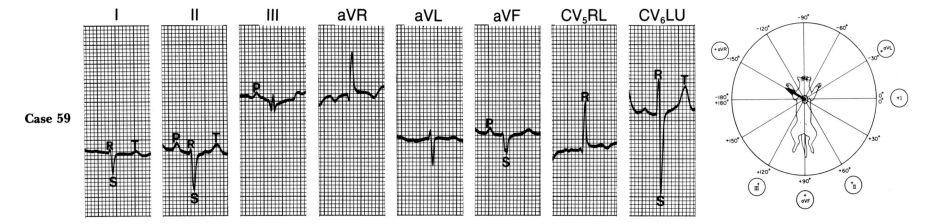

Case 59

Answer. Right ventricular enlargement. (Refer to Chapter 5.) There is a right axis deviation of $-150°$ (lead III isoelectric, aVR positive). S waves are present in leads I, II, III, aVF, and CV₆LU and of large deflection in leads II and CV₆LU. Because the kitten is asymptomatic, a pulmonic stenosis should first be considered. A kitten with tetralogy of Fallot or AV canal will usually be cyanotic.

Case 60

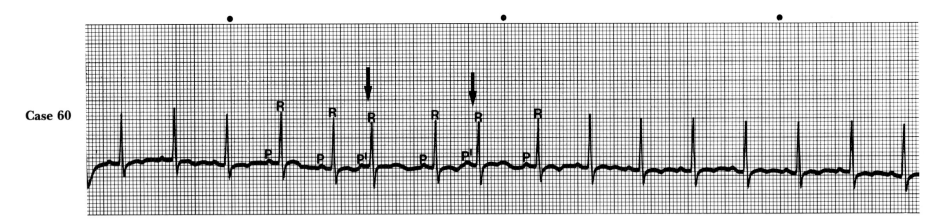

Answer. Atrial premature complexes (APCs) (arrows). (Refer to Chapter 7.) The QRS configuration is similar to that of sinus complexes, and the P′ waves and QRS complexes are premature. A noncompensatory pause follows each APC. The tall R waves indicate probable left ventricular enlargement. Hypertrophic cardiomyopathy was found later on further evaluation. APCs often lead to intermittent atrial tachycardia or atrial fibrillation. Propranolol in cats with hypertrophic cardiomyopathy is usually effective.

Case 61

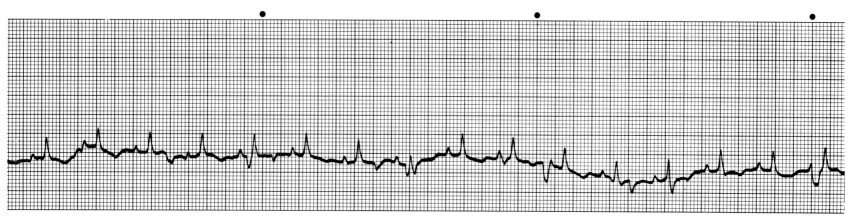

Question. This strip was obtained from a cat with no evidence of heart disease. What is your interpretation of the rhythm?

Case 62

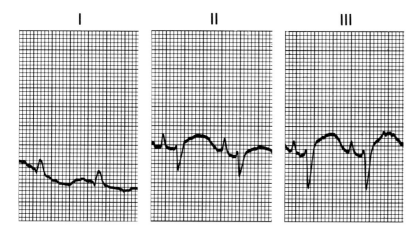

I   II   III

Question. These electrocardiographic strips were recorded from a cat with pulmonary edema. What is your interpretation? This electrocardiographic pattern is most often associated with what cardiac disease?

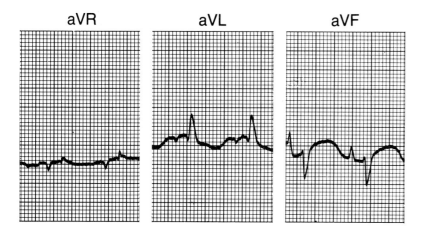

aVR   aVL   aVF

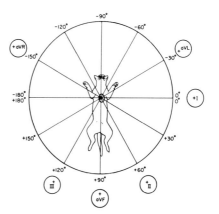

Case 61

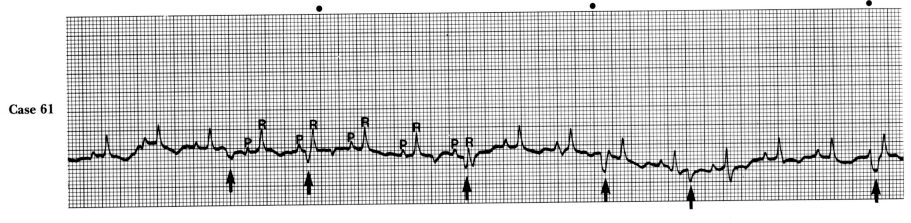

Answer. Sinus rhythm at a rate of 210 beats/min with artifacts (arrows) that happen to fall on the P-R-T complexes. (Refer to Chapter 7.) The artifacts are due to movements of the cat during the recording. They simulate ventricular ectopic complexes but do not interrupt the normal sinus rhythm.

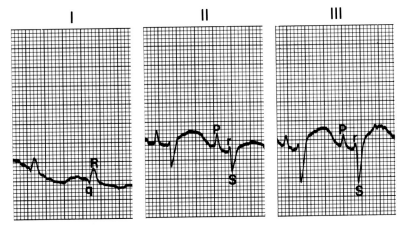

I   II   III

Answer. Left anterior fascicular block and right atrial enlargement. (Refer to Chapter 5.) There is a severe left axis deviation (−60°) (lead aVR isoelectric, perpendicular lead III negative) with a qR pattern in leads I and aVL and an rS pattern in leads II, III, and aVF. The electrocardiographic pattern of anterior fascicular block is commonly associated with hypertrophic cardiomyopathy. This pattern is compatible with an actual conduction defect and/or left ventricular hypertrophy. The tall peaked P waves indicate right atrial enlargement and probable right-sided hypertension from chronic passive pulmonary congestion.

Case 62

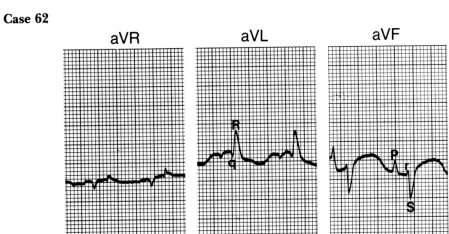

aVR   aVL   aVF

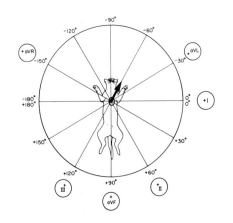

Case 63

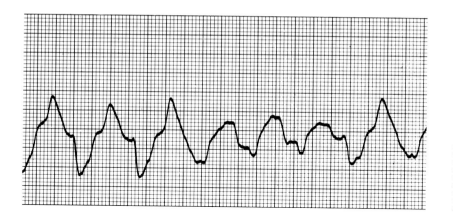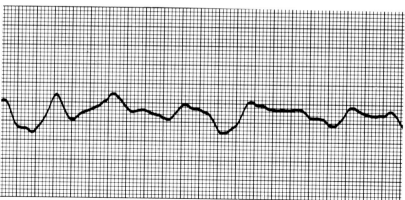

Question. These two strips were recorded from different cats in cardiac arrest. What is your interpretation? What treatment would you recommend?

Case 64

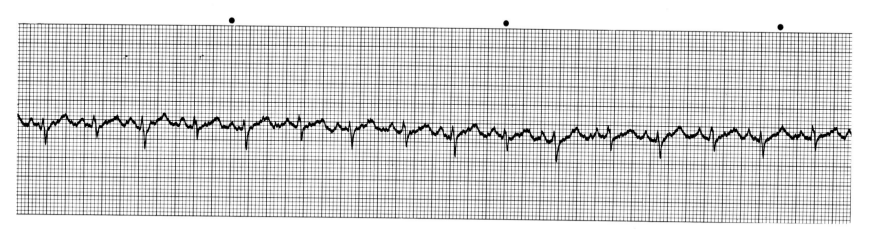

Question. This tracing was obtained from a cat with congestive heart failure and muffled heart sounds at auscultation. What is your interpretation? Name one cardiac condition associated with this electrocardiogram.

Case 63

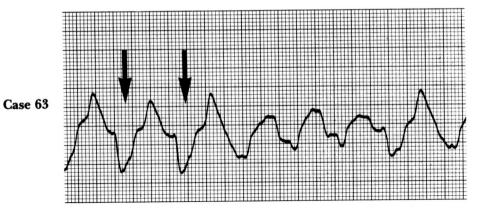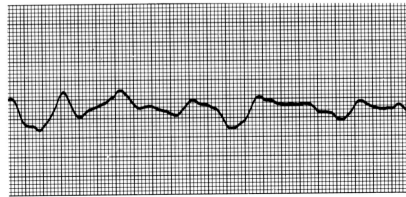

Answer. The strip on the left shows two bizarre ventricular complexes (arrows) with no associated P waves (ventricular tachycardia) followed by ventricular fibrillation. The bizarre complexes may represent the effect of hyperkalemia. (Refer to Chapter 7.) The strip on the right also reveals ventricular fibrillation. Treatment of ventricular fibrillation involves both prevention and resuscitation. Preventive therapy includes all the steps in the therapy of ventricular tachycardia. The "A-B-C-D-E" of resuscitation should be initiated. (Refer to Chapter 11.) Electroshock therapy or a sharp jolt to the precordial region may restore a sinus rhythm.

Case 64

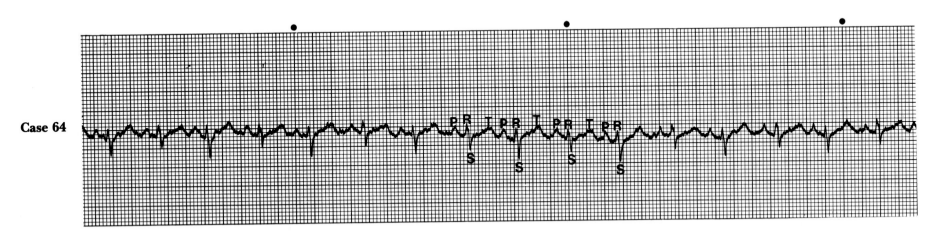

Answer. Electrical alternans. (Refer to Chapter 7.) The QRS-T complexes change their configuration and amplitude on every other complex. The heart rate is normal (210 beats/min). Pericardial effusion was later found on further evaluation. Other causes of electrical alternans are supraventricular tachycardia and alternating conduction in the ventricular conduction system. Ventricular bigeminy and the artifactual effects of respiration should not be confused with electrical alternans. The jagged baseline represents an artifact from poor contact of the clip electrodes with the skin.

Case 65

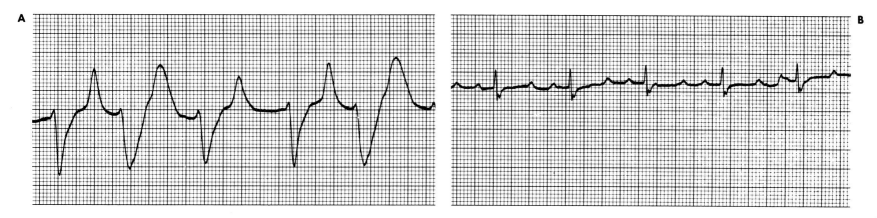

Question. Strip A was recorded from a recumbent and vomiting cat with urethral obstruction. What is your interpretation? What treatment was given to obtain strip B after a period of 15 minutes?

Case 66

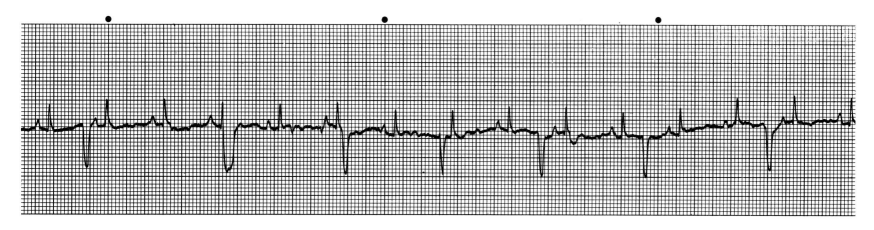

Question. This tracing was recorded from a cat that fell seven stories and fractured its humerus. What is your interpretation?

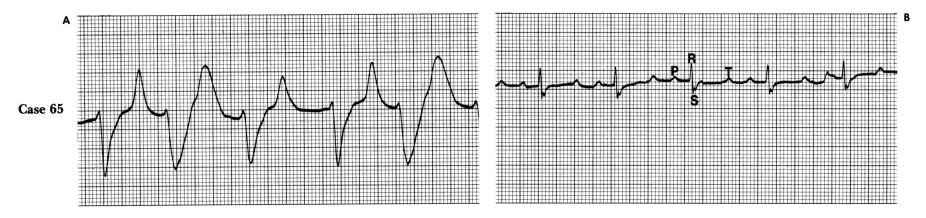

Case 65

Answer. Strip A shows atrial standstill (no visible P waves) and a sinoventricular rhythm. (Refer to Chapter 7.) The wide and bizarre QRS complexes indicate marked conduction delay in the ventricular conduction system. The serum potassium level was 9.0 mEq/L. Ventricular tachycardia should also be considered; but ventricular tachycardia is usually regular with a faster heart rate (above 150 beats/min), and P waves are often seen independent of the ventricular rate. The

severe hyperkalemia is not commonly associated with ventricular tachycardia. To obtain strip B, treatment included relief of urethral obstruction, intravenous fluid therapy, sodium bicarbonate, and 0.5 to 1 unit/kg regular insulin with 2 g dextrose per unit of insulin. Minor changes of hyperkalemia (serum potassium now 6.0 mEq/L) still exist; a prolonged P-R interval (0.10 sec; normal not greater than 0.09 sec), a wide S wave, and a long Q-T interval.

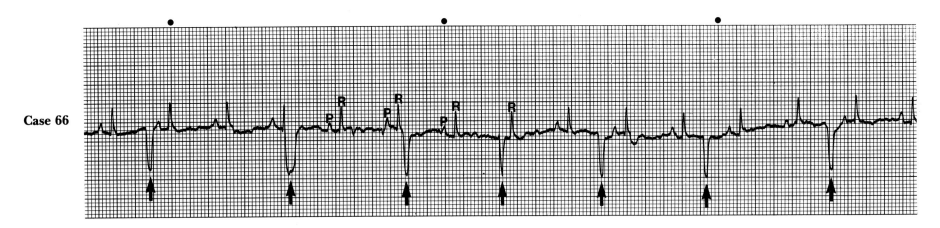

Case 66

Answer. Normal sinus rhythm with numerous artifacts (arrows) created when the cat intermittently jerked its leg. (Refer to Chapter 2.) The artifacts happen to fall before, within, and after the QRS-T com-

plexes and easily resemble ventricular ectopic complexes. They do not interrupt the sinus rhythm; some are too close to the sinus complexes to allow double depolarization of the ventricles.

Case 67

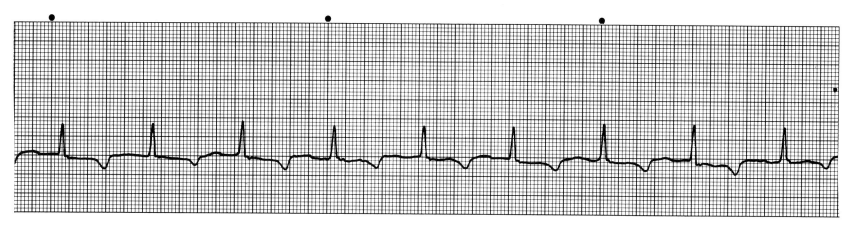

Question. This electrocardiogram was recorded from a Siamese cat with severe clinical signs of hypothermia, dyspnea, and marked lethargy. What is your interpretation? What is the likely underlying disorder?

Case 68

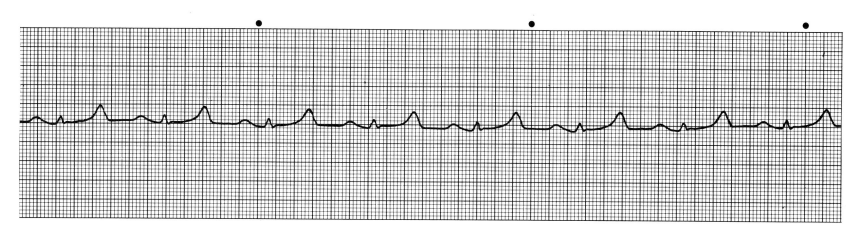

Question. This rhythm strip was recorded from a cat with vomiting. What is your interpretation? How should this condition be treated?

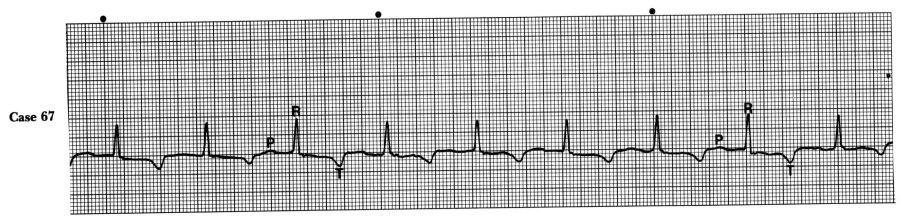

Case 67

Answer. Sinus bradycardia (refer to Chapter 7) (heart rate of 125 beats/min) with high normal QRS complexes (0.9 mv or 9 boxes) indicating possible left ventricular enlargement. The small P waves may indicate decreased atrial activity from disease involvement of the atrial myocardium. The dilated form of cardiomyopathy with severe atrial hypoplasia was found at necropsy. This syndrome is very common among the Siamese and Burmese.

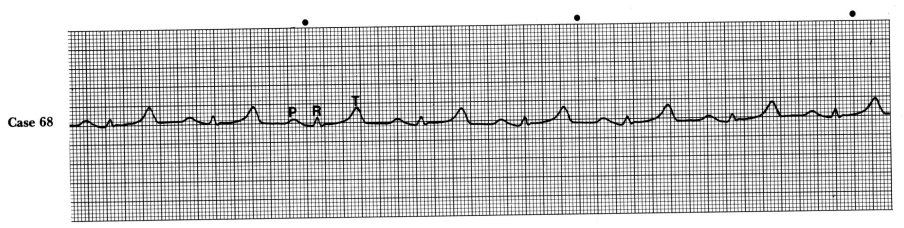

Case 68

Answer. Sinus bradycardia (heart rate 110 beats/min) with wide P waves (0.07 sec or 3 boxes) and large T waves. Differential diagnosis should first consider the common causes of hyperkalemia (refer to Chapter 7): urethral obstruction, renal insufficiency, and diabetic ke- toacidosis. Blood chemistries later confirmed renal insufficiency. With appropriate therapy, the P and T waves became smaller and the heart rate increased.

Case 69

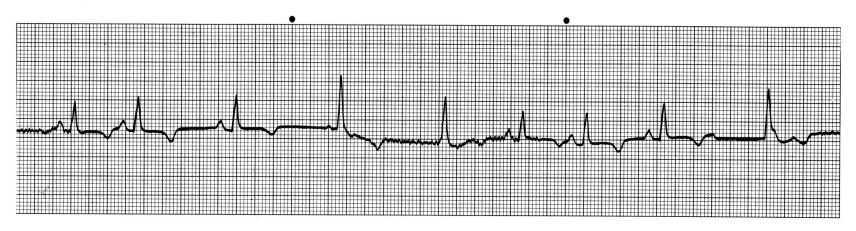

Question. This rhythm strip was recorded from a 16-year-old cat with severe vomiting. What is your interpretation?

Case 70

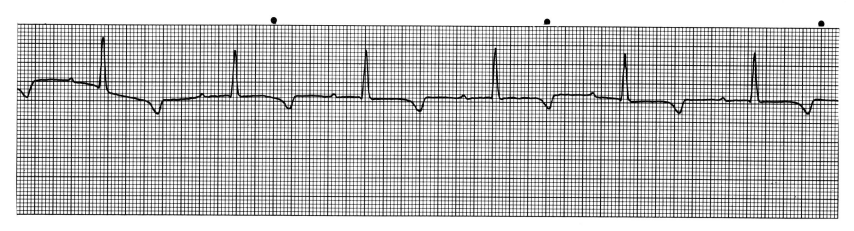

Question. This rhythm strip was recorded from a Siamese cat with dyspnea, hypothermia, and marked lethargy. Thoracic radiographs revealed cardiomegaly and pleural effusion. What is your interpretation? What is the differential diagnosis?

Case 69

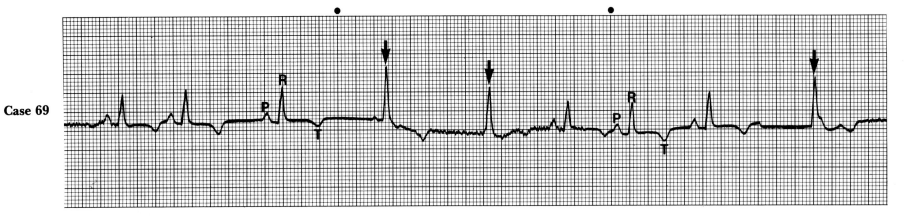

Answer. Sinoatrial block (or sinus arrest) with ventricular escape complexes (arrows). Electrical artifact is also present at various portions of the strip. The high normal QRS complexes (0.9 mv or 9 boxes) may be compatible with left heart enlargement, not uncommon in aged cats (often secondary to chronic renal disease and secondary hypertension). The sinoatrial arrest (or block) may indicate fibrotic changes in the SA node or may be secondary to increased vagal tone from the vomiting and gagging. A systemic metabolic disorder should also be considered.

Case 70

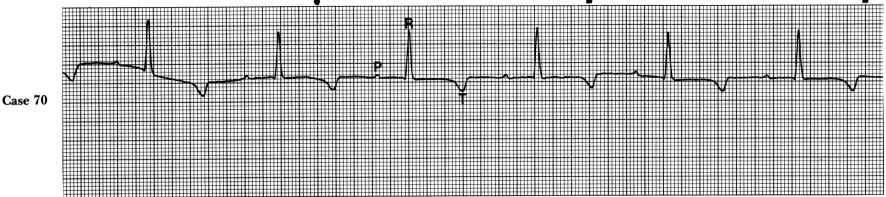

Answer. First-degree atrioventricular block (P-R interval 0.06 sec or 8 boxes; normal not greater than 0.09 sec or 4½ boxes), sinus bradycardia, and probable left ventricular enlargement (refer to Chapter 7). The Q-T interval may appear to be prolonged, but the interpreter should take into consideration the slow heart rate of 85 beats/min, since the Q-T interval varies inversely with the heart rate. The R wave is 1.2 mv or 12 boxes (normal not greater than 0.9 mv or 9 boxes). With these electrocardiographic abnormalities and the clinical evaluation, the dilated form of cardiomyopathy should first be considered. A systemic metabolic disorder should also be considered. Prognosis is guarded because of these major electrocardiographic abnormalities.

Case 71

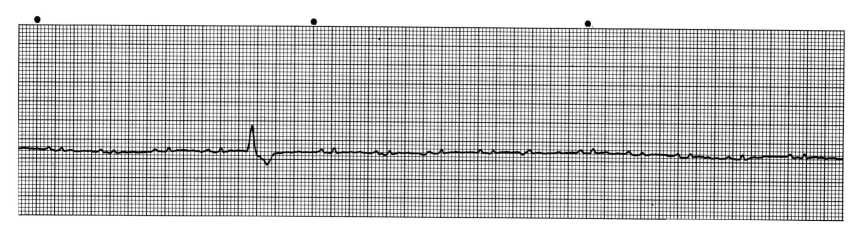

Question. This electrocardiogram was recorded from a 16-year-old cat with anorexia. Auscultation revealed no cardiac murmurs, but an arrhythmia was detected. What is your interpretation?

Case 71

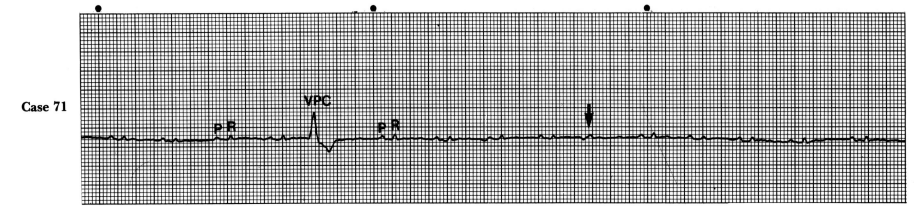

Answer. The most obvious abnormality is the one ventricular complex (VPC), as well as the small P-QRS complexes with no well-defined T wave. The one VPC can be of normal variation in the older cat, and the small complexes can also be normal in most cats. Pleural or pericardial effusion should be ruled out, however. The approximate sinus rate is 190 beats/min. The R-R interval does vary. The arrow points out a break in the rhythm due to a blocked P wave or a supraventricular premature complex. Precordial chest leads may be indicated to make it easier to see the P-QRS-T complexes.

Appendix A
THE NORMAL CANINE AND FELINE ELECTROCARDIOGRAM

Table A–1. CANINE

Rate
   70 to 160 beats/min for adult dogs
   Up to 180 beats/min for toy breeds
   Up to 220 beats/min for puppies
Rhythm
   Normal sinus rhythm
   Sinus arrhythmia
   Wandering SA pacemaker
Measurements (lead II, 50 mm/sec, 1 cm = 1 mv)
   P wave
      Width: maximum, 0.04 second (2 boxes wide)
      Height: maximum, 0.4 mv (4 boxes tall)
   P-R interval
      Width: 0.06 to 0.13 second (3 to 6½ boxes)
   QRS complex
      Width: maximum, 0.05 second (2½ boxes) in small breeds
               maximum, 0.06 second (3 boxes) in large breeds
      Height of R wave*: maximum, 3.0 mv (30 boxes) in large
                              breeds
                           maximum, 2.5 mv (25 boxes) in small
                              breeds
   S-T segment
      No depression: not more than 0.2 mv (2 boxes)
      No elevation: not more than 0.15 mv (1½ boxes)
   T wave
      Can be positive, negative, or biphasic
      Not greater than one fourth amplitude of R wave
   Q-T interval
      Width: 0.15 to 0.25 second (7½ to 12½ boxes) at normal
               heart rate; varies with heart rate (faster rates have
               shorter Q-T intervals and vice versa)
Electrical axis (frontal plane)
   +40° to +100°
Precordial chest leads (values of special importance)
   CV$_5$RL (rV$_2$): T wave positive
   CV$_6$LL (V$_2$): S wave not greater than 0.8 mv (8 boxes), R wave
      not greater than 2.5 mv (25 boxes)*
   CV$_6$LU (V$_4$): S waves not greater than 0.7 mv (7 boxes), R
      wave not greater than 3.0 mv (30 boxes)*
   V$_{10}$: negative QRS complex, T wave negative except in Chi-
      huahua
   *Not valid for thin deep-chested dogs under 2 years of age.

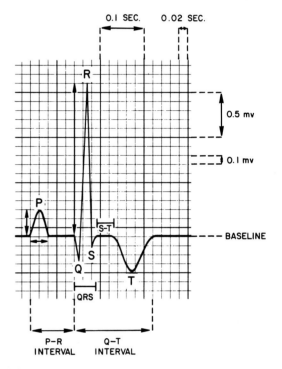

Fig. A–1. Close-up of a normal canine lead II P-QRS-T complex with labels and intervals. *P*, 0.04 second by 0.3 mv; *P-R*, 0.1 second; *QRS*, 0.05 second by 1.7 mv; *S-T* segment and *T* wave, normal; *Q-T*, 0.18 second.

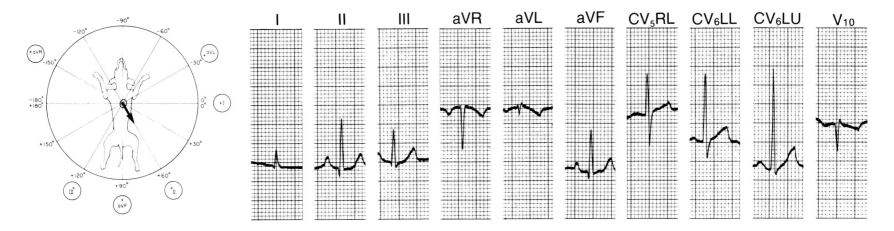

Fig. A–2. Normal canine electrocardiogram illustrating the bipolar standard leads *(I, II, III)*, the augmented unipolar limb leads *(aVR, aVL, aVF)*, and the unipolar precordial chest leads *(CV₅RL, CV₆LL, CV₆LU, and V₁₀)*. Mean electrical axis, +60°.

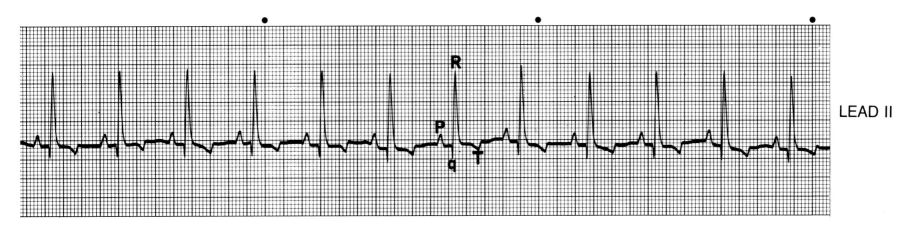

Fig. A–3. Normal sinus rhythm (lead II) at a rate of 167 beats/min. Paper speed, 50 mm/sec, standardization, 1 cm = 1 mv.

Table A–2. FELINE

Rate
  Range: 160 to 240 beats/min
  Mean: 197 beats/min
Rhythm
  Normal sinus rhythm
  Sinus tachycardia (physiologic reaction to excitement)
Measurements (lead II, 50 mm/sec, 1 cm = 1 mv)*
  P wave
    Width: maximum, 0.04 second (2 boxes wide)
    Height: maximum, 0.2 mv (2 boxes tall)
  P-R interval
    Width: 0.05 to 0.09 second (2½ to 4½ boxes)
  QRS complex
    Width: maximum, 0.04 second (2 boxes)
    Height of R wave: maximum, 0.9 mv (9 boxes)
  S-T segment
    No marked depression or elevation
  T wave
    Can be positive, negative, or biphasic; most often positive
    Maximum amplitude: 0.3 mv (3 boxes)
  Q-T interval
    Width: 0.12 to 0.18 second (6 to 9 boxes) at normal heart
      rate (range 0.07 to 0.20 sec, 3½ to 10 boxes); varies
      with heart rate (faster rates, shorter Q-T intervals; and
      vice versa)
Electrical axis (frontal plane)
  0 to +160°
Precordial chest leads
  No well-established normal values to date
  CV$_6$LU (V$_4$): R wave not greater than 1.0 mv (10 boxes)

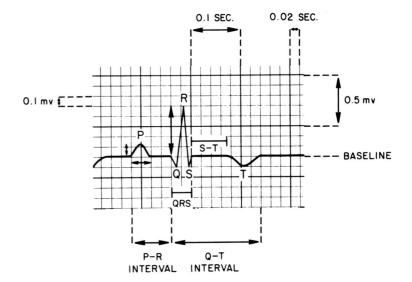

Fig. A–4. Close-up of a normal feline lead II P-QRS-T complex with labels and intervals.

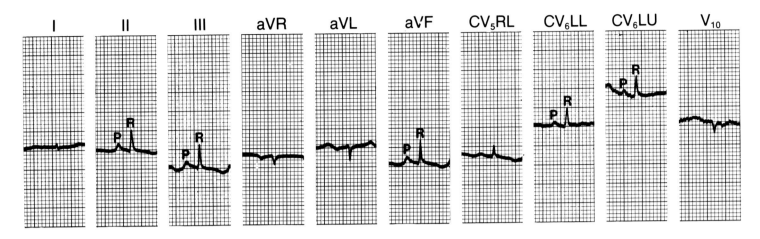

Fig. A–5. Normal feline electrocardiogram illustrating the bipolar standard leads *(I, II, and III)*, the augmented unipolar limb leads *(aVR, aVL, and aVF)*, and the unipolar precordial chest leads *(CV₅RL, CV₆LL, CV₆LU, and V₁₀)*. Mean electrical axis, +90° (isoelectric lead is I). Note the normal small amplitudes of complexes in all leads.

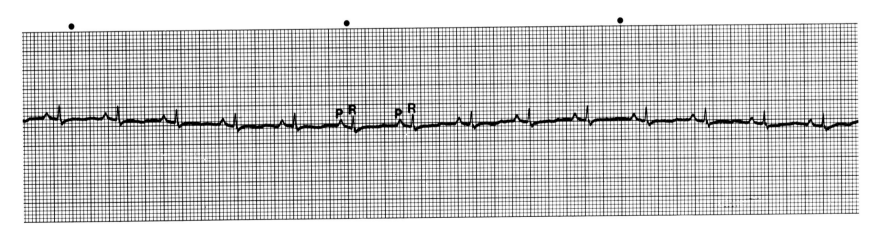

Fig. A–6. Normal sinus rhythm (lead II) at a rate of 188 beats/min. The heart rate is normally accelerated in cats because of excitement, which influences the sympathetic system. Paper speed, 50 mm/sec, standardization, 1 cm = 1 mv.

Appendix B
TABLES FOR DETERMINING THE FRONTAL PLANE MEAN ELECTRICAL AXIS*

*Adapted from the "Electrocardiographic Text Book", the American Heart Association, Inc., 1956. From Friedman, H.H.: *Diagnostic Electrocardiography and Vectorcardiography.* New York, McGraw-Hill, 1971, with permission of the American Heart Association, Inc.

Directions for using Tables B–1 through B–4 for determining the frontal mean electrical axis of the QRS complex:

1. Using amplitudes of deflections, calculate algebraic sum of positive and negative waves in lead I. If sum is positive, use Tables B–1 and B–2; if negative, use Tables B–3 and B–4.
2. Determine algebraic sum of positive and negative waves in lead III.
3. Plot values obtained under appropriate headings. Point of intersection of lead I and lead III columns gives electrical axis in degrees.
4. Normal axis is +40° to +100° (canine) and 0° to +160° (feline).

Table B–1. Frontal plane mean electrical axis (lead I positive, lead III positive)

Lead III Positive	Lead I Positive																					
	0.0	0.5	1.0	1.5	2.0	2.5	3.0	3.5	4.0	4.5	5.0	6.0	7.0	8.0	9.0	10.0	11.0	12.0	13.0	14.0	15.0	20.0
0.0		30	30	30	30	30	30	30	30	30	30	30	30	30	30	30	30	30	30	30	30	30
0.5	90	60	49	44	41	39	38	37	36	35	35	34	33	33	33	32	32	32	32	32	32	31
1.0	90	71	60	53	49	46	44	42	41	40	39	38	37	36	35	35	34	34	34	33	33	32
1.5	90	76	67	60	55	52	49	47	45	44	43	41	39	38	38	37	36	36	36	35	35	33
2.0	90	79	71	65	60	56	53	51	49	47	46	44	42	41	40	39	38	38	37	37	36	35
2.5	90	81	74	68	64	60	57	54	52	51	49	47	45	43	42	41	40	39	39	38	38	36
3.0	90	82	76	71	67	63	60	57	55	53	52	49	47	45	44	43	42	41	40	39	39	37
3.5	90	83	78	73	69	66	63	60	58	56	54	51	49	47	46	44	43	42	42	41	40	38
4.0	90	84	79	75	71	68	65	62	60	58	56	53	51	49	47	46	45	44	43	42	42	39
4.5	90	85	80	76	73	69	67	64	62	60	58	55	53	51	49	48	47	45	44	43	43	40
5.0	90	85	81	77	74	71	68	66	64	62	60	57	55	52	51	49	48	47	46	45	44	41
6.0	90	86	82	79	76	73	71	69	67	65	63	60	57	55	53	52	50	49	48	47	46	43
7.0	90	87	83	81	78	75	73	71	69	67	65	63	60	58	56	54	53	51	50	49	48	44
8.0	90	87	84	82	79	77	75	73	71	69	68	65	62	60	58	56	55	53	52	51	50	46
9.0	90	87	85	82	80	78	76	74	73	71	69	67	64	62	60	58	57	55	54	53	52	48
10.0	90	88	85	83	81	79	77	76	74	72	71	68	66	64	62	60	58	57	56	54	53	49
11.0	90	88	86	84	82	80	78	77	75	73	72	70	67	65	63	62	60	59	57	56	55	50
12.0	90	88	86	84	82	81	79	78	76	75	73	71	69	67	65	63	61	60	59	57	56	52
13.0	90	88	86	84	83	81	80	78	77	76	74	72	70	68	66	64	63	61	60	59	58	53
14.0	90	88	87	85	83	82	80	79	78	77	75	73	71	69	67	66	64	63	61	60	59	55
15.0	90	88	87	85	84	82	81	80	78	77	76	74	72	70	68	67	65	64	62	61	60	55
20.0	90	89	88	87	85	84	83	82	81	80	79	77	76	74	72	71	70	68	67	65	65	60

Table B-2. Frontal plane mean electrical axis (lead I positive, lead III negative)

Lead III Negative	Lead I Positive																					
	0.0	0.5	1.0	1.5	2.0	2.5	3.0	3.5	4.0	4.5	5.0	6.0	7.0	8.0	9.0	10.0	11.0	12.0	13.0	14.0	15.0	20.0
0.0		30	30	30	30	30	30	30	30	30	30	30	30	30	30	30	30	30	30	30	30	30
0.5	−90	−30	0	11	16	19	21	22	23	24	25	26	26	27	27	27	28	28	28	28	28	29
1.0	−90	−60	−30	−11	0	7	11	14	16	18	19	21	22	23	24	25	25	26	26	26	27	27
1.5	−90	−71	−49	−30	−16	−7	0	5	7	11	13	16	18	20	21	22	23	23	24	24	25	26
2.0	−90	−76	−60	−44	−30	−19	−11	−5	0	4	7	11	14	16	18	19	20	21	22	22	23	25
2.5	−90	−79	−67	−53	−41	−30	−21	−14	−8	−4	0	6	9	12	14	16	17	19	20	20	21	23
3.0	−90	−81	−71	−60	−49	−39	−30	−22	−16	−11	−7	0	5	8	11	13	15	16	17	18	19	22
3.5	−90	−82	−74	−65	−55	−46	−38	−30	−23	−18	−13	−6	0	4	7	10	12	14	15	16	17	21
4.0	−90	−83	−76	−68	−60	−52	−44	−37	−30	−24	−19	−11	−5	0	4	7	9	11	13	14	15	19
4.5	−90	−84	−78	−71	−64	−56	−49	−42	−36	−30	−25	−16	−9	−4	0	3	6	8	10	12	13	18
5.0	−90	−85	−79	−73	−67	−60	−53	−47	−41	−35	−30	−21	−14	−8	−4	0	3	6	8	9	11	16
6.0	−90	−86	−81	−76	−71	−66	−60	−54	−49	−44	−39	−30	−22	−16	−11	−7	−3	0	3	5	7	13
7.0	−90	−86	−82	−78	−74	−69	−65	−60	−55	−51	−46	−38	−30	−23	−18	−13	−9	−6	−3	0	2	10
8.0	−90	−87	−83	−80	−76	−72	−68	−64	−60	−56	−52	−44	−37	−30	−24	−19	−15	−11	−8	−5	−2	7
9.0	−90	−87	−84	−81	−78	−74	−71	−67	−64	−60	−56	−49	−42	−36	−30	−25	−20	−16	−13	−9	−7	3
10.0	−90	−87	−85	−82	−79	−76	−73	−70	−67	−63	−60	−53	−47	−41	−35	−30	−25	−21	−17	−14	−11	0
11.0	−90	−88	−85	−83	−80	−77	−75	−72	−69	−66	−63	−57	−51	−45	−40	−35	−30	−26	−22	−18	−15	−3
12.0	−90	−88	−86	−83	−81	−79	−76	−74	−71	−68	−66	−60	−54	−49	−44	−39	−34	−30	−26	−22	−19	−7
13.0	−90	−88	−86	−84	−82	−80	−77	−75	−73	−70	−68	−63	−57	−52	−47	−43	−38	−34	−30	−26	−23	−10
14.0	−90	−88	−86	−84	−82	−80	−78	−76	−74	−72	−69	−65	−60	−55	−51	−46	−42	−38	−34	−30	−27	−13
15.0	−90	−88	−87	−85	−83	−81	−79	−77	−75	−73	−71	−67	−62	−58	−53	−49	−45	−41	−37	−33	−30	−16
20.0	−90	−89	−87	−86	−85	−83	−82	81	−79	−78	−76	−73	−70	−67	−63	−60	−57	−53	−50	−47	−44	−30

Table B–3. Frontal plane mean electrical axis (lead I negative, lead III negative)

Lead III Negative	Lead I Negative																					
	0.0	0.5	1.0	1.5	2.0	2.5	3.0	3.5	4.0	4.5	5.0	6.0	7.0	8.0	9.0	10.0	11.0	12.0	13.0	14.0	15.0	20.0
0.0	−150	−150	−150	−150	−150	−150	−150	−150	−150	−150	−150	−150	−150	−150	−150	−150	−150	−150	−150	−150	−150	−150
0.5	−90	−120	−131	−136	−139	−141	−142	−143	−144	−145	−145	−146	−147	−147	−147	−148	−148	−148	−148	−148	−148	−149
1.0	−90	−109	−120	−127	−131	−134	−136	−138	−139	−140	−141	−142	−143	−144	−145	−145	−146	−146	−146	−147	−147	−148
1.5	−90	−104	−113	−120	−125	−128	−131	−133	−135	−136	−137	−139	−141	−142	−142	−143	−144	−144	−144	−145	−145	−147
2.0	−90	−101	−109	−115	−120	−124	−127	−129	−131	−133	−134	−136	−138	−139	−140	−141	−142	−142	−143	−143	−144	−145
2.5	−90	−99	−106	−112	−116	−120	−123	−126	−128	−129	−131	−133	−135	−137	−138	−139	−140	−141	−141	−142	−142	−144
3.0	−90	−98	−104	−109	−113	−117	−120	−123	−125	−127	−128	−131	−133	−135	−136	−137	−138	−139	−140	−141	−141	−143
3.5	−90	−97	−102	−107	−111	−114	−117	−120	−122	−124	−124	−129	−131	−133	−134	−136	−137	−138	−138	−139	−140	−142
4.0	−90	−96	−101	−105	−109	−112	−115	−118	−120	−122	−124	−127	−129	−131	−133	−134	−135	−136	−137	−138	−138	−141
4.5	−90	−95	−100	−104	−107	−111	−113	−116	−118	−120	−122	−125	−127	−129	−131	−132	−133	−135	−136	−137	−137	−140
5.0	−90	−95	−99	−103	−106	−109	−112	−114	−116	−118	−120	−123	−125	−128	−129	−131	−132	−133	−134	−135	−136	−139
6.0	−90	−94	−98	−101	−104	−107	−109	−111	−113	−115	−117	−120	−123	−125	−127	−128	−130	−131	−132	−133	−134	−137
7.0	−90	−93	−97	−99	−102	−105	−107	−109	−111	−113	−115	−117	−120	−122	−124	−126	−127	−129	−130	−131	−132	−136
8.0	−90	−93	−96	−98	−101	−103	−105	−107	−109	−111	−112	−115	−118	−120	−122	−124	−125	−127	−128	−129	−130	−134
9.0	−90	−93	−95	−98	−100	−102	−104	−106	−107	−109	−111	−113	−116	−118	−120	−122	−123	−125	−126	−127	−128	−132
10.0	−90	−92	−95	−97	−99	−101	−103	−104	−106	−108	−109	−112	−114	−116	−118	−120	−122	−123	−124	−126	−127	−131
11.0	−90	−92	−94	−96	−98	−100	−102	−103	−105	−107	−108	−110	−113	−115	−117	−118	−120	−121	−123	−124	−125	−130
12.0	−90	−92	−94	−96	−98	−99	−101	−102	−104	−105	−107	−109	−111	−113	−115	−117	−119	−120	−121	−123	−124	−128
13.0	−90	−92	−94	−96	−97	−99	−100	−102	−103	−104	−106	−108	−110	−112	−114	−116	−117	−119	−120	−121	−122	−127
14.0	−90	−92	−93	−95	−97	−98	−100	−101	−102	−103	−105	−107	−109	−111	−113	−114	−116	−117	−119	−120	−121	−125
15.0	−90	−92	−93	−95	−96	−98	−99	−100	−102	−103	−104	−106	−108	−110	−112	−113	−115	−116	−118	−119	−120	−125
20.0	−90	−91	−92	−93	−95	−96	−97	−98	−99	−100	−101	−103	−104	−106	−108	−109	−110	−112	−113	−115	−115	−102

Table B–4. Frontal plane mean electrical axis (lead I negative, lead III positive)

Lead III Positive	Lead I Negative																					
	0.0	0.5	1.0	1.5	2.0	2.5	3.0	3.5	4.0	4.5	5.0	6.0	7.0	8.0	9.0	10.0	11.0	12.0	13.0	14.0	15.0	20.0
0.0		−150	−150	−150	−150	−150	−150	−150	−150	−150	−150	−150	−150	−150	−150	−150	−150	−150	−150	−150	−150	−150
0.5	90	150	180	−169	−164	−161	−159	−158	−157	−156	−155	−154	−154	−153	−153	−153	−152	−152	−152	−152	−152	−151
1.0	90	120	150	169	180	−173	−169	−166	−164	−162	−161	−159	−158	−157	−156	−155	−155	−154	−154	−154	−153	−153
1.5	90	109	131	150	164	173	180	−175	−172	−169	−167	−164	−162	−160	−159	−158	−157	−157	−156	−156	−155	−154
2.0	90	104	120	136	150	161	169	175	180	−176	−173	−169	−166	−164	−162	−161	−160	−159	−158	−158	−157	−155
2.5	90	101	113	127	139	150	159	166	172	176	180	−174	−171	−168	−166	−164	−163	−161	−160	−160	−159	−157
3.0	90	99	109	120	131	141	150	158	164	169	173	180	−175	−172	−169	−167	−165	−164	−163	−162	−161	−158
3.5	90	98	106	115	125	134	142	150	157	162	167	174	180	−176	−173	−170	−168	−166	−165	−164	−163	−159
4.0	90	97	104	112	120	128	136	143	150	156	161	169	175	180	−176	−173	−171	−169	−167	−166	−165	−161
4.5	90	96	102	109	116	124	131	138	144	150	155	164	171	176	180	−177	−174	−172	−170	−168	−167	−162
5.0	90	95	101	107	113	120	127	133	139	145	150	159	166	172	176	180	−177	−174	−172	−171	−169	−164
6.0	90	94	99	104	109	114	120	126	131	136	141	150	158	164	169	173	177	180	−177	−175	−173	−167
7.0	90	94	98	102	106	111	115	120	125	129	134	142	150	157	162	167	171	174	177	180	−178	−170
8.0	90	93	97	100	104	108	112	116	120	124	128	136	143	150	156	161	165	169	172	175	178	−173
9.0	90	93	96	99	102	106	109	113	116	120	124	131	138	144	150	155	160	164	167	171	173	−177
10.0	90	93	95	98	101	104	107	110	113	117	120	127	133	139	145	150	155	159	163	166	169	180
11.0	90	92	95	97	100	103	105	108	111	114	117	123	129	135	140	145	150	154	158	162	165	177
12.0	90	92	94	97	99	101	104	106	109	112	114	120	126	131	136	141	146	150	154	158	161	173
13.0	90	92	94	96	98	100	103	105	107	110	112	117	123	128	133	137	142	146	150	154	157	170
14.0	90	92	94	96	98	100	102	104	106	108	111	115	120	125	129	134	138	142	146	150	153	167
15.0	90	92	93	95	97	99	101	103	105	107	109	113	118	122	127	131	135	139	143	147	150	164
20.0	90	91	93	94	95	97	98	99	101	102	104	107	110	113	117	120	123	127	130	133	136	150

Appendix C
CLIENT-EDUCATION CHARTS

THE NORMAL HEART AND HEART DISEASE
The normal heart

The heart is a hollow organ that serves as a double pump and is located approximately in the center of the chest cavity. Its walls consist of muscular tissue called *myocardium*. The pumping action of the heart causes blood to flow through the circulatory system, supplying oxygen and nutrients to the body tissue. Inside the heart a wall of tissue separates the heart into two sections of pumps: the "right heart" and the "left heart." Each side of the heart is made up of two hollow chambers: the upper chamber is the *atrium,* it receives blood; the lower chamber is the *ventricle,* it pumps blood from the heart. The cavities of the atrium and ventricle on each side of the heart communicate with each other, but the right chambers do not communicate directly with those on the left. Thus, right and left atria and right and left ventricles are distinct. Blood flow is directed by a series of valves that have nothing to do with the initiation of flow. The driving force for blood comes from the active contraction of cardiac muscles. The valves only prevent the blood from flowing in the opposite direction.

A drop of blood that is in the *right atrium* is first pumped through a valve into the *right ventricle.* The ventricle then pumps the droplet to the pulmonary artery and lungs. In the lungs, the blood takes on oxygen and gives up the carbon dioxide it was carrying. The oxygen-rich droplet is now ready to nourish cells of the body, but first it must return to the heart. This time the droplet enters the pulmonary veins and goes into the *left atrium.* The atrium pumps it through a valve into the *left ventricle.* The left ventricle then pumps it out to the cells of the body.

Heart disease

Heart disease is one of the most frequent problems in small animal medicine. The function of the heart is to maintain an adequate flow of blood at all times. Different diseases of the heart valves or heart muscle can eventually cause the heart to fail and cause inadequate blood flow. An electrocardiogram can be used to evaluate the status of the heart's conduction system, the status of the muscle, and, indirectly, the condition of the heart as a pump. The electrocardiogram is a graphic representation of the electrical activity of the heart muscle. Irregularities in the timing of the electrical activity (the cardiac rhythm) or how fast the heart is beating (the cardiac rate) can be identified by taking an electrocardiogram. The most common signs associated with heart disease are coughing, irregular and rapid respirations, weight loss, abdominal enlargement, and sometimes fainting.

Heart disease can be controlled, however, by use of oral medication, diet restriction, and exercise restriction. It is also important to have periodic check-ups to evaluate your dog's progress. How well your pet does at home will depend on how advanced the heart disease is and how well you are able to follow your veterinarian's instructions. By adhering to the professional advice of your veterinarian and with your own careful attention, your pet will be able to live a more comfortable and longer life.

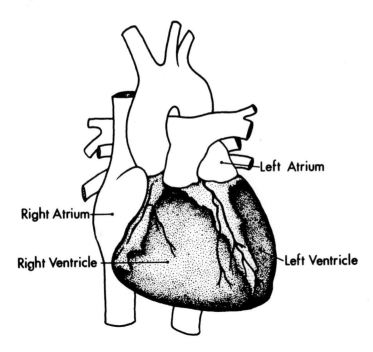

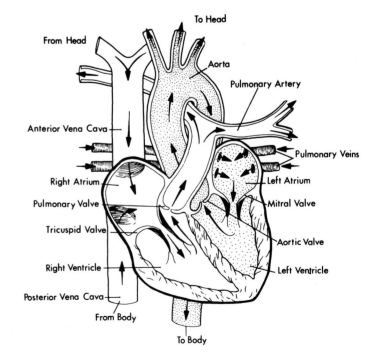

THE ELECTROCARDIOGRAM*
What is an electrocardiogram?

An electrocardiogram (ECG) is a test used widely to assess the condition of the heart. The ECG is used to evaluate the status of the heart's conduction system, the status of the muscle, and indirectly, the condition of the heart as a pump. The ECG is a graphical representation of the electrical activity (voltage) of the heart muscle and an ECG machine (electrocardiograph) is a recording voltmeter. The series of wavy lines represents the recording of the ECG machine that "reads" heartbeats and prints them out on a special pressure-sensitive paper. These readings are the veterinarian's tool for diagnosing cardiac abnormalities. The heart beats because a wave of electrical energy moves through the tissues of the chambers, starting in the atria and moving down to the ventricles. This electrical wave makes the muscle wall of these chambers contract, pumping out its contained blood.

The normal electrocardiogram

A spot of specialized tissue in the heart called the sinoatrial node sends out a short burst of electrical energy that follows the electrical conduction path of the heart. The small round wave "P" originates in the atria, while the large spike "R" originates in the ventricles. The P wave is caused by the depolarization and subsequent contraction of the atria. The R wave (called QRS complex) is the depolarization of the ventricles. The T wave is the repolarization of the ventricles, after which the heart muscle is ready for the next pulse from the sinoatrial node. If the heart beats 120 times per minute, there normally should occur 120 P-QRS-T complexes. Irregularities in the shape (morphology) of the P-QRS-T complex indicate heart muscle abnormalities.

The abnormal electrocardiogram

Irregularities in the timing of the wave forms (rhythm) either within one complex or between several complexes indicate abnormalities. Normal variations and medically important ECG conditions make the practice of diagnostic ECG interpretation a complex and hard-learned profession. A common change in rhythm is the premature beat, or *extra beat*. The extra, or ectopic beat comes soon after the normal beat like this: Beat Beat Beatbeat Beat. Many things can cause the cardiac tissue to become irritable: excitement, drugs, trauma, and, often, heart disease. If these extra beats come frequently, serious signs of heart disease can take place. *Paroxysmal tachycardia* can then result. Without any warning, the heart suddenly begins to race: Beat Beat Beatbeatbeatbeatbeatbeat and so on, for an indefinite period. This abnormality in rhythm can eventually cause the heart to fail and can cause an inadequate blood flow. Your veterinarian's instructions should be followed, since medication can be effective.

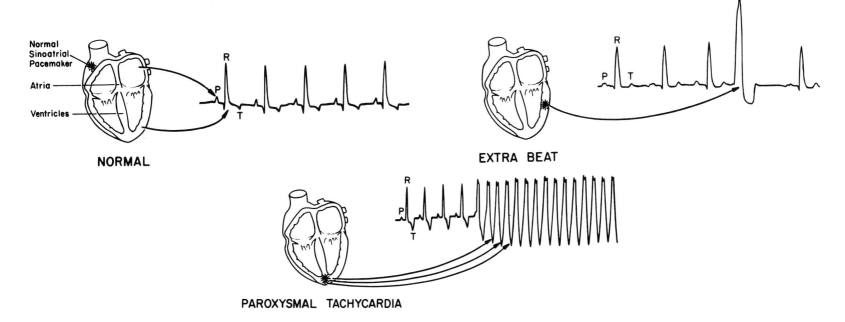

NORMAL

EXTRA BEAT

PAROXYSMAL TACHYCARDIA

---

*Adapted from "What is an electrocardiogram?" Hewlett-Packard. J., Oct. 1981, with permission.

Index

Page numbers in *italics* refer to figures; page numbers followed by t refer to tables.